WELLNESS
GUIDELINES FOR A HEALTHY LIFESTYLE

Brent Q. Hafen
Brigham Young University

Werner W. K. Hoeger
Boise State University

MP

Morton Publishing Company
925 W. Kenyon Avenue, Unit 12
Englewood, Colorado 80110

WELLNESS ▼ *Guidelines for a Healthy Lifestyle*

RA
776.9
.H34
1994

Copyright © 1994 by Morton Publishing Company

All rights reserved. No part of this publication may be reproduced, stored in a retrieval system, or transmitted, in any form or by any means, electronic, mechanical, photocopying, recording, or otherwise, without the prior written permission of the publisher.

Printed in the United States of America

10 9 8 7 6 5 4 3 2 1

ISBN: 0-89582-230-X

PREFACE

Why another health and wellness book? Health and wellness behavior have for too long been taught and studied almost exclusively through the physical or biological dimensions. Contemporary knowledge and ethical considerations suggest a broader approach to health behavior, involving the social, emotional, mental and spiritual natures and consequences. Ignorance of these aspects breeds myth, misconceptions and exploitation, all of which are avoidable through better understanding. Few books have explained, with support from the scientific literature, how each dimension contributes to wellness. In the pages that follow, you will learn what the research literature has to say about traditional health-related topics, as well as what we know about how emotions impact health and wellness. You'll see how nurturing "negative" attitudes, emotions, and relationships can hurt, and "positive" attitudes, emotions, and relationships, when nurtured, can enhance wellness, and even help to heal. What is written here will help you appreciate what we know about the mind/body connection and the tremendous healing power of your mind and heart.

Wellness - Guidelines for a Healthy Lifestyle is not a book about disease, but, rather, one that provides guidelines for preventing disease and enhancing health and wellness. There are self assessments in each chapter to help the student personalize and assess his or her own level of wellness, related to that particular dimension or concern. The assessments are followed by behavior-change guidelines that aid the reader in developing a prescription or strategy for behavior modification toward a more healthy lifestyle.

Self-responsibility is emphasized throughout the book with the realization that enhancing wellness requires personal decision making and realistic goal setting, with positive and optimistic follow through. The responsibility of enhancing health and wellness and developing a healthy lifestyle rests primarily with the individual. According to research literature, improving happiness, quality of life, and longevity is a matter of personal choice. The purpose of this book is not only to increase the reader's understanding about health and wellness, but to help assess his or her own personal attitudes and behavior, and where necessary, to make appropriate changes. The book has a strong emphasis on fitness, because the scientific evidence has clearly shown that one of the most effective ways to enhance wellness and longevity is to increase one's level of physical activity and fitness.

Wellness - Guidelines for a Healthy Lifestyle was developed for use in introductory health and wellness courses at the college level. The book provides a discussion of contemporary, personal health issues as a conceptual basis for intelligent, personal health decision and modes of behavior. The emphasis is shifted toward concepts, guidelines, and modes of behavior stressing health enhancement and healthy lifestyles, rather than health recovery.

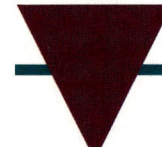

ACKNOWLEDGMENTS

We wish to express gratitude to Charles Scheer, Scott Whiles, Jamie Korte, Julie Wagner, Jennifer Blackman, Michelle Chupurdia, Monika Gangwer, Neil Edwards, Eric Heinz, Julie Hammons, and Brad Thompson who helped with the photography in this edition.

We also wish to thank Kathryn J. Frandsen for all her help.

CONTENTS

1 INTRODUCTION TO WELLNESS 1
Leading Health Problems in the United States 3
What Are Health and Wellness? 4
The Dimensions of Wellness 5
Risk Factors That Compromise Wellness 9
Wellness Challenges for the Next Century 11
A Personalized Approach to Health and Wellness 11

2 STRESS AND HEALTH 19
Stress and Disease 21
The General Adaptation Syndrome:
How the Body Reacts to Stress 23
How Stress Affects the Body Systems 23
Stress and the Immune System 24
Coping with Stress 27

3 THE MIND-BODY CONNECTION 45
The Science of Psychoneuroimmunology 46
Personalities and Health 49
Personality Traits and Health 56
The Disease-Resistant Personality 64

4 SOCIAL SUPPORT AND HEALTH 69
The Ties That Bind 72
Loneliness and Health 74
Marriage and Health 81
Families and Health 84
Grief, Bereavement, and Health 87

5 PERCEPTIONS, THE SPIRIT, AND HEALTH 93
Explanatory Style and Health 94
Locus of Control and Health 96
Self-Esteem and Health 98
Protecting Health With a Fighting Spirit 100
Spirituality and Health 101
Altruism and Health 104
The Healing Power of Faith 106
The Healing Power of Hope 107

6 FITNESS ASSESSMENT FOR WELLNESS 113
Fitness and Health 114
Benefits of a Lifetime Physical Fitness Program 115
The Fitness Challenge for the 21st Century 117
Personalized Fitness Programs 118
Health Screening Prior to Exercise Participation 118
Physical Fitness 118
Fitness Standards: Health Fitness
Versus Physical Fitness 119
Cardiovascular Endurance Assessment 120
Muscular Strength Assessment 123
Muscular Flexibility Assessment 127
Exercise Prescription 129

7 EXERCISE PRESCRIPTION FOR WELLNESS 133
Cardiovascular Endurance 134
Muscular Strength 140
Muscular Flexibility 145
Preventing and Rehabilitating Low Back Pain 147
Management of Exercise-Related Injuries 149
Exercise Intolerance 149
Leisure-Time Physical Activity 149
Tips to Enhance Exercise Adherence 151

8 NUTRITION AND WELLNESS 173

The Six Basic Elements of Nutrition 174
Energy (ATP) Production 190
Nutrient Supplementation 191
Recommended Dietary Guidelines for Americans 192
Food Labels: Reading Your Way to Better Health 193
Designing a Nutritional Plan for Wellness 195

9 BODY COMPOSITION ASSESSMENT 205

Essential and Storage Fat 206
Techniques for Assessing Body Composition 207
Waist-to-Hip Ratio 216
Body Mass Index 216
Determining Recommended Body Weight 217

10 WEIGHT MANAGEMENT, EATING DISORDERS, AND WELLNESS 221

The Dieting Myth 222
Eating Disorders 223
Principles of Weight Control 224
Relationship Between Lean Tissue and Metabolism 226
Exercise: The Key to Successful Weight Loss and Maintenance 227
Implementing a Sound and Sensible Weight Loss Program 230
Tips for a Lifetime Weight Management Program 232
In Conclusion 233

11 CARDIOVASCULAR WELLNESS 237

Incidence of Cardiovascular Disease 238
Coronary Heart Disease 239
Guidelines for Preventing Cardiovascular Disease 247
Resting and Stress Electrocardiograms 249
A Final Word 250

12 CANCER PREVENTION AND WELLNESS 251

Cancer Incidence and Risk Factors 252
Types of Cancer 256
Sites of Cancer 257
Guidelines for Preventing Cancer 264

13 ADDICTIVE BEHAVIOR AND WELLNESS 277

The Addictive Personality 279
The Risk Factors of Addiction 281

14 SEXUALLY TRANSMITTED DISEASE: PREVENTION AND WELLNESS 303

Chlamydia 305
Gonorrhea 306
Genital Warts 307
Herpes 308
Viral Hepatitis 309
Pelvic Inflammatory Disease 309
Pubic Lice and Scabies 310
Syphilis 311
HIV and AIDS 311
Guidelines for Preventing Sexually Transmitted Diseases 316

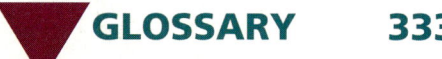 APPENDIX A NUTRITIVE VALUE OF SELECTED FOODS 321

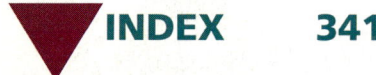 GLOSSARY 333

INDEX 341

Introduction to Wellness

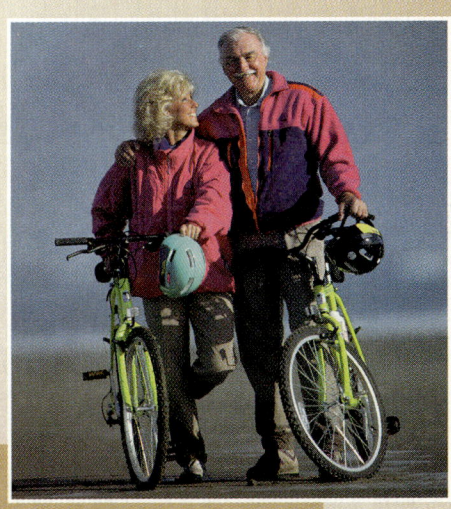

Objectives

- Identify 5 of the leading health problems in the United States.
- Define the characteristics of wellness.
- Identify at least 10 of the National Health Objectives for the year 2000.
- Identify and describe the 5 basic dimensions of wellness.
- Identify 6 risk factors that compromise wellness.

Most of us think of health or wellness merely as the absence of some physical disease, the absence of some specified illness with its range of clearly defined symptoms. Seen from that limited perspective, health is easy to assess. The silvered bulb of a thermometer is poked under a tongue, and the mercury that inches its way along a measured scale gives us the evidence we seek. The cold metal of the stethoscope probes for the faintly distinguishable rhythm. The drop of crimson blood is smeared beneath the powerful gaze of the microscope.

In reality, though, health and wellness in the truest sense are not easy to define. Some people believe they are almost impossible to measure. The World Health Organization, clutching at an elusive definition, earmarks health as "a state of complete physical, mental, and social well-being, and not merely the absence of disease or infirmity." The key word in that definition possibly is *well-being*, and true health actually may denote a condition in which we are able to avoid illness even if we are predisposed to it.

At the turn of the twentieth century, the most common "health problems" in the United States were infectious diseases — influenza, diphtheria, polio, and tuberculosis among them. Scientific advances enabled us to wipe out many of those diseases or, at the least, to reduce dramatically the deaths they caused. Unfortunately, those same scientific advances heralded an age of convenience chronicled by a sedentary lifestyle, more alcohol consumption, and a diet rich in fats and sugars. The result is America's *new* "health problem," chronic diseases — among them, heart disease, cancer, diabetes, emphysema, and cirrhosis of the liver.

The focus at the turn of the 20th century was treatment. Researchers confronted with infectious diseases searched, often with success, for a cure. Our focus on the eve of the 21st century must be on prevention. The health problems that face our nation are, in large measure, the result of lifestyle decisions. Emphatic statements released year after year by the U. S. Surgeon General's Office point out that the leading causes of premature death and illness in the United States could be prevented through positive lifestyle habits. The solution to those health problems, then, is largely within our control.

> You, the individual, can do more for your health and well-being than any doctor, any hospital, any drug, any exotic medical device.
>
> Joseph A. Califano,
> (former Secretary of Health, Education, and Welfare)

Until recently our health-care system has not reflected that focus. The American health-care system traditionally has not addressed prevention. Instead, it is in essence a sickness-care system. About $750 billion — more than a twelfth of the gross national product — is spent on the nation's health care, including hospitals, doctors, health maintenance organizations, pharmaceuticals, and other related companies. As a nation, the United States spends more per capita on health care than any other country in the world. The British, who spend a third what we do per person on health care, outlive us by an average of 3 years.

That's not all. Americans have a higher age-adjusted mortality rate and a higher infant mortality rate than a number of nations. Of twenty countries that researchers at Northwestern University Medical School in Chicago studied, the typical American diet was highest of all in the percentage of fat. Only a few nations ranked higher in the amount of artery-clogging cholesterol consumed. To top it off, the typical American diet is the lowest in dietary fiber. As a result, we are one of the fattest nations in the world.

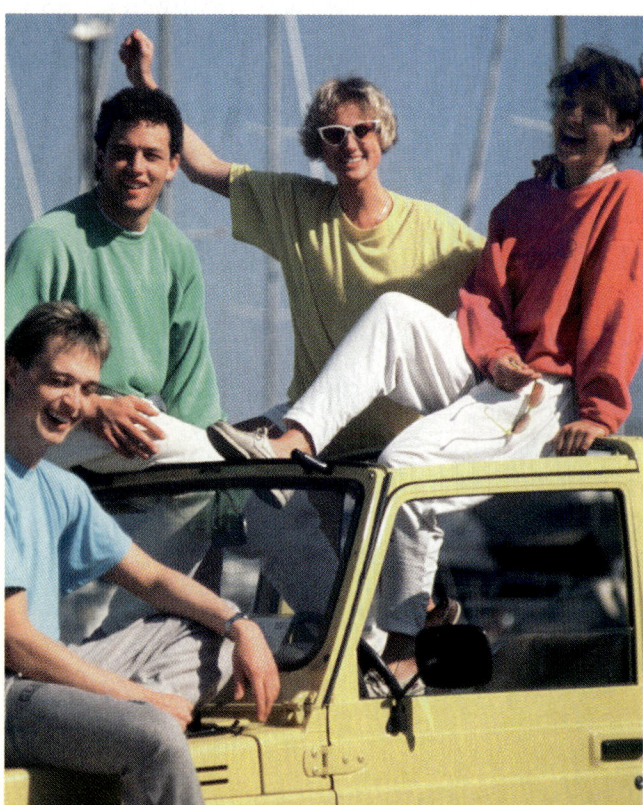

Health and wellness include physical, emotional, social, intellectual, and spiritual dimensions.

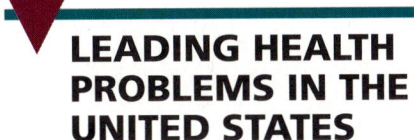

LEADING HEALTH PROBLEMS IN THE UNITED STATES

Approximately two-thirds of our middle-aged men are overweight, compared to only 3% of the middle-aged men in Japan.

There's more. Of the developed nations of the world, the United States has the highest rate of heart disease. We also have some of the highest rates in the world of cancer of the colon, rectum, breast, and lung.

Considering how much we as a nation spend on medical care, we should outshine the world in health and wellness, but we don't. Why? Because we have failed to make prevention a top priority.

Critical to a focus on prevention, say health-care experts, is a change in attitude by patients and health-care providers alike. Patients have to stop demanding medication for every ailment and hospitalization or surgery for every illness. Physicians, in turn, have to be more conservative in their approach to disease. According to Joseph A. Califano, former Secretary of Health, Education, and Welfare, America's doctors need to be "more skeptical in resorting to surgery and less promiscuous in dispensing pills."

The problem, in essence, lies with us, not with the medical establishment. Of all the people who die in this country every year, only 10% die because of inadequate health care. Only 20% die because of environmental or biological factors. The rest die as a direct result of an unhealthy lifestyle.

The importance of prevention is perhaps nowhere more apparent than in an analysis of the leading health problems in the United States today. About 83% of all deaths before age 65 could have been prevented. Almost half of all deaths among people of all ages is attributable to lifestyle factors. An additional 16% is caused by environmental factors. More than half of all disease is what researchers call "self-controlled"; we can control it through lifestyle changes and other preventive methods.

At the beginning of this century, almost one-third of all deaths in the United States resulted from tuberculosis, influenza, and pneumonia. Millions died of influenza in a 1918 epidemic. Fewer than 5% died from cancer, and only about 10% died from cardiovascular disease. Today, virtually no one dies of tuberculosis. Only 4% or 5% die from influenza and pneumonia. According to statistics recently released by the U. S. Department of Health and Human Services, approximately 70% of all deaths in the United States is from heart disease and cancer (see Figure 1.1). And, say the researchers, nearly 80% of those deaths could be prevented by

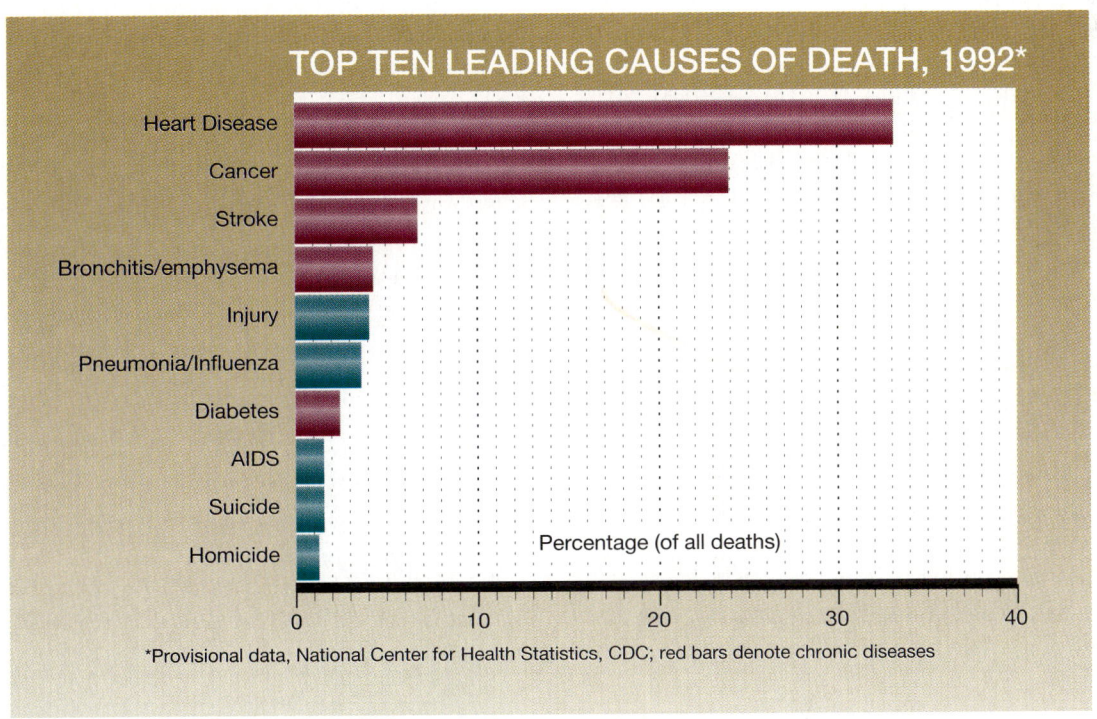

FIGURE 1.1 ▼ The top ten leading causes of death in the U.S., 1992.

making lifestyle changes — things as basic as eating a diet lower in fat, getting regular exercise, and quitting smoking.

Even the other top two causes of death — accidents and pulmonary disease — can be largely prevented. Many fatal accidents are the result of alcohol abuse, drug abuse, or failure to use seat belts. Most cases of chronic and obstructive pulmonary disease are caused by cigarette smoking. And, though our modern-day "epidemic" — AIDS — cannot be cured, it can be prevented by lifestyle choices.

▼ WHAT ARE HEALTH AND WELLNESS?

More than five decades ago health-care education pioneer Jesse Williams proclaimed that health is a condition that allows one to do the most constructive work, render the best possible service to the world, and experience the highest possible enjoyment of life. "Health as freedom from disease is a standard of mediocrity," he wrote. "Health as a quality of life is a standard of inspiration and increasing achievements."

Williams was ahead of his time. Most Americans have taken decades to catch on to his vision. A series of recent Gallup polls finally hinted at his much broader scope of health and wellness. In increasing numbers, however, Americans now are defining health as "the energy to do the things they care about."

The word *health* is derived from the Old English "hal," which means *whole*. Researchers on the cutting edge consider health to be a continuum, a perpetual but ever-changing balance of the various dimensions that make us whole: physical, mental, emotional, social, and spiritual.

Everything with which you interact — the place you live, the air you breathe, the food you eat, the job you have, the people you associate with — affects your position on the health continuum. The same series of Gallup polls shows that Americans are beginning to understand the influence of interactive factors. When ranking their "health priorities," their top concern was staying free of disease, but the third highest was "living in an environment with clean air and water."

And what about *wellness*? According to researchers, you can be well even if you are plagued by physical illness. Illness and health are opposite states, but you can be ill and still enjoy wellness if you have a purpose in life, a deep appreciation for living, a sense of joy.

People who are bound by the strictures of traditionally defined physical health wait until some disease has crept up on them, then consult a professional to evaluate their condition and prescribe treatment. Simply put, they turn over their physical health to someone else. Wellness, on the other hand, becomes a matter of self-evaluation and self-assessment. You continually work on learning and on making changes that will enhance your state of wellness. *You* take the reins. Rather than delegating your physical health to someone else, wellness requires a deep personal commitment.

Physical health is a fairly simple concept. Wellness, however, is a multifaceted and complex concept that involves much more than simple physical condition. Perhaps more important, physical health is something not available to everyone. On the other hand, everyone can enjoy wellness — despite physical limitations, disease, and handicap. Wellness fully

▼ Signs of Wellness

▼ Persistent presence of support network.

▼ Chronic positive expectations; tendency to frame events in a constructive light.

▼ Episodic peak experiences.

▼ Sense of spiritual involvement.

▼ Increased sensitivity.

▼ Tendency to adapt to changing conditions.

▼ Rapid response and recovery of adrenaline system as a result of repeated challenges.

▼ Appetite for physical activity.

▼ Tendency to identify and communicate feelings.

▼ Repeated episodes of gratitude, generosity, or related emotions.

▼ Compulsion to contribute to society.

▼ Persistent sense of humor.

If five or more of these indicators are present, you may be at risk for full-blown wellness.

Adapted from "Commentary," in *Brain/Mind*, (March, 1993, P.O. Box 42211, Los Angeles, CA 90042. Reprinted by permission.

integrates physical, mental, emotional, social, and spiritual well-being — a complex interaction of the factors that lead to a quality life.

If we are to accept a definition of wellness that goes beyond mere freedom from disease, we also must accept a notion that calls for a dramatic change in the way we deal with health. For centuries our emphasis has been on identifying bacteria, classifying viruses, and waging a determined war on devastating disease. We have concentrated on treatment. If we are to redefine health to reflect a condition of wellness, we also must redefine the ultimate goal of our health efforts: *to concentrate on a way of preventing disease.* Inherent in that task is the recognition that behavior — physical, mental, emotional, social, and spiritual — plays a key role not only in the development of disease but also in our ability to resist disease and maintain optimum health.

Embodied in a definition of wellness and behavioral health is a philosophy calling for consideration of the whole person, not a segmented fractionalization into separate parts. We need to consider ourselves as we interact in our environment, not separate complaints or body parts in a sterile laboratory or the unnatural environs of a physician's examining room. It stresses a conscious and active commitment by the individual, refusing to admit that optimum health is something that just happens. Most significantly, it calls for concentration on the factors that precede illness instead of concern solely with the anatomy of disease once it strikes.

▼ THE DIMENSIONS OF WELLNESS

Writing in *The History and Future of Wellness*, author Donald Ardell points out that living by the principles of wellness is considered a richer way to be alive. In optimum wellness five basic dimensions are balanced: physical, mental, emotional, social, and spiritual (see Figure 1.2).

PHYSICAL DIMENSION

Physical health, of course, is the kind most commonly associated with being healthy. A person who has good physical health eats a well-balanced diet, gets plenty of exercise, maintains proper weight,

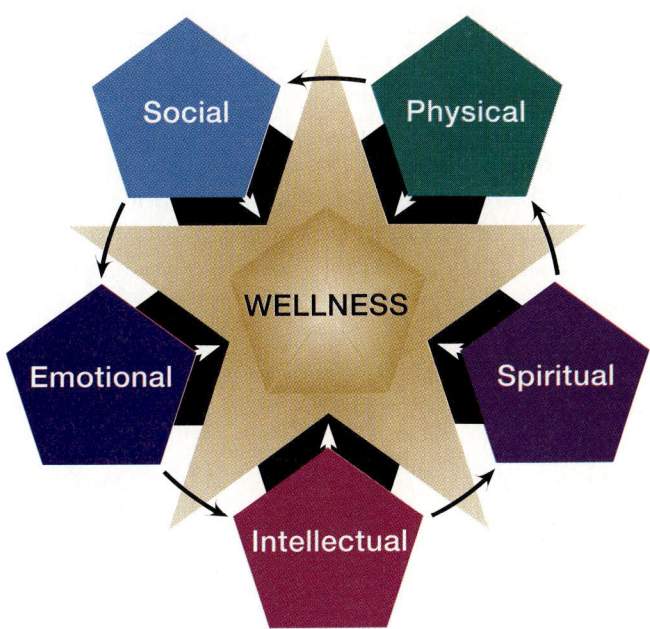

FIGURE 1.2 ▼ The dimensions of wellness.

avoids risky sexual behavior, tries to limit exposure to environmental contaminants, and restricts intake of harmful substances such as alcohol, tobacco, caffeine, and drugs. Physical wellness is characterized by good cardiovascular endurance, muscular strength and flexibility, and proper body composition.

A proper physical dimension of wellness involves taking steps to protect physical health: doing self-exams and getting a regular, thorough physical examination from a physician that includes appropriate screening tests. It also involves taking effective measures if you do become sick, such as seeking medical care and using medications conservatively.

Physical wellness entails confidence and optimism about one's ability to take care of health problems. These conditions don't prevent one from enjoying life. Physical wellness brings with it an almost remarkable resistance to disease. The right combination of nutrition and exercise renders healthy people capable of resisting the common colds and influenza that wipe out associates.

People who enjoy physical wellness are intelligent about their health. When they *do* develop an unusual or irritating symptom, they do what is necessary to relieve it. If symptoms persist, they check with a doctor.

Whether healthy individuals are or are not muscular, they usually are physically powerful. Exercise attunes their muscles and endows them with a high level of physical coordination and self-confidence. Instead of shying away from a physical challenge, they accept it with enthusiasm, confident they can make their body work for them. Reaction time is good, strength is obvious, and endurance is high.

People characterized by physical wellness have an active lifestyle. They love to be outdoors. They enjoy a fast-paced bicycle ride along a roadside choked with apple blossoms or a vigorous game of touch football on a crisp autumn afternoon. They have the energy they need to do the things they enjoy, and the energy they need to complete a demanding task at work, breeze through final exams on a wink of sleep, or clear all the debris out of last year's vegetable garden.

People with physical wellness respect and like their own bodies. They have a natural grace and ease. You can see their health in the way they move. Beauty in the traditional sense of the word has little to do with it. People with physical wellness make the most of their body, and they delight in it.

MENTAL DIMENSION

Just as the physical dimension of wellness embodies much more than the mere absence of disease, so, too, is the mental dimension characterized by signs of positive wellness. Pioneers in the field of psychoneuroimmunology are proving scientifically what philosophers such as Homer, Plato, and Aristotle speculated more than five thousand years ago: The mind has a striking influence on the body (and, therefore, on health and wellness).

Education shouldn't stop with commencement exercises. A sound mental dimension of wellness involves unbridled curiosity and ongoing learning. This dimension of wellness implies that you can apply the things you have learned, that you create opportunities to learn more, and that you engage your mind in lively interaction with the world around you.

People who are mentally well can think clearly, are quick to pick up new concepts, and rapidly catch on to new ideas. Instead of being intimidated by facts and figures with which they are unfamiliar, they embrace the chance to learn something new. Their confidence and enthusiasm enable them to approach any learning situation with eagerness that leads to success.

Mental wellness breeds creativity. Whereas some people seem burdened with the task of getting a job done, mentally well people seem to be able to approach the same task in a new way. They don't seem restricted by what they always have done before. They are willing to tackle the chore from a different angle, one that lets them exercise creativity and initiative.

Logic is a basic attribute of mental wellness. People who are confronted suddenly with an unfamiliar situation tend to experience mild panic. Mental wellness brings with it common sense and logic that enable them to reason their way through.

A genuine sense of curiosity leads mentally well people into a world that is always new and challenging. Where others accept what life has to offer with quiet resolve, mentally well people grasp each aspect of life with a desire to understand. They are the people who know why the surface of a lake is so blue, how a newspaper is printed, how a robin can tell that spring has arrived. Why? Because they ask. Some people pass a flowering hedge and notice that it is beautiful; healthy people want to know why the blooms are so pink, what kind of hedge it is, how they can grow one like it.

Along with alertness and brightness, mental wellness brings with it stimulation and capability. Mentally well people have a good memory and use it to their greatest advantage. They are skilled in their chosen area of expertise, and they usually are the ones who are open to new ideas and suggestions. They relish the chance to improve themselves or learn something new.

Mental wellness brings with it vision and promise. More than anything else, mentally well people are open-minded and accepting of others. Instead of being threatened by those who are different from them, they show respect and curiosity without feeling they have to conform. They are faithful to their own ideas and philosophies but do not hesitate to allow others the same privilege. Their self-confidence guarantees that they can take their place among others in the world without always having to give up part of themselves and without requiring others to do the same.

EMOTIONAL DIMENSION

We know that emotions involve both the mind and the body, and, as a result, they can bridge the gap between the mind and the body. We know that our emotions are extremely complex and that they can make us desperately ill. Emotions are a contributing factor in a number of diseases, such as rheumatoid arthritis, bronchial asthma, peptic ulcer, ulcerative colitis, hypertension, and dermatitis.

What, then, constitutes emotional wellness? Foremost is probably the ability to understand your own feelings, to accept your limitations, and to achieve emotional stability. Understanding and accepting your own feelings helps you understand and accept the emotions of others, which leads to the ability to maintain intimate relationships with other people. Emotional wellness also implies the ability to adjust to change, to cope with stress in a healthy way, and to enjoy life despite its occasional disappointments and frustrations.

The hallmark of emotional wellness is a deep and abiding happiness, not a happiness that depends on some frail set of circumstances but, rather, a happiness that stems from a powerful inner contentment. Instead of being dependent on a certain income or status in life, the happiness that signals real wellness is an emotional anchor that gives meaning and joy to life.

In penning the Declaration of Independence, Thomas Jefferson promised three things to all Americans: the rights to life, liberty, and the pursuit of happiness. He did not promise happiness itself, because he knew that the government could not deliver it. Why? Happiness is not a fleeting emotion tied to a single event. It is a long-term state of mind that permeates the various facets of life and influences our outlook. We can experience true happiness and temporary unhappiness at the same time. Happiness may seem to vanish temporarily, giving way to bursts of depression or disappointment, but it returns. As Harry Emerson Fosdick stated, "One who expects to completely escape low moods is asking the impossible. Like the weather, life is essentially variable, and a healthy person believes in the validity of his high hours even when he is having a low one."

No one has ever come up with a simple recipe for producing happiness, but researchers agree that certain ingredients seem universal among those who have the kind of true, abiding happiness characteristic of emotional wellness. Those who are happy usually are part of a family. They are partners, parents, or children. They love others, and they feel loved themselves. Healthy, happy people enjoy friends, work hard at something fulfilling, get plenty of exercise, and know how to enjoy play and leisure time. They know how to laugh, and they do it often. They give of themselves freely to others and seem to have found deep meaning to life.

An attitude of true happiness signals freedom from the tension and depression so many people suffer. Emotional wellness obviously is subject to the same kinds of depression and unhappiness that plague all of us once in a while, but the difference lies in the ability to bounce back. Well people take minor setbacks in stride and have the uncanny ability to enjoy life despite it all. When something unhappy happens, they put it behind them. They don't waste energy or time recounting the situation, wondering how they could have changed it, or dwelling on the past.

The spirit of optimism basic to healthy, happy individuals enables them to focus their energy on the present. They recognize that the past can hold powerful lessons, but they do not let it control the here and now. Instead of worrying about what they should have done differently back then, they concentrate with enthusiasm and energy on what they can do today.

In addition to avoiding the pitfalls of the past, they avoid the temptation to pin all their hopes and dreams on the future. They are goal-oriented and ambitious, but they have the ability to enjoy themselves today. They aren't waiting until they graduate from college, until they get married, until they pay off their home, or until they are the president of a company. Instead, they are happy today in the circumstances they are in. They may aspire to graduate with honors, marry their sweetheart, pay off the mortgage, or gain the top spot at the firm, but they are happy regardless. They know that happiness is not related to some *thing* but instead is a *condition*.

Part and parcel of happiness is acceptance of self. Happy people value themselves as having something to contribute and being worthwhile. Healthy people enjoy a sense of success — not as measured traditionally by the world but as measured against their own standards. They know what is important to them, and they are confident they can achieve it. They are in touch with self to the point that they have a clear definition of their own needs.

Emotional wellness brings with it a certain stability, an ability to look both success and failure squarely in the face and to keep moving along a predetermined course. When success is evident, the emotionally well person radiates the expected joy and confidence. When failure seems evident, the emotionally well person responds by making the best of circumstances and moving beyond the failure. Wellness enables us to move ahead with optimism and energy instead of spending time and talent worrying about failure. We learn from it, identify ways to avoid it in the future, and then go on with the business at hand.

Emotional wellness also embodies the ability to get in touch with your own feelings. Because healthy people have a good self-image, they do not worry about showing their feelings or sharing them with others. They are not concerned with what others think of them. They do not feel the need to prove themselves to others, nor do they feel they have to force others to accept their point of view. They quietly, peacefully accept themselves and are able to move freely beyond that to accept others.

Sensitive yet independent, emotionally well people accept themselves to an extent that they are able to be extremely insightful about themselves and others. Emotional wellness brings with it a necessary frame of mind that allows involvement with other people. A truly healthy person is one who enjoys others and who is not threatened by what other people might do or say.

Emotional wellness also brings with it a maturity that allows the individual to forgive others. Emotionally well people accept responsibility for their own happiness instead of blaming others when they are unhappy. They are free from anger and resentment because they recognize that anger is almost always destructive. By accepting responsibility for their own emotional well-being, they free themselves to achieve it.

More than dictating happiness and optimism, emotions play a profound part in physical health and avoiding disease. Biobehavioralist Norman Cousins maintained that what you think, what you believe, and how you react to experiences can impair or aid the workings of the body's immune system.

Studies of terminally ill cancer patients reveals that those who survive have one characteristic in common: their utter refusal to give up hope. Cousins said:[1]

> Nothing is more wondrous about the fifteen billion neurons in the human brain than their ability to convert thoughts, hopes, ideas, and attitudes into chemical substances. Every emotion, negative or positive, makes its registrations on the body's systems. . . . The most important thing I have learned about the power of belief is that an individual patient's attitude toward serious illness can be as important as medical help. It would be a serious mistake to bypass or minimize the need for scientific treatment, but that treatment will be far more effective if people put their creative hopes, their faith, and their confidence to work in behalf of their recovery.

Harvard-trained surgeon Bernie Siegel, who has spent his medical career working with cancer victims, remarked:[2]

> I can say from my own experience that patients who have given up, who have come to me feeling defeated and desperate, feeling that nothing can possibly help them, have often made their own predictions come true. The fighter-type patients who are willing to try anything that has a chance to help them, who have real faith in their survival, always do better.

SOCIAL DIMENSION

The social dimension of wellness, with its accompanying self-image, endows us with the ease and confidence to be outgoing, friendly, and affectionate toward others. Social wellness involves not only a concern for the individual but also an interest in humanity and the environment as a whole.

One of the hallmarks of social wellness is the ability to relate to others, to reach out to other people, both within the family unit and outside it. Healthy people are honest and loyal. Their own balance and sense of self allow them to extend respect and tolerance to others. They are confident of themselves and don't feel threatened by opening up to others.

People who are socially healthy can be intimate but are not promiscuous. They organize themselves in family groups and are loyal and faithful to family members. They are trustworthy and loyal to those outside the family unit and have the ability to make and keep friends. They treat others with fairness and respect.

Social wellness brings with it the ability to master social graces. Socially healthy people are affectionate, polite, and helpful toward others, can handle conflict without exploding, and are true to their ideals and beliefs while allowing others to be true to theirs. They do not interpret a difference of opinion as the basis for destruction. Instead, they are tolerant and secure. They can say "no" when they should and are sensitive in responding to others' needs without sacrificing their own.

Socially well people love themselves. This is not a vain, self-centered kind of love that causes them to develop an overinflated image of themselves. Instead, it is the kind of love that enables individuals to feel secure enough, confident enough, and good enough about themselves to reach out to others. Before you can love others, you must be able to love yourself.

The socially well person relishes touch, especially hugging, as a vital, irreplaceable means of communicating caring and concern for others. Long-term research by experts in a variety of disciplines has confirmed that touch is critical to well-being. San Diego psychologist James Hardison wrote: "It is through touching that we are able to fulfill a large share of our human needs and, in doing so, to attain happiness. By touching someone, we can affirm our friendship or approval, communicate important messages, promote health, and bring about love."

Unfortunately, Hardison continues, too many people put up barriers to the language of touch, equating "touching with either sex or violence. Consequently many people avoid the simple acts of touching — pats on the back, heartfelt handshakes, cordial hugs — that affirm goodwill."

Socially well people — whether at home, in the classroom, or at work — develop a spirit of teamwork with those around them. They do not view others with suspicion, jealousy, or contempt. They find no satisfaction in the thought of outdoing, putting down, or getting ahead of others. They find great joy in cooperation, mutual support, and working together to accomplish something of lasting value for all.

Ten Qualities of the Super-Well

- Deeply committed to a cause outside themselves.
- Physically able to do whatever they want with intensity and great energy; seldom sick.
- Caring and loving; a person others can lean on in a crisis.
- In tune with the spiritual; a clear sense of purpose and direction.
- Intellectually sharp; able to handle information; an ever-curious mind; good sense of humor.
- Well-organized and able to accomplish a lot of work.
- Able to live in and enjoy the present rather than focusing on the past or looking toward the future.
- Comfortable with feeling the full range of human emotions.
- Accepting of limitations, handicaps, and mistakes.
- Able and willing to take charge of their life, to practice positive self-care, and to be assertive when necessary.

Ten Qualities of the Super Well: Structured Exercises in Wellness Promotion. Vol. 1, pg. 16.

SPIRITUAL DIMENSION

Spiritual wellness — composed of the ethics, values, and morals that guide us — gives meaning and direction to life. Every human being needs the sense that life is meaningful, that life has purpose and direction, and that some power (nature, science, or religion) brings all of humanity together.

Spiritual wellness embodies commitment to a worthwhile purpose, faith and peace, and an undaunted comfort with life and its outcome. It is characterized by faith and optimism, by a hope that sustains through whatever life has to offer. It entails developing the inner self and identifying a purpose to life. Optimum spiritual wellness happens when you are able to *act* on that purpose.

Spiritually well people have the unique ability to see beyond the isolated event, to envision the whole picture. A spiritually well person sets realistic goals and goes about reaching them with hope, enthusiasm, and determination. Those goals are never the end result, though. They are part of the whole, cogs in the larger machine in life. Healthy people are enthused about what lies ahead, not merely content with what they have accomplished in the past.

That's not to say that spiritually well people never experience disappointment. Spiritually healthy people, however, are able to bridge the gap from one success to another, able to develop the fortitude necessary to keep going. Healthy individuals don't dwell on discouragement. They mobilize their inner resources to reach the next pinnacle. Instead of envisioning disappointments or setbacks as craggy stone walls, spiritually well people see them as smooth stepping stones, inviting them to keep going, inviting them to make their way, carefully but securely, to the other side.

RISK FACTORS THAT COMPROMISE WELLNESS

Now you've got a fairly clear picture of what wellness means, but what are the risk factors that affect wellness? More than half consists of lifestyle factors you can control! That means you can take an intelligent, well-planned approach to eliminating risk factors that may compromise your health and well-being. A graphic illustration lies in the top ten causes of death. Of the ten leading causes of death in 1900, six of them — tuberculosis, diarrhea, intracranial lesions, nephritis, senility, and diphtheria — have been all but eliminated as causes of premature death, thanks to medical breakthroughs.

Today's top killers all have something in common: They are caused largely by the lifestyle factors we choose to adopt. Among the leading risk factors are a diet high in fats and cholesterol and low in dietary fiber, cigarette smoking, and inactivity.

According to the American Council on Science and Health in a landmark report on America's health, five of the leading causes of death — heart disease, cancer, cerebrovascular disease, accidents, and chronic obstructive pulmonary disease — claimed the lives of nearly one and a half million Americans in a recent year. Almost one-third of these deaths, the Council claims, could have been prevented by modifying just three risk factors: smoking, hypertension, and alcohol abuse (see Figure 1.3).

Behavioral health, the role of lifestyle in health, brings with it solutions that seem simple in comparison to the array of scientific tests, the complex chemical formulas, the powerful lens of the microscope, and the elaborate array of available treatments. Researchers have found that a few simple lifestyle habits can add significantly to longevity:

▶ Sleeping 7 to 8 hours each night.
▶ Eating breakfast every day.
▶ Maintaining an ideal weight.
▶ Drinking only moderate amounts of alcohol or no alcohol at all.
▶ Exercising regularly.
▶ Not smoking cigarettes.

Researchers also have found that five common factors directly or indirectly cause seven of the ten major killers in this country, and that all five of those factors are behavioral, well within our control. What are they?

▶ Eating foods high in fats.
▶ Smoking.
▶ Not exercising regularly.
▶ Drinking too much alcohol.
▶ Failing to take prescribed medication for hypertension.

According to the American Council on Science and Health, four of the five leading causes of death are related directly to cigarette smoking. Smoking is responsible for an estimated 30% of all cancer deaths, 30% of all heart disease fatalities, 85% of all deaths from chronic bronchitis and emphysema, and it is an "unquantifiable risk factor" for cerebrovascular disease.

According to the Council, infant and fetal mortality also could be reduced substantially by less cigarette smoking. Smoking is responsible for higher rates of spontaneous abortion and stillbirth and accounts for up to 14% of all premature births in the United States.

The official position of the World Health Organization on smoking is clear: "The control of cigarette smoking could do more to improve health and prolong life in developed countries than any other single action in the whole field of preventive medicine." And, according to the U.S. Surgeon General, cigarette smoking is the number-one preventable cause of death and disease in the United States.

In a nutshell, here's what the risk factors to wellness prescribe for a healthy lifestyle: Eat a well-rounded diet low in fats and cholesterol and high in dietary fiber, and make sure you eat a good breakfast every day. Maintain recommended weight. Get at least 30 minutes of moderate exercise at least three times a week. Get a good night's sleep. Surround yourself with a supportive network of friends and family. Implement personal safety measures — things as simple as wearing seat belts. Stay informed about the environment, and avoid potential contaminants whenever you can. Take any medication your doctor prescribes, and be consistent in following precise directions. Above all, stop smoking and limit your intake of alcohol.

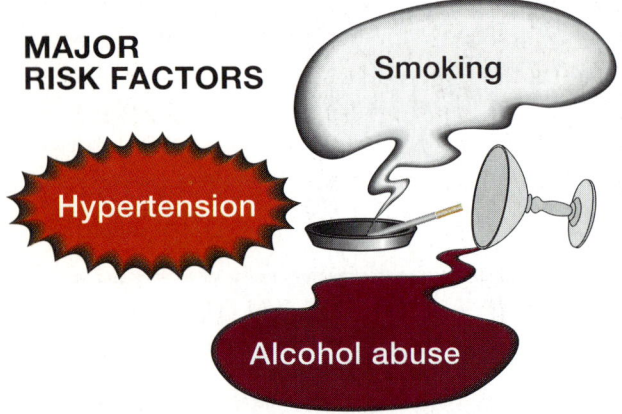

FIGURE 1.3 ▼ Major risk factors for five of the leading causes of death in the United States.

WELLNESS CHALLENGES FOR THE NEXT CENTURY

With the landmark 1979 publication of *Healthy People,* the U.S. Surgeon General's report on health promotion and disease prevention, the government embarked on a plan of establishing broad national goals intended to promote wellness among all Americans. Those goals were converted into specific health objectives a year later, with a precise list of measurable goals we hoped to attain by the year 1990.

We were successful at some; we failed at others. After assessing what had been achieved and what still had to be done, the U.S. Public Health Service in 1987 began to conduct hearings across the nation with health professionals from a variety of settings. The result is the *Year 2000 National Health Objectives,* a set of goals aimed at taking Americans into the 21st century with a higher level of health and wellness. The health objectives, which are aimed at protection, promotion, and prevention, fall under the umbrella of three main goals: to increase the span of healthy life for all Americans; to reduce health disparities among Americans; and to achieve access to preventive health services for all Americans.

Priorities for *protecting* health fall into the areas of improving food and drug safety, protecting environmental health, improving oral health, boosting occupational safety and health, and reducing the incidence of unintentional injuries. The priorities for *promoting* health fall into the areas of educational and community-based programs that foster healthier choices regarding nutrition, physical fitness, family planning, violent and abusive behavior, mental health, and tobacco, alcohol, and other drugs.

Perhaps most exciting are the priorities dealing with *preventive* services. The national objectives encompass measurable goals to provide services that will help reduce the incidence of maternal and infant mortality, heart disease and stroke, cancer, diabetes, HIV infection, sexually transmitted diseases, and a host of chronic disabling conditions. Part of that effort includes a national commitment to clinical preventive services and a national emphasis on immunization and the prevention of infectious diseases.

Experts who were instrumental in formulating the national objectives point to the commitment of the government toward achieving wellness goals. They also invite the commitment and involvement of each American in accepting responsibility for health and wellness.

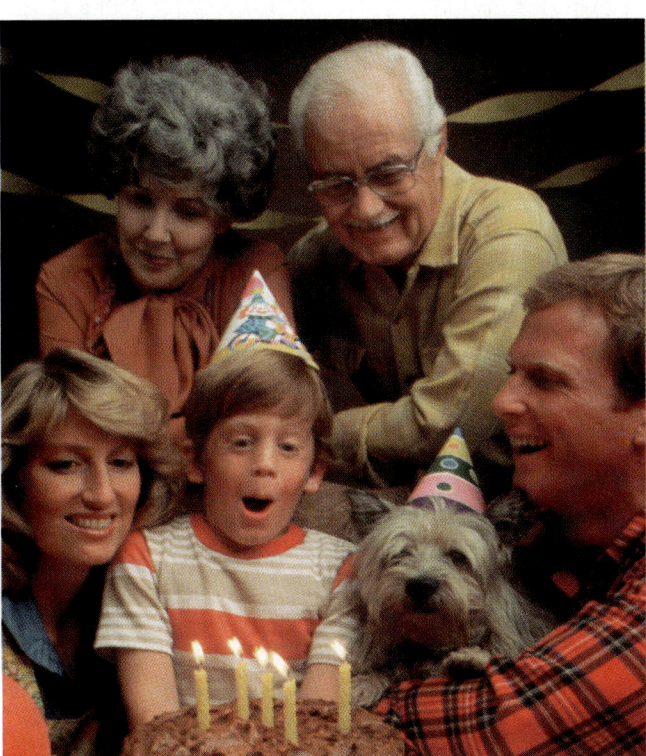

Objectives for enhancing health and wellness are aimed at protection, promotion, and prevention.

A PERSONALIZED APPROACH TO HEALTH AND WELLNESS

Vital to achieving health and wellness is your willingness to take personal responsibility for your behaviors and choices. We know enough about disease and premature death that we can formulate a set of goals that applies to the nation as a whole. How you achieve those goals, however, requires a personal decision. It entails careful, intelligent planning. How you apply the principles you'll learn in this book has to be highly personalized. What will work for someone else won't necessarily work for you.

As you study the information in this book on achieving wellness, try to take the following personalized approach:

▶ If you're smoking now, determine how you are going to stop. Find out what community resources are available to help you. If you need to,

Health Objectives For The Year 2000

I. Physical Activity and Fitness
1. Increase the proportion of people who engage regularly, preferably daily, in *light* to *moderate* physical activity for at least 30 minutes per day.
2. Increase the proportion of people who engage in *vigorous* physical activity that promotes the development and maintenance of cardiorespiratory fitness 3 or more days per week for 20 or more minutes per occasion.
3. Increase the proportion of people who regularly perform physical activities that enhance and maintain muscular strength, muscular endurance, and flexibility.
4. Reduce the proportion of people who engage in no leisure-time physical activity.
5. Reduce overweight to a prevalence of no more than 20% among people aged 20 and older and no more than 15% among adolescents aged 12 through 19.
6. Increase to at least 50% the proportion of overweight people aged 12 and older who have adopted sound dietary practices combined with regular physical activity to attain an appropriate body weight.

II. Nutrition
1. Reduce dietary fat intake to an average of 30% of calories or less and average saturated fat intake to less than 10% of calories among people aged 2 and older.
2. Increase complex carbohydrate and fiber-containing foods in the diets of adults to 5 or more daily servings for vegetables and fruits, and to 6 or more daily servings for grain products.
3. Increase calcium consumption in the diet.
4. Reduce iron deficiency among children 1 through 4 and women of childbearing age.
5. Decrease salt and sodium intake in the diet.
6. Increase to at least 85% the proportion of people aged 18 and older who use food labels to make nutritious selections.

III. Chronic Diseases
1. Increase years of healthy life to at least 65 years.
2. Reduce coronary heart disease deaths.
3. Reduce the mean serum cholesterol level among adults to no more than 200 mg/dL.
4. Increase the proportion of adults with high blood cholesterol who are aware of their condition and are taking action to reduce their blood cholesterol to recommended levels.
5. Increase the proportion of people with high blood pressure whose blood pressure is under control.
6. Increase the proportion of people with high blood pressure who are taking action to help control their blood pressure.
7. Reverse the rise in cancer deaths.
8. Slow the rise in lung cancer deaths.
9. Reduce the rate of breast cancer deaths.
10. Reduce colorectal cancer deaths.
11. Reduce diabetes-related deaths.
12. Reduce the proportion of people with asthma who experience activity limitation.
13. Reduce deaths from cirrhosis of the liver.
14. Reduce hip fractures among older adults.
15. Reduce activity limitation due to chronic back conditions.
16. Reduce the proportion of people who experience a limitation in major activity due to chronic conditions.

IV. Mental Health and Disorders
1. Reduce the prevalence of mental disorders.
2. Reduce the suicide rate.
3. Reduce the proportion of people who experience adverse health effects from stress.
4. Decrease the proportion of people who experience stress who do not take steps to reduce or control their stress.

V. Tobacco
1. Reduce the incidence of cigarette smoking.
2. Reduce the initiation of cigarette smoking by children and youth.
3. Reduce the proportion of children who are regularly exposed to tobacco smoke at home.
4. Reduce smokeless tobacco use.
5. Increase the proportion of worksites with a formal smoking policy that prohibits or severely restricts smoking at the workplace.

VI. Alcohol and Other Drugs
1. Reduce the proportion of young people who have used alcohol, marijuana, and cocaine.
2. Reduce the proportion of high school seniors and college students engaging in recent occasions of heavy drinking of alcoholic beverages.
3. Reduce alcohol consumption by people aged 14 and older to an annual average of no more than 2 gallons of ethanol per person.
4. Increase the proportion of high school seniors who associate risk of physical or psychological harm with the heavy use of alcohol, occasional use of marijuana, and experimentation with cocaine.
5. Reduce the proportion of male high school seniors who use anabolic steroids.
6. Reduce deaths caused by alcohol-related motor vehicle crashes.
7. Reduce drug-related deaths.
8. Increase the proportion of all intravenous drug abusers who are in drug abuse treatment programs.
9. Increase the proportion of intravenous drug abusers not in treatment who use only uncontaminated drug paraphernalia ("works").

VII. AIDS, HIV Infection, and Sexually Transmitted Diseases
1. Confine annual incidence of diagnosed AIDS cases to no more than 98,000 cases.
2. Confine the prevalence of HIV infection to no more than 800 per 100,000 people.
3. Increase the proportion of sexually active, unmarried people who used a condom at last sexual intercourse.
4. Reduce the incidence of gonorrhea.
5. Reduce the incidence of Chlamydia.
6. Reduce the incidence of primary and secondary syphilis.
7. Reduce the incidence of genital herpes and genital warts.
8. Reduce the incidence of pelvic inflammatory disease.
9. Reduce the incidence of sexually transmitted hepatitis B infection.

VIII. Family Planning
1. Reduce the number of pregnancies that are unintended.
2. Reduce the proportion of adolescents who have engaged in sexual intercourse.
3. Increase the proportion of sexually active, unmarried people aged 19 and younger who use contraception, especially combined method contraception that both effectively prevents pregnancy and provides barrier protection against disease.

IX. Unintentional Injuries
1. Reduce deaths caused by unintentional injuries.
2. Increase use of occupant protection systems, such as safety belts, inflatable safety restraints, and child safety seats among motor vehicle occupants.
3. Increase use of helmets among motorcyclists and bicyclists.

---

* Adapted from the U.S. Department of Health and Human Services, Public Health Service. *Healthy People 2000: National Health Promotion and Disease Prevention Objectives.* Boston, Jones and Bartlett Publishers, 1992. Refer to this publication for further information on these objectives.

talk to your doctor. Outline a specific course of action that will work for you.

▶ If you have a drinking problem or a drug dependency, find out specifically where you can get help. Make an appointment. Follow through. Start by figuring out *why* you started using drugs or alcohol to begin with. Your personal motives have a lot to do with your ability to kick the habit.

▶ If you have a weight problem, get help. With guidance from your doctor or another health-care professional, outline specifically how you are going to change your eating and exercise habits so you can lose weight safely and permanently. In essence, write your own weight-loss program geared to your situation, your preferences, and your abilities. Then make it work!

▶ Increase your level of physical activity. Before you do, however, take a critical look at your situation and determine whether you need a doctor's okay. If you do, schedule an appointment for a thorough physical examination, discuss your objectives with your physician, and get the go-ahead for a safe, effective fitness program. Then design a program that works for you, based on your situation and preferences. If you hate running, try bicycling or swimming instead. If you can't afford the fees at the racquetball court, challenge a group of friends to an equally demanding but less expensive competition a couple of times a week.

▶ Pinpoint your individual sources of stress. You probably can eliminate some of them. You can respond to others differently. If you have a particularly difficult class, for example, get on top of things by scheduling an extra hour every day to study that subject or talk to the professor about getting individualized help from a teaching assistant. Stress has a major impact on disease. A wellness plan demands that you handle stress with determination and commitment.

At the center of wellness is self-responsibility. No one else can make you eat better, exercise more

The Benefits of Wellness

Wellness reaps benefits not only to the physical body but to the soul as well. Achieving a high level of wellness helps you:

▼ Delay the aging process.
▼ Reduce your risk of chronic illness.
▼ Be self-confident.
▼ Boost your muscle strength, endurance and flexibility.
▼ Identify and meet your needs.
▼ Function better.
▼ Increase your energy.
▼ Do better at school and on the job.
▼ Maintain optimism and hope.
▼ Get good nutrition.
▼ Look better.
▼ Stay stimulated intellectually.
▼ Bounce back faster after illness or injury.
▼ Raise your level of cardiovascular health.
▼ Look at problems as challenges, not stumbling blocks.

regularly, stop smoking, use alcohol in moderation, or cope with stress. It's up to you. Accepting the challenge to achieve wellness implies that you are willing to make lifelong lifestyle changes. Wellness doesn't happen in a day. It involves an ongoing process of healthy choices throughout the rest of your life.

The information that follows can help you get started. It offers a concrete way to measure your own wellness and to identify risks you might have. It can be the impetus for making changes, for identifying what you need to do to improve your own odds for a long, satisfying life of wellness. As you read, follow the suggestions. Do what you can to eliminate risks. Take charge of yourself — the first step toward achieving your own high level of wellness and an essential step in realizing the wellness goals of an entire nation.

NOTES

1. Norman Cousins, *Head First: The Biology of Hope* (New York: E. P. Dutton, 1989).

2. Bernie Siegel, cited in *The Complete Book of Cancer Prevention* (Emmaus, PA: Rodale Press, 1986).

Health Assessment

Assessing mental health and stress is a complex task and difficult to do in limited space. The following assessment instruments represent a sampling of stress and mental-health indicators.

Self-Esteem Assessment

For each item write *a* in front of each statement that describes you and *b* in front of each statement that does not describe you.

_____ 1. People generally like me.
_____ 2. I am comfortable talking in class.
_____ 3. I like to do new things.
_____ 4. I give in easily.
_____ 5. I'm a failure.
_____ 6. I'm shy.
_____ 7. I have trouble making up my mind.
_____ 8. I'm popular with people at school.
_____ 9. My life is all mixed up.
_____ 10. I often feel upset at my home, room, or apartment.
_____ 11. I often wish I were like someone else.
_____ 12. I often worry.
_____ 13. I can be depended on.
_____ 14. I often express my views.
_____ 15. I think I am doing okay with my life.
_____ 16. I feel good about what I have accomplished recently.

Scoring/Interpretation

Determine how many matches you have with the following key. Total that number.

1. a	5. b	9. b	13. a
2. a	6. b	10. b	14. a
3. a	7. b	11. b	15. a
4. b	8. a	12. b	16. a

From the total number of matched, interpret as follows:

   12-16 high self-esteem
   8-11 moderately high self-esteem
   4-7 moderately low self-esteem
   0-3 low self-esteem

Depression Assessment

Indicate which of the following reflect what you do or how you feel. Indicate by marking an *X* in the space provided if it is like you.

_____ 1. I use drugs to relax or have fun.
_____ 2. I need to see a professional about how sad I feel.
_____ 3. I have trouble making it to class.
_____ 4. I think I would be better off dead.
_____ 5. My life seems hopeless.
_____ 6. I have thought through how I would kill myself.
_____ 7. People around me would be better off if I were gone.
_____ 8. I change my moods often.
_____ 9. I'm not interested in much anymore.
_____ 10. I can't seem to concentrate.
_____ 11. I feel unloved and unwanted.
_____ 12. I have a quick temper.
_____ 13. I feel guilty.
_____ 14. I take things too hard.
_____ 15. I have been thinking a lot about death lately.

Scoring/Interpretation

If you have marked number 2, 4, 5, 6, 7, or 11, you should talk with someone right away about your feelings and needs. You may want to talk to your instructor about where to go for help.

If you have marked any of the other responses (number 1, 3, or 8-13) in conjunction with number 15, then you should also talk with someone about how you feel.

If you have marked three or more of the remaining statements (number 1, 3, or 8-13), you also may want to seek help.

Assertiveness Assessment

Indicate what you would do in the following situations by circling *a*, *b*, or *c*.

1. A professor gives you a grade that is lower than you had expected.
   a. Ask the professor to recalculate the grade because you feel he or she is in error.
   b. Complain to the professor but accept the grade.
   c. Say nothing.
2. In a cafeteria line after waiting some time to get something to eat, a group of people recognize the person in front of you and crowd in line.
   a. Ask them to please move to the back of the line and wait like everyone else.
   b. Make a comment but not ask them to move back.
   c. Say nothing.
3. Someone near you is smoking in a nonsmoking section.
   a. Ask him or her to notice the no smoking sign and please put out the cigarette.
   b. Make a comment like, "Can't you read?" but don't ask him or her to put it out.
   c. Say nothing.
4. You have waited for ten minutes at a department secretary's office to get course information, and she is obviously making a personal call.
   a. Get her attention and say, "Can you help me?"
   b. Sigh heavily and give frustrated looks.
   c. Wait patiently.

Scoring/Interpretation

Assign the following number of points to each of your answers. Total your points.

   a = 4   b = 2   c = 0

Interpret as follows:
   12-16 assertive
   6-11 moderately assertive
   0-6 unassertive

(continued)

From Clint E. Bruess and Glenn E. Richardson, *Healthy Decisions*. Copyright © 1994 Wm. C. Brown Communications, Inc., Dubuque, Iowa. All Rights Reserved. Reprinted by permission.

Health Assessment (continued)

Stress Index

To identify the types and degrees of stress you are experiencing, complete the following index. Circle the number that corresponds to your reaction to each statement. Total the numbers in each column and add them to arrive at a subtotal for each section

	Always	Often	Sometimes	Rarely	Never
1. I get upset when I have to wait in lines.	5	4	3	2	1
2. I work by the clock to see how much I can get done in a short time.	5	4	3	2	1
3. I get upset if something takes too long.	5	4	3	2	1
4. I make almost every activity I do competitive with myself or others.	5	4	3	2	1
5. I feel guilty when I'm not working on something.	5	4	3	2	1

Section subtotal _____

6. I get upset when I can't do something my way.					
7. I get upset when my accomplishments depend on others' actions.	5	4	3	2	1
8. I get anxious when my plans become disrupted.	5	4	3	2	1
9. All good things are worth waiting for.	1	2	3	4	5
10. When I set a goal I can't reach, I simply alter it.	1	2	3	4	5

Section subtotal _____

11. I have been given too much responsibility.	5	4	3	2	1
12. I get depressed when I think of everything I have to do.	5	4	3	2	1
13. People demand too much of me.	5	4	3	2	1
14. I often find myself without enough time to complete my work.	5	4	3	2	1
15. Sometimes I feel that my head is spinning, or I get confused because so much is happening.	5	4	3	2	1

Section subtotal _____

16. I succeed in most things and try even when the task is difficult.	1	2	3	4	5
17. I am comfortable being with members of the opposite sex.	1	2	3	4	5
18. I am generally comfortable around teachers, bosses, and other superiors.	1	2	3	4	5
19. I prefer that others make decisions for me.	5	4	3	2	1
20. I don't think I have too much going for me.	5	4	3	2	1
21. I'm most relaxed when I'm busy.	5	4	3	2	1
22. I throw away old clothes, toys, and other mementos.	1	2	3	4	5
23. I enjoy being alone.	1	2	3	4	5
24. I feel the need to belong to a social group.	5	4	3	2	1
25. I get homesick easily.	5	4	3	2	1

Section subtotal _____

26. I often feel my stomach knotting, my mouth getting dry, and my heart pounding when I get nervous.	5	4	3	2	1
27. When I get nervous, I can feel my muscles tense, my hands and fingers shake, and my voice become unsteady.	5	4	3	2	1
28. After a crisis I relive the experience over and over in my mind, even though it is resolved.	5	4	3	2	1
29. I know I must resolve a crisis or it will bother me for a long time.	5	4	3	2	1
30. When I'm nervous, I imagine the worst possible outcomes of the original crisis.	5	4	3	2	1

Section subtotal = _____

Total = _____

Scoring/Interpretation

By summing all the subtotals on the index, you estimate your overall susceptibility to stress based on social situation and personality. Interpret your score as follows:

100 or higher – High stress   50-99 – Moderate stress   49 or below – You are doing well for now; keep it up

The Wellness and Longevity Potential Test

CHANGEABLE LIFE-STYLE FACTORS

1. **Tobacco**
   (1 pipe = 2 cigarettes, 1 cigar = 3 cigarettes)
Never smoked	+20
Quit smoking	+10
Smoke up to one pack per day	−10
Smoke one to two packs per day	−20
Smoke more than two packs per day	−30

   Pack-years smoked (number of packs smoked per day, times number of years smoked):
7-15	−5
16-25	−10
Over 25	−20

2. **Alcohol**
   (1 beer or 1 glass of wine = 1.25 oz. alcohol)
1.25 oz. per day or less	+10
Between 1.25 and 2.5 oz. per day	−4
−1 more for each additional 1.25 oz. per day	−___

3. **Exercise**
   (20 min. or more moderate aerobic exercise)
3 or more times per week	+20
2 times per week	+10
No regular aerobic activity	−10
Work requires regular physical exertion or at least 2 miles walking per day	+3
+1 more for each additional mile walked per day	+___

4. **Weight**
Maintain ideal weight for height	+5
5-10 lbs. over ideal	−1
11-20 lbs. over ideal	−2
21-30 lbs. over ideal	−3
−1 more for each additional 10 lbs.	−___
Yo-yo dieting	−10

5. **Nutrition**
Eat a well-balanced diet	+3
Do not eat a well-balanced diet	−3
Regularly eat meals at consistent times	+2
Do not regularly eat meals at consistent times	−2
Snack or eat meals late at night	−2
Eat a balanced breakfast	+2
Eat fish or poultry as primary protein source (totally replacing red meat)	+5
Do not eat grains and fish as primary protein source	−2
Eat at least 5 servings of green leafy vegetables per week	+3
Eat at least 5 servings of fresh fruit or juice	+3
Try to avoid fats	+5
Do not try to avoid fats	−5

   For each of the following foods eaten 2 or more times per week:
Beef, veal or pork	−1
Bacon or sausage	−1
Luncheon meat or hot dogs	−1
Fast food	−1
Fried food	−1
Processed food/TV dinners	−1
Eggs	−1
Cheese	−1
Butter	−1
Whole milk or cream	−1
Pastries, doughnuts, muffins	−1
Candy, chocolate	−1
Pretzels, potato chips	−1
Ice cream	−1

Eat some food every day that is high in fiber (whole-grain bread, fresh fruits and vegetables)	+3
Do not eat some food every day that is high in fiber	−3
Take a daily multivitamin/mineral supplement	+10
Women: Take a calcium supplement	+5
Subscribe to health-related periodicals	+2

   Subtotal: ___ A   ___ G

FIXED FACTORS

1. **Gender**
Male	−5
Female	+10

2. **Heredity**
Any grandparent lived to be over 80	+5

   Average age all four grandparents lived to:
60-70	+5
71-80	+10
Over 80	+20

3. **Family history**
Either parent had stroke or heart attack before age 50	−10

   −5 for each family member (grandparent, parent, sibling) who prior to age 65 has had any of the following:
Hypertension	−___
Cancer	−___
Heart disease	−___
Stroke	−___
Diabetes	−___
Other genetic diseases	−___

   Subtotal B: ___ +___

   (continued)

This test was developed for the average healthy person. If you already have a serious health condition, such as heart disease, diabetes, cancer or kidney disease, ask your physician for a health-risk assessment designed especially for you.

Reproduced by permission of Longevity, ©1990, Longevity International, Ltd.

The Wellness and Longevity Potential Test (continued)

PARTIALLY FIXED FACTORS

1. Family income
- 0–$5,000   −10
- $5,001–$14,000   −5
- $14,001–$20,000   +1
- +1 for each additional $10,000, up to $200,000   +___

2. Education
- Some high school (or less)   −7
- High school graduate   +2
- College graduate   +5
- Postgraduate or professional degree   +7

3. Occupation
- Professional   +5
- Self-employed   +6
- In the health-care field   +3
- Over 65 and still working   +5
- Clerical or support   −3
- Shift work   −5
- Unemployed   −7
- Possibility for career advancement   +5
- Regularly in direct contact with pollutants, toxic waste, chemicals, radiation   −10

4. Where you live
- Large urban area   −5
- Near an industrial center   −7
- Rural or farm area   +5
- Area with air-pollution alerts   −5
- Area where air pollution has curtailed normal daily activities   −7
- High crime area   −3
- Little or no crime area   +3
- Home has tested positive for radon   −7
- Total commuting time to and from work:
  - 0–1/2 hour   +3
  - 1/2 hour–1 hour   +0
  - −1 for each 1/2 hour over 1 hour   −___
- Within 30 miles of major medical/trauma center   +3
- No major medical/trauma center in area   −3

Subtotal C: ___ +___

CHANGEABLE HEALTH STATUS AND MAINTENANCE FACTORS

1. Health status
- ▼ Present overall physical health:
  - Excellent   +15
  - Good   +12
  - Fair   +5
  - Poor   −10
- ▼ Normal or low blood pressure   +5
  - High blood pressure   −10
  - Don't know   −5
- ▼ Low cholesterol (under 200)   +10
  - Moderate cholesterol (200–240)   +5
  - High cholesterol (over 240)   −10
  - Don't know   −5
- ▼ HDL cholesterol 29 or less   −25
  - 30–36   −20
  - 37–40   −5
  - 41–45   +5
  - Over 45   +10
  - Don't know   −5
- ▼ Have medical insurance coverage   +10
  - Able to use physicians of your choice   +5

2. Preventive and therapeutic measures
- Physical exams (every 3 to 4 years before age 50, every 1 to 2 years over 50)   +3
- Women:
  - Yearly gynecological exam and Pap smear   +2
  - Monthly self breast exam   +2
  - Mammogram (35–50, every 3 years; over 50, every year)   +2
  - Smoke and use oral contraceptives   −5
- Men:
  - Genital self-exam every 3 months   +2
  - Rectal or prostate exam (yearly after age 30)   +2
- All:
  - Current on mumps, measles, rubella, diphtheria and tetanus immunizations   +2
  - Tested for hidden blood in stool (over 40, every 2 years; over 50, every year)   +2
- If over age 50:
  - Yearly sigmoidoscopy of the lower bowel   +2
- All:
  - Regularly use sunscreen and avoid excessive sun   +2
  - Actively involved in a life-extension, prevention, or comprehensive wellness program   +10

3. Accident control
- Always wear seat belt as driver and passenger   +7
- Do not always wear seat belt as driver and passenger   −5
- Never drink and drive or ride with a driver who has been drinking   +2
- −10 for each arrest for drinking while under the influence of alcohol in the past 5 years   −___
- −2 for every speeding ticket or accident in the past year   −___
- For each 10,000 miles per year driven over 10,000 (national average)   −1
- Primary car weighs more than 3,500 lbs.   +10
- Subcompact   −5
- Motorcycle   −10
- −2 for every fight or attack you were involved in, or witness to, in the past year   −___
- Smoke alarms in home   +1

Subtotal D: ___ +___

(continued)

The Wellness and Longevity Potential Test (continued)

CHANGEABLE PSYCHOSOCIAL FACTORS

Married or in long-term committed relationship	+5
Satisfying sex life	+3
Children under 18 living at home	+3
For each 5-year period living alone	−1
No close friends	−10
+1 for each close friend (up to 5)	+___
+2 for each active membership in a religious community or volunteer organization (up to 4)	+___
Have a pet	+2
Regular daily routine	+10
No regular daily routine	−10
Hours of uninterrupted sleep per night:	
Less than 5 hours	−5
5-8 hours	+5
8-10 hours	−7
−1 for each additional hour over 10	−___
Not consistent	−7
Regular work routine	+5
No regular work routine	−5
−2 for every 5 hours worked over 40 in a week	−___
Take a yearly vacation from work (at least 6 days)	+5
Regularly use a stress-management technique (yoga, meditation, music, etc.)	+3
Subtotal E:	___+___

CHANGEABLE EMOTIONAL STRESS FACTORS

N = Never **R** = Rarely **S** = Sometimes
A = Always (or as much as possible)

	N	R	S	A
Generally happy	−2	−1	+1	+2
Have and enjoy time with family and friends	−2	−1	+1	+2
Feel in control of personal life and career	−2	−1	+1	+2
Live within financial means	−2	−1	+1	+2
Set goals and look for new challenges	−2	−1	+1	+2
Participate in creative outlet or hobby	−2	−1	+1	+2
Have and enjoy leisure time	−2	−1	+1	+2
Express feelings easily	−2	−1	+1	+2
Laugh easily	−2	−1	+1	+2
Expect good things to happen	−2	−1	+1	+2

	A	S	R	N
Anger easily	−2	−1	+1	+2
Critical of self	−2	−1	+1	+2
Critical of others	−2	−1	+1	+2
Lonely, even with others	−2	−1	+1	+2
Worry about things out of your control	−2	−1	+1	+2
Regret sacrifices made in life	−2	−1	+1	+2

Subtotal F: ___ + ___ + ___ + ___

SCORING

A+B+C+D+E+F=_____ (Subtotal, up to 200*)

Subtotal + G = Total

Divide total by 2. This gives your chance (in %) of living to or beyond average life expectancy of a person your age.

Total: _____ ÷ 2 = _____ %

If you scored 100%, congratulations. But don't rest on your laurels. Keep looking for ways to improve your good health. And if you didn't score as well as you would have liked, it's never too late to begin improving your longevity potential.

*If this number is higher than 200, use 200 as your subtotal. Maintain those healthy habits that allowed you to score much higher than the average person (around 50%), and try to turn any of the negatives in section G (e.g., smoking) into positives. You have the very best chance of living a long and healthy life, because these factors are totally in your control. — Linda Addlespurger

STRESS AND HEALTH

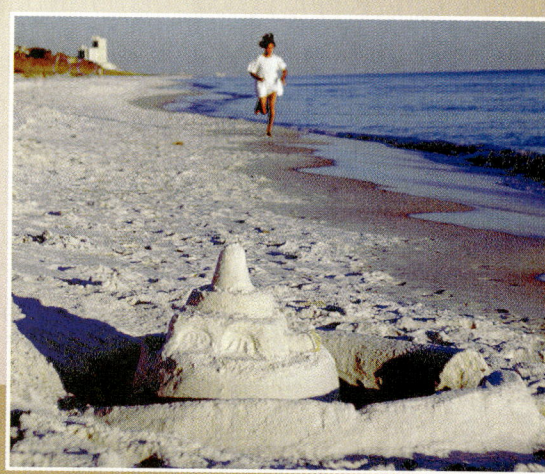

Objectives

- ▼ Learn the definition and characteristics of stress.
- ▼ Understand the relationship between stress and illness.
- ▼ Recognize the signs and symptoms of stress.
- ▼ Identify the body systems affected by stress.
- ▼ Gain strategies for coping with and reducing stress.
- ▼ Recognize the importance of diet in relation to stress.
- ▼ Recognize the importance of regular exercise in stress reduction.
- ▼ Understand the role of rest and sleep in stress.
- ▼ Be introduced to some effective time management guidelines.
- ▼ Define burnout and learn how to help prevent it.
- ▼ Learn the specific steps involved in meditation, progressive relaxation, autogenics, and biofeedback, and the philosophy of yoga.

The 1949 Conference on Life and Stress and Heart Disease provided the first formal recognition that stress could precipitate chronic disease. Practitioners who gathered at that conference also were among the first to formally define stress by stating that it is "a force which induces distress or strain upon both the emotional and physical makeup."[1]

Our understanding of stress has come a long way in the last four or five decades. Today, we understand that stress is anything in the environment that causes us to adapt, and that a stressful situation can be either happy (such as the birth of a baby) or sad (such as the death of a loved one). Stress isn't the same as frustration, anxiety, or conflict, though it can lead to all of those emotions.

Stress is no respecter of persons or situations. It can happen at home, in the classroom, on the job, in families, between friends or associates, and even between us and our surroundings, in the form of extreme heat or cold, noise, pollution, or overcrowding. Stressors can be physical (such as fatigue or a bacterial infection), emotional (such as pent-up anger or hostility), social (such as rejection or embarrassment), intellectual (such as confusion), and spiritual (such as guilt).

We also understand that stress isn't limited to what goes on in our thoughts. We know that stress is "a nonspecific automatic biological response to demands made upon an individual."[2] Scientifically speaking, stress is "any challenge to homeostasis,"[3] or the body's internal sense of balance. Stress is a biological and biochemical process that begins in the brain and spreads through the autonomic nervous system, causing the release of hormones and exerting eventual influence over the immune system.

Stress does not have to be a major, cataclysmic event. Some of the most pervasive stressors are what researchers call *hassles* — the seemingly minor, irritating annoyances that happen every day, such as losing the car keys, getting stuck behind a dimwitted shopper in a grueling grocery-store line, waking up to a miserable snowstorm, being kept waiting for an appointment, or getting stuck in a traffic jam. In his now-famous work *Future Shock*, researcher Alvin Toffler listed problems such as rising consumer prices, yard work, losing things, and having too many things to do as among the top ten reported hassles. Researchers now believe that these seemingly trivial problems actually are more damaging to health and wellness than are major stressors, partly because they eat away at us constantly, piling up until no end is in sight.

Stress does not do the same thing to all people, and it can be altered by perceptions and outlook. You may react to some stress in a negative way. Then it becomes *distress*, a type of anxiety that leads to illness. You may handle other stress in a positive way. Then it becomes *eustress*. For example, when confronted by the stress of a final exam in a particularly difficult class, you may react either by becoming extremely anxious and unable to study (distressed) or by taking on the challenge of studying twice as long and enlisting the help of study companions (eustressed). These differences in outlook are illustrated beautifully by the Chinese symbol for stress; it combines two different characters, one representing "danger" and one representing "opportunity."

According to Austrian-born Dr. Hans Selye, considered the father of stress research, eustress is "desirable" stress, the stress that keeps life interesting and provides opportunity for growth (such as marriages, births, new jobs, and exciting vacations). Eustress, says Selye, also is the physiological stress that is essential for maintaining life (such as the churning of the digestive tract or the rhythmic contractions of the heart). Distress, on the other hand, is an overload of stress — too much stress in a brief time, chronic stress over a long time, or a combination of stressors (even good ones) that eventually throw you out of balance. How much stress is too much varies from one person to another, and even from one time to another for the same person, depending on how the person perceives the stress.

Plenty of evidence confirms that the way you perceive stress has a lot to do with how stress affects you. The president of the American Institute of Stress, Paul Rosch, likens stress to a ride on a roller coaster:[4] "There are those at the front of the car, hands over head, clapping, who can't wait to get on again," he points out, "and those at the back cringing, wondering how they got into this and how soon it's going to be over." Or, to put it another way, one roller coaster passenger "has his back stiffened, his knuckles are white, his eyes shut, jaws clenched, just waiting for it to be over. The wide-eyed thrill-seeker relishes every plunge, can't wait to do it again."

Some stress even promotes curiosity and exploration. Some stressful situations are challenging, stimulating, and rewarding. Competitive sport is an excellent example. To gear up for a football game, worry about winning, and then pound across the field for 3 hours in an attempt to do it is extremely stressful, both physically and emotionally. Many believe the rewards and the thrill are well worth the stress — and millions of fans couldn't agree more.

No one is free of stress. According to figures from New York's American Institute of Stress, published in *Time* magazine, 90% of all American adults have high stress levels one or two times a week and a fourth of all American adults are subject to crushing levels of stress nearly every day. The only way to be completely free of stress is to be dead.

Stress is costly. Researchers at the American Institute of Stress estimate that 75% to 90% of all visits to health care providers result from stress-related disorders. Just among the nation's executives, an estimated $10 to $20 billion are lost each year through absence, hospitalization, and early death, much of this as a result of stress. The National Council on Compensation Insurance states that stress-related claims account for almost one-fifth of all occupational disease.[5] Fully one-fourth of all Worker Compensation claims are for stress-related injuries, and researchers estimate that 60% to 80% of all industrial accidents are related to stress. Stress-related symptoms and illnesses are costing industry a conservatively estimated $150 billion a year in absenteeism, company medical expenses, and lost productivity.

STRESS AND DISEASE

Stress has been shown to affect almost all body systems, resulting in cardiovascular disease, neuromuscular disorders, respiratory and allergic disorders, immunologic disorders, gastrointestinal disturbances, dermatologic diseases, dental problems, and a host of other disorders. Because most diseases are caused by a variety of factors instead of only one, stress probably does not *cause* illness, but various studies have pointed to a strong link between stress and the onset of disease.

Signs and Symptoms of Stress

Cardiovascular
Pounding of the heart
Racing of the heart
High blood pressure
Irregular heartbeat
Chest pain
Cold, sweaty hands

Mental
Inability to concentrate
Lack of creativity
Loss of memory
Low self-esteem

Respiratory
Shortness of breath
Rapid breathing
Asthma attacks

Sleep Disorders
Insomnia
Fatigue
Nightmares

Emotional
Nervousness
Unexplained fearfulness
Anxiety
Emotional instability
Impulsive behavior
Depression
Irritability
Forgetfulness
Severe mood swings
Tearfulness
Urge to hide
Difficulty in completing tasks
Changes in eating/-
    smoking/drinking
Increased dependence on drugs

Skin
Acne
Excessive dryness of skin
Rashes
Excessive perspiration

Gastrointestinal
Dryness of the mouth and throat
Difficulty swallowing
Grinding of the teeth
Indigestion
Nausea or queasiness
Vomiting
Loss of appetite
Excessive appetite
Diarrhea or constipation
Abdominal pain
Increased cravings
Frequent urination

Musculoskeletal
Twitching or shakiness
Neck or back pain
Headache, including migraine
Stiffness of the muscles

Stress has been shown to be a risk factor in a number of disease conditions, including the following:

- ▶ **Cardiovascular diseases.** While recognizing that other factors — such as cigarette smoking and blood cholesterol levels — are certainly important, stress seems to play a significant role in heart disease because of the specific effects it has on the cardiovascular system (discussed later in this chapter). Friedman and Rosenman, who pioneered the concept of the Type A coronary-prone personality, believe that stress is the major cause of heart disease. High blood pressure, which afflicts approximately a third of all American adults, also has been linked to stress, as has stroke, which often is caused directly by high blood pressure. Other researchers believe that coronary artery disease and congestive heart failure both are partly caused by or aggravated by stress.

- ▶ **Gastrointestinal diseases.** Ulcers in the stomach and the small intestine have been induced in mice subjected to psychological stress. And the link between human stress and our own ulcers is strong and undisputed. Stress also has been shown to have tremendous effect on the colon, producing diarrhea, constipation, and ulcerative colitis (deterioration of the membranes lining the colon). Stress even can affect the way we eat, causing severe loss of appetite in some people and eating disorders or obesity in others.

- ▶ **Musculoskeletal disorders.** One of the most common results of stress is the tension headache, caused by chronic tension in the muscles of the scalp and neck. Another type of headache — the migraine, in which the blood vessels of the scalp become dilated and exert extreme pressure — is also caused by stress. Interestingly, migraines often occur once the stress is relieved instead of during the stressful incident or period. Other musculoskeletal disorders associated with stress include rheumatoid arthritis, chronic muscle tension, and low back pain.

- ▶ **Respiratory distress.** Asthma and hay fever, both signs of allergic reaction, are both strongly linked to stress. Significant emotional stress often precipitates an attack of asthma or hay fever, even in the absence of the "allergen."

Stress also has been shown to be a factor in a number of skin conditions (such as hives, eczema, and psoriasis), metabolic disorders (such as thyroid malfunctions or diabetes), menstrual irregularity, and gout. Some researchers are even finding convincing evidence that stress plays a significant role in the development of some cancers.

THE GENERAL ADAPTATION SYNDROME: HOW THE BODY REACTS TO STRESS

When the body becomes stressed, regardless of the source of the stress, it undergoes what scientists now recognize as the stress response: the "fight or flight" response primitive people used when facing the various threats in their environment. It is the collection of physiological changes that occurred in rapid-fire succession when a cave-dweller was confronted by a saber-toothed tiger. The body systems sped up, and hormones started surging through the bloodstream. The senses sharpened, and levels of energy were high. Everything combined to enable cave-dwellers to conquer their enemies or run for their life.

Even though society has become more civilized, our bodies have not. A student giving an oral presentation to a classroom full of sleepy students and an unthreatening professor has the same physiological response as the cave-dweller who faced the saber-toothed tiger. Unfortunately, that kind of response usually isn't appropriate in today's world. As Boston University psychiatrist Peter Knapp pointed out, "When you get a Wall Street broker using the responses a caveman used to fight the elements, you've got a problem."

With stress as an enemy, the body has powerful and intricate weapons to summon in response. "The problem is that many of our battleship's weapons are beautifully designed," one writer commented, "but for the wrong war. The enemy has changed greatly. Our stress responses were programmed for life in the primitive state, thousands of years before we became 'civilized.' No longer are our stresses a simple matter of life and death threats; they now involve much more intricate and complex challenges."

The "stress response" has been termed the *general adaptation syndrome*. This reaction occurs in three general stages: alarm, resistance, and exhaustion. (See Figure 10.1)

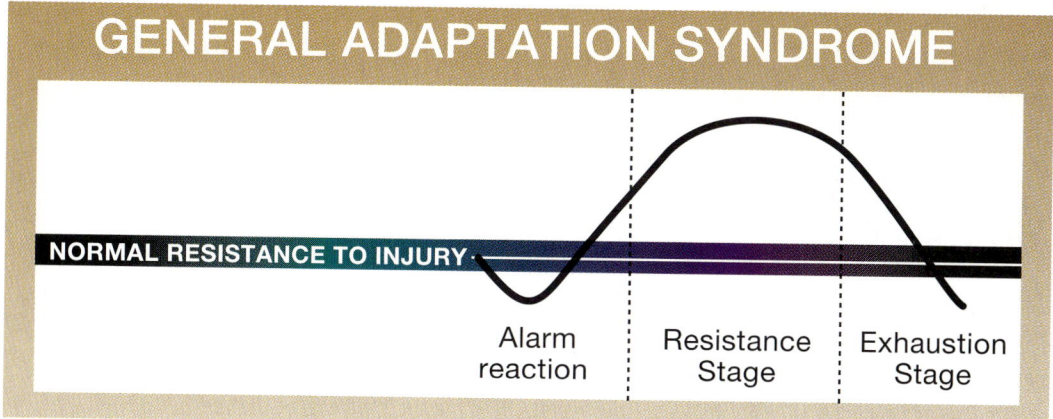

FIGURE 2.1 ▼ Stages of the General Adaptation Syndrome.

ALARM

The stress response begins the second the brain perceives any kind of stress or threat. The initial reaction is an emotional one, but physical reactions follow rapidly in the classic fight-or-flight syndrome. The mouth gets dry, and the palms get sweaty. Adrenaline and other hormones are pumped throughout the body, speeding the heart to deliver oxygen-rich blood; digestion shuts down so much-needed blood is not diverted to the stomach. The muscles get tense, prepared for a workout. The senses — sight, hearing, smell, and taste — become acute, ready to identify any "danger."

During the alarm stage, a person can exhibit "super-human" strength. The physiological reactions of the alarm stage are what enable a small woman to lift a car weighing several tons off the chest of a toddler.

RESISTANCE

During the second stage of the stress response, resistance, you actually meet the perceived challenge. Basically, the adrenal glands continue to release adrenaline, the thyroid pumps out thyroid hormones, the hypothalamus releases endorphins (the body's natural painkillers), and the adrenal releases fewer sex hormones (again, to prevent the possibility of any diversion). Glucose and cholesterol are released into the bloodstream, providing instant energy and endurance. Heart and breathing rates increase to boost the supply of oxygen to the body. The blood thickens; the skin "crawls," pales, and sweats. All told, during the alarm and resistance stages of the stress response, the body has more than 1,400 known physicochemical reactions.

The resistance stage of the stress response is ideally suited to meeting the challenges of short-term stress. Simply stated, the body tries to *adapt*, to once again achieve the balance (homeostasis) that existed before the stress occurred. The body is "on guard," trying to resist the ill effects of the stress. If the stress is short-term, the body generally is able to adapt and return to a state of balance. If the stress becomes chronic, however, the body eventually loses the ability to adapt.

EXHAUSTION

Although most people experience the alarm and resistance stages of the stress response frequently, only those with chronic stress experience exhaustion, a stage in which the body's resources are depleted and its adaptive abilities are lost. Many of the events of the alarm stage occur again as the body attempts to adjust to higher levels of stress, but the resulting wear and tear knock out the immune system, injure body systems and organs, and lead to illness and disease. The exhaustion stage is when long-term effects of stress occur.

HOW STRESS AFFECTS THE BODY SYSTEMS

The brain usually is the first body system to recognize a stressor. The brain then reacts with split-second timing to instruct the rest of the body how to adjust to the stressor. The latest research shows that the brain continues to stimulate the stress reaction as long as 72 hours after a traumatic incident occurs.

The brain is not a discriminator of stressors. It reacts the same whether the stress is physical (you are almost hit by a car) or emotional (your boss calls you in for another one of his "talks"). The result is a virtual cascade of hormones and brain chemicals that take their toll. The latest research reveals that elevated levels of stress hormones kill off significant numbers of vitally important brain cells. When researchers at the University of Kentucky exposed rats to prolonged stress, the rats showed reduced electrical activity in the hippocampus after only 3 weeks. When examined in autopsies at the end of 6 months, the rats that had been exposed to stress lost twice as many brain cells — 50% of the total brain cells — as same-aged rats who had been spared the stress.[6]

The brain isn't the only thing that suffers as a result of chronic stress. The endocrine system works overtime, pumping out excesses of hormones that increase blood pressure, damage the lining of the heart and blood vessels, inhibit vitamin D activity, cause a loss of calcium, increase the risk of diabetes, and suppress the immune system.

Stress impacts every aspect of the gastrointestinal system. The mouth stops producing saliva. The regular rhythmic contractions of the esophagus are disrupted, making swallowing difficult. The stomach slows down and becomes bathed in gastric acid (leading to ulcers), and its lining becomes fragile and engorged with blood. The liver overproduces glucose, and the pancreas becomes chronically inflamed. Increased production of hydrochloric acid and disruption of normal peristaltic action throughout the intestinal tract lead to duodenal ulcers and chronic diarrhea or constipation.

The cardiovascular system reacts with increased heart rate, higher blood pressure, damaged blood vessels, and a boost in serum cholesterol levels, all of which lead to greater risk of cardiovascular disease. Research efforts have shown a strong link between stress and all kinds of cardiovascular disease, including deaths attributed to cardiovascular disease. Maryland psychologist David Krantz[7] summarizes heart disease as "some interaction of mind, body, and behavior. Your coronary risk probably depends on how your body reacts, and how often your behavior leads you into stressful situations."

Stress can cause blood pressure to go up, resulting in permanent hypertension if stress persists over time. Men and women react differently to stress. In women, blood pressure soars with much less negative stress. The effects of stressors on high blood pressure for both men and women are intensified by caffeine (though the dose does not seem especially important) and by a family history of high blood pressure.

For people with existing heart disease, stress may be as hard on the heart as an intense physical exertion is. In both physical stress tests and mental stress tests, the mental stress test caused the heart to slow down — with a resulting significant decrease in blood flow to the heart — in more than half the heart disease patients in a UCLA School of Medicine study. The reason is that stress causes blood vessels to constrict (grow smaller) instead of expand, reducing the amount of blood that can be circulated. One question asking the heart disease patients to list their own shortcomings caused almost as much stress on the heart as did an intense workout on a stationary bicycle.

Stress may even be a strong contributing factor to heart disease. A number of studies have shown that stress causes the body to release cholesterol into the bloodstream. Well-documented evidence proves that high blood cholesterol level is a leading risk factor for the development of coronary artery disease. When the bloodstream carries too much cholesterol or other fats, fatty deposits build up on the walls of the coronary arteries, narrowing them and restricting blood flow to the heart. If the arteries eventually become too clogged, blood flow to a certain part of the heart stops, that part of the heart muscle dies, and the victim suffers a heart attack.

The effects of stress don't stop there. As part of the fight-or-flight reaction (the alarm stage of the stress response), the blood thickens. As a result, it coagulates more easily. Blood platelets build up along fatty deposits in the coronary arteries, worsening existing arteriosclerosis.

STRESS AND THE IMMUNE SYSTEM

Perhaps the greatest effect of stress is on the immune system. During the forty some years that scientists have been taking a hard look at the immune system, other researchers have become sophisticated at studying the effects of stress on immunity and disease. In one series of studies, reported by Dr. Sheldon Cohen, British volunteers from all walks of life agreed to expose themselves to the common cold virus to see who would get sick. The researchers found that subjects judged to have been under stress before the study were more than twice as likely to come down with colds than those who were not.[8]

Herpes viruses such as Epstein-Barr offer a helpful model for studying the effects of stress on immunity: the viruses are common, and, unlike some other viruses, herpes viruses are never completely wiped out by the immune system but simply are held in check by immune response. Diseases caused by herpes viruses often come and go as the virus advances and retreats. Specific herpes viruses are responsible for recurring oral cold sores and genital ulcers, as well as for chicken pox, and for its recurring form, known as shingles.

Having more herpes antibodies, or lower immunity, has been associated with many kinds of stress. For example, studies have indicated that students show more herpes antibodies while undergoing exams than they do after summer vacation.

Research provides strong evidence that microorganisms alone do not cause infectious disease. The condition of the person exposed to the microorganism also matters. Scientists are studying, more exactly, how stress might affect the immune systems of people at different stages of life and, in turn, how these immune changes might affect health and disease.

As research continues into the link between stress and the immune system, scientists have come up with a veritable shopping list of conditions caused or aggravated by stress: coronary heart disease, arteriosclerosis, atherosclerosis, high blood pressure, coronary thrombosis, stroke, angina, respiratory ailments, ulcers, irritable bowel syndrome, ulcerative colitis, gastritis, pancreatitis, diabetes, migraine headache, myasthenia gravis, epileptic attacks, chronic backache, kidney disease, chronic tuberculosis, allergies, rheumatoid arthritis, systemic lupus erythematosus, psoriasis, eczema, cold sores, shingles, hives, asthma, Raynaud's disease, multiple sclerosis, cancer, and an entire spectrum of endocrine and autoimmune problems, to name just a few. Physicians caution that few of these diseases are caused or triggered solely by stress, that other factors also must be considered. Continuing research, however, is clear: Stress plays a moderate to major role in a whole Pandora's box of disease conditions.

Stress is a leading factor in disease because, many researchers believe, it compromises the immune system, making the body less capable of fighting disease and infection. Stress can, in fact, literally shut down the immune response. Simply stated, stress suppresses the immune system's ability to produce and maintain lymphocytes (the white blood cells necessary for killing infection) and natural killer cells (the specialized cells that seek out and destroy foreign invaders), both vital in the fight against infection and disease. And that's not all. Stress affects all the key players in immunity, from the levels of interferon to the organs vital to immune system functioning (such as the thymus).

A number of studies shows that stress increases the risk of suffering allergic reactions, contracting infectious diseases, and developing autoimmune diseases (such as rheumatoid arthritis). One reason is the tendency of stress to suppress the body's production of T lymphocytes, the immune cells that fight bacterial and viral infections, fungi, and cancer cells.

Apparently, stress doesn't have to be chronic to compromise the immune system. In one study conducted by researchers at the University of Rochester, mice were separated into three groups. One group was not stressed at all; a second group was stressed just once; and a third group was stressed every other day for about 2 weeks. Researchers found that the mice exposed to stress just once showed a drop in natural killer cells.[9]

"We live in a world of uncertainties," says cardiologist Herbert Benson, "everything from the nuclear threat to job insecurity to the near assassination of the President to the lacing of medicines with poisons." Those stressors can accumulate enough to result in chronic stress and, if an individual isn't resilient enough, the final product is illness.

The good news is that stress doesn't have to knock you out. Some people manage to be resilient to stress; others exhibit what scientists call "hardiness," an ability to resist the ill effects of stress. City University of New York researcher Suzanne Kobasa, a pioneering scientist who studied a group of AT&T executives during an 8-year period of extreme stress — the largest corporate reorganization in history — found that even through debilitating stress, some of the executives didn't get sick. In fact, they suffered less than half the number of illnesses as their co-workers who were under the same amount of job stress. Kobasa and her colleagues determined that the healthy executives had the ability to withstand the negative effects of stress. She coined the term *hardiness* to denote this quality.

Kobasa boiled down the hardiness concept to what she called *the three Cs: commitment, control, and challenge.* The executives who withstood the stress had a strong commitment in their lives. That commitment (to families, work, religious faith, friendships) gave them something to strive toward and work for. They also believed they had some amount of control over their lives, that even when negative things were happening, they were not completely out of control. They trusted that they could get enough information to make intelligent decisions, and that those decisions could help them maintain command. They also saw stressful events as an exciting challenge that tested their creativity and resources instead of a debilitating threat that could wipe them out.

▼ Stress Affects Susceptibility

Ever wonder why tense times are often accompanied or followed by a cold, sore throat, or flu? Stress lowers resistance to infection by temporarily inhibiting some facets of the immune response. Keeping stress under control likewise may have positive results in a person's resistance against enemies such as cancer, heart disease, and accidents.

Listen to Your Body!

Some people become so accustomed to chronic stress that they fail to recognize the symptoms as abnormal. Consider stopping and listening. Your body is "talking" to you all the time about how you manifest stress. It is important to understand your own responses to pressure so you can take advantage of the positive ones and minimize the ones that work against you.

Recognizing your body symptoms and signs is a good first step to knowing your stress strengths and susceptibilities. It will also cue you to select skills and strategies that best address your needs. Complete the Symptoms of Stress activity below before reading on.

THE ART OF LISTENING TO YOUR BODY: THE SYMPTOMS OF STRESS

Circle the number that most accurately describes how often you experience each of the following symptoms or behaviors in response to stress.

1 = Rarely   2 = Sometimes   3 = Frequently

Listen To Your Body		Observe Your Actions		Listen To Your Emotions	
Change in breathing	1 2 3	Yelling	1 2 3	Worrying	1 2 3
Rapid or abnormal pulse	1 2 3	Crying	1 2 3	Depression	1 2 3
Muscle tension	1 2 3	Hostility	1 2 3	Impatience	1 2 3
Headaches	1 2 3	Decreased productivity	1 2 3	Loneliness	1 2 3
Upset or queasy stomach	1 2 3	Use of alcohol	1 2 3	Powerlessness	1 2 3
Fatigue	1 2 3	Use of drugs	1 2 3	Boredom	1 2 3
Dry throat or sweaty palms	1 2 3	Increased smoking	1 2 3	Poor self-esteem	1 2 3
Difficulty sleeping	1 2 3	Eat more/eat less	1 2 3	Frustration	1 2 3
Frequent colds or flu	1 2 3	Forgetfulness	1 2 3	Overwhelmed	1 2 3
Total _____		Total _____		Total _____	

If your total in any category is greater than 10, or your total for all categories is greater than 20, there's a good chance that your symptoms and actions are controlling you. Most of us are somewhere along a spectrum: our symptoms neither totally control us, nor do we totally control our symptoms. Because it tells us where we stand, symptom recognition is one of the most important steps in gaining control over stress.

Reprinted from *Pathways: A Success Guide for a Healthy Life*, by Donald W. Kemper, Jim Giuffre, and Gene Diabeski. Healthwise, Inc., P.O. Box 1989, Boise, Idaho, 83701.

Ohio State University psychologist Janice Kiecolt-Glaser, known for her work in immune studies, says, "Just because your immune function goes down during a stressful period doesn't mean you are going to get sick. Where stress seems to have the greatest impact on health is on individuals who already have poor immune function because of age or diseases that impair the immune system, or on individuals who have already been chronically stressed for reasons other than health."[10]

Yale oncologist and surgeon Bernie Siegel is one of the nation's foremost researchers of the link between behavior and disease. He pointed out, in *Love, Medicine, and Miracles,* that "stresses that we *choose* evoke a response totally different from those we'd like to avoid but cannot. Helplessness is worse than the stress itself. That is probably why the rate of cancer is higher for blacks in America than for whites, and why cancer is associated with grief and depression."[11]

Epidemiologist Leonard Sagan reported that "whether altered conditions are viewed as threatening or challenging, and whether the consequences contribute to personal growth or apathy and despair is the result of the interaction of two factors: the magnitude and quality of the external stressor and the capacity of the individual to cope."[12]

▼ COPING WITH STRESS

Capacity to cope depends not only on inherent qualities, such as the qualities exhibited in hardiness, but also in astute coping strategies, such as eating right, getting plenty of exercise, getting enough rest, changing the way you think about stress, practicing good time management, preventing burnout, and using relaxation techniques. Successfully coping with stress isn't something that just happens. It's something you have to plan for and work at. Sometimes it involves changing attitudes, ideologies, values or goals. It may even require making gradual but significant lifestyle changes to eliminate debilitating sources of stress when you can't find any other solutions. Often it requires strategies you develop ahead of time, strategies that help you manage stressful situations.

GENERAL GUIDELINES

As you develop an arsenal of coping strategies, you should remember that *these strategies are designed to reduce the amount and extent of stress in your life*, not to cause you more stress. To reach that goal:

▶ Don't try to incorporate too many strategies at once. Changing old habits and developing new ways of dealing with things require time. If you load on too much at once, you'll end up feeling frustrated and stressed. Too much change, even if it's positive, can translate into stress.

▶ Before you decide on the strategies you want to use, consider your own strengths and skills. Think about which you would *enjoy*. Assess what kind of social support you'll have. Those kinds of considerations can help you choose the most workable strategies for you.

▶ Keep in mind that what works for you won't necessarily work for someone else — and won't even work for you in all situations. Be flexible, be willing to change your coping strategies, and never stop assessing.

▶ Do not expect a single coping strategy to provide you with enough coping power, just as the same strategy won't work for you in all situations. Don't overload by trying everything at once. Several coping strategies will be required to do the trick.

▶ Recognize that even negative stress can have a positive outcome if you meet it head-on and use it as an opportunity for learning and growth. Even a stressful situation can give you insights or help you become more prudent.

A BALANCED DIET

One of the most effective stress-busters is diet. A poor diet not only increases your susceptibility to disease in general but also increases your susceptibility to the negative effects of stress. Certain things in your diet can even exaggerate your stress by making you more uptight. Overeating, undereating, or eating the wrong foods can upset your body's balance, making all your systems more apt to suffer the ill effects of stress.

Stress may change your nutritional requirement, too. Chronic stress may influence your body's stores

Take Your Stress Temperature

How stressed are you?
Let's play 20 questions. Check "yes" or "no" for the following: YES   NO

1. Do you prefer to do everything yourself rather than let people help you?
2. For you, is there only one right way to do things?
3. Do you find it hard to make decisions?
4. Do you forget to laugh?
5. Do you never have time to daydream?
6. Is it important to you that everyone likes you?
7. When little things go wrong, does it ruin your whole day?
8. Do you constantly feel exhausted?
9. Have you had problems with insomnia?
10. Do you grind your teeth?
11. In the last year have you had three or more illnesses that could have been triggered by stress — headaches, diarrhea, colds, flus?
12. Do you hate it when the plan changes?
13. Do you get upset when you have to wait in line?
14. Are you easily bored?
15. Do you find it hard to say no?
16. Do you hate the shape your body is in but can't seem to do anything about changing it?
17. Does your life feel out of control?
18. Are you resentful that so many people make demands on your time?
19. Have you moved, broken up with a boyfriend/girlfriend, lost a parent, or gone through any other big changes in the last year?
20. Was the last time you had a vacation over a year ago?

Count one point for each "yes." The closer your total is to 20, the higher your stress level. If you rate 10 or above, be sure you do *something* because, with this level of stress in your life, you have a high risk of getting sick unless you learn to manage it.

From *Shape*, April 1992.

Stress may change your nutritional requirement, too. Chronic stress may influence your body's stores of important vitamins and minerals. It also can increase the amount of fats in your bloodstream, requiring you to eat a diet lower in fats and may boost your protein requirements. If you're under chronic stress, you may need more than the normal amount of protein. You also may need more calories, as stress makes your body cells less capable of metabolizing the energy released from the food you eat and causes you to burn up your food more quickly.

You should concentrate on eating three sensible meals a day containing foods low in fat and high in fiber. Most of your calories should come from complex carbohydrates: grains, pastas, vegetables, and fruits. If you are under chronic stress, you should boost your protein intake with the leanest protein sources possible: fish, poultry, lean cuts of beef, and low-fat or skim dairy products.

Follow these specific dietary guidelines:

▶ Cut back on sugar and foods containing sugar. The stress response changes your metabolism, which leads to higher levels of sugar in the bloodstream. Check labels. Corn syrup, corn sweeteners, sucrose, and honey are examples of sugars in processed foods. Even though sugar provides calories for energy, it may be followed by a "crash" as the rapid effects of the sugar wear off.

▶ Avoid all products containing nicotine: cigarettes, cigars, pipes, chewing tobacco, snuff. Nicotine is a stimulant that can make you high-strung and irritable.

▶ Cut back on or eliminate caffeine, a stimulant that increases your sensitivity to stress. Caffeine is found not only in coffee and tea but also in cola drinks, chocolate, and a number of both prescription and over-the-counter medications.

▶ Reduce the amount of salt in your diet. Major culprits are processed foods, including some that don't even taste salty, such as canned soup and powdered gelatin and salad mix.

REGULAR EXERCISE

The stress response is characterized by the fight-or-flight syndrome, a collection of physical reactions that prepare the body for intense physical activity. To dissipate the effects of stress, start moving! Regular aerobic exercise eases the muscle tension caused by stress and reduces the amount of adrenaline circulating through the bloodstream. Exercise decreases the intensity of stress, lessens the effects of stress, cuts down the time to recover from stress, and even minimizes the physiological reactions of the stress response. Regular exercise reduces the risk of getting sick, even for those under severe or chronic stress.

Various tests have proven how much exercise can reduce the effects of stress. In one, University of Washington psychologist Jonathon Brown studied

---

Stress Management Skills: What Do You Do?

For each skill, circle the number that corresponds to your typical skill use.

I use the following skills . . .	never	rarely	occasionally	regularly
Personal Management Skills: Organizing Yourself				
Valuing: Investing self appropriately	1	2	3	4
Planning: Moving toward goals	1	2	3	4
Commitment: Saying yes and sticking to it	1	2	3	4
Time Use: Setting priorities	1	2	3	4
Pacing: Controlling the tempo	1	2	3	4
Relationship Skills: Changing The Scene				
Contact: Reaching out	1	2	3	4
Listening: Tuning in to others	1	2	3	4
Assertiveness: Saying no	1	2	3	4
Fight: Standing your ground	1	2	3	4
Flight: Leaving the scene	1	2	3	4
Nest-Building: Creating a home	1	2	3	4
Outlook Skills: Changing Your Mind				
Relabeling: Turning a spade into a diamond	1	2	3	4
Surrendering: Saying goodbye	1	2	3	4
Faith: Accepting your limits	1	2	3	4
Imagination: Laughing, creativity	1	2	3	4
Whispering: Talking nicely to oneself	1	2	3	4
Physical Stamina: Building Your Strength				
Exercise: Fine-tuning your body	1	2	3	4
Nourishment: Feeding your body	1	2	3	4
Gentleness: Wearing kid gloves	1	2	3	4
Relaxation: Cruising in neutral	1	2	3	4

Look down the column of 1's. These are your underdeveloped skills. Underline the ones you would like to use more often. **Look at the column of 4's.** These are probably your skills of habit. Mark those you tend to overuse. Which three individual coping skills do you use most often? For what kinds of stressors? As you identify your pattern of skill use, what insights and observations strike you?

Reprinted with permission from *Kicking Your Stress Habits*, copyright 1981, 1989. Donald A. Tubesing. Published by Whole Person Associates Inc., PO Box 3151, Duluth, MN 55803, (218) 728-6807. Used by permission.

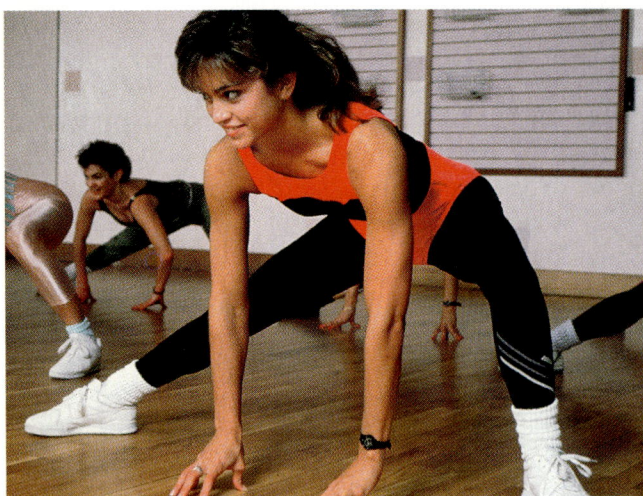
Exercise buffers the effect of stress.

stress levels among students there. He found that those suffering the highest levels of stress were also those most likely to develop a wide range of medical problems. He also found something unexpected: Those who exercised regularly reported far fewer visits to the university student health center, even when under extreme stress.

To get the maximum stress-reducing benefit from your exercise routine:

▶ Choose a form of exercise you *like*. Not only will you be more prone to stick with it, but you'll enjoy yourself, too — an essential factor in alleviating stress.

▶ Try to find an activity suited to your personality. Consider whether you'd like an exercise that requires keen concentration or one that allows you to daydream; whether you want some time alone or want to exercise with a partner or as part of a team; and whether you'd rather engage in a competitive or a noncompetitive exercise.

▶ Consider how much equipment the exercise requires. Walking takes nothing more than a good pair of shoes, whereas golf requires a set of clubs, a handful of tees, and plenty of fresh balls. Consider, too, where you'll have to go to exercise. Walking and bicycling can be done almost anywhere. But you'll have to go to a pool if you want to swim. Consider options for different climates and weather conditions. You can walk in almost any weather, but you'll need certain seasons and conditions for skiing, golfing, or swimming outdoors. For greatest versatility, choose a variety of activities so you won't be limited by locale, weather, and equipment needs.

▶ Don't feel limited to what you can do already. If you think fencing sounds like fun, take a class. If you think golf sounds challenging and enjoyable, sign up for lessons.

▶ Don't overlook team sports as a good form of exercise. Not only do you get to vent your stress, frustrations, and aggression, but you'll also enjoy some good social support — another proven stress-buster. Team sports don't have to involve competition; you might join a group of classmates in an informal football contest every Saturday or play some "parking lot basketball" just for fun.

▶ If you haven't been exercising, start slowly. If you try too much at first, you're likely to get injured, or, at the least, stiff and sore. The resulting discouragement might keep you from exercising at all. If you're just starting out, take it easy; try 10 to 15 minutes at a time, then work up as you get more conditioned. Challenge yourself, but don't overdo it.

▶ Consider aerobic exercises that help condition your heart and lungs. Try walking, jogging, running, bicycling, swimming, or racquetball.

▶ Exercise regularly. Experts think four to five times a week is ideal.

▶ Consider exercising more often for shorter periods. Dr. Irving Dardik, a founding chairman of the U.S. Olympic Sports Medicine Council, has found that exercising in 5-minute chunks followed by relaxation techniques (what he calls "recovery") can be more beneficial in relieving stress than a continuous 30-minute workout.

▶ Don't overdo it. People who get "addicted" to exercise are vulnerable to injury, fatigue, and overexertion, all of which can lead to depression and anxiety instead of stress relief. If you start to feel anxious about your exercise, cut back and ease off until you find you're enjoying yourself again.

PLENTY OF REST

Sleep is essential to coping with stress. If you've had your rest, it's easier to face almost anything. Sleep offers other, not-so-obvious benefits, too, including the relaxation so important to minimizing the effects of the stress response.

If you're feeling fatigued:

▶ Try to establish a sleep pattern. Go to bed at about the same time every night and wake up at the same time every morning instead of skimping on sleep during the week and sleeping until noon on weekends.

▶ If you really need to, take a *short* nap during the day; 20 minutes is an optimal time. Shorter than that doesn't give you enough sleep, and longer than that can make you drowsy.

▶ If you're having trouble falling asleep at night, avoid napping during the afternoon, eat a light dinner, and avoid caffeine after 6 p.m.

▶ Use your bedroom only for sleeping. Don't watch television, study, or do work in bed. You need to associate your bed and your bedroom with sleep.

▶ Most people need 6 to 8 hours of sleep a night to function well and feel refreshed, but that requirement can vary from one person to another. To discover how much sleep you *really* need, go to sleep at the same time every night, then sleep until you wake up. It will take a couple of weeks to determine what you need. Once you've figured it out, discipline yourself and set a goal to get the rest you need.

REFRAMING THOUGHTS

Reframing entails changing the way you look at things, learning to be an optimist instead of a pessimist. The way you think often determines what really happens, and under stress it can help change the way stress impacts your body. In Suzanne Kobasa's study of AT&T executives, the ones who didn't get sick were the ones who had a positive perspective on the situation, who saw it as a unique opportunity for meeting a challenge instead of a life-altering change that would destroy them and their careers.

To help reframe your own thinking:

▶ Listen carefully to the words you use to describe yourself and your situation. Are they positive or negative? Make it a point to listen for a few weeks. Then, if you need to, use different phrases and descriptions.

▶ Try role playing, either by yourself or with a friend. Start by relating a stressful situation you have experienced lately; tell how you reacted. Then come up with some different ways in which you could have reacted to the situation. If you're role playing with a friend, ask for feedback or suggestions. Next, imagine some plausible stressful situations and outline how you'd handle them. Concentrate on positive responses.

▶ For one week, look for the good in every person and every situation you encounter. It can be tough, but you always can find something! This kind of exercise is like conditioning your attitudes. Before long, it can become a habit.

▶ Avoid words that signal defeat: *always, never, should have, ought to*. Replace them with more benign choices. Instead of saying, "I *always* fail quizzes in class," change your statement to, "I'm *sometimes* unprepared when the teacher springs a quiz on us."

EFFECTIVE TIME MANAGEMENT

One of the leading sources of stress is simply too much to do in too little time. We are living in the fastest-paced society of this century, and the mere speed at which we move can be a significant stressor. Learning to manage the time you have can alleviate stress and reduce anxiety.

To better manage your time:

▶ Figure out how you're spending your time: Keep a diary for 2 weeks. You might be stunned to find out how much time you're spending on the phone or in front of the television. You can't outline realistic goals until you know what you're really doing.

▶ Try to figure out your peak time. Are you a "morning person," or do you get your second wind when most people are quitting for the day? Try to plan your most demanding tasks — studying, working — for the time you're at your peak. If you have to take a particularly challenging class and you're generally sluggish in the morning, see if you can schedule it for the afternoon, or find out if it's offered at night.

▶ Before you schedule anything else on your daily calendar, schedule time for a break. Plan on several periods for doing what you *want* to do — soaking in a hot tub, reading a good book, watching a football game on TV, or talking to a friend. Knowing you can look forward to a few breaks can help you more easily face the more stressful periods of your day.

▶ Learn to prioritize. Not every demand is a top priority. You usually can split up tasks into those that are essential, important, and unimportant or trivial. Spend your time and attention on the ones that are essential and important. If you have time left over, you can go for the trivial ones.

▶ Try attacking things one at a time. If you are faced with a number of things to do, don't try to accomplish everything at once. Instead, decide on a course of action that lets you move through the list calmly.

▶ Learn to judge realistically how long a task will take. Most people underestimate by about 50%, so get into the habit of adding 50% to the time you think it will take. Once you learn how to realistically estimate the time different tasks take, you can stop overcrowding your day with too much to handle.

▶ Before you go to bed each night, write down your schedule for the next day. Think through what *has* to be done — classes you need to attend, your part-time job, a commitment at the community crisis center. Prioritize. Figure out which are most important, and make the time for those. Include times for leisure.

▶ Learn to set realistic goals. Write them down, and break them up into chunks you can more readily accomplish. Keep track of your progress, and reward yourself for a job well done.

▶ Don't feel guilty if you have to say "no" to a request. You can do only so much in a single day. If you start to get overwhelmed, back off. Going to the movies with a few friends might be fun, but not if you have to stay up half the night to study for an exam in exchange. If you can, delegate some tasks to others, freeing up your time for something more important.

▶ Protect against boredom. Set a satisfying, realistic goal, and do something toward it every day.

BURNOUT PREVENTION

Stress — especially chronic stress — can quickly lead to *burnout*, a state of physical and mental exhaustion with few remaining resources. Accompanying physical symptoms may include headache, indigestion, fatigue, and muscle soreness. Mental symptoms might be depression, apathy, or loss of enjoyment in life.

To prevent burnout:

▶ Surround yourself with a strong network of social support. Have at least one friend in whom you can confide.

▶ Distract yourself from your routine by developing a new interest, trying a new hobby, or volunteering for something new. Two hours a week telling animated stories to a group of captivated preschoolers at the local library might be just what you need to get a fresh perspective on things.

▼ Burnout Quiz

Take a look at all three aspects of your life: career (school), personal, and relationships, and ask yourself the following questions. If the answer is an emphatic *yes*, score 5 points. If it's definitely no, give yourself 0 points. If you're in between, score 1 to 4 points, depending on your level of discomfort.

1. I feel more negative than positive lately.
2. I feel more fatigued than energetic.
3. I work harder and harder and accomplish less and less.
4. Joy is elusive, and I'm often invaded by a sadness I can't explain.
5. I'm increasingly irritable and choosing not to be with people.
6. I suffer from physical complaints (legs feel heavy, backache, headache, lingering colds).
7. I'm unable to laugh at a joke about myself.
8. I feel a loss of self-esteem, confidence and can-do attitude.
9. Sex seems like more trouble than it's worth.
10. I'm increasingly judgmental, short-tempered, and disappointed in the people around me.

SCORING

0-15:	You're doing fine.
16-25:	Oops! There are things you should be watching.
26-35:	You're a candidate for burnout.
36-45:	You're burning out.
46 and over:	Take special note. There are distinct threats to your health and well-being.

From *Shape*, May 1991.

▶ Take the time to have fun. With all the demands of everyday life, a person can get bogged down in things that aren't always enjoyable. Go fly a kite, go wading in a ditch, or have a picnic in the middle of a downtown park. Aim for fun, silly things you can laugh over at least once a day.

▶ If you've got a strenuous class load, take a class just for fun. Go for something you've always wanted to do — maybe a watercolor class, or a bowling class.

RELAXATION TECHNIQUES

One of the best and most *immediate* ways of breaking the stress response is to employ a relaxation technique. This may be any one of a host of techniques that bring on what Harvard Medical School researcher Herbert Benson calls "the relaxation response, an inborn bodily reaction that counteracts the harmful effects of stress."

Invoking the relaxation response not only breaks up stress, but it also gives you a more positive mental outlook, eases anxiety, and brings on a sense of control (essential to overcoming the negative aspects of stress). Regular relaxation exercises can reduce stress, increase resistance to stress-induced illness, minimize the symptoms of illness (such as headache), lower your blood pressure, and alleviate pain.

Of the number of relaxation exercises, some are based on deep relaxation with a myriad of benefits, and others (such as deep breathing or a quick massage) reduce stress and are a good way of leading into more extensive relaxation exercises. As with physical exercise, learning about various relaxation exercises takes some time. Before you decide which ones to try, you should consider your likes and dislikes, your personality, and your situation. You can learn some of them on your own, but you will need some training for others. The techniques include, among others, meditation, progressive relaxation, autogenics, deep breathing, biofeedback training, and yoga.

Meditation

Simply stated, meditation is an exercise that lets you get control over your thoughts. During meditation, you focus on some thought or object and banish all other thoughts from your mind. During meditation, heartbeat and breathing slow down, blood pressure drops (often for 12 to 24 hours after the meditative period), and the body's metabolism slows, decreasing its need for oxygen and other nutrients. As relaxation occurs, blood flow to the arms and legs increases, which helps to ease muscle tension. Laboratory studies have shown that people who meditate have fewer blood lactates, enzymes associated with stress and anxiety.

Meditation originated in India and Tibet and first became popular in the United States during the 1960s, when the Maharishi Mahesh Yogi introduced it as *transcendental meditation* (TM). The exercise got its name because of the practitioner's ability to effortlessly "transcend" (go beyond) everyday thought. Today, meditation is recognized as one of the most effective ways to reduce stress. More than 700 scientific studies have proven that meditation induces the relaxation response and alleviates the harmful physiological effects of stress. Whereas basic meditation requires little training, TM is a little more specialized. TM classes are taught throughout the country and usually require several sessions.

The most essential element of meditation is something to focus on: a word or phrase you silently repeat (a *mantra*) or an unchanging object on which you can focus. To be effective, meditation has to be done in a comfortable position in a quiet place, free of distractions. No specific posture is required for meditation. To begin:

1. Find a quiet room as free from distraction as possible. Lighting and temperature are a matter of individual preference. Just make sure you're comfortable. Turn off the phone. Alert others that you don't want to be disturbed.

2. Loosen your clothing if it is tight, especially at the wrists, neck, and waist. Get in the most comfortable position you can, in a chair or on a couch. Some recommend a straight-backed chair to prevent you from falling asleep. Place your feet flat on the floor, and rest your hands in your lap.

3. Inhale slowly and deeply through your nose, hold your breath briefly, then exhale slowly. As you begin to breathe deeply, let the tension flow out of your body. Don't force it or concentrate on it. Just let it happen.

4. If you are concentrating on an unchanging object, partially close your eyes so the object is blurred. Softly focus on it without bringing in any of the

sharp details. If you are focusing on a mantra, begin repeating it silently and rhythmically as you breath in and out. Repeat the word *slowly* with the rhythm of your breathing. Gradually focus all your attention on that object or mantra. Do not let any other thoughts invade your meditation.

5. Continue meditating for approximately 20 minutes. Don't worry about the exact time. You'll probably have to work up to it at first. Learning to sit still for 20 minutes at a time takes practice, especially when you are so intensely focusing on a single object or phrase, so give yourself plenty of practice. For maximum effects, experts recommend meditating 20 minutes at a time, twice during the day.

6. When you are finished meditating, give yourself time to readjust. Open your eyes, focus on various objects around the room, and gradually return to your normal rate and pattern of breathing. While still seated, stretch your arms, legs, back, shoulders, and neck. Finally, stand up slowly.

For the best meditative effects, you should avoid any stimulants — cigarettes, coffee, tea, cola drinks — during the hour or two before you meditate. The best times to meditate are early in the morning (before breakfast) and before dinner. Eating a meal just before you meditate diverts blood flow to your stomach and makes it difficult to achieve the relaxation response.

Progressive Relaxation

Progressive relaxation was pioneered by Edmund Jacobson, a physician who wanted to help patients suffering from muscle tension associated with stress. He showed patients how to recognize muscle tension and how to differentiate it from muscle relaxation. His three-step technique was simple: Patients first contracted (tensed) a small muscle group, then relaxed the muscle group, and finally concentrated on determining how different the two sensations felt.

Progressive relaxation is simple. In essence, you contract, then relax the muscles of the body. You can design your own routine — working from your head to your toes, for example, or from your feet to your head — as long as all major muscle groups in the body are eventually relaxed. When you initially start doing progressive relaxation, you should first tense the muscles as hard as you can, then relax them. Once you become practiced, you can relax the muscles easily and effortlessly without having to first contract them.

Unlike meditation, in which you should *not* think about what's happening to your body, progressive relaxation requires you to *concentrate on what's happening to your muscles*. For the best results, you need to be acutely aware of the relaxed condition of your body.

As mentioned, you can design your own routine. Regardless of your routine:

1. Practice progressive relaxation while lying on your back in the most comfortable position possible. Take off your shoes, and loosen any restrictive clothing. Close your eyes, rotate your ankles outward, and put your arms at your sides.

2. Make sure you move to all major muscle groups in the body. Don't forget your face, including your forehead, eyes, nose, mouth, cheeks, and tongue.

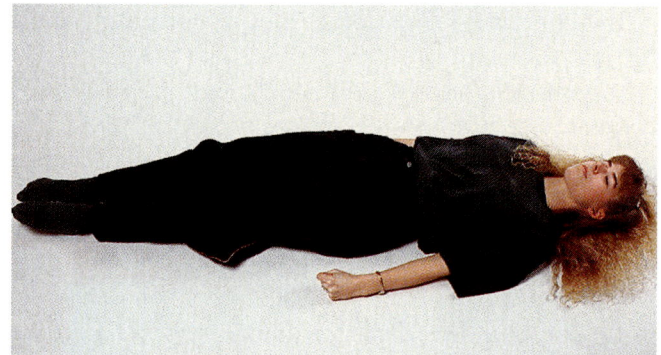

Practicing progressive muscle relaxation can elicit the relaxation response.

3. As you move to each muscle group, contract the muscles as tightly as you can and hold the contraction for 20 or 30 seconds. If you experience pain or cramping, immediately release the contraction.

4. Concentrate on the dramatic difference in feeling between a tensed muscle and a relaxed one. With practice, you'll be able to achieve relaxation "on demand."

Breathing Techniques

Breathing exercises also can be an antidote to stress. These exercises have been used for centuries in the Orient and India as a means to develop better mental, physical, and emotional stamina. In breathing exercises, the person concentrates on "breathing away" the tension and inhaling fresh oxygen to the entire body. Breathing exercises can be learned in only a few minutes and require considerably less time than other forms of stress management.

As an example of a breathing exercise:

1. Sit in a comfortable position with hands folded over your abdomen, just over your navel.
2. Keeping your eyes open, imagine a balloon lying beneath your hands.
3. Begin to slowly inhale through your nose, concentrating on the warm air entering your nose and slowly filling the balloon. When the balloon is full (this should take 3 to 4 seconds initially), slowly exhale to empty the balloon, feeling your chest and abdomen relaxing.
4. Repeat the entire process two or three times.
5. When finished, sit quietly for a few minutes before rising. If you feel dizzy at any point, stop the procedure.[13]

Autogenics

Similar to progressive relaxation, autogenics is self-induced relaxation that causes all major muscle groups in the body to feel relaxed, heavy, and warm. It begins with a routine that relaxes all the major muscles (much like that of progressive relaxation), followed by imagery (vivid mental visualization) that extends the relaxed state. Developed by German psychiatrist Johannes Shultz, it involves both progressive relaxation and self-hypnosis.

The benefits of autogenics exceed those of progressive relaxation. It goes a step further to invoke the relaxation response. According to research, autogenics and the associated imagery reduce heartbeat and breathing rates, ease muscle tension, and increase the brainwaves associated with deep relaxation.

Autogenics requires time, commitment, and practice. Commercial tapes are available to guide you through the relaxation exercises. You also can make your own tape, or simply repeat the phrases aloud as you move through the exercises. As with progressive relaxation, you can design your own routine.

1. In a quiet room with mild temperature, free of distractions, sit in the most comfortable position you can. Experts recommend sitting in a straight-backed but comfortable chair with your feet flat on the floor, your head hanging loosely forward, your eyes closed, and your hands in your lap with your palms turned upward. Loosen any restrictive clothing.
2. Imagine you have just had a strenuous workout. You might begin with your legs. As you inhale and exhale deeply and slowly, repeat "My legs are so tired. My legs are so heavy. My legs are very heavy and warm." As you repeat these phrases, feel the heaviness and warmth in your legs. With practice, your legs should become so heavy and relaxed that you can lift them only with considerable struggle.
3. Move to other muscle groups — buttocks, abdomen, chest, arms, shoulders, and so on. You even might imagine your internal organs, such as your stomach and your heart, relaxed and warm.
4. Concentrate on how cool your forehead feels. For you to feel refreshed and alert, your forehead must feel cool.
5. Once your entire body is relaxed, visualize an image you find relaxing. It might be waves lapping against a sandy beach, a cloud drifting lazily across the afternoon sky, an eagle soaring silently across a ravine. The image is different for everyone, but it should lead you to total relaxation.

For the greatest benefit, experts recommend that you practice autogenics twice a day for 10 minutes at a time. As with other kinds of relaxation exercises, autogenics requires practice, starting out slowly, then working up to a 10-minute period of visualization and relaxation.

Biofeedback Training

Essentially, biofeedback training is a method of measuring physiological functions you're not normally aware of (such as skin temperature and blood pressure). This information is converted into something meaningful to you so you can control your responses.

Unlike some other forms of relaxation exercises, you can't learn biofeedback training on your own. It requires that you be monitored by extremely sensitive equipment, then taught to regulate your own physiological responses. Biofeedback training is extremely valuable as a stress management technique, as it allows you to control your body's responses to stress. Most people can learn effective biofeedback techniques in a few sessions from a trained therapist using sensitive biofeedback equipment.

Biofeedback training is extremely effective. Within a few sessions most people are able to competently control physiological effects of stress such as higher blood pressure, increasing heart rate, and muscle contraction. An obvious disadvantage is the necessity of using expensive machinery and trained therapists. Most people, however, quickly gain the ability to control their own physiological responses without the biofeedback machinery.

Yoga

Yoga, an ancient exercise technique known to induce calm and invigorate the mind, has been shown in scientific studies to reduce the biological effects of stress. In addition, yoga is an excellent exercise for improving strength, flexibility, and endurance.

Unlike other relaxation exercises, you can't design your own technique or routine in yoga. It is composed of precise postures done in a specific sequence combined with an exact breathing rhythm designed to reduce tension and inflexibility.

The yoga postures are difficult and complex and require training and practice. Few people can assume the postures at first, and you may not be able to complete the sequence properly for as long as 3 months. A number of good yoga instruction books are on the market, and yoga classes are taught throughout the United States. Most experts recommend practicing yoga for 15 to 45 minutes a day in a place free of distraction. Many people sign up for classes, where they actually perform yoga daily.

Checkmate For Stress

Like improving your game of chess, you can develop strategies to put stress in check. Based on years of researching why some people stay cool while others buckle, Salvatore Maddi, professor of psychology at the University of California, Irvine, founded The Hardiness Institute in Irvine, which offers training courses throughout the country. Here are three key techniques for "hardy coping":

1. *Situational reconstruction:* When a stressful event occurs, replay it in your mind to gain understanding and pinpoint where the anxiety is coming from. If you've had an argument, what contribution did you make? What did the other person do? Next, get some perspective by imagining both how the situation could get worse and how it could get better. Finally, ask yourself what you could do to increase the likelihood of it getting better, and put your answer into action.

2. *Focusing:* If you can't get your imagination going in the first exercise, the situation may be evoking emotions you're not acknowledging. For example, you assumed you are angry when, in fact, you're frightened. In this case, let your body cue you in. Try focusing on your center, the chest-abdomen area, and ask yourself, "What is it about this situation that stands in the way of my feeling good?" If you come up with an answer that seems familiar, put it aside, refocus, and ask the question again. When an unexpected thought or feeling pops into your mind, that's probably the information you've been burying; acknowledge it, and try the first step again.

3. *Compensatory self-improvement:* When you can't think of anything you could do to make the situation better, you may be confronting something you can't change. That's rarely the case, but if it is, accept the facts gracefully without falling into bitterness and self-pity. One way to do this is by choosing another problem related to the first one and work on that instead. Rather than feeling victimized or overwhelmed, say to yourself, "I may not be able to fix everything, I can improve some things."

In short, start with yourself. There are few situations that can't be improved by working on your own personal changes. For example, try seeking greater understanding by identifying with the people who are causing you the stress. In this way they become human again, no longer monsters. They'll also be more likely to listen to you and to help find a solution that will ease your stress.

NOTES

1. Marc K. Lewen and Harold L. Kennedy, "The Role of Stress in Heart Disease," *Hospital Medicine*, August 1986, pp. 125–138.
2. Ari Kiev, "Managing Stress to Achieve Success," *Executive Health*, 24:1 (October, 1987), 1–4.
3. Ari Kiev.
4. Paul Rosch, "Good Stress: Why You Need It to Stay Young," *Prevention*, April 1986, p. 29.
5. Ruthan Brodsky, "Identifying Stressors is Necessary to Combat Potential Health Problems," *Occupational Health & Safety*, pp. 30–32.
6. "Workplace Warning: Stress May Speed Brain Aging." *New Sense Bulletin* 16:11, Aug. 1991, p. 1.
7. Peter Knapp, cited in John Tierney, "Stress Success and Samoa" *Hippocrates*, May/June, 1987, p. 84.
8. Brendan O'Regan, Caryle Hirshberg, Nola Lewis, Barbara McNeill, and Winston Franklin, *The Heart of Healing* (Atlanta: Turner Publishing, 1993).
9. Nan Silver, "Long Term Stress: Does Your Body Fight Back?" *American Health*, May 1986, p. 20.
10. Betty Weider, "The Stress-Free Personality," *Shape*, July 1990, p. 18.
11. Bernie S. Siegel, *Love, Medicine, and Miracles* (New York: Harper and Row, 1986).
12. Leonard A. Sagan, *The Health of Nations* (New York: Basic Books, 1987).
13. Adapted from Daniel A. Girdano, George S. Everly, and Dorothy Dusek, *Controlling Stress and Tension*, 3d ed. (Englewood Cliffs, NJ: Prentice Hall, 1990), p. 219.

Scoring Your Stress:
A Test to Pinpoint What's Eating You

How stressed are you?
The answer depends in part on what's going on in your life. But it also depends on some other factors — like what your *attitudes* are about those events and how much control you feel over what happens.
The first step in managing stress, of course, is to *identify* it — and the test below will help you do just that. It's simple: read each question, then circle the number that most closely describes your situation or attitude. If you're completely neutral, circle **5**; if a question doesn't apply to you at all, skip it.
Ready?
Sharpen your pencil, and go to work:

1 How often do you suffer stress-related physical symptoms, such as headaches, jaw pain, neck pain, back pain, indigestion, abdominal pain, diarrhea, loss of appetite, excessive perspiration, fatigue, or a pounding in your chest?

Rarely or never   Every day
1   2   3   4   5   6   7   8   9   10

2 Do you wash your hands before you eat?

Always   Rarely or never
1   2   3   4   5   6   7   8   9   10

3 Do you take measures to keep your food safe, such as cooking it adequately, storing it properly, and avoiding obvious contaminants?

Almost always   Rarely or never
1   2   3   4   5   6   7   8   9   10

4 How often do you eat fresh fruits, fresh vegetables, whole grains, and foods high in fiber?

Every day   Rarely or never
1   2   3   4   5   6   7   8   9   10

5 How often do you eat high fat or high-sugar foods — including candy, pastry, soft drinks, and food from fast-food restaurants?

Occasionally   Every day
1   2   3   4   5   6   7   8   9   10

6 How often do you exercise?

Every day   Rarely or never
1   2   3   4   5   6   7   8   9   10

7 How many hours of sleep do you get each day?

Eight or more   Less than four
1   2   3   4   5   6   7   8   9   10

8 How many cups of coffee or caffeinated soft drinks do you drink each day?

None   Five or more
1   2   3   4   5   6   7   8   9   10

(continued)

9 How often do you use alcohol, tobacco, over-the-counter drugs, or prescription drugs to relieve stress?

Never   Every day

1   2   3   4   5   6   7   8   9   10

10 If you have a relationship with a significant other, how would you describe that relationship?

Mutually satisfying in many ways   Marked by jealousy or insecurity

1   2   3   4   5   6   7   8   9   10

11 How do you feel when you have to say "no" to a request for your time, energy, talents, or money?

Confident and at ease   Anxious and guilt-ridden

1   2   3   4   5   6   7   8   9   10

12 How would you characterize your support system?

Broad-based, many sources   Limited or no sources

1   2   3   4   5   6   7   8   9   10

13 What kinds of friendships do you have?

At least several close friends/confidants   No close friends

1   2   3   4   5   6   7   8   9   10

14 What do you do if you have a problem you can't solve on your own?

Seek help immediately   Suffer on my own

1   2   3   4   5   6   7   8   9   10

15 How many major changes (such as entering or ending an intimate relationship, the death of a family member, a change in your financial status, moving, starting a new job, a change in sleeping habits, a change in living conditions, or a change in the number of arguments you have with roommates) have occurred in your life during the last year.

None   Many

1   2   3   4   5   6   7   8   9   10

16 How do you react when confronted with a problem or stressful situation?

Put it aside to gain perspective,   Feel overwhelmed
then focus on solutions   or panic-stricken

1   2   3   4   5   6   7   8   9   10

17 How often do you "retreat" temporarily when you start to feel overwhelmed by stress?

Most of the time   Never

1   2   3   4   5   6   7   8   9   10

18 How do you normally feel at the end of the day?

I got the important things done   I didn't accomplish anything

1   2   3   4   5   6   7   8   9   10

19 How many "hassles" do you have in a typical day?

A few   A lot

1   2   3   4   5   6   7   8   9   10

(continued)

20 How much noise are you exposed to every day?

Not very much   Most of the day is noisy

1   2   3   4   5   6   7   8   9   10

21 How comfortable is your environment? (Consider temperature extremes, humidity, crowding, and environmental pollutants.)

Very comfortable   Very uncomfortable

1   2   3   4   5   6   7   8   9   10

22 Overall, how satisfying is your life?

Very satisfying   Very disappointing

1   2   3   4   5   6   7   8   9   10

Scoring

Time to take a look at your stress level. This exercise will tell you *two* things: first, it will indicate your general stress level. Then it will help pinpoint the specific things that are causing you stress.

First, total up your score by adding every number you circled. Now divide it by the number of questions you answered. This is one test on which you don't want a high score: The closer your average creeps toward 10, the higher your stress level is likely to be. (By the way, it's important to "average" your stress score this way; a high level of stress in a few areas won't cause your *general* stress level to skyrocket.

Next, go back and isolate what's causing you problems. Look back through your responses. Find those in which you circled a number higher than 5. Simple — you've found your problem areas.

Finally, determine some stress-busting strategies. Check out your problematic question number, then find the corresponding number among the tips below. The rest is up to you!

Stress-Savvy Tips

1 Obviously, stress-related physical symptoms are just that: related to stress. The best way to get rid of them is to get rid of the stress that causes them? In the meantime, there are a few things you *can* do to manage your most troublesome symptoms. **For headaches:** keep a "headache diary"; it will help you identify what triggers your headaches, a first step in prevention. Until you can do that, try deep breathing, relaxation, stretching muscles to relieve tension in your neck and jaw, or a warm bath. **For back pain:** try deep breathing combined with gentle stretching exercises, soaking in a warm bath, or meditation. **For irritable bowel syndrome:** stay away from high-fat foods, avoid caffeine (including chocolate), add fiber to your diet (eat plenty of whole grains), and try relaxation exercises. **For indigestion:** eat smaller meals more often during the day; stick to foods that are mild and easy to digest. Watching what you eat can also ease **fatigue** — eat foods rich in vitamins, potassium, calcium, iron, and zinc.

2 Washing your hands before you eat dramatically reduces your chance of picking up an infection — an obvious stressor. Other simple things you can do: Keep your hands out of your mouth, don't share eating utensils or drinking glasses, avoid contact with people you know are ill, limit sexual contact and use safe sexual practices, and make sure your immunizations are up to date.

3 You can avoid the physical stress of food-borne illness by scrubbing fruits and vegetables thoroughly; preparing raw meat on surfaces that can be easily cleaned; preparing raw meats separate from other foods; avoiding raw or rare meats or fish; cooking hamburger until it's no longer pink; boiling canned foods before you eat them; refrigerating leftovers immediately; avoiding foods that contain raw eggs; avoiding foods that are obviously spoiled; and avoiding wild nuts, berries, mushrooms, and plants unless you are certain they are edible.

(continued)

4 Stress robs your body of certain nutrients — if you're under stress from *any* source you need an extra shot of certain vitamins and minerals. Especially important are the B vitamins (found in nuts, seeds, beans, peas, meat, and whole grains), vitamin C (found in citrus fruits, green peppers, dark-green vegetables, strawberries, and tomatoes), calcium (found in milk and dairy products, citrus fruits, dark-green leafy vegetables, and dried beans), and protein (found in meat, fish, poultry, dairy products, and eggs). Don't forget that you can get a "complete" protein by combining certain plant foods — rice with legumes, wheat with soybeans, or legumes with corn, rice, wheat, or oats, for example.

5 Stress robs your body of some vital nutrients, and sugars and fats speed up the process! Sugars, in fact, tend to strip out certain B vitamins and actually make you more *susceptible* to stress. Concentrate on eating a balanced diet of foods low in fats and sugars; check labels, and steer clear of foods that list sugar in any form as the first or second ingredient. Avoid skipping meals; eat a hearty breakfast and light supper; drink plenty of water; and check with your physician about nutritional supplements if you're under a lot of stress.

6 Research proves that regular exercise diminishes the effects of stress — even stress you can't avoid. The best kind of stress-busting exercise is continuous, rhythmic, aerobic exercise — walking, running, bicycling, swimming, or cross-country skiing are good choices. To avoid injury, make sure you allow for warm-up and cool-down time. And if your joints are a little creaky from inactivity, start slowly and build up gradually. Wear light-colored clothing in the summer, and several light layers of dark-colored clothing in the winter. Drink plenty of fluid before and after you exercise. You should feel energized, not tired, when you finish exercising; you're pushing too hard if you feel a heaviness in your arms or legs, soreness in your muscles or joints, or extreme fatigue.

7 Sleep relieves stress. How? While you're asleep, you breathe more deeply, your heart slows down, your blood pressure drops, and your muscles relax. To get better sleep, review the suggestions earlier in this section; in a nutshell, try to relax for an hour or so before you go to bed, do your best to stick to a regular sleep schedule, avoid eating a big meal right before you go to sleep, and do what you can to make your sleep environment comfortable.

8 Caffeine actually *increases* your sensitivity to stress by stimulating the central nervous system, charging up the autonomic nervous system, and lowering your ability to tolerate stress. Avoid caffeine or use it only in moderation. Remember, too, that caffeine is found in more than just coffee and cola drinks — cut back on chocolate, cocoa, and over-the-counter medications that contain caffeine, too. Try drinking decaffeinated coffee, or switching to a soothing herbal tea.

9 Alcohol might relax you at first — but research shows that, over the long term, alcohol actually *increases* stress by causing your body to churn out stress-related hormones. Keep a diary of your alcohol intake for a few weeks; if you're drinking too much (more than an occasionally drink, or more than 12 ounces of beer or 4 ounces of wine at a time), take measures to stop. Find some other ways to relieve stress, and try substituting another kind of drink for alcohol — exotic fruit juices or sparkling mineral water can be fun.

And don't forget tobacco: we know that smoking causes a long list of health problems. What you may not know is that smoking *combined with stress* escalates the situation. Take measures to stop; ask your doctor or the college health center about local problems that can help you quit.

10. The least stressful relationship is one in which your combination is also your *friend* — someone with whom you share your feelings, triumphs, disappointments, goals, and dreams. If appropriate, healthy sexual expression should be part of that relationship; aside from being a way to communicate within a committed relationship, the physiological processes involved in sex work to relieve stress and tension. Finally, remember that no matter how well matched you are, no two people can fill *every* need for each other; maintain separate friends and interests to avoid becoming too dependent on each other.

(continued)

11. The ability to assert yourself means you usually meet your own needs without destroying interpersonal relationships. Assertive behavior allows you to protect your own rights — essential to avoiding stress. If you're not very assertive now, start by respecting yourself. You're responsible for yourself, and others need to live with your decisions. If you need to say "no," just say it; don't feel obligated to offer excuses. And remember the nonverbals that go along with it: speak in a firm, steady voice without hesitation, stand straight, and look at the other person directly in the eye.

12. The larger your network of support the better you will be able to manage stress. Ideally, your network of support should be broad, stemming from your family, church, neighborhood, school, social and political organizations, and friends. Try organizing or joining a study group (students in a class or within a major area of study), service group, sports team, hobby group, campaign team, social group, or simply a group of friends who share a favorite activity — bicycling, kite-flying, or watercolors, for example. Remember — the most valuable type of social support from groups like these often happens from the informal contacts, such as riding to a meeting with someone or getting together for dinner after the meeting.

13. Research shows that one of the best ways to prevent stress-related illness is to have good friends — people you can really talk to, people with whom you can share your joys, concerns, apprehensions, and love. If you need to expand your circle of friends, start by expanding your contacts: in other words, go where the people are? Draw people into conversation, invite people to informal get-togethers, show people you care, and get involved with others.

14. An important part of social support — and stress reduction — is your willingness to seek help when you need it *and* the assurance that there are people who can help you. Close friends can act as confidants, but you should also know that there are others in your support network to whom you can turn — a clergyman, school counselor, or therapist.

15. Research has shown that your chance of developing a stress-induced illness increase with the number of "life crises" you have during any given time. (Check the list of specific crises earlier in this section for an idea of what we're talking about.) Whenever you can, avoid too many changes at once: If you've just ended an important relationship, for example, don't move to a new apartment and start a part-time job, too. For the best coping strategy, try to anticipate likely changes — then slow down your pace, be gentle on yourself, avoid as many new commitments as you can, and stay flexible. Still another strategy is called *stress-inoculation*: in essence, you imagine —vividly — the worst thing that could happen, then map out how you'd handle it. Then, no matter what happens, you know you can do *something* to cope.

16. Your ability to *adapt* to situations and problems directly affects your ability to manage stress. Boost your odds by trying the following: Put the problem aside long enough to get perspective — what long-range effects will it have? Who does it involve? Then focus in on what you can do to solve the problem, and try to come up with several different alternatives. (Having several different plans for confronting the situation gives you flexibility and removes the anxious possibility of your *only* plan failing.) Above all, relax and keep a sense of humor; and, when you've successfully met the challenge, reward yourself for succeeding!

17. There's nothing wrong with retreat — it's a coping skill that can help you buffer the effects of stress. Don't run away from problems or avoid responsibility — that's not what we're talking about. But when you're feeling overwhelmed, buy yourself some breathing space by going for a long walk, taking in a new movie, putting together a challenging puzzle, going to lunch with a friend, reading a favorite book, or taking a nap. The key is to get a mini-escape or time-out: something that will divert your thoughts and recharge your batteries. You'll go back to the problem renewed and strong enough to handle the challenge!

(continued)

18 If you want to manage stress, learn to manage your time. There are some excellent pointers earlier in this section. One of the most important tactics is prioritizing: figure out which tasks are most important, then *do those things first.* It helps to make a list of everything you need to do — then assign each a "priority" (for example, **1** for things you *must* get done today if you want to avoid problems, **2** for things that *must* be done but that could wait, and **3** for things you'd like to do but that are not essential). Start out with the things that are the highest priority; get them done first. Then move to the second category;. If you have time left over, start on the last category — but, if not, no big deal. For maximum effectiveness, schedule your time, delegate things that someone else could do for you, limit the number of interruptions you have, and plan for some breaks.

19 *Hassles* are defined as the irritants and annoyances — most of them fairly minor — that all of us encounter on a daily basis. Simply stated, they're part of living. Hassles can include things like having to wait for someone, getting caught in traffic, not being able to find a parking space, having to stand in lines, being bothered by a fly, not being able to find the book you need at the library, conflicts with a roommate, having to endure a boring professor, sleeping in and missing breakfast, or not having enough change to do laundry. One or two aren't bad. But when your day gets filled with hassles, your stress skyrockets.

There's not a lot you can do to prevent hassles — but you *can* work smart to defuse them. Think ahead; anticipate what you can. If you think you might get stuck in traffic, leave fifteen minutes early. If you know the parking on campus is a nightmare, ride the bus, ride your bike, walk, or join a carpool. If it's laundry day, stop at the bank on the way home and buy a couple of rolls of quarters. If you've had trouble finding resource materials for a paper, start early. For the rest — those things you can't circumvent — try to change your expectations. Don't expect to avoid traffic problems; don't expect to get your groceries without standing in line. If you learn to look at things differently, you'll be able to wait patiently, sit calmly, and think of something pleasant instead of getting uptight.

20 Everyone knows that noise is irritating. But did you know that *noise actually increases stress*? How? It boosts the heart rate, increases blood pressure, tenses the muscles, and causes the body to secrete stress-related hormones. At certain decibels (a jet plane engine, a pneumatic riveter, a guitar amplifier), noise can permanently damage hearing; if you're trying to concentrate on a difficult task, even a little noise can be stressful. The most stressful is noise that constantly changes in intensity, frequency, or pitch.

There's a lot you can do to reduce your stress from noise. If you can, choose an apartment away from a busy street, a convenience store, a fast-food restaurant, or an industrial area. Look for a carpeted apartment — you at least want carpet in the rooms that are directly adjacent to other units. Choose upholstered instead of hard-surfaced furniture, heavy drapes instead of aluminum blinds. Put a small foam pad under noisy appliances, such as blenders. Turn down the TV and the stereo. And, if you're exposed to chronic noise, use cotton or ear plugs to protect your ears and filter out some of the sound.

21 The environment you live in can either soothe you or add to your stress. You can't control some things — like air pollution — but you *can* clean up clutter, keep your room at the most comfortable temperature, and use adequate lighting, for example. Do whatever you can to limit your exposure to pollutants, insecticides, pesticides, food additives, gasoline exhaust, industrial wastes, and glazes or paints that contain lead.

22 You'll do best at coping with stress if you are generally satisfied: you feel some control over your life, you are able to set and meet goals, you have aspirations you believe you'll fulfill, the people closest to you are affectionate and caring, you feel valued, and you are able to make a meaningful contribution. Generally, satisfaction leads to optimism — and optimists suffer fewer symptoms of stress. If you're not optimistic and satisfied, try to figure out why. Change the things you can. Work to accept the things you can't change. Most importantly, learn to concentrate on your successes and use what you learned from them to meet your challenges head-on.

The Mind-Body Connection

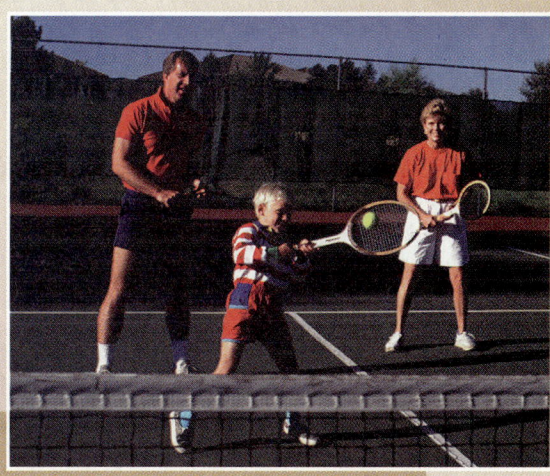

Objectives

▼ Understand the physiological manifestations of specific emotions.

▼ Define psychoneuroimmunology and its emphasis on links between the mind, the brain, and the immune system.

▼ Identify the connection between disease and personality.

▼ Learn the characteristics of the coronary-prone personality and Type A personality traits.

▼ Become acquainted with the Type C personality.

▼ Understand the differences between anger and hostility and the health effects of each.

▼ Understand the health effects of depression.

▼ Identify the disease-resistant personality and the "three C's".

In a pronouncement that at first rocked the medical community if not the lay public, one practitioner proclaimed that an estimated 90% of all physical problems have emotional roots. He followed up by saying his estimate was, at best, "conservative." A growing body of evidence indicates that virtually every illness known to modern humanity — from arthritis to migraine headaches, from the common cold to cancer — is influenced for good or bad by our emotions.

What we have learned from the most recent research in the exciting new field of psychoneuroimmunology is this: Illnesses don't just happen to us. Many are caused by bacteria, viruses, fungi, or other microbes. But what factors determine whether we will fall ill when introduced to these microscopic trouble-makers? What determines our immunity?

To a profound extent, emotions impact our susceptibility and immunity. The American Medical Association has estimated that half of all disease is preventable. An analysis of the leading causes of death among Americans shows that at least half are related to behavioral factors, such as our response to stress. The way we react to what comes along in life can determine in great measure how we will react to the disease-causing organisms that come along. A growing body of evidence indicates that the way we emote — the feelings we have and the way we express them — can either boost our immune system or weaken it.

There's a physiological reason why emotions can influence health. Certain parts of the brain are associated with specific emotions and specific hormone patterns. The release of certain hormones is associated with various emotional responses, and those hormones affect health.

Many researchers also believe that the *inability* to express emotions may be an even greater cause of disease. Loyola University Medical Center professor of psychiatry Domeena Renshaw maintains that emotions have to be expressed somewhere, somehow. If they are suppressed repeatedly, and there is conflict about controlling them, they often reveal themselves through physical symptoms. Research bears out her theory: In a series of studies, breast cancer patients who showed little emotion were the ones to die early on. The survivors were the ones who felt and openly expressed emotions.

One of the reasons strong emotions can cause illness — even infectious disease — is that they may weaken the immune system over time. The classic fight-or-flight response to emotional distress gradually weakens the immune system. And a growing body of evidence suggests that emotions send chemical messages to the brain that alter involuntary physiologic responses. This may affect the way the brain responds to messages from the immune system in the presence of disease. Emotions have been linked to a wide variety of conditions, including allergies, asthma, angina, heart disease, high blood pressure, arthritis, back pain, cancer, dental cavities, diabetes, gastric ulcers, insomnia, irritable bowel syndrome, and a variety of skin problems.

A number of scientists agree that it's not the emotion but the way we react to it that can help determine health. In an address to the Institute for the Advancement of Health, Rachel Naomi Remen advised that perhaps there is a positive way to feel *all* emotions. Perhaps it is not so much the emotions themselves as the way we deal with them that is or is not life-affirming.[1]

▼ THE SCIENCE OF PSYCHONEUROIMMUNOLOGY

The scientific investigation of how the brain affects the body's immune system can be affected by behavior is called *psychoneuroimmunology*, a term coined in 1964 by Dr. Robert Ader, director of the division of behavioral and psychosocial medicine at New York's University of Rochester. The science of psychoneuroimmunology (PNI) focuses on the links between the mind, the brain, and the immune system. As a science, it has received the endorsement of the National Institutes of Health.

Although controversy still surrounds the science itself and some skepticism about the concepts behind it, PNI researchers are proving that the way we think and feel influences our immune system. One report hails PNI as "the hottest and most promising area of medical research today."[2]

Proponents cite solid examples that support the theories of PNI. One is the late Norman Cousins, former editor of the *Saturday Review* and member of the UCLA medical faculty, who twice intrigued both the medical community and the public by overcoming usually fatal conditions — once a massive heart attack, and once an advanced case of ankylosing spondylitis (a degenerative spinal disease). Cousins followed his physicians' regimen each time but also infused himself with vast doses of positive emotions and laughter. According to Cousins himself, he was healed not only by the miracle of modern medicine but also by the healing emotions of love, hope, faith, confidence, and a tremendous will to live.

The theories behind PNI aren't new. Chinese physicians noted more than four thousand years ago that physical illness often followed episodes of frustration. Some of the world's greatest physicians and philosophers — including Hippocrates, Galen, and Descartes — believe that a fundamental link exists between the body and the mind. Only in the 1980s, however, did immunologists finally begin to seriously consider the possibility of anatomical links between the brain, the nervous system, and the immune system. Based on overwhelming evidence, they found that the brain literally "talks" to the cells of the immune system.

Today, brain research is booming. Even though psychoneuroimmunology is still considered to be in its infancy, a number of medical schools already have integrated it into their curricula and a host of federal grants is underwriting its increased research. Almost every important conference on immunology now includes at least one seminar on the relationship between the brain and the immune system, and an increasing number of physicians is acknowledging that the way a patient thinks and feels can be a powerful determinant of physical health.

THE BRAIN

The brain is a privileged organ. The heart supplies it with blood; the lungs supply it with oxygen; the intestines supply it with nutrients; and the kidneys remove poisons from its environment. The most important part of the nervous system, it is the focal point of organization. For the body to survive, the brain must be maintained. All other organs undergo sacrifice to keep the brain alive and functioning when the entire body is under severe stress.

The brain masterminds nerve impulses that are carried throughout the body. It controls voluntary processes, such as the direction, strength and coordination of muscle movements; the processes involved in smelling, touching, and seeing; and other processes over which you have conscious control. The brain also controls many automatic, vital functions in the body, such as breathing, heart rate, digestion, control of the bowels and bladder, blood pressure, and release of hormones (see Figure 3.1).

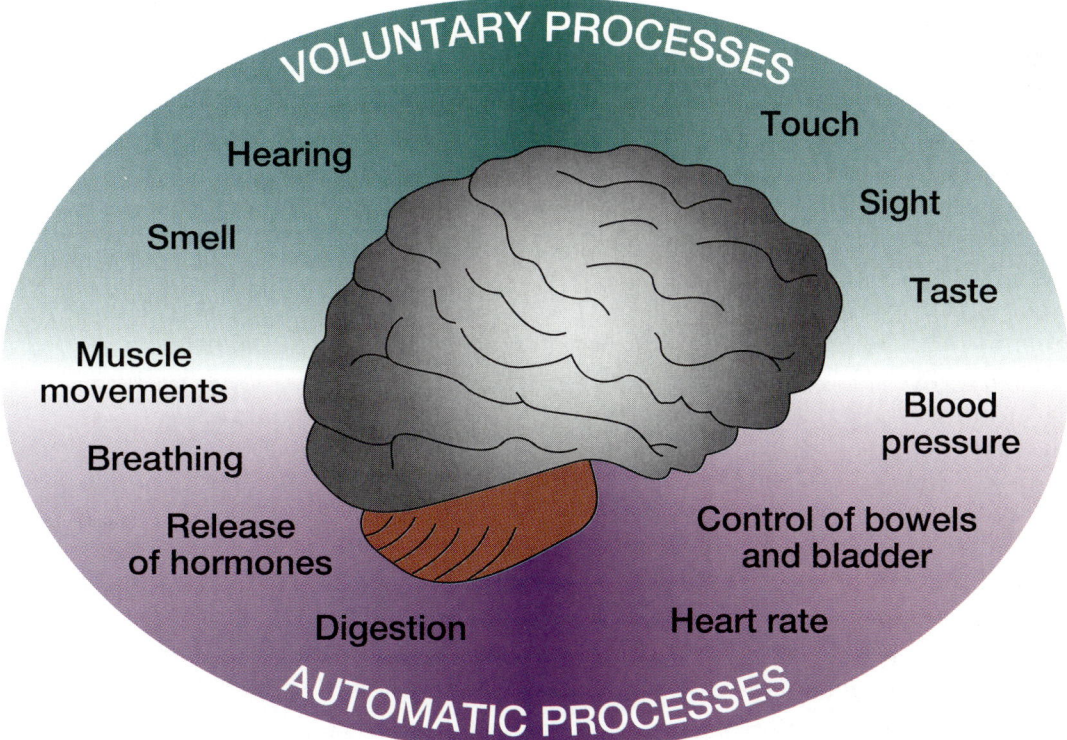

FIGURE 3.1 ▼ The brain controls voluntary and automatic processes throughout the body.

Finally, the brain is the cognitive center of the body, the place where ideas are generated, memory is stored, and emotions are experienced. Thus it is that the emotions that so affect the body originate in the brain, and this process explains the brain's powerful influence over the body, as well as its link to emotions and the immune system. That link is extremely complex. One California neuroscientist summed up the process neatly by comparing the manufacture of emotion to a television set. There are individual tubes, he points out, and you can say what they do, but if you take out even one tube, the television doesn't work.[3]

The emotions the brain produces are, in a real sense, a mixture of feelings and physical responses. And every time the brain manufactures an emotion, physical reactions accompany it. Scientists have found that the brain's natural chemicals, such as endorphins and peptides, form literal communication links between the brain, its thought processes, and the cells of the body, including those of the immune system.

THE IMMUNE SYSTEM

The immune system patrols and guards the body against attackers, both from without and from within. It is a complex system consisting of about a trillion cells called *lymphocytes* and about a hundred million trillion molecules called *antibodies*. According to Dr. Steven Locke, associate director of Psychiatry Consultation Services at Beth Israel Hospital in Boston, the immune system does not operate within a biological vacuum; it is sensitive to a number of influences. One of those seems to be the brain.

Various studies have shown a real connection between the central nervous system and the immune system, a connection that allows the mind to influence either susceptibility or resistance to disease. A number of immune system cells — including those in the thymus gland, spleen, bone marrow, and lymph nodes — are laced with extensive networks of nervous system cells.

Further, the cells of the immune system seem to be equipped to respond to chemical signals from the central nervous system. For example, the surface of the lymphocytes has been found to contain receptors for a variety of central nervous system chemical messengers, such as catecholamines, prostaglandins, serotonin, endorphins, sex hormones, the thyroid hormone, and the growth hormone. National Institutes of Mental Health researchers discovered that certain white blood cells are equipped with the molecular equivalent of antennas tuned specifically to receive messages from the brain.

▼ Do You Have an Immune-Competent Personality?

Consider the following questions as a probe to help you determine whether you have the elements of an immune-competent personality. Questions to which you answer "no" represent areas that need your attention, except for the last two, which need attention if you answer "yes." The questions are based on Dr. George Solomon's research and ideas about the effects of personality, coping, and emotions on our immune systems.

1. Do I have a sense of meaning in my work, daily activities, family, and relationships?
2. Am I able to express anger appropriately in defense of myself?
3. Am I able to ask friends and family for support when I am feeling lonely or troubled?
4. Am I able to ask friends or family for favors when I need them?
5. Am I able to say no to someone who asks for a favor if I can't or don't feel like doing it?
6. Do I engage in health-related behaviors (exercise, diet, meditation, etc.) based on my own self-defined needs instead of someone else's prescriptions or ideas?
7. Do I have enough play in my life?
8. Do I find myself depressed for long periods, during which time I feel hopeless about ever changing the conditions that cause me to be depressed?
9. Am I dutifully filling a prescribed role in my life (that is, wife, husband, parent, boss, nice guy) to the detriment of my own needs?

Reprinted with permission from *Natural Health*, 17 Station St., Box 1200, Brookline Village, MA 02147.

Because of these receptors on the lymphocytes, physical and psychological stress alters the immune system. Stress causes the body to release several powerful neurohormones, including catecholamines, corticosteroids, and endorphins, which bind with the receptors on the lymphocytes and alter immune function. Corticosteroids, in fact, have been found to have such a powerful influence in suppressing the immune system that they are used widely as drugs in treating allergic conditions (such as asthma and hay fever) and autoimmune disorders (such as rheumatoid arthritis and preventing the rejection of transplanted organs). These corticosteroids and other brain chemicals are unleashed by the hypothalamus and have profound effects on the immune system.

According to the latest scientific studies, the link between the mind and the immune system has gained a new dimension with the growing evidence that psychosocial factors directly affect immune function and, thus, potentially influence a wide range of disorders, including allergies, infections, autoimmune disorders, and even cancer. As one practitioner put it, "The human body can be conceived of as a five-million-year-old healer, with an internal pharmacopoeia of neuropeptides, neuroendocrine secretions, and immunological restoratives that maintain and enhance health."[4]

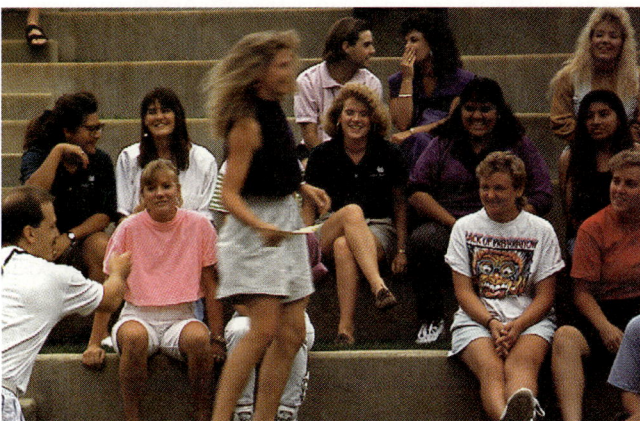

New findings suggest personality may play a role in health and wellness.

▼ PERSONALITIES AND HEALTH

Howard Friedman, psychologist and clinical professor of community medicine at the University of California, wrote, "I have never seen a death certificate marked 'Death due to unhealthy personality.' But maybe pathologists and coroners should be instructed to take into account the latest scientific findings on the role of personality in health."[5]

Personality is *the whole of your personal characteristics*, the group of behavioral and emotional tendencies that make you up. It is the way your habits, attitudes, and traits combine to make the person that is uniquely you. Because of your personality, you act in a similar way from one day to the next, and, when you are placed in various situations, you still tend to act in a generally consistent way. Your personality, in essence, is *the pattern of behavior that distinguishes you from everybody else*. Personality depends partly on biology and genetics (the unique set of genes you inherited from your parents) but also is shaped heavily by the family you grow up in, the environment that surrounds you, and the culture and subcultures that influence you.

The theory that personality impacts health is, as world-renowned psychologist Hans Eysenck put it, a theory based on centuries of observations made by keen-eyed physicians. The notion that a certain personality type leads to heart disease dates back more than 2,000 years to Hippocrates, and the belief that a certain "personality" is associated with cancer goes back several centuries. What *is* new is the flood of scientific data that now seems to be substantiating those notions.

When we explore the link between disease and personality, two important issues have to be addressed. At first, they may seem at odds. Even when people accept blame for an illness, to assume that they brought it on themselves may be a mistake. This viewpoint may lead to inhumanity and a lack of compassion for people who need it the most. On the other hand, we must study the links that we know exist between personality and disease, because we know we can do a great deal to protect and preserve our own health. It won't work all of the time for all of the people in all circumstances, but a fair share — a majority, in fact — can help themselves stay healthy. And a fair share of those who become ill can help themselves recover.

Most people, whether they realize it or not, associate certain personality types with certain illnesses.

Workaholics have heart attacks. Worriers get ulcers. People who get too uptight have asthma attacks. In reality, can they be so neatly categorized?

Not yet, but researchers have made tremendous strides in proving that personality *does* have an impact on health. They have found that the way we look at things, as determined by our personality, may actually contribute to illness or help keep us well.

Numerous studies show a link between personality and health. In one, University of California psychologists Howard Friedman and Stephanie Booth-Kewley analyzed 101 studies that had been conducted over four decades (from 1945 to 1984). They concluded that strong links exist between personality and health.[6] Based on their analysis of the studies, the two say, they are not sure there is a specific "personality" for an individual disease, but they are convinced that there may well be a "generic disease-prone personality." Personality may function like diet: Imbalances may predispose one to all sorts of diseases.

Other researchers say that certain personalities or personality traits can be linked specifically to certain diseases. Most prominent in research has been the *coronary-prone personality*, characterized by the hard-driving and competitive Type A personality who also is hostile, angry, and suspicious. Also prominent in current research is the *cancer-prone personality* characterized by people who demonstrate little emotion, are ambivalent toward self and others, and were not close to their parents.

Researchers even have been able to ascribe certain personality traits to highly specific illnesses. Dr. Arnold Levy, vice-president of the American Digestive Disease Society, says that young women who are characteristically self-demanding and high achievers are the most likely candidates for irritable bowel syndrome.[7] Psychologist Ross Vickers, Jr., of the Naval Health Research Center in San Diego, says people who are neurotic — especially if neurosis is coupled with depression — are particularly prone to upper respiratory tract infection.[8]

A third group of researchers believes a specific personality may make a person susceptible to a "cluster" of disease conditions, not just a specific disease. Some of the longest-standing research in this area has been conducted by Caroline Bedell Thomas and her co-workers at the Johns Hopkins School of Medicine. Based on her extensive research beginning in 1947, she believes that people can be categorized into three broad personality types that can determine whether a person is most apt to become ill or stay healthy.[9]

Still other researchers group people with similar personalities into "personality clusters." Georgia State University researchers Douglas Stanwyck and Carol Anson identified five clusters of personalities based on their study of 194 different groups of people who had taken the well-respected Minnesota Multiphasic Personality Inventory (MMPI). The clusters range from people who are most prone to staying well (those who scored closest to "normal" on the MMPI) to those most prone to getting sick (those characterized by depression, indecision, hopelessness, chronic fatigue, physical weakness, and severely low self-esteem).[10]

The link between personality and health has become the subject of a number of aggressive studies, and researchers are beginning to attempt to duplicate long-term studies. Most now accept the notion of an "immune-prone personality," in which hardiness enables resistance to the ravages of stress without becoming ill. The notion that certain personality traits are linked to illness, however, does not have such widespread acceptance.

When Marcia Angell, pathologist and senior deputy editor of the *New England Journal of Medicine*, editorialized in 1985 that too much credit is given to personality and emotions in relationship to physical health — saying that "our belief in disease as a direct reflection of mental state is largely folklore"[11] — the journal was flooded with letters from physicians and former cancer patients, disputing the editorial's claims. The 60,000-member American Psychological Association (APA) issued a statement attacking Angell's piece as "inaccurate and unfortunate." In the succeeding years, the debate has raged.

Keeping in mind that controversy exists among researchers and the medical profession regarding the personality/health link, we also must realize that a host of new research is slowly unraveling the mystery behind the effect of personality. The bulk of the research is centering on the existence of a generic "disease-prone personality," one that creates a tendency toward illness. Research continues into the classic "coronary-prone personality." Other research is directed at the possible existence of a "cancer-prone personality," which some researchers have called the Type C personality. Still others have looked at personality traits that predispose a victim to rheumatoid arthritis or ulcers.

THE CORONARY-PRONE PERSONALITY

In a summary of research printed in *Psychology Today*, a writer editorialized, "By treating the heart as an unfeeling pump, surgeons have been able to create pacemakers and work their way up to the ultimate in high-tech medicine: the artificial heart. But even as Barney Clark and other courageous patients were testing the electronic pumps, scientists were using chemistry, psychology and hard data to discover that trouble in the heart may come in part from sickness of the soul."[12]

That "sickness of the soul" began three decades ago as a notion called the Type A personality; today, it has evolved into a more broad-based concept that entails not so much a distinct personality as a behavior pattern. For ease of discussion, however, we will refer to that pattern by the name most researchers prefer: the Type A personality.

The Type A personality does *not* equate with stress, cautions cardiologist Ray Rosenman — who, with colleague Meyer Friedman, originated the theory of Type A personality three decades ago. The Type A behavior pattern, he says, does not imply a stressful situation or a distressed response. The Type A person is not necessarily anxious, depressed, worried, fearful, or neurotic. Type A refers to the behaviors of an individual who reacts to the environment with characteristic gestures, facial expressions, a fast pace of activities, and the perception of daily events and stresses as challenges, all leading to an aggressive, time-urgent, and impatient style of living.[13]

No one knows for sure how many Type A personalities exist. One researcher conservatively estimated that 40% of all Americans are Type A.[14] And, though original research focused on men, more recent studies show that women and children also can be Type A's. Researchers believe the Type A personality can result from a number of influences including genetic and environmental factors, most prominent of which is a hostile, angry, nonsupportive family environment. And, although some aspects of Type A personality are linked definitely to the development of heart disease, other facets of the behavior pattern may not be harmful to health.

According to researchers, Type A personalities never slow down. Type A has been dubbed the "hurry sickness." These people try to do two or more things simultaneously, have a sense of time urgency, are extremely competitive and tend to "keep score" of even trivial situations, are aggressive, have forceful, rapid, or "staccato" gestures, are insecure about their status, and sometimes harbor an unconscious drive to self-destruct. According to Friedman, these traits add up to "joyless striving" — but they actually are the least detrimental to health.

Instead, the traits that are most detrimental to health, the most predictive of coronary disease, are the "harmful" Type A traits, a "toxic core" consisting of anger, cynicism, suspiciousness, and excessive self-involvement. Probably the most detrimental trait of the toxic core is free-floating hostility, a permanent, deep-seated anger that hovers quietly until some trivial incident causes it to erupt in a burst of hostility. Important and still-controversial studies have made a startling conclusion about the hostility factor: Apparently a person can have many of the characteristics typically associated with Type A personality — such as competitive drive, an aggressive personality, and impatience — without running the risks of a heart attack *as long as the person is not hostile.* The hostility component is more accurate in predicting coronary heart disease than the more general notion of Type A behavior.

How does the hostility-laden Type A personality affect the body? According to prominent Duke University researcher Redford Williams,[15] the Type A personality is in a chronic state of "vigilant observation," a constant fight-or-flight state. The hormones that are continually released cause an increase in serum cholesterol and fat levels, leaching of blood platelets, overworking of the heart and arteries, excessive insulin secretion, and suppression of the immune system.

The result is a higher risk for heart disease. In one long-term study, researchers found that Type A personalities were more than twice as likely to develop heart disease; among those aged 39 to 49, the risk leaps to six times as high.[16] If Type A personality exists alongside two other risk factors for heart disease (such as cigarette smoking or high blood pressure), the risk for developing coronary heart disease is eight times greater.[17] Researchers also have found that Type A personality increases the risk for developing other diseases, including ulcers, headache, cancer, genital herpes, and vision problems.

As Williams points out, not all components of the Type A personality are harmful to health. Type A's don't necessarily have to slow down — as long as they are not driven by hostility. People who have many of the Type A traits without the toxic core that

Hostility Could Harm Your Heart

Experts now conclude that feelings of hostility increase your risk of heart disease. Dr. Redford Williams, Duke University Medical Center, has designed a questionnaire to help you determine whether you have a hostile personality. Circle the answer that most closely fits how you would respond to the given situation:

1. **A teen-ager drives by my yard blasting the car stereo:**
   A. I begin to understand why teen-agers can't hear.
   B. I can feel my blood pressure starting to rise.

2. **A boyfriend/girlfriend calls at the last minute "too tired to go out tonight." I'm stuck with two $15 tickets:**
   A. I find someone else to go with.
   B. I tell my friend how inconsiderate he/she is.

3. **Waiting in the express checkout line at the supermarket where a sign says "No More Than 10 Items Please":**
   A. I pick up a magazine and pass the time.
   B. I glance to see if anyone has more than 10 items.

4. **Most homeless people in large cities:**
   A. Are down and out because they lack ambition.
   B. Are victims of illness or some other misfortune.

5. **At times when I've been very angry with someone:**
   A. I was able to stop short of hitting him/her.
   B. I have, on occasion, hit or shoved him/her.

6. **When I am stuck in a traffic jam:**
   A. I am usually not particularly upset.
   B. I quickly start to feel irritated and annoyed.

7. **When there's a really important job to be done:**
   A. I prefer to do it myself.
   B. I am apt to call on my friends to help.

8. **The cars ahead of me start to slow and stop as they approach a curve:**
   A. I assume there is a construction site ahead.
   B. I assume someone ahead had a fender-bender.

9. **An elevator stops too long above where I'm waiting:**
   A. I soon start to feel irritated and annoyed.
   B. I start planning the rest of my day.

10. **When a friend or co-worker disagrees with me:**
    A. I try to explain my position more clearly.
    B. I am apt to get into an argument with him or her.

11. **At times when I was really angry in the past:**
    A. I have never thrown things or slammed a door.
    B. I've sometimes thrown things or slammed a door.

12. **Someone bumps into me in a store:**
    A. I pass it off as an accident.
    B. I feel irritated at their clumsiness.

13. **When my spouse (significant other) is fixing a meal:**
    A. I keep an eye out to make sure nothing burns.
    B. I talk about my day or read the paper.

14. **Someone is hogging the conversation at a party:**
    A. I look for an opportunity to put him/her down.
    B. I soon move to another group.

15. **In most arguments:**
    A. I am the angrier one.
    B. The other person is angrier than I am.

Score one point for each of these answers: 1. B, 2. B, 3. B, 4. A, 5. B, 6. B, 7. A, 8. B, 9. A, 10. B, 11. B, 12. B, 13. A, 14. A, 15. A. If you scored 4 or more points you may be hostile. Questions 1, 6, 9, 12 and 15 reflect anger. Questions 2, 5, 10, 11, 14, reflect aggression. Questions 3, 4, 7, 8, 13 reflect cynicism. If you scored 2 points in any category, you should work on that area of your personality.

From *Anger Kills* by Redford Williams and Virginia Williams. Copyright © 1993 by Redford B. Williams, M.D. and Virginia Williams, Ph.D. Reprinted by permission of Times Books, a division of Random House, Inc.

How to Change a Type A Personality

▼ Make a contract with yourself to slow down and take it easy. Put it in writing to up your odds of actually making the changes you need to. Post it in a conspicuous spot, then stick to the terms you set up. Be specific; abstracts ("I'm going to be less uptight") don't work. Work on only one or two things at a time. Wait until you change one habit before you tackle the next one.

▼ Eat more slowly, and eat only when you are relaxed and sitting down.

▼ Stop smoking.

▼ Cut down on your caffeine intake; it increases the tendency to become irritated and agitated.

▼ Take regular breaks throughout the day, even as brief as 5 or 10 minutes. Totally change what you're doing. Get up, stretch, get a drink of cool water, walk around the yard for a few minutes.

▼ Work on fighting your impatience. If you're standing in line at the grocery store, study the interesting things people have in their carts instead of getting upset.

▼ Work on controlling hostility. Keep a written log. When do you flare up? What causes it? How do you feel at the time? What preceded it? Look for patterns, and figure out what sets you off. Then do something about it. Either avoid the situations that cause you hostility or practice reacting to them in different ways.

▼ Plan some activities just for the fun of it. Load a picnic basket in the car and drive to the country with a friend; after that stressful physics class, stop at a theater and see a good comedy.

▼ Choose a role model, someone you know and admire who does not have a Type A personality. Observe the person carefully, then try out some new techniques.

▼ Simplify your life so you can learn to relax a little bit. Figure out which activities or commitments you can eliminate right now, then get rid of them.

▼ If morning is a problem time for you, set your alarm clock half an hour earlier.

▼ Learn to relax. Take time out during even the most hectic day to do something truly relaxing. Because you won't be used to it, you may have to work at it at first. Begin by listing things you'd really enjoy that would calm you. Include some things that take only a few minutes: Watch a sunset, lie out on the lawn at night and look at the stars, call an old friend and catch up on news, take a nap, saute a pan of mushrooms and savor them slowly.

▼ If you're under a deadline, take short breaks. Stop and talk to someone else for 5 minutes, take a short walk, lie down with a cool cloth over your eyes for 10 minutes.

▼ Pay attention to what your own body clock is saying. You've probably noticed that every 90 minutes or so, you lose the ability to concentrate, get a little sleepy, and have a tendency to daydream. Instead of fighting the urge, put your work down and let your mind wander for a few minutes. Use the time to imagine, and let your creativity run wild.

▼ Learn to treasure unplanned surprises: a friend dropping by unannounced, a hummingbird outside your window, a child's tightly clutched bouquet of wildflowers.

▼ Savor your relationships. Think about the people in your life. Relax with them and give yourself to them. Give up trying to control others, and resist the urge to end relationships that don't always go as you'd like them to.

---

harms health, Williams reminds us, are driven by a positive, enthusiastic approach to the world — a characteristic that can be protective, not harmful.

THE CANCER-PRONE PERSONALITY

One of the most controversial notions medical researchers are exploring today is the "cancer personality" — a set of personality traits that disposes a person to cancer. The exact effect of personality on cancer is difficult to assess. People can be exposed unwittingly to carcinogens that may be a factor, and the number of factors between the time of prognosis and the time of diagnosis can be vastly different. Nonetheless, more and more physicians believe in a link between personality and cancer, and this gives a new and pressing direction to medical research.

Researchers became keenly interested in the possibility of a cancer-prone personality during the 1950s, when psychologist Eugene Blumberg began noticing a "trademark" personality in cancer patients in a Long Beach veterans' hospital. He wrote: "We

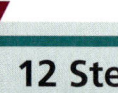

12 Steps To a Trusting Heart

The following behavior modification program will help you develop a more trusting, less hostile heart.

1. **Monitor your destructive thoughts.** Keep a log of incidents that trigger your anger so you learn to recognize and arrest them.
2. **Share your hostility problem with someone.** Let your spouse, or a close friend, know that you recognize you have a problem with hostility, and that you hope he or she will support your efforts to change.
3. **Stop those hostile thoughts.** As soon as you realize you are having cynical thoughts, say loudly to yourself, "STOP!" Those thoughts will stop, and the anger may cease also.
4. **Reason with yourself.** Because you are a rational being, try to reason with yourself.
5. **Put yourself in the other person's shoes.** Empathy and anger are incompatible.
6. **Learn to laugh at yourself.** Humor is an excellent strategy to deflect cynical mistrust and defuse your anger.
7. **Learn to relax.** [The relaxation techniques presented in Chapter 2 may be helpful.]
8. **Practice trust.** Trusting others makes them feel good about you and in turn allows you to feel good about them.
9. **Learn to listen.** By not interrupting others, you will learn to value their opinion, and they, in turn, will value you and your ideas.
10. **Learn to be assertive.** A measured response to injustice is more effective than a hostile one.
11. **Pretend today is your last.** Which would you rather be remembered for — angry feelings and aggressive acts, or joyful feelings and acts of kindness?
12. **Practice forgiving.** By letting go of resentment, you may find the weight of anger lifting, helping you to forget the wrong.

Executive Health Report, Vol. 26, No. 5, February, 1990, p. 5. Used by permission. Developed by Dr. Redford Williams.

---

were impressed by the polite, apologetic, almost painful acquiescence of the patients with rapidly progressing disease as contrasted with the most expressive and sometimes bizarre personalities of those who responded brilliantly to therapy with remissions and long survival.[18]

To figure out whether there was any connection, Blumberg administered psychological tests to the cancer patients. He found that the patients with the fastest-growing tumors were consistently serious, overly cooperative, overly nice, overanxious, painfully sensitive, passive, and apologetic. Furthermore they had been that way all their lives. The patients with the slow-growing tumors, on the other hand, were the ones who had developed a way of coping with life's stresses.

At about the same time, physicians at San Francisco's Malignant Melanoma Clinic were gaining interest in the same thing. They had noticed a disturbing pattern in the personalities of patients with melanoma, a particularly virulent form of skin cancer. These patients were nice — too nice. They were passive about everything, including their cancer.

Mindful that these traits could be a coincidence, the physicians asked University of California School of Medicine psychologist Lydia Temoshok to talk to the patients and determine whether a personality pattern would emerge. After talking in detail to 150 of the clinic's melanoma patients, Temoshok declared that a distinct pattern was present. The cancer patients were, indeed, very, very nice. They never seemed to express any negative emotion — not fear, or sadness, or anger, or denial, or any of the other emotions common to a patient struggling with a terminal disease. The researchers characterized these patients as the rock of stability for their families. Even in the face of cancer, they maintained this composure. When one of them was diagnosed, she might say, "I'm doing fine, but I'm really worried about my husband. He takes things so hard."[19]

The results of this and other research led Temoshok to coin the term Type C personality, and other researchers have looked at the same thing. One of the scientists most prominent in the study of a cancer personality is psychologist Lawrence LeShan, who interviewed 250 patients hospitalized for cancer and compared them with interviews of patients hospitalized for other diseases. Based on his study, LeShan identified specific life events that seemed common to the cancer patients:[20] (a) They had a "bleak" childhood characterized by a tense or hostile relationship with one or both parents and feelings of loneliness and isolation; and (b) as young adults, they made a strong, central emotional commitment to someone or something and then something happened to remove the source of the emotional investment. Six to eight months later, LeShan says, these people were diagnosed with cancer.

According to researchers, the hallmark of the cancer personality is the *nonexpression of emotion* Even when they are experiencing tremendous despair, they characteristically "bottle it up." Although other people often describe cancer patients as kind, sweet, and benign, this sweetness is really a mask they wear to conceal their feelings of anger, hurt, and hostility. Other personality traits that seem common in cancer victims are loneliness (in one study, "loners" developed cancer 16 times more often) and an attitude of helplessness and hopelessness (those who have this attitude usually fare the worst).

In this area, as in almost all other areas of medical research, research findings are inconsistent. Not every study finds a link between cancer and personality, and a few have found no relationship at all between the two. Others find that personality may play a role in either — but not both — developing cancer or its progression once the disease is established. Even with these inconsistencies in mind, however, leading researchers believe enough evidence exists for a link between cancer and personality that they need to take a hard look at the possibility.

As a caveat, Harvard psychologist Joan Borysenko cautions that the very presence of cancer can create physiological changes that could affect personality — such as attacking the central nervous system or skewing the delicate internal balance of hormones. Certain tumors are known to secrete hormones, some of which alter behavior or moods.

PERSONALITY AND RHEUMATOID ARTHRITIS

Of all the forms of arthritis, rheumatoid arthritis clearly is the most crippling and most devastating. It's an autoimmune disease (the immune system actually turns against the body) in which the immune system begins attacking the collagen, the connective tissues in the joints.

Could there be a set of personality traits that is characteristic of rheumatoid arthritis? Researchers think so. One of the most convincing studies began in the 1960s when a team of researchers from the University of Rochester studied eight pairs of female identical twins, one who had rheumatoid arthritis and the other who did not. By using identical twins for the study, the possibility of a genetic factor was eliminated.

A distinct pattern emerged. The women with arthritis actually seemed to seek out stress. The healthy twins felt free to express criticism and argue. They also described their marriages as happy, whereas the arthritic twins spoke poorly of their husbands and apparently put up with considerable abuse in their marriages. The healthy women described themselves as people who liked people; they said they were easy to get acquainted with, active, constantly busy, productive workers, and enjoyed life in general. The self-image of the arthritic twins was just the opposite. They described themselves as moody and easily upset, nervous, tense, worried, depressed, and high-strung. Other research has shown similar findings. One researcher who studied more than 5,000 rheumatoid arthritis patients found that, in a high percentage of cases, the patients suffered from worry, work pressures, marital disharmony, and concerns about relatives immediately prior to onset of disease.[21]

Still other researchers have found that people who have rheumatoid arthritis are more likely to have emotional disturbance, and that they tend to be perfectionistic, chronically anxious, depressed, hostile, and introverted. The disease seems to become the most severe when the arthritic person has the following traits: self-sacrificing, masochistic, conforming, self-conscious, shy, inhibited, perfectionistic, interested in sports, nervous, tense, worried, moody, depressed, and fearful of marital rejection.[22] Those with the poorest prognosis are more anxious and depressed, more isolated, introverted, alienated, and least able to suppress anger over time.

PERSONALITY AND ULCERS

The physiology behind gastric ulcer is simple: The person with an ulcer secretes too much gastric acid. A number of factors have been identified as causing an increase in gastric acid, including tobacco, alcohol, caffeine, and aspirin, as well as certain emotions such as frustration, hostility, and resentment.

Recent research has identified an "ulcer personality" that either may cause ulcers or may determine how severe existing ulcers become. The ulcer personality is characterized by excessive dependence on others; far less social support than normal; excessive worry, annoyance, and fear of common situations or circumstances; and frequent crises. Ulcer patients show a fairly consistent quality: Whereas other people are able to bend with stress, an ulcer patient tends to "break." Researchers at the University of Texas Health Science Center in Dallas theorize that ulcer patients have the same number of stressful situations as people who don't have ulcers, but the ulcer patients *perceive* the situations as being far more negative than do other people.

▼ PERSONALITY TRAITS AND HEALTH

ANGER

What exactly is anger? It is a temporary emotion that combines physiological arousal with emotional arousal. It can range in severity all the way from intense rage to "cool" anger that doesn't really involve arousal at all (and might be defined more accurately as an "attitude," such as resentment). The terms *anger* and *hostility* often are used interchangeably to describe a set of negative emotions, but they are not the same. Unlike anger, hostility is not a temporary emotion but, rather, an attitude expressed in aggressive behavior motivated by animosity and hatefulness.

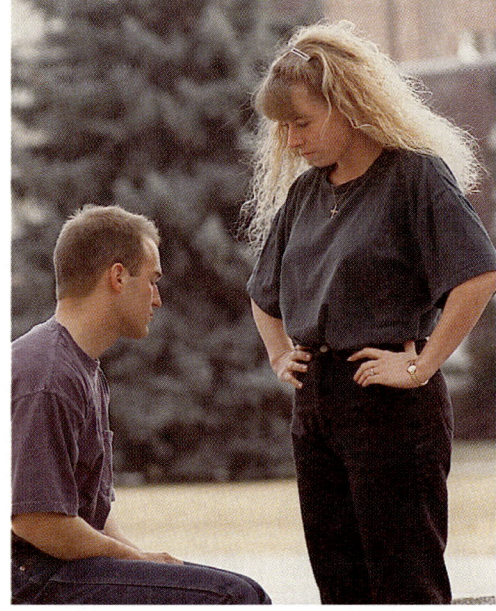

Some personality styles may harm health.

Research has shown that, to be healthy, people need to express anger. It is a mandate to confront the things that are making us angry and to work through the anger. Problems arise when anger is misdirected, when anger is expressed through miscommunication, emotional distancing, escalation of conflicts, endless rehearsals of grievances, assuming a hostile disposition, acquiring angry habits, making a bad situation worse, loss of self-esteem, and loss of the respect of others. Misdirected anger buries the real problem and creates more problems along the way.

According to researcher Carol Tavris, "The purpose of anger is to make a grievance known, and if the grievance is not confronted, it will not matter whether the anger is kept in, let out, or wrapped in red ribbons and dropped in the Erie Canal."[23]

Even more serious problems derive from suppressed anger. Preliminary research has shown that bottling up anger can lead to many health consequences — among them, heart disease, cancer, rheumatoid arthritis, hives, acne, psoriasis, peptic ulcer, epilepsy, migraine, Raynaud's disease, and high blood pressure. But expressing anger is healthy only if the expression itself is healthy. Tavris adds that "ventilating is cathartic only when it restores our sense of control, reducing both the rush of adrenaline that accompanies an unfamiliar and threatening situation and the belief that you are helpless and powerless."[24] According to one scientist, "medical research shows that no matter how many times you work out at the gym or how careful you are to eat correctly, you're putting yourself at risk if you don't manage your anger effectively."[25]

To understand the broad consequences of anger, consider the wide range of physiological reactions that accompany anger: changes in muscle tension, scowling, grinding of teeth, glaring, clenching of fists, flushing, goosebumps, chills and shudders, prickly sensations, numbness, choking, twitching, sweating, losing self-control, feeling either hot or cold. Common reactions associated with anger include fatigue, teeth clenching, pain in the neck or jaw, ringing in the ears, lowered skin temperature, excessive sweating, redness, hives, acne, itching, severe headache, migraine headache, belching, hiccupping, peptic ulcers, chronic indigestion, diarrhea, constipation, intestinal cramping, loss of appetite, and frequent colds.

Chronic repression of anger has physical effects similar to those of chronic stress. One of the major physiological effects is the release of chemicals and hormones, principally adrenaline and noradrenaline, which impact proper heart functioning and the amount of constriction or dilation of the arteries. It's a situation, according to Friedman, that is chiefly responsible for the development of arterial diseases.[26]

According to data published in the *New England Journal of Medicine*, mismanaged anger is perhaps the main factor involved in predicting cardiovascular

▼
Temper Test

Directions: A number of statements that people have used to describe themselves are given below. Read each statement and then circle the appropriate number to indicate how you generally feel. There are no right or wrong answers. Do not spend too much time on any one statement, but give the answer that seems to describe how you generally feel.

	Almost Never	Sometimes	Often	Almost Always
1. I am quick-tempered	1	2	3	4
2. I feel annoyed when I am not given recognition for doing good work	1	2	3	4
3. I have a fiery temper	1	2	3	4
4. I feel infuriated when I do a good job and get a poor evaluation	1	2	3	4
5. I am a hotheaded person	1	2	3	4
6. It makes me furious when I am criticized in front of others	1	2	3	4
7. I get angry when I'm slowed down by others' mistakes	1	2	3	4
8. I fly off the handle	1	2	3	4
9. When I get mad, I say nasty things	1	2	3	4
10. When I get frustrated, I feel like hitting someone	1	2	3	4

Total Points: _____

Scoring
Add the points from each item (1-4) together to get your total score, somewhere between 10 and 40. A man who scores 17, or a woman who scores 18, is just about average. If you score below 13, you're well down into the safe zone. A score above 20 means you may be a hothead — scoring higher than three-quarters of those tested.

American Health © 1983 by Charles D. Spielberger.

disease.[27] A number of major studies now have definitely linked anger to heart disease, and the evidence continues to mount. In addition to heart attack, anger also leads to a much higher risk for high blood pressure.

Studies conducted as early as four decades ago also show a link between anger and cancer. Researchers who studied the life patterns of approximately 400 cancer patients during the 1950s found a common thread among them: Many seemed unable to express anger or hostility in defense of themselves. The same patients could get angry in the defense of others or even in the defense of a cause, but not in defense of themselves.[28]

Other studies of cancer victims, especially women with breast cancer, indicate that the style of expressing anger (or the ability to express it at all) seems to have considerable impact on the development and spread of cancer. In one study of women with breast disease, those who were diagnosed later as having breast cancer had an entirely different style for expressing anger than those who had benign breast disease. The cancer victims were much more likely to suppress their anger and then finally "explode" with anger when they could no longer hold it in. Many didn't express anger at all.[29]

In a separate study, researchers found a big difference in the way the cancer victims expressed anger. Women in normal health tended to get angry and then forget about it. Those with benign disease tended to get angry and stay angry. Those with cancer got angry but either didn't express it or apologized for it, even when they were in the right.[30]

HOSTILITY

Hostility comes from the Latin word *hostis*, which means "enemy." Enemies seem to abound for people. They are everywhere: at the office, in the elevator, in the grocery store checkout line, on the freeway, in the house on the corner. Because of the health-damaging effects of hostility, hostile people become their own enemies.

Hostility is an ongoing accumulation of anger and irritation. As psychologist Robert Ornstein and physician David Sobel put it, hostility is a permanent resident kind of anger that shows itself with ever greater frequency in response to increasingly trivial happenings.[31] Tavris says that "into each life come real problems that people should be angry about. But hostile personality types get equally angry about cold soup and racial injustice. They're walking around in a state of wrath." Finally, Williams — whose research on hostility is making medical

▼
Blowing Off Anger the Healthy Way

▼ Recognize the anger for what it is. Don't be afraid of it or try to suppress it.

▼ Figure out what made you so angry, then figure out whether it's really worth being so upset over. Chances are that it's really a minor irritation or hassle.

▼ Stop before you act. Calm down first. Count to 10, take a deep breath, mentally recite the words to a favorite verse, or some other distracting and relaxing activity. *Then* get ready to deal with the anger.

▼ If you're ticked off at somebody else, use calm tact to say why, without ripping into the other person. Tell the person how *you're* feeling, and try to negotiate to change things.

▼ Be generous with the other person. Maybe he just failed an exam. Maybe she just heard bad news from home. Maybe he's having a rotten day. Listen carefully to her side of things, and try as much as you can to understand.

▼ When all else fails, forgive the other person. Everyone makes mistakes. Carrying a grudge is going to hurt *you* worse than it hurts the other person.

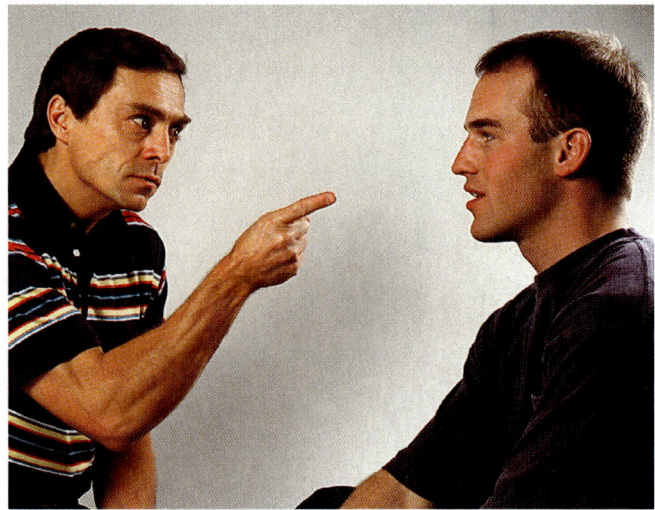

Anger and hostility can be a health risk factor.

history — claims that hostility is a basic lack of trust in human nature, in human motives; it's a belief that people are more bad than good, and that they will mistreat you.[32] Generally, a hostile person has an orientation toward hurting other people, either physically or verbally.

Victims of free-floating, generalized hostility usually have the following characteristics:

▶ Even when they're smiling, they look uptight and tense; they appear ready to jump into a fight at a second's notice.

▶ They have an intense need to win in sports and in games, even when other people are playing just for relaxation or fun.

▶ They are extremely sensitive to any perceived criticism against them but are loudly critical of others, and of themselves.

▶ They argue incessantly, even over trivial issues. Every conversation gets turned into an angry debate, and they refuse to lose an argument.

Although almost everyone occasionally exhibits one or more of these traits, victims of free-floating hostility exhibit them continuously. Life has become a sordid battle, and they charge into the fray armed with anger and irritation.

Williams, who has spent his professional career as a physician trying to determine the role hostility plays in disease, believes that not all components of hostility are equally risky. Through his research, he has isolated what he believes are the most toxic traits associated with hostility: cynical beliefs that others are inherently bad, selfish, mean, and not to be trusted; frequent angry feelings when these negative expectations are fulfilled; and overtly expressing those angry feelings in aggressive acts directed toward others.[33]

The effects of hostility are especially devastating to the body for two reasons:

1. Hostility causes the constant, unending release of stress hormones that destroy health in a variety of ways.

2. Hostility weakens the branch of the nervous system designed to calm down the body after an emergency.

To understand why hostility is so harmful to health, let's explore what happens in both of these scenarios.

Strategies for Beating Hostility

If you're a hostile person, can you change? Evidence says *yes*, and you can work to overcome a hostile attitude in a number of ways:

▼ This sounds too simplistic, but when you realize you're feeling hostile, tell yourself to *stop*. You might have to shout it out at first. Later, as you get better at it, you can change to a silent command.

▼ Talk to yourself about how you're feeling. Evaluate the situation. Figure out why you're so upset. Figure out whether your anger and hostility are justified. If they aren't, give them up. If they *are* (and in many cases they are), figure out another way to respond to the situation, one that won't fuel your fire.

▼ Don't let yourself get trampled. If your anger is justified, deal with it calmly and rationally, but deal with it. Stand up for yourself. Work to correct a wrong. If a classmate fails to recognize your contribution on an important final project, for example, don't just blow up and seethe with hostility. Talk to the professor, set the record straight, and spell out what you did toward the project. Then confront your classmate *calmly*, and express your feelings. Ask for a specific commitment (that he or she will explain to the professor what you did to help).

▼ Learn to trust other people. This might be hard at first, and, strange as it sounds, you might have to practice. Start with a minor situation in which you usually take control. Then let someone else be in charge. As you learn that others can do it, too, you gradually can learn to trust what other people can do.

▼ Be tolerant and nonjudgmental of others. The source of anger and hostility often is our response to someone else. Put yourself in the other's shoes. Consider the situation from the other's point of view. Even if you still think you're right, you might have gained empathy for that person that will allow you to deal with the situation free of hostility.

▼ Cut down on things that speed up your system, cause your body to churn out hormones, and lead to physical stress. These include sugar, caffeine, and nicotine, and the hidden sources of caffeine such as soft drinks, chocolate, and many over-the-counter and prescription drugs.

▼ If all else fails, distract yourself. If you're standing in a long line at a grocery store, read — and laugh at — the tabloid headlines; then mentally create your own bizarre stories. If you're caught in traffic, turn on the radio. Start singing. Visualize the last concert you went to. Do anything you can to take your thoughts off the situation that is getting you all riled up.

Hostility and Hormones

In essence, chronic hostility causes a reaction in the body much like that of stress. The difference is that a hostile person goes throughout the entire day in a stressed condition. Many hostile people don't even get relief at night while sleeping. Stress hormones are secreted throughout the night and eliminated in the urine around the clock.

To begin with, hostility causes the body to release corticotropin, which kicks into gear the whole sequence of stress hormones. The body secretes, among other hormones, epinephrine, norepinephrine, cortisol, prolactin, and testosterone. Blood pressure increases, the heart beats harder and faster, blood volume increases, blood moves from the skin and organs to the brain and muscles, the liver releases stored sugar, and breathing speeds up. Those reactions in themselves wouldn't be so bad, *if* they were to happen only occasionally and if the body were to have a way to physically overcome the reaction. With hostility, neither is the case.

Difficulty with Calming Down

The autonomic nervous system has two main branches: the "emergency branch," which pumps out hormones and prepares the body to respond in case of emergency; and the "calming branch" (the parasympathetic branch), which switches the hormones back off when the emergency is over. The calming branch literally calms and soothes the body, preventing it from remaining too long in an aroused state — which, as discussed, can result in disease.

Hostility weakens the parasympathetic branch of the nervous system. It can't do its job effectively any more. The body can't bounce back from the surge of stress hormones, no calming takes place, and the body remains in a state of prolonged arousal.

One of the most pronounced effects is heart disease. Hostility, one of the components of Type A behavior, now is known to be an independent risk factor for coronary heart disease. Williams says "we have strong evidence now that hostility alone damages the heart."[34]

Heart-harming hostility is characterized by anger-proneness, resentment, and suspicion. It also is marked by explosive and vigorous vocal mannerisms, competitiveness, impatience, and irritability.

A study of more than 400 patients at Duke Medical Center showed that more than 80% of the men who were classified as Type A and who *also* measured high in hostility had seriously diseased coronary arteries; only half of the other men did. The risk for women was even more significant.[35]

Hostility has been shown, in large-scale and long-term studies, to cause coronary blockages, coronary heart disease, and coronary death, to contribute significantly to a second heart attack, and to lead to the premature death of people with existing heart disease. In one study spearheaded by Williams and his colleagues, more than 2,280 Duke University Medical Center patients were studied for signs of Type A behavior and for the trait of hostility. The researchers found that they could predict which patients would be diagnosed with coronary heart disease simply by pinpointing which ones were hostile, and that hostility served as well as or better than Type A as a predictor.[36]

In a smaller but still convincing study, more than 250 physicians were tested for personality traits and then followed for 25 years. The death rate from heart disease and from all causes in general was six times greater for the physicians who measured high in hostility.[37]

Researchers with the Recurrent Coronary Prevention Project in San Francisco found that hostility is a significant factor in determining which heart attack patients will have a second heart attack. In addition, people who are more retributional in their hostility (people who want to get back at others) are much more likely to have another myocardial infarction than are hostile people who are less retributional.[38]

A number of researchers who have attempted to pinpoint the health effects of hostility have found that it contributes to premature death from many causes, including cancer. In one study, students in law school were given a battery of psychological tests intended to measure hostility. In a 25-year follow-up, researchers found that only 4% of the non-hostile lawyers died from any cause, but 20% of the hostile attorneys died during the 25-year period.[39]

WORRY, ANXIETY, AND FEAR

According to clinical psychologist Thomas Pruzinsky of the University of Virginia, worry is a state in which we dwell on something so much it causes us to become apprehensive. It differs from the far stronger emotion of fear, which causes physical changes such as a racing pulse and fast breathing. Worry is the thinking part of anxiety.[40]

When people convert emotions such as worry, anxiety, or fear into physical complaints — they actually *feel* something — these physical changes can impair the immune system and result in physical illness. Worry has been shown to affect the heart and the circulatory system as a whole, causing arrhythmias (irregular heartbeat), high blood pressure, and various abnormalities involving the arteries. Scientific tests also show that worry causes the body to produce the chemical acetylcholine, which causes the airways to contract and results in asthma.

One specific kind of worry, *uncertainty*, has been shown to create a particularly devastating kind of stress. Uncertainty keeps a person in a constant state of semiarousal, putting an extreme burden on the body's adaptive resources and resistance systems. The result is often disease — most particularly, gastrointestinal disease.

When worry escalates, the outcome is fear. Fear causes the heart to race, the head to spin, the palms to sweat, the knees to buckle, and the breathing to become labored. The level of arousal is similar to that of stress, and the human body can't withstand it indefinitely. Fear causes the body to secrete epinephrine, or adrenaline, with a resulting powerful effect on the heart. Both the rate and the strength of contractions increase, and blood pressure soars. The body is stimulated in turn to release other hormones. If the fear is intense enough, all systems can be overloaded fatally.

▼ A Simple Strategy for Beating Fear

- ▼ First, admit you're afraid. List the things that cause you fear. As you mentally recreate those fears, try to imagine them *without* the emotion of fear. It takes some practice, but you can do it!

- ▼ Next, confront your fear. Do whatever it is you're so afraid of. *Realize that your fear will intensify as you face it*, but do it anyway. Go back to your mental pictures, and try to imagine that the situation is not fearful.

- ▼ Do whatever it is that you're so afraid of at least three times. Chances are, you'll be less afraid each time. Chances are even better that you were afraid because you were *unsure*.

- ▼ As you confront your fear, call it something else — excitement or a thrill, for example.

The physical effects of fear are the same whether the fear is totally understandable or illogical. "The messages from the brain to the body are the same," one researcher pointed out, "whether you're teetering on the edge of a cliff, about to fall, or standing safely at the foot of a mountain, fearful of climbing to the top."[41]

When dogs are injected with catecholamines, the hormones released in response to fear, they die. Autopsies reveal certain characteristic lesions on the surface of their hearts, presumably an effect of the catecholamines. The same lesions are visible under microscopic examination on the hearts of 80% of all victims of sudden cardiac death.

DEPRESSION

Depression is much more than an occasional sad mood. It generally involves quitting or just plain giving up. A depressed person "goes on strike" from life, doing less and less, losing interest in people, abandoning hobbies, and giving up at work. One reason depression is so difficult to define is its evasiveness. Steven Paul, chief of clinical neuroscience at the National Institute of Mental Health, says depression is "like a fever, in that it's often an unspecific response to an internal or external insult. Like fever, it has a number of origins and

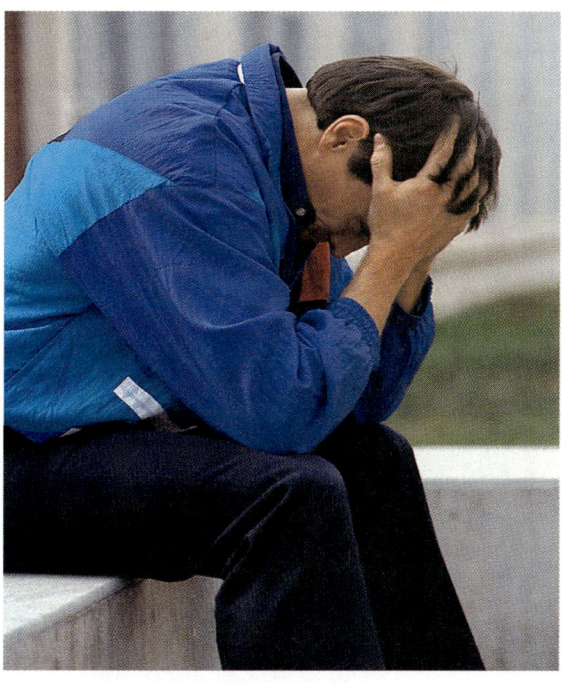

Worry may trigger or increase the stress response.

treatments."[42] Most experts estimate that between 10 and 14 million Americans suffer from depression. One study says the percentage of teenagers with clinical depression has increased more than fivefold over the past 40 years.

Depression often is caused by loss — of something valued or someone important. Under those circumstances, feeling sad or discouraged is normal. In some cases, though, depression is caused by biological factors — a chemical imbalance in the brain, a physical illness, a disturbance in the nervous system or neurotransmitters, or an injury involving brain tissue.

Frederick Goodwin, scientific director of the National Institute of Mental Health, says depression is the richest, most striking example in psychiatry — and possibly in all of medicine — of the relationship between the mind and the body.[43] Some of the depression's effects on the body are obvious. For example, a depressed person might not have the energy to get out of bed in the morning.

Other changes aren't so obvious but can have even more profound effects. Researchers have learned that during depression the body undergoes hormonal and chemical changes similar to those of stress — mostly, says National Institute of Mental Health psychiatrist Phillip Gold, because the mechanisms that normally regulate the stress response fail in depressed people.[44] In addition to having high levels of the hormones usually associated with stress, depressed people have significantly lower levels of three important brain chemicals: norepinephrine, dopamine, and serotonin, the chemicals that make us feel good.

Depression can increase mortality in some obvious ways. Severe depression, for example, can lead to suicide. Depression also can worsen the plight of people who already are ill with a medical problem. They tend to become sicker, need more medication, and spent more days in the hospital. Worst of all, depression can actually shorten life. Even among people who are not ill, depression can cut life short.

Epidemiological studies of depressed people show that people who are depressed have significantly higher mortality rates than people who are not depressed. One study following up on 1,593 patients hospitalized for depression at a care facility in Iowa showed that, when compared to a control group, death rates for the depressed patients soared for the first 2 years following hospitalization and remained higher than average throughout the 14 years of the study.[45]

Depression itself can become a potent risk factor in determining whether a person will die sooner than expected, either of natural causes or of underlying disease. Depression also becomes a significant risk factor for mortality among elderly people, people with health impairments, people who have preexisting immune system problems, and people who have been exposed to an infectious agent or a carcinogen. Depression even has been linked to sudden death in a number of studies.

Depression and the Immune System

Depression seems to have a significant impact on the immune system in a variety of ways, one of the most significant being the impact on the natural killer cells, the immune cells that assist the body in its surveillance against tumors and its resistance to viral disease. A number of studies shows that natural killer cell activity is lower in people who are depressed, and the more severe the depression, say researchers at the University of California at San Diego, the greater is the impairment in natural killer cell activity.

Other components of the immune system are crippled by depression as well. Studies have found that depression causes a striking reduction in white blood cells, an upset in the ratio of helper and suppressor cells, a reduction in the number of T cells, and an overall suppression of immune function.

Depression and the Heart

Depression causes irregularities in the nervous system. When those irregularities become severe enough, heart rate and blood pressure go awry, leading to cardiac problems. A number of impressive studies has shown a definite link between depression and heart disease. In several studies the effect of depression on the heart has been so profound that researchers were able to predict who would have a heart attack based solely on the presence of depression.

Perhaps some of the most profound influences of depression are on people who already have coronary artery disease or other cardiac problems. A striking example was provided in a study conducted at the Washington University School of Medicine in St. Louis, in which 52 people with coronary artery disease were studied for one year following their diagnosis.[46] Researchers found that 18% of the people in

Symptoms of Depression

When someone is depressed, that person has several symptoms nearly every day, all day, which last at least two weeks.

Use the chart to check off any symptoms you have had for two weeks or more.

- ❏ Loss of interest in things you used to enjoy, including sex.*
- ❏ Feeling sad, blue, or down in the dumps.*
- ❏ Feeling slowed down or restless and unable to sit still.
- ❏ Feeling worthless or guilty.
- ❏ Changes in appetite or weight loss or gain.
- ❏ Thoughts of death or suicide; suicide attempts.
- ❏ Trouble concentrating, thinking, remembering or making decisions.
- ❏ Trouble sleeping or sleeping too much.
- ❏ Loss of energy or feeling tired all of the time.

Other symptoms include:

- ❏ Headaches.
- ❏ Digestive problems.
- ❏ Other aches and pains.
- ❏ Sexual problems.
- ❏ Feeling pessimistic or hopeless.
- ❏ Being anxious or worried.

If you have had five or more of these symptoms **including at least one of the first two symptoms marked with an asterisk (*)** for at least two weeks, you may have major depressive disorder. See your health care provider for diagnosis.

Even if you have only a few depressive symptoms, you should also tell your health care provider. Sometimes a few symptoms can go on to become major depressive disorder. Some forms of depression are mild, but if symptoms are persistent or chronic, you may need treatment.

National Depressive and Manic-Depressive Association, 730 North Franklin St., Suite 501, Chicago, IL 60610, 312/642-0049 or 800/642-7243 (800-82-NDMDA) has adapted this checklist from the U.S. Dept. of Health and Human Services booklet, "Depression is a Treatable Illness, A Paient's Guide."

> ### How to Relieve Depression
>
> If your depression is caused by biological factors, you need medical help. Consult a physician if you have been depressed for a long time or your depression is unusually severe. If your depression is mild or your physician rules out biological factors, try these coping measures:
>
> - Start by admitting you are depressed, then try to figure out why. Once you have identified a cause, you might be able to eliminate it.
>
> - As much as you can, stick to your normal routine. Change — even positive change — is a source of stress and can intensify depression.
>
> - If you can, plan some quiet times each day when you can relax, pamper yourself, do something you enjoy, or just get away from stresses you might feel. If you've been feeling depressed for a while, you might need to start by actually making a list of things you'd like to do — read the newest book on the best-selling list, take a watercolor class, travel to a new area.
>
> - Find a confidant, someone you can talk to about your feelings. If you're lucky, you'll find someone who can listen without judging or giving advice. Whatever you do, don't choose another depressed person as your confidant. You'll only end up dragging each other down.
>
> - Do something you're good at: Write an essay for a literary magazine, enter a local bicycle race, volunteer to play the piano at a local retirement center, ask your landlord if you can plant flowers around your apartment building. You'll get an immediate boost, something that helps banish depression.
>
> - Get regular exercise. Studies have shown that exercise is one of the best ways to conquer depression. For starters, exercise causes the body to produce endorphins, a natural painkiller that results in a "high" for people who exercise longer than 30 minutes. Plan an activity you enjoy, something you can do regardless of the weather, and something for which you have the equipment.
>
> - Whatever you do, don't try to get rid of depression with alcohol or drugs. They only make things worse.

the study were seriously depressed,[47] compared to only 4% of all Americans and fewer than 3% of all people in the St. Louis area.[48] Major depression was found to be the best single predictor of serious problems and complications among the heart patients, an even stronger predictor than factors such as age, smoking, severity of artery damage, and levels of cholesterol in the bloodstream. Of the depressed patients, 78% had some cardiac event during the 12 months following their diagnosis, and one died. Only a third of the nondepressed patients had problems. The results of this and other studies show that heart patients who are happier, rather than depressed, are less likely to have heart attacks, bypass surgery, and other heart-related problems.

People who are depressed tend to magnify their medical problems. They are apt to have multiple chronic medical illnesses, as well as more aches and pains. They may not do as well in surgery, either. According to a study published in the *American Journal of Public Health*, depressed elderly women who had hip fractures did much more poorly following surgery than did the same type of patients who were not depressed.[49]

THE DISEASE-RESISTANT PERSONALITY

Too often we ask ourselves why someone got ill instead of how someone managed to stay well. Friedman noted that tendency when he wrote, "Each week the prestigious *New England Journal of Medicine* publishes a 'Case Record of the Massachusetts General Hospital,' detailing the pathology of an unusual or informative patient's case. There is no corresponding 'Case History of a Person Who Remained Well Throughout a Long Life.'"[50]

Researchers have long known that certain groups of people enjoy remarkably good health and longevity. Among them are "Mormons, nuns, symphony conductors, and women who are listed in *Who's Who*. This suggests that something in the way these people live, possibly even such abstractions as faith, pride of accomplishment, or productivity, plays a role in diminishing the ill effects of stress."[51]

Volumes of research have proved that stress is devastating to health. Fortunately, some things have been identified as *stress buffers*, factors that alleviate the deleterious effects of stress. Although controversy surrounds some of these findings, researchers have generally shown that social support, a sense of control, physical fitness, a sense of humor, self-esteem, optimism, advantageous coping styles, and hardiness all help to buffer stress.

How Hardy Are You?

Evaluating hardiness requires more than this quick test, but this simple exercise should give you some idea of how hardy you are.

Directions: Write down how much you agree or disagree with the following statements, using this scale:

0 = Strongly Disagree   2 = Mildly Disagree   3 = Mildly Agree   4 = Strongly Agree

- [ ] **A.** Trying my best at work [or school] makes a difference.
- [ ] **B.** Trusting to fate is sometimes all I can do in a relationship.
- [ ] **C.** I often wake up eager to start on the day's projects.
- [ ] **D.** Thinking of myself as a free person leads to great frustration and difficulty.
- [ ] **E.** I would be willing to sacrifice financial security in my work if something really challenging comes along.
- [ ] **F.** It bothers me when I have to deviate from the routine or schedule I've set for myself.
- [ ] **G.** An average citizen can have an impact on politics.
- [ ] **H.** Without the right breaks, it is hard to be successful in my field.
- [ ] **I.** I know why I'm doing what I'm doing at work [school].
- [ ] **J.** Getting close to people puts me at risk of being obligated to them.
- [ ] **K.** Encountering new situations is an important priority in my life.
- [ ] **L.** I really don't mind when I have nothing to do.

These questions measure control, commitment, and challenge. For half the questions, a high score (such as 4, "strongly agree") indicates hardiness; for the other half, a low score (disagreement) does.

To get your scores on control, commitment, and challenge, first write the number of your answer — 0, 1, 2, or 3 — above the letter of each question on the score sheet below. Then add and subtract as shown. (To get your score on "control," for example, add your answers to questions A and G; add your answers to B and H; and then subtract the second number from the first.)

Add your scores on commitment, control, and challenge together to get a score for total hardiness.

Total Scores: **10-18:** a hardy person;   **0-9:** moderate hardiness;   **Below 0:** low hardiness

Control Scores............................ ☐ + ☐ = ☐   MINUS   ☐ + ☐ = ☐   EQUALS   ☐
                                                         A   G   B   H   +

Commitment Scores.............. ☐ + ☐ = ☐   MINUS   ☐ + ☐ = ☐   EQUALS   ☐
                                                           C   I   D   J   +

Challenge Scores.................... ☐ + ☐ = ☐   MINUS   ☐ + ☐ = ☐   EQUALS   ☐
                                                         E   K   F   L   EQUALS

TOTAL HARDINESS SCORE: ☐

American Health, © 1984 by Suzanne Ouellette.

Perhaps most important is hardiness, a concept introduced in Chapter 2. Suzanne Ouellette Kobasa, who teaches psychology in the City University of New York's graduate school and is the acknowledged pioneer of the hardiness concept, defined the personality traits of hardiness as the three C's: commitment, control, and challenge. We will expand on the three C's here.

COMMITMENT

Commitment entails a commitment to yourself, your work, your family, and the other important values in your life. This is not a fleeting involvement. It is a deep and abiding interest. People who are committed are greatly involved with their work and their families, have a deep sense of meaning, and have a pervasive sense of direction in their lives. In one study involving students at Harvard Medical School, students who were best able to withstand stress were personally committed to a goal of some kind.[52]

A perfect example is Mohandas Ghandi, a man who by all standards was a driven workaholic. He went on countless fasts, depriving himself of nourishment, and spent months in prison — one of the most stressful scenarios possible. Yet he was strong and healthy until his assassination at age 77. Many believe it was because of his unwavering commitment to become one of the world's great leaders and to win political freedom for his homeland.

CONTROL

As defined by psychologist S. C. Thompson, control is *a belief that one has at one's disposal a response that can influence the aversiveness of an event*. It is a belief that you can cushion the hurtful impact of a situation by the way you look at it and react to it. The kind of control that keeps a person healthy is the opposite of helplessness. It is the firm belief that you can influence how you will react and the willingness to act on that basis. It is the refusal to be victimized.

It is not the erroneous belief that you can control your environment, your circumstances, or other people. That kind of an attitude leads to illness, not health. The control that keeps you healthy is a belief that you can control yourself and your reactions to what life hands you.

In the Harvard Medical School study, the healthiest students were the ones who approached problem-solving with a sense of control; the least healthy were the ones who were passive.[53] The healthiest and hardiest people are those who focus on what they can control, ignoring the rest. They believe every problem has a solution, through skill, planning, and diligent attention to detail.

CHALLENGE

Challenge means the ability to see change as an opportunity for growth and excitement. Excitement is crucial, because boredom puts people at high risk

▼ How to Improve Hardiness

- ▼ Figure out what is causing you stress. Make a list. Then divide your list into two columns: things you can control, and things you can't control. Map out a strategy to help you change the things you *can control*. Then map out a strategy to help you *overcome* — ignore, move away from — the things you can't control. Don't waste a lot of time and energy pounding against something you can never change.

- ▼ Look back on ways you've handled your stress in the last month. Again, it helps to write it down. Summarize the situation, then write down the way you handled it. Now evaluate. Did you respond appropriately? How could you have done it better? Finally, describe how you could have better dealt with the stress. Use that alternative as your blueprint for the future.

- ▼ Do a little self-examination a couple of times a day. Are you uptight? Is your stomach tied up in knots? Are you clenching your fists or grinding your teeth? Take a minute and ask yourself why. Then relax. Learn some meditation or relaxation techniques, and use them to *take control*.

- ▼ Learn to change your attitude. When you're confronted with a problem, intentionally tell yourself that it's a *challenge* instead. Try to see some excitement in it. Try to find some pleasure.

- ▼ Do whatever you can to create some situations in your life when you *are* in control: paint your room, direct a play, take charge of a simple class project. Keeping control over some things in your life reassures you that you *can* be in control and hones your skills for the times you're not so sure of yourself.

for disease.[54] People who are challenged constructively are more healthy. A German philosopher mused that one of the two biggest foes of human happiness is boredom.

A person who is not healthy and hardy views change with helplessness and alienation. A healthy, hardy person can face change with confidence, self-determination, eagerness, and excitement. Change becomes an eagerly sought-after challenge, not a threat. Joan Post-Gorden, psychologist at the University of Southern Colorado, says healthy people don't even *see* the negatives, because they thoroughly *expect* a positive outcome.

In a comprehensive, year-long study of college students, researchers at Boston University School of Medicine concluded that illness is preceded by a definite sequence of events.[55] First, a person perceives a distressing life situation. For whatever reason, he or she is not able to resolve the distressing situation effectively. As a result, the person feels helpless and anxious. Those feelings of helplessness weaken the immune system and resistance to disease, and the person becomes more vulnerable to disease-causing agents that are always in the environment.

The traits of a disease-resistant personality interrupt this cycle and, therefore, help prevent illness. Healthy people and ill people look at things in entirely different ways. For example, healthy people tend to maintain reasonable personal control in their lives. If a problem crops up, they look for resources and try out solutions. If one doesn't work, they try another one. People who are frequently ill, on the other hand, leave decisions up to others and try to get other people to solve their problems. Their approach tends to be passive.

"One reason people can undergo tremendous stress and not get sick," says Yale surgeon Bernie Siegel, "has a lot to do with meeting your own needs, expressing your own feelings, learning to say 'no' without guilt. Now, I'm not suggesting that people blame themselves for an illness. Rather, they should see the illness as a message to redirect their life accordingly — to resolve conflicts with other people, express anger and resentment and other negative emotions they've been bottling up inside, to begin looking out for their own needs. And, in so doing, the immune system becomes stimulated and healing takes place."[56]

▼ NOTES

1. Rachel Naomi Remen, "Feeling Well: A Clinician's Casebook," *Advances*, 6:2, 43-49.
2. Gina Maranto, "Emotions: How They Affect Your Body," *Discover*, November 1984, p. 35.
3. Erica E. Goode, "Accounting for Emotion, *U.S. News and World Report*, June 27, 1988, p. 53.
4. Maureen Groër, "Psychoneuroimmunology," *American Journal of Nursing*, August 1991, p. 33.
5. Howard S. Friedman, *The Self-Healing Personality* (New York: Henry Holt and Company, 1991), p. 1.
6. Grossarth-Maticek's studies are described in Eysenck, pp. 30-31.
7. "How Your Personality Affects Your Health," *Good Housekeeping*, June 1983.
8. Clive Wood, "The Cold Character," *Psychology Today*, April 1988, p. 13.
9. Joann Rodgers, "Longevity Predictors: The Personality Link," *Omni*, February 1989, p. 25.
10. Douglas J. Stanwyck and Carol A. Anson, "Is personality Related to Illness? Cluster Profiles of Aggregated Data," *Advances*, 3:2 (Spring 1986), pp. 4-15.
11. Marcia Angell, "Disease as a Reflection of the Psyche," *New England Journal of Medicine*, 312 (1985), 1570-1572.
12. T. George Harris, "Heart and Soul," *Psychology Today*, p. 50.
13. Ray Rosenman, "Do You Have Type 'A' Behavior?" *Health and Fitness '87*, supplement, pp. S-12–S-13.
14. S. I. McMillen, *None of These Diseases*, revised edition (Old Tappan, New Jersey: Fleming H. Revell Company, 1984).
15. Redford Williams, *The Trusting Heart: Great News About Type A Behavior* (New York: Times Books, Division of Random House, Inc., 1989) p. 120.
16. R. M. Suinn, "The Cardiac Stress Management Program for Type A Patients," *Cardiac Rehabilitation*, 5 (1975), pp. 13-15.
17. Marcia Angell, "Disease As a Reflection of the Psyche," *New England Journal of Medicine*, 312:24 (1985), pp. 1570-1572.
18. Steven Locke and Douglas Colligan, *The Healer Within: The New Medicine of Mind and Body* (New York: E. P. Dutton, 1986), p. 140.
19. Locke and Colligan.
20. Locke and Colligan, p. 134.
21. Barbara Powell, *Good Relationships Are Good Medicine* (Emmaus, Pennsylvania: Rodale Press).
22. Redford Williams, "The Trusting Heart," *New Age Journal*, p. 26.
23. Carol Tavris, "On the Wisdom of Counting to Ten," pp. 170-191 in P. Shaver, editor, *Review of Personality and Social Psychology*, 5 (Sage, 1984).

24. Carol Tavris, *Anger: The Misunderstood Emotion.* (New York: Touchstone, 1982)
25. Hendrie Weisinger, "Mad? How to Work Out Your Anger," *Shape*, January 1988, pp. 86-93.
26. Barbara Powell, *Good Relationships are Good Medicine* (Emmaus, Pennsylvania: Rodale Press, 1987), pp. 158-159.
27. Weisinger.
28. Emrika Padus, *The Complete Guide to Your Health and Your Emotions* (Emmaus, Pennsylvania: Rodale Press, 1986).
29. Padus.
30. Padus.
31. Robert Ornstein and David Sobel, *The Healing Brain* (New York: Simon and Schuster, 1987), p. 181.
32. Emrika Padus, *The Complete Guide to Your Emotions and Your Health* (Emmaus, Pennsylvania: Rodale Press, 1986), p. 595.
33. "Is Yours a Hostile Heart?" *Men's Health*, 5:7/8 (August/September 1989), p. 1.
34. Redford B. Williams, Jr., "Neurocardiology."
35. Carl E. Thoresen, "The Hostility Habit: A Serious Health Problem?" *Healthline*, April 1984, p. 5.
36. Redford B. Williams, Jr., "Hostility, Anger, and Heart Disease," *Drug Therapy*, August 1986, p. 43.
37. Thoresen; and Williams, "Neurocardiology."
38. Thoresen.
39. Kathy A. Fackelmann, "Hostility Boosts Risk of Heart Trouble," *Science News*, 135 (January 28, 1989), p. 60.
40. Amy H. Berger, "Are You a Chronic Worrier?" *Complete Woman*, October 1987, p. 58.
41. Emrika Padus, *The Complete Guide to Your Emotions and Your Health* (Emmaus, Pennsylvania: Rodale press, 1986).
42. Winifred Gallagher, "The Dark Affliction of Mind and Body," *Discover*, May 1986, pp. 66-76.
43. Gallagher.
44. Christopher Vaughan, "The Depression-Stress Link," *Science News*, 134 (September 3, 1988), p. 155.
45. D. W. Black, G. Winokur, and A. Nasrallah, "Mortality in patients with primary unipolar depression, secondary unipolar depression, and bipolar affective disorder: A comparison with general population mortality," *International Journal of Psychiatric Medicine*, 17 (1987), 351-360.
46. R. M. Carney, M. W. Rich, K. E. Freedland, J. Saini, A. TeVelde, C. Simeone, and K. Clark, "Major Depressive Disorder Predicts Cardiac Events in Patients With Coronary Artery Disease," *Psychosomatic Medicine*, 50 (1988), pp. 627-633.
47. Mia Adessa, "Sad Hearts," *Psychology Today*, August 1988, p. 23.
48. "Hearts and Minds," *Longevity*, April 1989, p. 14.
49. Jana M. Mossey, Elizabeth Mutran, Kathryn Knott, and Rebecca Craik, "Recovery After Hip Fractures: The Importance of Psychosocial Factors," *Advances*, 6:4 (1989), pp. 23-25.
50. Howard S. Friedman, *The Self-Healing Personality* (New York: Henry Holt and Company, 1991), p. 99.
51. Claudia Wallis, "Stress: Can We Copy?" *Time*, June 6, 1983, pp. 48-54.
52. Raymond B. Flannery, "The Stress-Resistant person," *Harvard Medical School Health Letter*, February 1989, pp. 1-3.
53. Flannery.
54. Friedman, p. 111.
55. M. A. Jacobs, A. Spilken, and M. Norman, "Relationship of Life Change, Maladaptive Aggression, and Upper Respiratory Infection in Male College Students," *Psychosomatic Medicine*, 31:1 (1969), pp. 31-44.
56. Bernie Siegel, "Mind Over Cancer," *Prevention*, March 1988, pp. 61-62.

Social Support and Health

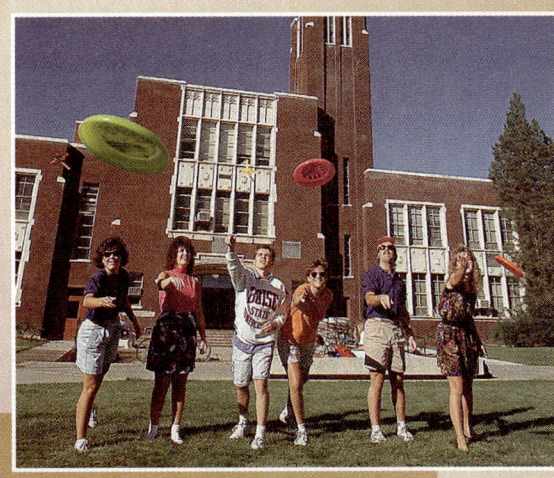

Objectives

▼ Illustrate how social support systems contribute to health and well-being.

▼ Point out the benefits of friends, confidants, and mates.

▼ Understand the differences between loneliness and aloneness.

▼ Know the connection between loneliness and health, including impacts on longevity, immune system functioning, heart health, and cancer.

▼ Learn how family life can contribute to the health of its members, including children.

▼ Become familiar with the health hazards of divorce.

▼ Compare the health of divorced people with those who are unhappily married.

▼ Learn the benefits of marriage as related specifically to coronary heart disease, cancer, immune system functioning, and life expectancy.

A group of researchers went to Alameda County, California, and gathered data on more than 7,000 people over a 9-year period. At the end of the study, they found the common denominator that most often led to good health and long life: the amount of social support a person enjoys.

Researchers who conducted the study concluded that people with social ties — regardless of their source — lived longer than people who were isolated. And people who have a close-knit network of intimate personal ties with other people seem to be able to avoid disease, maintain higher levels of health, and in general deal more successfully with life's difficulties.[1]

The people in the study with many social contacts — a mate, a close-knit family, a network of friends, church or other group affiliations — lived longer and had better health. People who were socially isolated had poorer health and died earlier. Actually, those who had few ties with other people died at rates two to five times higher than those with good social ties.[2] The link between social ties and death rate help us regardless of gender, race, ethnic background, or socioeconomic status.[3]

Some well-loved people fall ill and die prematurely, the researchers concluded, and some isolates live long and healthy lives. These occurrences are infrequent, though. For the most part, people tied closely to others are better able to stay well.[4]

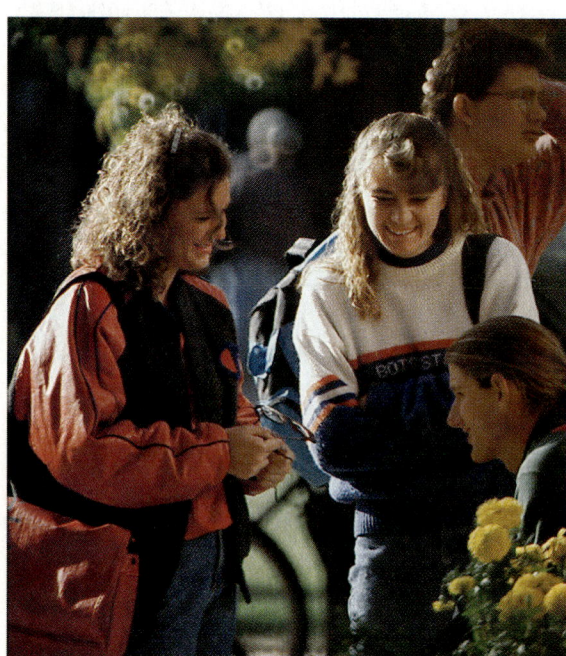

A network of social support can enhance and protect health.

Sidney Cobb, president of the Society of Psychosomatic Medicine, claims the notion of social support as an element of health is not new. What is new, he says, is the collection of hard evidence that proves the case — proof positive that social support can indeed protect people in crises from a wide variety of diseases.

As most researchers define it, social support is the extent to which a person's basic social needs are met through interaction with other people. It's the resources — both tangible and intangible — that other people provide. It's a person's perception that he or she can count on other people for help with a problem or in time of crisis.[5]

According to University of Michigan researchers James House and Robert Kahn, three factors comprise social support:[5]

1. *Social network*, the size, density, durability, intensity, and frequency of your social contacts.

2. *Social relationships*, the presence of relationships, number of relationships, and type of relationships.

3. *Social support*, the type, source, number, and quality of your resources.

The resources your social network provides may come in the form of tangible, instrumental aid — lending you money, driving you to your doctor's appointment, doing your grocery shopping, helping assume responsibility for your children while you are sick. Another kind of resource is equally as important, though. It's the emotional, "intangible" kind of help — affection, understanding, acceptance, esteem.

No one knows for certain how social support works to protect health, but some theories by prominent researchers who have done the most specialized work in the field of social support seem to be standing up to close scrutiny. One is that *social support enhances health and well-being no matter how much stress a person is under*. The enhancement may result from an overall positive feeling and a sense of self-esteem, stability, and control over one's environment. A second theory is that *social support acts as a buffer against stress* by protecting a person from the diseases that stress often causes.

Besides the buffering effects of stress and protecting health, strong social ties might give people still another edge in good health. The range of problems people bring to friends and neighbors is much broader than those brought to doctors, says Dr. Eva Salber, professor emeritus of Duke University's School of Medicine. Less than 5% of all physician visits are for psychological problems, she says, because we learn that if we want a doctor's attention, we must focus on a physical symptom. A woman might tell her doctor, for example, that she has a bladder infection, but she'll tell a friend that she's lost her job, had a fight with her husband, and has a bladder infection. What it boils down to, says Dr. Salber, is that most human ills are never seen by a doctor. The real primary care is provided by one's family, close friends, and neighbors.[6] These natural helpers — friends, family, and neighbors — may prove to be our most important untapped resource.

Regardless of *how* social support protects health, we know it does. Early researchers who struggled to determine what sort of patient has disease found striking similarities in the circumstances of people with conditions as diverse as depression, tuberculosis, high blood pressure, multiple accidents, and even complications in pregnancy. The people who were ill usually lacked a strong supportive network or had experienced a recent disruption in their traditional sources of social support.

Unfortunately, the number of people in that category seems to be increasing, not decreasing. In comparing people in the United States today with those of earlier generations, a disturbing trend is evident. People today are more likely to live alone, less likely to be married, and less likely to belong to a social organization. The result is a generation of people with weaker social ties — and poorer health.

One widely acclaimed study conducted by graduate students and faculty members at the University of California at Berkeley School of Public Health demonstrates exactly how important social support is to people who deal with "battle stress" in their lives. Called The Tenderloin Senior Outreach Project,[7] it was a 10-year study that delved into San Francisco's seedy Tenderloin District — a cluster of low-priced, single-room-occupancy hotels crammed with the poverty-stricken elderly. The district was characterized by skyrocketing crime rates, deteriorating housing conditions, poor access to food — and remarkably bad physical and mental health among its residents.

For the study, the Berkeley group organized weekly support groups for the elderly residents of the district. They organized "Safehouse Project," in which more than eighty stores and agencies in the neighborhood became places of refuge where residents could flee in case of emergency. The students acted as leaders in organizing groups of hotel residents. Buoyed by each other's strength, the residents themselves soon began working on their problems.

The results were dramatic. Several resident groups formed "mini-markets" in the lobbies of their hotels so that residents could get access to fresh fruit and vegetables. Other groups successfully blocked attempts to increase rents. Others were able to get food service restored to several of the hotels. And still others succeeded in getting the city to enhance public transportation access to the district.

In the 18 months following initiation of the project, crime dropped by a startling 26%. Nutritional status of hotel residents improved dramatically. So did their physical and mental health.

The sense of control and the social networking that came out of the project has been studied and acclaimed for their health-enhancing benefits. Researchers delight in making an example of one elderly resident, who had habitually checked himself into mental institutions every month or so for

▼ Is a Support Group Right for You?

If you're longing for social ties but having a tough time finding them, you might consider joining a support group — one that mirrors your interests, provides education about specific topics, helps you change your perspectives, or provides support for people with certain illnesses (physical or emotional).

You can locate a support group through your physician, psychologist, or health-care worker; through local chapters of national organizations; or through newspaper ads. To determine if a group is right for you:

▼ Attend one of the meetings; check out who is there and whether you feel welcome and free to participate.

▼ Decide whether you feel free to express your own ideas and thoughts. A good group should provide for open discussion without judgment or criticism. Some groups, though, want to foster only positive ideas and frown on anyone who brings up negatives.

▼ Even if you disagree with some of the ideas presented or discussed, you should leave the group feeling uplifted and helped. If not, the group is probably not right for you.

"reality orientation." After two years of involvement with the program, his monthly visits stopped altogether. When researchers asked him about it, he quipped, "I'm a co-leader of my hotel support group, a founder of the anticrime project, and a member of the Mayor's Task Force on Aging. I don't have time for reality!"

▼ THE TIES THAT BIND

Social ties — good friendships, good relationships with family members, the presence of people we know we can lean on — play an important role in our good health. A scientific panel convened by the U. S. government found that social support not only reduced mortality but was a key to protecting health as well. According to the panel, the number and strength of an individual's close relationships are closely related to an individual's health and longevity.[8]

Dr. James Lynch, a specialist in psychosomatic medicine at the University of Maryland's School of Medicine and a well-known researcher in the field of social support, concludes that individuals who lack the comfort of another human being may very well lack one of nature's most powerful antidotes to stress.[9] In summing up the results of his research, Lynch remarked, "The mandate to *love your neighbor as you love yourself* is not just a moral mandate. It's a physiological mandate. Caring is biological. One thing you get from caring for others is you're not lonely; and the more connected you are to life, the healthier you are."[10]

In one long-term study, nearly 3,000 adults in Tecumseh, Michigan, were studied for 10 years. At the beginning of the study, each adult was given a thorough physical examination to rule out any existing illness that would force a person to become isolated. Researchers then watched these people closely for the next 10 years, making special note of their social relationships and group activities. Those who were socially involved were found to have the best health. When social ties were interrupted or broken, the incidence of disease increased significantly. Researchers particularly noticed that certain conditions seemed related to marginal social ties. Among them were coronary heart disease, cancer, arthritis, strokes, upper respiratory infections, and mental illness. In fact, researchers concluded, interrupted social ties actually seemed to suppress the body's immune system.[11]

Those who conducted the study called close personal relationships a safety net. They stated that people without such a safety net are vulnerable to a wide variety of diseases at far greater frequencies than people who are surrounded by the comfort of good social relationships.

The results of these and a host of other studies show the strong influence of social support. It can help buffer the effects of disease through some of the worst stresses in life, such as unemployment, relocation and disruption, pregnancy, and even the stress of battle.

LOVE STRONGER, LIVE LONGER!

The results of a variety of studies prove that if we want to live longer, we need to surround ourselves with at least a few good people as friends and confidants. That finding has consistently held true across the board, regardless of how the studies have been set up or what population was studied.[12]

In the Alameda County study discussed at the beginning of this chapter, the residents initially were studied for 9 years. People were categorized into two groups: those who lived lonely lives (without many friends or relatives) and those who had rich

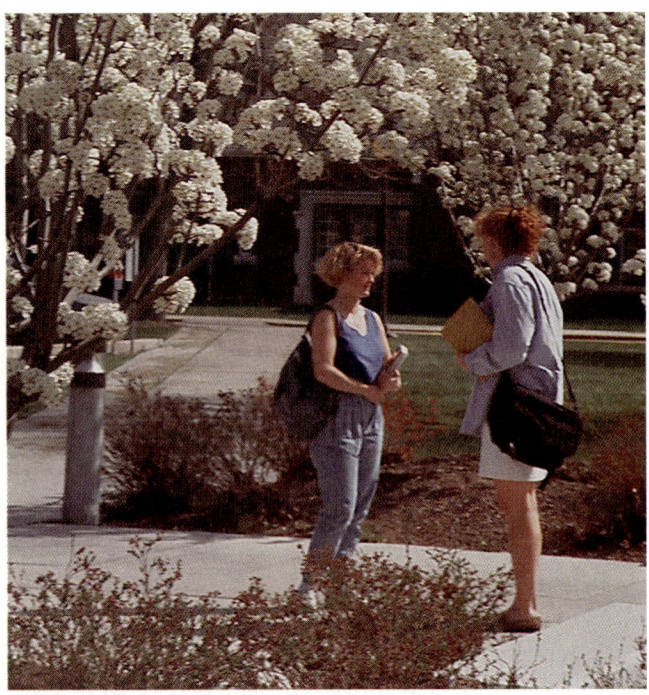

Social ties play an important role in good health.

resources of family and friends. During the next 9 years, researchers sifted through medical records, death certificates, and other data. The results were convincing: The people who had been classified as lonely and isolated were dying at three times the rate of those who had stronger social ties. The same finding held true during the next 8 years — for a total of 17 years — of the Alameda study.

A similar finding stemmed from the Tecumseh, Michigan, study. During the 10 years of the study, those who were the most socially isolated had four times the mortality rate of those who were more socially involved.

Other studies have confirmed these findings. Large-scale studies in North Carolina, Sweden, and Japan found that those with the highest mortality rates were those who were most socially isolated. Research from various studies shows, in essence, that people who are socially isolated — unmarried, divorced, widowed, people with few friends, and people who have few church or social contacts — are three times as likely to die of a wide variety of diseases than those who have happy, fulfilling social lives.

SOCIAL CONNECTIONS AND THE HEART

Social support — even the most simple social support — seems to have a particular effect on the heart, as was shown in a landmark study in the close-knit Italian-American community of Roseto, Pennsylvania. Researchers who studied the Roseto residents for years found that its residents had average incidence of exercise, cigarette smoking, obesity, high blood pressure, and stress. In addition, their diets were higher in fat, cholesterol, and red meat than the average American diet. The men in Roseto, however, had only about one-sixth the incidence of heart disease and deaths from heart disease as random population groups in the United States. The rates for Roseto's women were even better.

Researchers concluded that the protective factor was the people's strong sense of community and their strong social ties. Stewart Wolf, a professor of medicine at Temple University School of Medicine in Philadelphia and one of the study's researchers, said, "More than any other town we studied, Roseto's social structure reflected old-world values and traditions. There was a remarkable cohesiveness and sense of unconditional support within the community. Family ties were very strong. And what impressed us the most was the attitude toward the elderly. In Roseto, the older residents weren't put on a shelf; they were promoted to 'supreme court.' No one was ever abandoned."[13]

As researchers continued to watch the residents of Roseto, they found that when the younger generations started changing — moving away, marrying "outsiders," severing the close emotional ties to the "old neighborhood" — their physical health began to deteriorate. By the mid 1970s, the mortality and heart disease rate of the Rosetans was comparable to that in surrounding Pennsylvania communities.

When community members had tremendously strong social ties, their hearts were protected. When those social ties started to vanish, so did the protection. "The experience clearly demonstrates that the most important factors in health are the intangibles — things like trust, honesty, loyalty, team spirit," Wolf concluded. "In terms of preventing heart disease, it's just possible that morale is more important than jogging or not eating butter."[14]

Studies in the United States, Sweden, and Finland show that social support may even help reduce or modify risk factors for heart disease, including the Type A personality. In one study, researchers used coronary angiography to determine the health of the coronary arteries. They found that the Type A men who had strong social support were on an even par with the Type B men when it came to coronary health.[15]

Social support is such a powerful factor in mortality that it even lowers mortality among those who are *unhealthy* (such as survivors of heart attacks). One reason may be its effect on the immune system. Well-documented studies show that stress generally decreases the number and function of natural killer cells and reduces the percentage of T-lymphocytes. Strong interpersonal relationships, however, protect the functioning of the immune system, even in the face of stress.

Obviously, social support is a crucial factor in determining how well you fare when illness strikes. According to David Spiegel, a professor of psychiatry and behavioral sciences and director of Stanford University School of Medicine's Psychosocial Treatment Laboratory, says that what matters is *how* people interact with a sick person — how often they visit the hospital, how much they show they care about what happens. According to Spiegel, four basic steps can provide much-needed support for someone who is sick:[16]

1. Be honest. Communicate directly and openly with family members and close friends about the seriousness of the illness. This kind of openness fosters intimacy and lets others join in support for the patient.

2. Explain what's going on to children, and let them help. Even young children often understand more than we give them credit for. Being honest is especially important for *their* well-being. Children often fear *they* are the cause for any mishap, and unless you explain otherwise, they may be convinced that the illness is punishment for some wrongdoing on their part.

3. Don't think you have to explain every detail to everyone who comes along. Be selective. Realize that some relationships will become even richer through an illness, and others will deteriorate. That's fine. Invest yourself emotionally with the relationships that are thriving, and don't worry about relating all the details of the illness to people who just don't matter.

4. If people want to help, let them, and give them concrete suggestions about *how* they can help. You might need a ride to a doctor's appointment; your family might need the boost of a good meal; or maybe you need someone to come to your home to cut your hair. Maybe you need someone to walk your dog, do your laundry, pick up your medications, or go with your child to the dentist. You'll find that many people are more than willing to help out, if they simply know what to do.

TOUCH: A CRUCIAL ASPECT OF SOCIAL SUPPORT

As important as social support is to health, perhaps one of its most powerful components is also one of its simplest: People who touch others and are touched enjoy the best health!

Observations researchers made nearly four decades ago as they watched groups of monkeys provided us some of the best information we have on the power of touch. University of Wisconsin researchers Harry and Margaret Harlow compared monkeys that were raised together in cages to monkeys whose only social contact came through hearing, seeing, and smelling other monkeys.[17] The

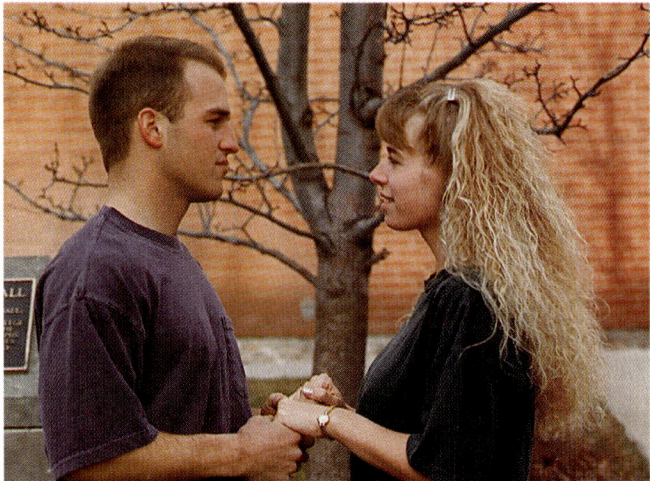

Touch can be an important part of the health benefits of social support.

Harlows found that the monkeys that did not touch or have actual body contact with other monkeys grew up with a variety of emotional abnormalities. While young, the monkeys seemed especially prone to self-mutilation. As they grew older, their self-aggression turned into aggression against other monkeys. Perhaps most striking was the way mothers behaved toward their young. The mothers that grew up without touch showed less warmth and affection toward their offspring. Some even killed their own babies.

Numbers of studies are showing the same result today: People who enjoy regular, satisfying touch — a pat on the back, a hug — enjoy health benefits as a result. The good health that emanates from touch is both psychological and physical. Those who are touched have stronger hearts, lower blood pressure, lower stress levels, and less overall tension.

▼ LONELINESS AND HEALTH

Loneliness has been characterized as *an unpleasant experience that occurs when a person's network of social relationships is significantly deficient in either quality or quantity.*[18] Loneliness is not necessarily a consequence of living alone. When more than 22,000 American adults responded to a survey in five major newspapers, researchers found that almost a fourth of the survey respondents who lived alone fell into the "least lonely" category.[19] On the other hand, loneliness can be present even when we're surrounded by people. According to research at Kent State University, loneliness is associated less with the number of people in our lives than the satisfaction with those relationships. Loneliness sets in when our current relationships fall short of our ideal.[20]

Feelings of loneliness are worse when the lonely person is surrounded by people who don't seem to be lonely — people who seem to have secure interpersonal attachments — or when the lonely person suffers from a sense of low self-esteem. And, though loneliness can stem from lack of attachment to someone else, loneliness can be just as intense if the person has a sense of not belonging within an accepting community.

According to researchers, factors that help determine when someone who is alone is also lonely are general attitude, boredom, and attitude toward self. Anne Morrow Lindbergh wrote, in *Gift From the Sea*, "I find there is a quality to being alone that is incredibly precious. Life rushes back into the void, richer, more vivid, fuller than before. It is as if in parting one did actually lose an arm. And then, like starfish, one grows it anew; one is whole again, complete and round — more whole, even, than before, when the other people had pieces of one."

Even though being alone doesn't necessarily mean people are lonely, many people who are alone *are* lonely. And more people than ever are living alone — more than 20 million in the United States alone. Between 1950 and 1980, the figure rose by 385%. The most radical change has been in the number of men living alone — twice as many now as 10 years ago.[21] More than 35 million households in the United States now are headed by singles. Estimates are that sometime during the first few years of the 1990s, almost as many American households will be headed by divorced, separated, and widowed people as by married ones. Trends include a rising divorce rate, fewer and later-in-life marriages, smaller household sizes, and increasing mobility.

THE HEALTH CONSEQUENCES OF LONELINESS

Loneliness carries with it a big risk for health problems. Lynch says loneliness is "the greatest unrecognized contributor to premature death in the United States."[22] Loneliness, and the stress that accompanies

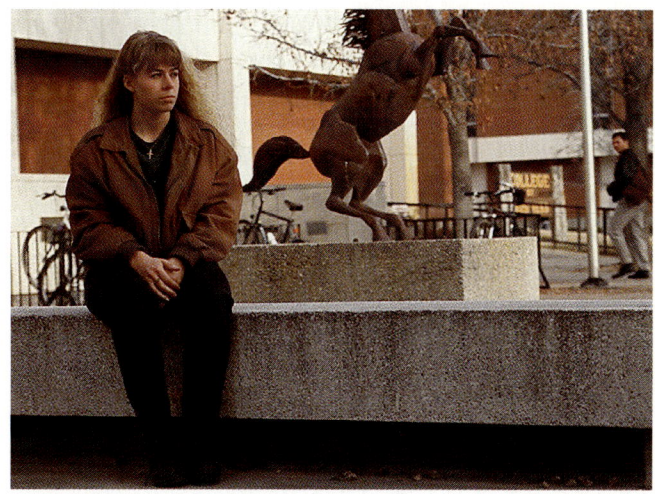

Loneliness is a factor that may increase the risk of disease and health problems.

it, has been connected not only to premature death but to a host of physical and mental disorders as well. Loneliness has been definitely linked to disease. People who are not lonely have a better chance of staying healthy or recovering from disease than people who are lonely.

Researchers Louise Bernikow reports, "Loneliness can, indeed, make you sick. Heart disease and hypertension are now generally thought of as loneliness diseases, exacerbated by a person's sense of abandonment by the world, separation from the rest of humanity. Most addictions also are considered loneliness diseases, which the medical profession is beginning to recognize but which recovering alcoholics, drug addicts, even smokers have been long aware of. Most addicts admit that their best friends have been booze, drugs, or tobacco."[23]

In a comprehensive study that shed light on the health impact of loneliness, Dr. Caroline Thomas and Dr. Karen Duszynski of the Johns Hopkins School of Medicine examined more than a thousand medical students over almost two decades and then followed their progress. The physicians who eventually committed suicide or had to be hospitalized for mental illness or developed malignant tumors shared a common denominator: They had significantly greater problems with interpersonal relationships and suffered significantly more from loneliness.[24]

Other studies verify that loneliness impacts physical health greatly. When a woman gives birth, loneliness even impacts labor and delivery. In one fascinating study, researchers compared a group of women who went through labor and delivery alone with those who had the companionship of an untrained woman previously unknown to the participant. The support the untrained women provided varied from mere companionship to holding hands, talking, or rubbing the mother's back during labor. The results were striking. Among the mothers who underwent labor alone, 75% developed complications during labor or birth, including induced labor, fetal distress, stillbirths, or caesarean section deliveries. Only 12% of the mothers with companions developed complications. The supported mothers were in labor an average of less than half as long as the unsupported mothers. The differences continued after birth. During the first hour after the babies were born, the supported mothers were more awake and alert, talked to their babies more, stroked their babies more, and smiled more at their babies.[25]

Loneliness and Longevity

According to James Lynch, all available data from hundreds of in-depth studies point to several factors — among them, lack of human companionship, chronic loneliness, and social isolation — as among the leading causes of premature death.[26] And, says Lynch, though the effects of human loneliness are related to virtually every disease, they are particularly strong in heart disease, the leading cause of death in the United States. Samuel Silverman, associate clinical professor of psychiatry at Harvard University, claims a person can add as many as 15 years to life simply by reducing two "emotional aging factors." One of them is loneliness.[27]

In the Tecumseh study, women who were lonely and isolated were one and a half times more likely to die prematurely than women with strong social ties. For men, the risk was double.[28] In the Alameda County study, loneliness was still a major risk factor for premature death, but the gender risk seemed to switch: Lonely women had a nearly three times greater risk, and lonely men had a doubled risk, of illness and premature death than men and women who had close ties with family and friends.

Loneliness and Immune Function

A host of studies has shown that loneliness has a considerable effect on immune system function. In one, researchers at the University of Denver showed that baby monkeys separated from their mothers had later immune system problems, including lower levels of both B-cell and T-cell activity.[29] In another, Harvard Medical School students who scored as lonely on a psychological test had significantly below-par functioning of the immune system, including less active natural killer cells and an inability to fight off the Epstein-Barr virus.[30]

Apparently the reduction in immune system functioning has a medical reason. Lonely people secrete an excessive amount of the hormone cortisol, which suppresses the immune system. And when loneliness is coupled with stress — another condition that stimulates cortisol production — the results can be particularly crippling.

Loneliness and Heart Function

The brain's perception that a person is lonely apparently has significant effect on the individual's heart. In the largest study yet attempted on the impact of loneliness on cardiac health, researchers from the Karolinska Institute in Sweden and the Johns Hopkins School of Public Health studied more than 17,000 Swedes for more than 6 years. Those who said they were lonely had a 40% greater risk of dying from cardiovascular disease than the rest of the people in the study.[31] When the researchers followed up with a second study spanning 10 years, they found an actual physiological link between loneliness and heart disease.[32] Apparently, loneliness creates neuroendocrine changes that lead to atherosclerosis.[33]

Researchers at three hospitals in New York state followed 1,200 heart-attack survivors to see whether their living arrangements affected their health. They found that patients who lived by themselves were nearly twice as likely as those with companions to have another attack — or die of one — within 6 months.[34]

The researchers reported that none of the known risk factors for second heart attacks — advanced age, low socioeconomic status, and severe heart damage — accounted for the ill health of subjects who lived alone. Nearly 16% of that group had another heart attack within 6 months. Only 9% of the patients who shared living quarters were stricken.

The researchers, led by Dr. Robert Case of Manhattan's St. Luke's-Roosevelt Hospital, suggest that human contact may subtly affect heart function, or it simply may improve one's chances of getting quick medical attention in an emergency. In any case, they didn't live alone.

Other studies support the apparent associations between heart function and loneliness. In one aggressive study that followed more than 50,000 former students from the University of Pennsylvania and Harvard University, researchers carefully looked at the records of those who had died of coronary heart disease. Nine factors characterized the men who died of heart disease. Several of these — including early parental death, absence of siblings, and nonparticipation in sports — were indicators of loneliness. Researchers found that those who were loneliest and most socially isolated were at greatest risk for dying of heart disease.[35]

Loneliness and Cancer

A number of studies has correlated loneliness with the unusually high incidence of cancer. Researchers now believe the higher cancer rate among the lonely may have something to do with the reality that loneliness cripples the immune system.

A significant study showing the link between loneliness and cancer was conducted at the Johns Hopkins University School of Medicine. Between 1948 and 1964, researchers collected psychological data on nearly 1,000 male medical students who attended Johns Hopkins. The men were divided into five groups based on their personality traits. After collecting medical records each year through 1987, the researchers examined the records carefully. They found that only 1% of the "acting out/emotional" cluster — the group consisting of members who were anxious, easily upset, and prone to depression — developed cancer during the years of the medical follow-up; but nearly one in five of the "loner" cluster — a group of men who felt lonely and faced the world with a bland, unemotional exterior — developed cancer.[36]

THE IMPORTANCE OF GOOD FRIENDS

Close friendships clearly buffer stress and help overcome the health effects of loneliness. In the Alameda County study, researchers concluded that a "larger network size and greater frequency of contact was related to decreased mortality for both men and women at all ages," even when other factors were taken into account.

In some cases, the support of close friends may be even more important than the support of family. One study looked at people aged 55 and older in three North Carolina communities. The researchers first determined who had the greatest satisfaction with life, those who were the happiest, healthiest, and generally most satisfied. Then they searched to determine what kinds of social support seemed to contribute most to that satisfaction. For this older population, at least, the frequency and satisfaction of contacts with family weren't what made people happiest in life. Contact with close friends that made the biggest difference.[37]

Probably one of the best examples of the health benefits of close friends is provided by Japanese culture. Dr. Leonard Syme, an epidemiologist with the School of Public Health at the University of California at Berkeley, has spent years studying the health of Japanese immigrants to the United States. What he has found at first puzzled researchers — and then served as a brilliant demonstration of the health benefits of close friends.[38]

Japan has both the good and bad features of an advanced, industrialized nation in the twentieth century — and, by all accounts, its residents should have more than their share of health problems. According to Syme, air pollution is "horrendous" in and around the large cities. Smoking is widespread. The diet includes highly pickled foods. The pace of life in the great urban centers is as hectic as in any American city — and, in fact, 6-day work weeks are common. All the earmarks of severe stress are present. Yet, the Japanese have among the highest life expectancies in the world.

Researchers were puzzled. At first, they proposed that the Japanese had some sort of genetic superiority. But that notion was quickly abandoned when they studied Japanese who had moved to the United States. Those who arrived on American shores, adopted American lifestyles, and started eating like Americans do began dying from heart disease and cancer at the same rate as native-born Americans — and it all happened within a single generation.

Then researchers noticed that some Japanese who immigrated to America were smoking heavily and eating the high-fat foods characteristic in American diets — but they were escaping the diseases and the premature deaths we suffered as a result. After studying 17,000 Japanese — both here and in Japan — researchers concluded that Japan's emphasis on "the group" was the key to health and long life. Traditionally, Japanese are very tied to family and friends; they honor and respect their elderly, and

Do You Have the Qualities of Friendship?

Friendship is a two-way business. To make friends, you have to be a friend. The better friend you are, the more friends you are likely to have. This questionnaire lists some of the qualities of friendship.

Check "yes" or "no" to the questions. Then look at the scoring key at the end.

YES   NO

☐   ☐   1. Are people able to depend on you to keep your word?
☐   ☐   2. Can they rely on you to respect their confidences?
☐   ☐   3. Do you keep the friends you make?
☐   ☐   4. Do you often put yourself to trouble and inconvenience to oblige other people?
☐   ☐   5. Suppose they want to do something you are not particularly keen on. Would you go along with them and do what they want to do?
☐   ☐   6. Are you quick to pay your share of the expenses?
☐   ☐   7. Are you generous with your praise and appreciation?
☐   ☐   8. Do you show affection when you feel it?
☐   ☐   9. Is it easy for you to forgive and forget?
☐   ☐   10. Do you readily give people the benefit of the doubt and make allowances?
☐   ☐   11. In a sharp difference of opinion, would you speak first?
☐   ☐   12. Do you own up when you are wrong and say you are sorry?
☐   ☐   13. You may like somebody very much, but would you feel the same if he or she were to become unpopular?
☐   ☐   14. Are you quick off the mark to give sympathy and practical help when people need it?
☐   ☐   15. Do you like to see others praised and fussed over?
☐   ☐   16. Can you agree to differ and stay on the best of terms?
☐   ☐   17. Are you an attentive and sympathetic listener?
☐   ☐   18. Are you always the same, not full of welcome today and too busy to bother tomorrow?
☐   ☐   19. Do you mind people having other friends and interests that you do not share?
☐   ☐   20. Can you say you are much more interested in other people than in yourself?

SCORING

Count 5 points for every "yes." A score of 70 or over is good, and 60-70 is satisfactory. Under 60 is not satisfactory. You are not likely to be a good friend. Usually, when we are like this, we're wrapped up in ourselves. We like only the individuals who notice us and make a fuss over us and dislike anybody who is not interested in us or who will not do what we want. If you desire to be a good friend, you will have to be more interested in other people than in yourself and put them first.

Adapted from Singer Communications, Inc., Anaheim, California

---

they place a high priority on developing life-long friendships.

It was the Japanese in this country who retained their culture — who used the language, generally resisted Westernization, and kept tightly-knit group ties and friendships — who did so well healthwise. Those who kept close to their lifelong friends and their families had significantly lower incidences of heart disease, cancer, and diseases of all kinds. Surprisingly, other factors — such as genetic traits, age, gender, social class, and even health habits — seemed to have little effect, especially when compared to the factor of keeping their Japanese friendships alive.

Friends contribute to health by providing all the functions of the family. In some cases, friends may be closer confidants than family members are. And people who are able to build close relationships with friends have greater health protection against stress.

In one of the Johns Hopkins studies, researchers developed an inkblot test and a method for scoring it. They then showed more than 1,000 graduates the test and evaluated them psychologically based on test results. In the ensuing years, the graduates who developed cancer were the ones who were withdrawn. The ones who remained cancer-free were judged to be congenial, more easily able to interact with others and make friends, and better able to express affection to their friends.[39]

According to a study conducted by the California Department of Mental Health, close, confiding personal relationships — good friends — were found to buffer not only the stress from life's major changes but from life's daily hassles as well. People in crisis, whether it's from a major life change or from an accumulation of daily hassles, have higher morale, fewer physical symptoms, and less illness if they have support from and contact with close friends.[40]

James Pennebaker, a professor of psychology at Southern Methodist University, Dallas, believes that confiding — having a confidant — forges a powerful and lasting bond and can provide many of the health benefits discussed here. Pennebaker warns, however, of some risks involved in confiding and urges that you consider the following before you begin to confide in someone.[41]

▶ Realize that your relationship may be at risk. In most cases, confiding in someone helps the two of you grow closer. Your friend, however, might feel threatened or hurt by what you say, changing the nature of the relationship.

▶ Realize that your own traumas may traumatize the listener, too. If the information you divulge is upsetting enough, the listener may be so burdened by what you say that he or she, in turn, may need to share it. This is known as gossip; but, in this case, there's a real need for your confidant to unload the burden.

▶ Realize that you're opening yourself up for potential social blackmail. Your confidant is in a powerful position and, if the relationship sours, may use that power against you.

▶ Realize that what you say and how you say it depends on how your confidant reacts to you. In the best possible situation, your friend will allow you to freely express all your feelings and frustrations without judging or criticizing you.

▶ Realize that you might have a twisted motive for confiding in a certain person. A surprising number of people confide out of revenge. "You hurt me, so I am going to hurt you," Pennebaker

How to Develop a Lasting Friendship

Some of the best social support possible comes from good friends, and you can do plenty of things to develop a lasting friendship with someone you care about:

▼ Start with someone you feel close to or *want* to feel close to.

▼ Be willing to share your most personal thoughts and feelings, as well as your time, your possessions, and other things that are important to you.

▼ Spend plenty of time together. That's what helps you develop closeness. If you have to, adjust your schedule so you can spend time together.

▼ Be a good listener. It's easy to pick a friend to talk to as a confidant; remember that your friend needs one, too.

▼ Learn to trust. It's tough to face the possible rejection when you let someone in on your deepest secrets, but a true friend will love and accept you regardless of your flaws.

writes. You know why you should choose someone as a confidant. Revenge, anger, and hurt are *not* good reasons.

▶ Realize that there might be a better way to solve a problem than disclosing or confiding. You might be able to take direct action, for example. If so, do it. Don't spend your time and energies discussing your grievances instead.

THE IMPORTANCE OF PETS

Research into the health benefits of pet ownership has shown beyond a doubt that comfort does not always have to come only from people. Pets fulfill a variety of needs for their human owners. They provide a chance for interaction with another living thing and fulfill the natural craving for emotional relationships. They meet our need to care and our desire to be loved. As anyone who owns a pet knows, pets also give love in return.

Researchers have conducted studies showing that pets alleviate loneliness and thereby enhance immune function. The University of Pennsylvania's Center for Interaction of Animals and Society showed that coronary disease patients with pets have one-third the death rate of people who do not have pets. The researchers discovered at least one reason for this: Patients actually had lower heart rates when they were with their pets. They concluded that "even small reductions in the heart rate repeated thousands of times per week could provide direct health benefits by decreasing the frequency of arterial damage, and thus slowing the arteriosclerotic process."[42]

Subsequent research has shown that pets also reduce blood pressure, help hospitalized patients recover more quickly, speed recovery from surgery, and alleviate the effects of stress. To test the latter notion, researchers at the University of Oklahoma studied the role of pets in one of life's most stressful situations: death of a spouse. When researchers compared a group of widows who had pets to a group of widows who did not have pets, the widows with pets were healthier, had fewer illnesses and physical complaints, and were able to interact better with others. Those without pets had more persistent fears, headaches, and feelings of panic, and they took more medication than did the pet owners.[43]

The health benefits of pets are obvious, but that doesn't mean you should rush into pet ownership without weighing the pros and cons. Owning a pet is a tremendous commitment, and you need to be in a position to handle it before you take on the care of a pet.

What is the down side to owning a pet? Consider some of the following:

▶ Pets cost money. There's the initial expense of purchasing the pet, plus bills for food and for veterinarian expenses (inoculations, neutering or spaying, and inevitable illnesses). Added to those are the expenses of licensing your pet and purchasing any related paraphernalia, such as food bowls, collars, and leashes.

▶ Pets also can cause indirect expense by ruining carpets and furniture, digging up flowers or shrubs, and damaging other personal goods.

▶ Some pets are difficult to housebreak. You can overcome this objection by purchasing a pet that already is housebroken, but you should expect some minor accidents as the pet adjusts to its new surroundings.

▶ A pet can interfere with *your* independence. If you have a dog, for example, and want to travel for a week, you have to take the dog with you or

Choosing the Right Pet

Pets provide plenty of rewards and healing interaction, but they also require plenty of attention! Before you choose a pet, carefully consider your schedule and the demands on your time. You can expect the following from these pets:

▼ **Birds, fish, hamsters, guinea pigs.** These and other similar pets require much less time and direct care. You have to make sure they have food, and you have to clean their cages or bowls, usually a few times a week. Although these kinds of pets require less care, they also provide less intense interaction.

▼ **Cats.** Cats require more care than the pets listed above, but less care than dogs. You can leave a large amount of water and dry food if you are gone for quite a while, and a cat will do just fine. You also can train cats to use an indoor litter box, so cats can adapt to staying indoors. Cats preen themselves, so they do not need grooming and do not require you to provide exercise. Cats can adjust to even a small apartment. Although they provide a lot of interaction, they also can be independent.

▼ **Dogs.** Dogs offer the most intense interaction but also require the most care. They must be fed at the same time each day, exercised twice a day, and groomed several times a month. Larger dogs need space for exercise, and you must clean up after dogs.

pay to board the dog at a kennel or pay someone to come to your home and care for the dog every day.

▶ While they provide health benefits, pets also can cause anxiety and concern. Many pet owners fear their pets will be injured or kidnapped. Pets also eventually die, which means a period of bereavement as you grieve the loss of your pet.

Those are some of the down sides, but owning a pet has tremendous benefits in addition to the health benefits already discussed.

▶ Certain pets, such as dogs, can contribute to your safety.

▶ If you choose a pet that needs exercise, you'll find that your own exercise increases, too. You're the one who has to walk the dog twice a day.

- Pets bring cheerfulness, play, and laughter to your life. There's nothing like watching a cat get intoxicated on a catnip mouse!
- Pets help boost your self-esteem. After a hard day away from home, when all the world seems to be against you, a bounding greeting from your dog is quite a treat.

MARRIAGE AND HEALTH

Marriage — a good one, that is — can help protect people from illness and disease, help them bounce back more quickly if they do get sick, and even help people live longer. If current research is accurate, divorced people and those who are unhappily married don't fare nearly as well in terms of health and long life.

What does "happily married" mean? The editors of *Prevention* magazine identified seven characteristics of a happy marriage, characteristics you can use as a barometer for your own relationship:

1. The partners find their prime source of joy in each other, but they maintain separate identities. They are independent; they have outside interests and hobbies that don't depend on their partner.
2. They are generous and giving out of love, not because they expect repayment or are keeping score.
3. The partners enjoy a healthy and vigorous sexual relationship.
4. The partners fight — that's right! — in a constructive way. For people in a healthy marriage, verbal fighting offers a chance to air feelings and frustrations without implying that the other person is wrong or at fault.
5. The partners communicate with each other openly and honestly. There's a risk in it, but experts claim it's worth the risk.
6. The two partners in the marriage trust each other. Even after a lapse in the relationship, trust can be reestablished if both work at it.
7. Both partners talk about their future together, a future they will share because they *want* to. They may dream about a house on the beach, a vacation to Europe, or a child they want to have late in their 30s. This kind of planning and talking indicates that both people intend to be together later on — again, because they want it more than anything else.

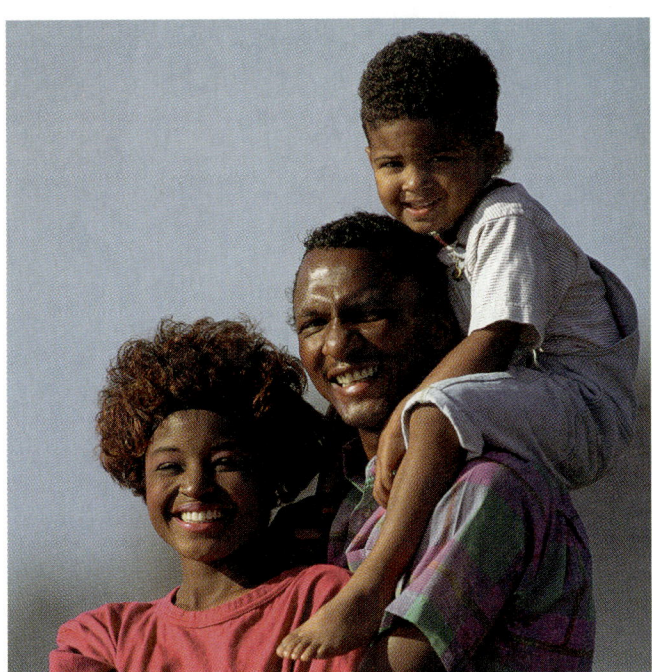

A happy marriage can help provide protection from illness and disease.

Factors Leading to a Happy Marriage

The *attitudes* you have about marriage helps determine how happy you'll be. Your marriage will more likely be happy if you *both* want the marriage to succeed and you share with your partner the following attitudes about marriage:

- Marriage is a long-term commitment ("we're in this for good").
- Marriage is a spiritual, sanctified institution between two people.

The *person* you marry has a bearing on how happy the marriage will be. Your chances for success are highest if you marry:

- Your best friend.
- Someone you genuinely like as a person.
- Someone who grows more interesting to you as time goes on.
- Someone who shares your basic dreams, goals, and aspirations.

THE HEALTH HAZARDS OF DIVORCE

As a country, the United States has the highest divorce rate in the world, approaching 50%. According to statistics, the parents of more than 1 million children divorce in the United States each year. Those same statistics tell us that 30% of America's white children and 40% of black children spend at least part of their formative years in post-divorce, single-parent families. Increasingly, too, children are being subjected to a second divorce during their childhood. A child born in 1983 has a 40% chance of experiencing a parent's second divorce by the time he or she is 18 years old.

A number of factors lead to divorce in today's society. Consider the following:

- Divorces are easier to get today than ever before. Many states have no-fault divorces, in which one partner does not have to prove the other to be at fault. In some states, "do-it-yourself divorce kits" enable couples to split property and even custody without the assistance of an attorney.
- The strong social stigma against divorce three or four decades ago is no longer there.
- Many people go into marriage without the proper preparation. The resulting unrealistic expectations can make adjustment to marriage extremely difficult. An amazing number of couples, for example, think they should never argue, when in reality constructive fighting is a characteristic of a healthy relationship. As a result, they abandon the marriage when they begin fighting.
- Large percentages of women work outside the home, making them less financially dependent on their husbands and making divorce a less devastating option.

Perhaps because of the emotional repercussions, divorce seems to pose particular health hazards. Several studies, involving thousands of men and women, have found that men and women who are separated or divorced have poorer physical health than do comparable widowed, married, or single adults. Of all these groups, the divorced have the most medical complaints, limiting chronic medical conditions, and overall disability, even when age, race, and income are taken into account.

Every major study agrees that people who are divorced — and others who are separated from their mates — experience more mental and physical illness than those who are married. Psychologically, in-depth studies have shown that divorce is significantly related to depression, alcoholism, increased incidence of traffic accidents and accidental deaths, higher rates of admission to psychiatric facilities, and more suicides and homicides. Most therapists further agree that divorced people have higher rates of cancer, heart disease, diabetes, pneumonia, and high blood pressure than do married, single, or widowed persons.

Various studies provide insight into the specific health hazards of divorce. In one, divorced caucasian men under age 70 who lived alone had twice the death rate from heart disease, stomach cancer, and cirrhosis of the liver, and three times the incidence of high blood pressure. James Lynch, who has done extensive research into the phenomenon of divorce and loneliness, says the findings apply to men and women alike of all ages.[44]

How to Negotiate an Argument

If you find yourself in an argument with someone important to you, try the following negotiation tactics to avoid a knock-down drag-out:

- State your needs or wants clearly. If you've already given up something, say so.
- Ask your partner to do the same. Communication should be open and honest.
- Listen carefully and honestly until your partner is ready to listen *you*.
- Figure out whether your needs or wants are compatible. If they are, the argument is over. If not, you have four choices:
    1. Both of you can maintain your positions. That's okay, as long as it doesn't happen all the time, OR
    2. You can compromise. Both of you get a little of what you want, OR
    3. Both of you get *all* of what you want, but you take turns. You might get everything you want tonight, and your partner might get everything he or she wants tomorrow night, OR
    4. You can *freely* give up on your position in deference to the other person. That's okay, too, as long as you're doing it freely and as long as it doesn't happen all the time either.

Research has shown that divorce actually can compromise the immune system, which helps explain why illness and death rates are higher among the divorced. Immune system compromise is especially apparent the first year following divorce. A study of divorced or separated women during the first year following divorce or separation showed that they had poor cellular immune function, a lower number of natural killer cells, and a deficit in the ability to fight disease with responsive lymphocytes.[45]

Risks for disease in almost every category soar with divorce. And divorce affects longevity, clearly evidenced by the fact that the state of Nevada had the second highest death rate from all causes in the United States during the years when it was the "divorce capitol" of the nation.[46]

Children of divorce, we must point out, are often the ones who suffer the most profoundly. Divorce is one of the most disruptive of all life events for children, and it leads to changes in biological health. Children almost universally experience divorce as a profound personal, familial, and social loss. In addition to health problems, most children involved in divorce suffer emotional and behavioral changes that also can impact health.

Children of divorce visit health clinics and physicians more often. Some childhood cancers and other alterations in physical health as a result of injury have been strongly associated with divorce. Divorce is particularly damaging to a child's emotional and physical health if it involves a move.

THE DIVORCED VERSUS THE UNHAPPILY MARRIED

New evidence shows that unhappily married people may be the worst off in terms of good health and long life. Research results from a number of cross-sectional studies are all saying the same thing: Unhappily married people have poorer health than their single counterparts, even the ones who are divorced.[47]

Studies now offer preliminary evidence that actual physical changes occur during marital conflict. Marital conflict apparently causes a sharp increase in blood pressure, a much higher risk for all kinds of illness, and reduced functioning of the immune system. Interactions characterized by hostility, sarcasm, and blame — refusing to take responsibility and demeaning the other partner — seem most damaging.

Not surprisingly, marital satisfaction has a real bearing not only on physical, but also mental, health. Researchers have found a definite relationship between depression and dissatisfaction with one's marriage. One long-term study conducted at Vanderbilt University showed that people who said they were "not too happy" or "not at all happy" in their marriages were in poorer mental health than were people who were single, divorced, or widowed.[48] In a separate, extensive study involving more than 5,000 people, those who were unhappy or dissatisfied with their marriages were in poorer mental health than any of the people who were single — whether they had never married, had divorced, or had been widowed.

THE HEALTH BENEFITS OF A HAPPY MARRIAGE

The greatest benefits regarding health and long life come to those who are happily married. Those who are happily married seem healthier, overall, than any other group, according to government researchers with the National Center for Health Statistics. The Center, which recently completed a survey of 122,859 people in more than 47,000 families nationwide found that married people have fewer health problems than unmarried people.[49]

The health benefits of marriage may be attributable to a number of factors, including better integration into the community, social support, the tendency to eat more regular and nutritionally balanced meals, and better economic status.

Coronary Heart Disease

Detailed studies done by several researchers indicate that marriage is a protecting factor. Coronary heart disease deaths in the United States per 100,000 population are 176 among the married and 362 among the divorced. Death rates for single, divorced, and widowed individuals are significantly higher than the rates for married individuals. One researcher who has specialized in the study of heart disease says death rates in the nonmarried groups sometimes exceed the rates of married groups as much as *five times*. Among those under age 35, the death rate of those who are not married exceeds that of the married *tenfold*.[50]

Married men and women also are 20% less likely to have high blood pressure than people who are single, separated, divorced, or widowed. Married people also are more likely to seek treatment for high blood pressure when they discover it. According to a University of Texas epidemiologist, married people with high blood pressure were 59% more likely to be receiving treatment for it, and 78% more likely to have it under control.[51]

Cancer

Research has shown that marriage has an influence on survival rates from cancer. In one energetic study, researchers collected data on 27,779 cases of cancer on file at the New Mexico Tumor Registry, part of the National Cancer Institute's surveillance program. In analyzing the results, unmarried status was associated with a lower survival rate for patients diagnosed with cancer. The percentage of individuals surviving at least 5 years was greater for married people than for unmarried people in almost every category of age, gender, and stage of cancer.[52] Among those in the study, all three categories of unmarried people — single (never married), divorced/separated, and widowed — were more likely to develop cancers that had spread beyond a local site, were less likely to receive definitive treatment, and had poorer survival rates after the diagnosis of cancer.

The most controversial finding of the study was this: Even when the disease was diagnosed at a more advanced stage, the best odds for survival seemed to lie with those who were married. James Goodwin, director of the study, summed it up by stating that the protective impact of being married affected every stage of cancer.

A study of women with breast cancer, conducted at the M. D. Anderson Hospital and Tumor Institute in Houston, showed that widowed patients were less likely to survive than married patients with similar histories. According to the researchers, marital status was the strongest predictor of survival in the breast cancer patients.[53]

Immune System Function

A number of tests and careful studies have shown that marriage helps keep the immune system strong — one possible reason why married people enjoy better health. In one study, researchers at Ohio State University compared the immune function of 38 separated or divorced women with that of 38 married women. They found that women within the first year of separation had significantly poorer immune function. Among the married, those who described their marriage as being better also had better immune function, and the longer women had been separated or divorced, the better the immune system was working.[54]

In a separate study involving men, the same research team found that separated or divorced men had significantly weaker immune systems than those who were married. Among the married men, the ones who were happy with their marriages had the strongest immune functioning, and those who were unhappily married had lower ratios of T helper cells to suppressor cells (a characteristic of weakened immunity).[55]

MARRIAGE AND LIFE EXPECTANCY

As study results have poured in, researchers have reached the same conclusion: Happy marriage dramatically increases life expectancy. A man who marries can expect to automatically add about 9 years and 7 months to his life. In one large-scale study of Swedish men, married men had a mortality rate of only 9% during the 3 years of the study. Their divorced counterparts had a rate of 20%.[56]

In one recent study, unmarried middle-aged men and women faced twice the risk of dying within 10 years as did those still living with their mates. Marriage itself, the researchers concluded, seems to be the key factor.[57]

Researchers agree that unmarried people have higher death rates from all causes. According to one researcher who has specialized in the study of heart disease and other causes of death, some of the increased death rates in unmarried individuals are "astounding," rising as high as 10 times the rates for married individuals of comparable ages.[58]

FAMILIES AND HEALTH

The term *family* describes *a unique cluster of people who enjoy a special relationship by reason of love, marriage, procreation, and mutual dependence.* A family is a group that shares common goals and values and works together to achieve those goals. A family may be a dual-career family, a single-parent family, or a "binuclear family" (in which the father and mother no longer live together but both provide a place for the children). And what goes on in a family — the network of relationships between its members — can have a profound effect on the health and longevity of its members.

The health of family members can be influenced profoundly by a number of factors. Health is affected by the early influence of parents (research shows that the influence is present from the moment of birth), parental styles (especially regarding styles of discipline), parental loss, and the involvement and attachment of parents to children. How children are perceived in the family can have great impact, even on physical growth. According to researcher Leonard Sagan, "Children raised in an affectionate environment grow more rapidly and reach greater size as adults. On the other hand, there is ample evidence that emotional deprivation can have a deleterious effect on growth."[59]

One study at the University of Massachusetts clearly shows the tremendous influence a parent can have on a child — even a baby as young as 3 months. Researchers Jeffrey Cohn and Edward Tronick wanted to find out how a mother's depression might affect her 3-month-old baby. The mothers and babies were divided into three groups. Mothers were told to imagine being deeply depressed — to think of some time in their lives when they were extremely sad, discouraged, or disappointed. The first group of mothers started out acting depressed for 3 minutes, and then switched to acting normal for a second 3-minute period. During the time they were acting depressed, they spoke in a monotone, avoided much contact with their babies, and kept their faces relatively expressionless. The second group of mothers started out normal and became depressed. The third group of mothers — the control group — remained normal during both 3-minute intervals.

The babies definitely reacted to their mothers' depression, and they did not like it. During the period in which the mother was depressed, the baby reacted both behaviorally and verbally. Most babies cried, made writhing movements, arched their backs, grimaced, fussed, or made negative facial expressions. Some reacted with extreme soberness and concern. Even if the baby played for a few seconds, he or she would return quickly to a negative countenance. After the mothers started acting "normal," the babies continued to be upset and depressed. The effect was longer lasting on the child; the child had a more difficult time "recovering" from the mother's bout of depression than she did.

HEALTH PROBLEMS IN WEAK OR STRESSED FAMILIES

Health problems can be traced to weak or stressed families, and many of those families have characteristics in common that help us identify them. The major signs of tension and distress in a family are physical symptoms of stress in its members, such as stuttering, bed-wetting, and nail-biting; burnout, in which the family becomes a burden instead of a joy; lack of communication between family members; "controlled" arguments in which disagreements are buried in silence; too-tight or too-loose construction of the family; lack of affection; and sexual infidelity.

According to researchers, the top 10 stressors for today's families are economics; children's behavior, discipline and sibling fighting; insufficient couple time; lack of shared responsibility within the family; communicating with children; insufficient "me" time for individual members; guilt for not accomplishing more; poor spousal relationships; insufficient family play time; and an overscheduled family calendar. Marital stress and tension, troubled family life, and other problems in the family unit can be a direct cause of illness and stress in individual family members.

One basic problem researchers have uncovered is the tendency for "learned" pain: North Dakota State University psychologist Patrick Edwards believes pain can be something children learn, something parents help them "rehearse." Children who grow up in pain-plagued households are more likely to experience pain themselves, and girls seem to be influenced more by the way other family members feel than boys are.[60]

Other researchers have found that families can either encourage or discourage physical distress and suffering. They believe a family's response to a family member's complaints influences how sick a family member feels, the way the family member feels about the symptoms, and, in the end, even how disabled the family member becomes.

Families have other definite impacts on health. One team of researchers at Harvard Medical School found that members of chronically stressed families had more frequent strep infections and that their infections turned into illness four times more often than in families without chronic stress.[61]

Other studies indicate that the emotional rigidity characteristic of many cancer patients may be a result of their upbringing. In one study, cancer patients at Jefferson Medical College in Philadelphia described their parents as "aloof, cold people."[62] Cancer patients who were asked about childhood traumas tended to gloss over the death of a parent or sibling; some had to be prodded to even remember that a parent had died when they were very young. In a number of studies, cancer patients described themselves as "emotionally detached" from their parents, and they described their parents as having been disagreeable to each other.[63]

Problems in the family may contribute to asthma. Studies of people with asthma reveal that many consider their parents to be rejecting or overbearing. In one study, researchers sent the parents of asthmatic children on paid vacations and left trained observers to care for the children. Without any other treatment, about half of the children improved.[64]

Also, stressed family conditions apparently can influence diabetes. A study conducted almost 20 years ago by a psychiatrist at the Albert Einstein College of Medicine in New York showed that well over two-thirds of the adolescent diabetics studied had a disturbed family life (involving serious illness of a parent, parental fighting, chaotic atmosphere, and so on) or the loss of a parent. Only about one-fifth of the diabetes-free control group had experienced similar family problems.[65] The same pattern seems to hold true for victims of anorexia nervosa, a malady considered by some professionals to be closely related to abnormal patterns of interaction between the patient and the family, mostly involving overly restrictive or suffocating relationships.

In general, a study conducted at Duke University Medical Center indicated that people from weak families tend to have weak health. The findings showed that families that were weak in structure and support produced people with more symptoms, impaired physical health, and weakened emotional health.[66]

THE HEALTH BENEFITS OF STRONG FAMILIES

Just as weak or stressed families can contribute to illness, strong families can contribute to good health and long lives. And just as weak families show signs of distress, healthy families have characteristic signs.

Strong families show positive listening and communication; strong feelings of affirmation and support; respect for all family members; high levels of trust; great enjoyment of each other; positive and equal interaction; plenty of leisure times together; shared responsibility among family members; a strong sense of right and wrong; traditions and rituals; a strong religious core; respect for the privacy of all family members; service, both within and outside the family circle; and the ability to solve problems.

Individuals in a healthy family have lower stress levels, significantly less illness, and the ability to recover from illness and disease much more rapidly. In a special Gallup poll commissioned by *American Health* magazine, Americans credit much of their health, and most of their positive health changes, to the influence of the family.[67]

A host of studies has proved that stress causes disease. A number of separate studies have shown that a strong family helps an individual cope with stress, reducing the risk of illness and disease. Evidence of the buffering effect of healthy families abounds. Because children experience less stress from hospital visits when parents are there, many hospitals now allow parents to stay in the room with sick infants and children. People in strong families recover more quickly from surgery, tend to follow medical instructions, maintain treatment recommendations, take prescribed medications, and get better more quickly with fewer complications. People in strong families also tend to manage chronic illness better.

Studies have shown that people with strong families are more likely to survive a heart attack and less likely to develop heart disease, even when standard risk factors are present. People in strong families tend to live longer than people in weak families or people without children. Finally, people in strong families are twice as likely to be alive at any given age.

Should your family include children? That's a difficult question that depends on you, your partner, your lifestyle, and your goals. Before you decide whether to have children:

▶ Talk openly and honestly to your partner. Is your relationship healthy? Do you both want a child? If one partner wants a child and the other doesn't, but caves in from pressure or a desire to make the other person happy, problems could result.

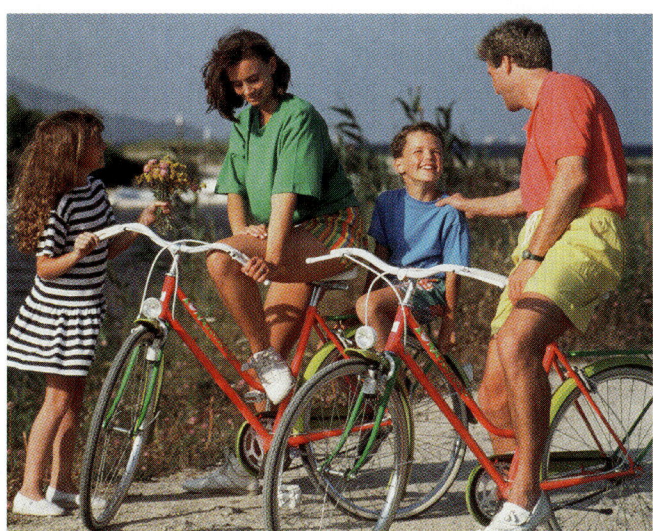
Strong families can enhance health.

▶ Discuss your philosophies about children. You should share pretty much the same views about disciplining children and techniques for rearing children. What about religion? Do you share the same religious views? If not, in which church will the child be reared?

▶ Consider *why* you want to have a child. If you want to share your life with someone and want to share your love, that's fine. It's not so fine to hope to realize a goal or dream through a child that you couldn't realize on your own, or to have a child because you're being pressured. Worst of all is to have a child because you hope the child will make you happy or take care of you.

▶ Consider your lifestyle carefully. If you're both working, do you both want to keep working after you have a child? How will that impact you? If one of you decides to quit, can you get along on just one income? If you both decide to keep working, can you afford day care, and how will you work it out? If you're going to school, will having a child interfere with your education? Are you ready to give up some of your freedom and independence in making a commitment to a child?

▶ Assess your personal characteristics. How do you express yourself when you're angry? Would you take it out on a child? Are you a person who gives love easily? Can you share? Do you enjoy teaching other people? Do you get along pretty well with your parents and your brothers and sisters? Most important, do you *like* children? If you've been miserable around children, you might need to take a hard look at your own decision to become a parent.

▼ Why Having Children Makes You Healthy:

▼ They protect against loneliness.
▼ They provide love, companionship, happiness, and joy.
▼ They boost creativity.
▼ They provide a sense of meaning and immortality.
▼ They help convince you that you've done something great!

▼ GRIEF, BEREAVEMENT, AND HEALTH

For more than 2,000 years people have recognized that grief — the overwhelming sorrow that follows a loss — can make people sick. Even longer ago, philosophers and physicians knew that grief alone could kill. Today, loss and the grief that follows it still are recognized as a precursor to distress, depression, and disease. Loss has even been implicated as a factor in premature death.

In one study, Dr. Arthur Schmale studied 42 patients admitted consecutively to the Rochester Memorial Hospital with conditions as diverse as cardiovascular disease and skin problems. He interviewed each regarding the events that led up to the illness and found a common thread: loss. Approximately three-fourths of the patients had developed their disease within one week after the loss of a loved one. The loss led to feelings of helplessness and hopelessness, and illness followed.[68]

Loss has been shown to be a factor in a variety of illnesses, but it seems to have particular influence in some — notably, cancer. A vast number of long-range studies points to loss and the grief that follows it as a contributing factor in cancer. Renowned general and pediatric surgeon Bernie Siegel, who has become well-known for his work with cancer patients, said, "One of the most common precursors of cancer is a traumatic loss or a feeling of emptiness in one's life. When a salamander loses a limb, it grows a new one. In an analogous way, when a human being suffers an emotional loss that is not properly dealt with, the body often responds by developing a new growth. It appears that if we can react to loss with personal growth, we can prevent growth gone wrong within us."[69]

Some kinds of loss are especially devastating. For the elderly, loss of possessions places them at particular risk for illness. Parents who lose children are at risk, as are children who lose parents. The loss of a parent through death, separation, or divorce can lead to later health problems. From what researchers can determine, *early* loss of a parent is associated with both physical and psychological illness. One study of cardiac patients in Philadelphia revealed that a significant number of the coronary disease patients had lost their fathers, most of them between the time they were 5 and 17 years old.[70]

Grieving is hard work, but it's essential when suffering a significant loss. If you don't go through the stages of grieving, you can get stuck in a stage and suffer what researchers call abnormal grief. The result can be serious illness and premature death. Researchers recommend three important steps in grieving:

1. The earliest stage of grief is *denial*. You literally can't believe the loss has occurred. That kind of denial should last only a few days. After that, it's necessary to face up to the loss. Admit that the loss happened. In the case of death, attending a funeral service can be helpful in that you may be able to view the body and hear tributes to the person's life, both of which help you accept the reality of the death.

2. Even though you probably will always have pleasant memories of a person who was important to you, you need to do something tangible to help break the bonds with the person. If the person lived with you, for example, you might box up or give away shoes, clothing, and personal possessions. Fill the empty dresser drawers with your things.

3. Grieving saps a tremendous amount of emotional and physical strength. As soon as you can, get active in something you really enjoy. If you need to, develop a new interest or hobby. It helps you "move on" and gives you something pleasant to look forward to every day.

THE HEALTH CONSEQUENCES OF BEREAVEMENT

Because it's a process of healing, grief is necessary. Most experts agree that for grief to progress

▼ Some Tips for Coping With Bereavement

If you lose someone you love, you may feel overwhelmed at first. The human spirit has an innate ability to bounce back from loss and despair, though. You can do some things to help you through this difficult time:

▼ Try to keep things in your life as *status quo* as possible. The death of a loved one is a major source of stress, so cut down on other things that could cause stress right now — a new job, a vacation, moving to a new house or apartment, for example.

▼ If you can, postpone making decisions that can wait until later, when you'll be thinking more clearly and won't be reacting under duress.

▼ Keep in touch with other people. Social support is especially important now. Let other people express their concern and help you out.

▼ Avoid the temptation to use drugs or alcohol to ease your feelings of grief. They only make things worse, and you'll have to adjust eventually anyway.

▼ Believe in yourself and your ability to recover. You have the right to go through the stages of grief, so don't be too hard on yourself.

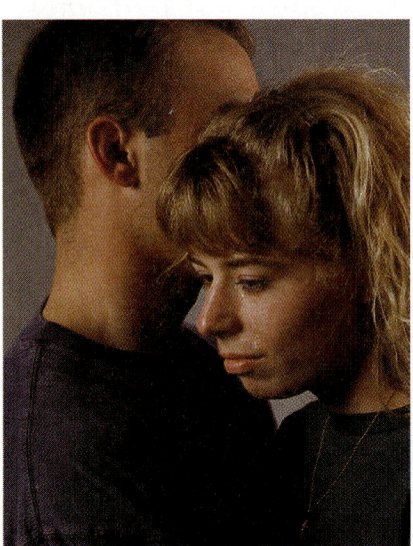

Grieving increases our vulnerability to illness but social support can lessen the chances of a negative physical response to loss.

"normally," a person needs to systematically pass through a series of stages, identified as denial, then anger, then bargaining, then depression, then acceptance, and, finally, hope for the future. Those stages don't occur in rapid-fire succession. The average recovery time from a major loss ranges from 18 to 24 months.

Even though grief is normal and natural and necessary, it can cause illness because it involves intense emotions and because it is so inseparably connected to loss. A special kind of grief is *bereavement*, the process of "disbonding" from someone who played an important role in one's life and now is gone. The intense and significant grief involved in bereavement has been shown to pose significant health risks, ranging all the way from immune system disorders to suicides, sudden deaths, and increased death rates from all causes.

A decade ago, a prominent psychologist maintained that every death has at least two victims and that the surviving "victim" is the one who hurts the most deeply. The impact of bereavement on health has been shown in several studies to depend on a variety of factors, including how often the bereaved person talks about the death, how much the bereaved person thinks about the death, what caused the death, how swiftly the person died, and how old the bereaved person was at the time of death.

The profound health effects of widowhood and bereavement are no respecter of persons. Men and women alike have significantly higher risk for a number of diseases, as well as premature death. Widowhood, however, seems to have an especially profound effect on the well-being of men, who apparently are harder hit healthwise than women who lose a mate. In one large-scale study, researchers found a significant difference in illness and death among widowed men, especially men who did not remarry, when compared to the rates of illness and premature death among widowed women.

A host of symptoms and illnesses strike the bereaved with greater frequency. These include heart disease, immune system dysfunction, and sudden deaths, as well as deaths in general.

Heart Disease

Data published by the National Office of Vital Statistics show that people widowed under the age of 35 are more than ten times as likely to die from several leading causes of death, including arteriosclerotic heart disease, a disease that is unusual in a young person. Apparently bereavement hastens a disease process that usually develops at an imperceptibly slow pace over decades.[71]

A number of studies indicate that bereavement wreaks havoc on the heart. In one persuasive study, researchers found that a high number of surviving spouses died during the first 6 months of bereavement. Three-fourths of them fell prey to either arteriosclerosis or coronary thrombosis.[72]

Immune System Function

Researchers say there's a logical reason why the bereaved have greater health problems than usual: The process of bereavement compromises the immune system. Many studies confirm that notion. In one, physicians from Florida's Veterans Administration Medical Center and the University of Miami School of Medicine studied a group of men who had experienced serious illness or the death of a close family member during the previous 6 months. In each case, the men had a lower activity level of lymphocytes, cells vital to immune system functioning.[73]

In other tests involving both men and women, bereaved individuals reveal a number of immune system problems. These include a lower activity level

---

▼ How to Protect Your Immune System While You Grieve

Are you struggling to cope with a loss? Keep your immune system in shape by doing the following:

▼ Get plenty of rest. Take naps if you need them, and try to maintain your normal sleeping pattern at night.

▼ Eat a balanced diet. Maintain your normal eating patterns. You should eat three solid meals a day with choices from all four food groups. Eat low-fat snacks high in complex carbohydrates when you feel hungry in between meals.

▼ Get plenty of fluids, but not those that contain alcohol or caffeine. Avoid dehydration, as both alcohol and caffeine *increase* dehydration.

▼ Exercise regularly. Choose an activity you enjoy, and do it for at least half an hour at least three times a week. Bicycling, walking, swimming, and sports are good choices.

Above all, *stay connected to other people!* Social support is especially important during grief. It can help keep your immune system healthy.

of lymphocytes, diminished natural killer cell activity, and feeble T-cell strength, among others.

One source of immune system shifts during bereavement may be a simple hormone. During periods of active mourning, separation, depression, and high levels of uncertainty, corticosteroid levels increase vastly. In the bloodstream, corticosteroids put a damper on the immune system's antibody response, preventing the immune system from completely kicking into gear, lowering the immune response, and increasing susceptibility to all kinds of illnesses.

Sudden Deaths

Those who are mourning a loss have a higher than expected rate of sudden death. In one study, researchers investigated the sudden deaths among Eastman Kodak employees in Rochester, New York. In at least half of the sudden deaths studied, the deaths were preceded by the departure of the last or only child in the family for college or marriage.[74]

In another study, Dr. George Engle studied newspaper reports of sudden deaths in the Rochester area over a 6-year period. In more than half of the sudden deaths he investigated, he was able to document that the death was immediately preceded by some kind of interpersonal loss. In men and women alike, most of the deaths occurred after the collapse or death of a loved one, during acute grief (within 16 days of the loss), or during the threat of loss of a loved one. Many of the deaths were of young, apparently healthy people.[75] Several interesting studies involving twins have shown that when one twin dies, the other twin, though healthy, sometimes dies within minutes or hours.

General Mortality Rates

When considering all causes of death, bereaved people have a much higher death rate than people of the same age whose spouses are living. Although the exact statistics vary according to the specific study, the results are the same: People who are widowed are more likely to die early.

One broad-scale study in Finland showed that the rate of death from all causes was 6.5% higher than expected for age and gender among the bereaved. The increase was sharpest during the first months after the loss. During the first week alone, mortality rates doubled for both men and women.[76]

In a separate study done in England involving more than 4,000 bereaved men, death rates increased more than 40% during the first 6 months following the death of a mate. After 6 months, the mortality rates started to gradually decline until they reached the death rates for married men of the same age.[77]

In still another study, known as "the broken heart study," the death rate from cardiovascular disease was 67% higher among the men in the study than would have been expected[78] without the bereavement factor. And results of a study by the National Institute on Aging suggested that death rates are higher during the first 2 years after the death of a mate. The bereaved had a consistently higher death rate than those of the same age who were married.[79]

Although death rates are higher overall for bereaved people, studies consistently reveal unusually high death rates for certain conditions. Those differ between men and women and even somewhat with age. Bereaved women tend to die more often than expected from cancer, heart disease, tuberculosis, cirrhosis, and alcoholism. Bereaved women over age 60 have a higher death rate from accidents, suicide, and diabetes. Bereaved men have a higher risk of dying from heart disease, tuberculosis, influenza, pneumonia, cirrhosis, alcoholism, accidents, and suicide.

The best protection for the bereaved is good social support, strong religious beliefs, rituals, and the belief that one can control the bereavement. These factors all increase the odds of good health and long life.

NOTES

1. Emrika Padus, *The Complete Guide to Your Emotions and Your Health* (Emmaus, Pennsylvania: Rodale Press, 1986).
2. Meredith Minkler, "The Social Component of Health," *American Journal of Health Promotion*, Fall 1986, pp. 33-38.
3. Minkler.
4. Marc Pilisuk and Susan Hillier Parks, *The Healing Web* (Hanover, New Hampshire: University Press of New England, 1986).
5. Sheldon Cohen, "Social Support and Physical Illness," from *Advances*, 7:1 (1990); original source, *Health Psychology*, 7:3 (1988).
6. Tom Ferguson, "The Invisible Health Care System," January/February 1988.
7. Robert Ornstein and Charles Swencionis, editors, *The Healing Brain: A Scientific Reader* (New York: The Guilford press, 1990).
8. The Health of Nations, Leonard A. Sagan, New York, Basic Books Inc., Publishers, 1987.
9. James J. Lynch, *The Broken Heart: The Medical Consequences of Loneliness* (New York: Basic Books, 1977).
10. Brent Q. Hafen and Kathryn J. Frandsen, *People Who Need People Are the Healthiest People: The Importance of Relationships* (Provo, Utah: Behavioral Health Associates).
11. Hafen and Frandsen.
12. Cohen.
13. Hafen and Frandsen.
14. Hafen and Frandsen.
15. "Friendship: Heart Saver for Type A's," *Men's health*, November 1987, p. 4.
16. David Spiegel, "A Psychosocial Intervention and Survival Time of Patients with Metastatic Breast Cancer," *Advances*, 7:3 (Summer 1991), pp. 10-19.
17. Albert L. Huebner, "The Pleasure Principle," *East/West*, May 1989, pp. 14-19.
18. "Loneliness: A Healthy Approach," *Longevity*, April 1990, p. 22.
19. Boris Blai, "Health Consequences of Loneliness: A Review of the Literature," *JACH*, 37 (January 1989), p. 162.
20. Padus.
21. Louise Bernikow, *Alone in America* (New York: Harper & Row, Publishers, 1986).
22. Hafen and Frandsen, p. 33.
23. Bernikow.
24. James J. Lynch, *The Broken Heart: Medical Consequences of Loneliness* (New York: Basic Books, 1977).
25. Robert Ornstein and David Sobel, *The Healing Brain* (New York: Simon and Schuster, 1987), pp. 195-196.
26. Sharon Faelten, David Diamond, and the Editors of *Prevention* Magazine, *Take Control of Your Life: A Complete Guide to Stress Relief* (Emmaus, Pennsylvania: Rodale Press, 1988), p. 58.
27. Frances Sheridan Goulart, "How to Live a Longer, Healthier Life."
28. "Lack of Social Relationships Increases Risk of Illness and Death," *The Wellness Newsletter*, November/December 1988, p. 4.
29. Nan Silver, "Lonely Child, Sick Adult?" *American Health*, April 1986, p. 20.
30. Barbara R. Sarason, Irwin G. Sarason, and Gregory R. Pierce, *Social Support: An Interactional View* (New York: John Wiley & Sons, 1990), p. 256; and J. Stephen Heisel, Steven E. Locke, Linda J. Kraus, and R. Michael Williams, "Natural Killer Cell Activity and MMPI Scores of a Cohort of College Students," *American Journal of Psychiatry* 143 (November 1986), 1382-1386.
31. Alix Kerr, "Hearts Need Friends," from *Physician's Weekly*.
32. "Social Isolation Tied to Heart Attack Deaths," *Deseret News*, May 1, 1988, p. A10.
33. The Editors of *Prevention* Magazine, *Positive Living and Health: The Complete Guide to Brain/Body Healing and Mental Empowerment* (Emmaus, Pennsylvania: Rodale Press, 1990), p. 154.
34. "Living Alone Could Shorten Your Life," *Newsweek*, February 3, 1992.
35. Lynch.
36. Eleanor Smith, "Fighting Cancerous Feelings," *Psychology Today*, May 1988, pp. 22-23.
37. Sheldon Cohen and S. Leonard Syme, *Social Support and Health* (Orlando, Florida: Academic Press, Inc., 1985).
38. Steven Locke and Douglas Colligan, *The Healer Within* (New York: E. P. Dutton, 1986), pp. 88-90.
39. Dan Zevin, "Blotting Out Cancer with a Smile," *Health*, May 1987, p. 14.
40. Faelten and Diamond, p. 273.
41. J. W. Pennebaker, et al., *Psychosomatic Medicine*, 51 (September-October 1989), p. 577.
42. Title of an article by Shelley Levitt in *50 Plus*, July 1988, pp. 56-61.
43. Padus, pp. 660-661.
44. Brent Q. Hafen and Kathryn J. Frandsen, *People Need People: The Importance of Relationships to Health and Wellness* (Evergreen, Colorado: Cordillera Press, Inc., 1987), pp. 33-34.
45. Barbara R. Sarason, Irwin G. Sarason, and Gregory R. Pierce, *Social Support: An Interactional View* (New York: John Wiley and Sons, 1990), p. 257.
46. Barbara Powell, *Alone, Alive, and Well* (Emmaus, Pennsylvania: Rodale Press, 1985).
47. Sarason et al., p. 258.
48. Powell.
49. "Marriage and Wellness Linked," *Deseret News*, November 15, 1988, p. 4A.
50. Lynch.
51. Sally Squires, "Marriage—Good For the Heart," *American Health*, July 1987, p. 111.
52. James S. Goodwin, William C. Hunt, Charles R. Key, and Jonathan M. Samet, "The Effect of Marital Status on Stage, Treatment, and Survival of Cancer Patients," *Journal of the American Medical Association*, 258:21 (December 4, 1987), pp. 3125-3130.

53. Neale, Tilley, and Vernon, "Marital Status, Delay in Seeking Treatment, and Survival from Breast Cancer," *Social Science and Medicine*, 23:3 (1986), 305-312.
54. "Is Marriage Good For Your Health? An Interview with Janice Kiecolt-Glaser," *Mind/Body/Health Digest*, 1:2 (1987), p. 1.
55. Rick Weiss, "Worried Sick: Hassles and Herpes," *Science News*, 132 (December 5, 1987), p. 360.
56. A. Rosengren, H. Wedel, and L. Wilhelmsen, "Marital Status and Mortality in Middle-Aged Swedish Men," *American Journal of Epidemiology*, 129:1 (January 1989), pp. 54-64.
57. Morton Hunt, "Long-Life Insurance: For Men, It's Marriage," *Longevity*, February 1991, p. 10.
58. Lynch.
59. Leonard A. Sagan, *The Health of Nations* (New York: Basic Books, Inc., Publishers, 1987).
60. "Pain: Is It All in Your Family?" *Executive Fitness*, May 1987, p. 7.
61. Blair Justice, *Who Gets Sick: Thinking and Health* (Houston, Texas: Peak Press, 1987), pp. 37-38.
62. Steven Locke and Douglas Colligan, *The Healer Within: The New Medicine of Mind and Body* (New York: E. P. Dutton, 1986), p. 141.
63. Locke and Colligan, p. 145.
64. S. I. McMillen, *None of These Diseases*, revised (Old Tappan, NJ: Fleming H. Revell Company, 1984).
65. Locke and Colligan, p. 103.
66. G. R. Parkerson, Jr., J. L. Michener, L. R. Wu, et al., "Associations Among Family Support, Family Stress, and Personal Functional Health Status," *Journal of Clinical Epidemiology*, 42:3 (1989), pp. 217-229.
67. Sharon Faelten, David Diamond, and the Editors of *Prevention* Magazine, *Take Control of Your Life: A Complete Guide to Stress Relief* (Emmaus, Pennsylvania: Rodale Press, 1988), p. 273.
68. Lynch.
69. Bernie S. Siegel, *Love, Medicine, and Miracles* (New York: Harper and Row Publishers, 1986).
70. Lynch.
71. Lynch.
72. Lynch.
73. Justice, p. 189.
74. Lynch.
75. Justice, pp. 192-193.
76. Jaakko Kaprio, Markku Koskenvuo, and Heli Rita, "Mortality After Bereavement: A Prospective Study of 95,647 Widowed Persons," *American Journal of Public Health* 77 (March 1987): 283-287.
77. Lynch.
78. Cohen and Syme.
79. "If Surviving Spouse Endures 2 Years, Normalcy Returns," *Deseret News* and United Press International.

5

Perceptions, the Spirit, and Health

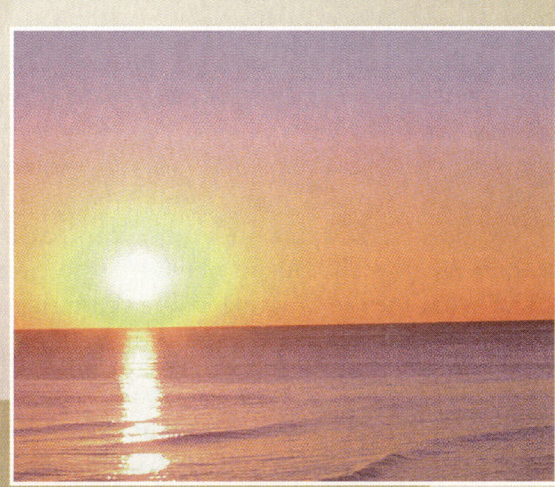

Objectives

▼ Define "explanatory style."
▼ Describe the differences between a pessimistic style and an optimistic style, and their effects on health.
▼ Learn specific ways to change a pessimistic style.
▼ Explain the differences between an internal locus of control and an external locus of control, together with their health effects.
▼ Understand the connection between self-esteem and health.
▼ Learn how to protect health with a fighting spirit.
▼ Understand the connection between spirituality and health, including the power of prayer, forgiveness, and faith.
▼ Describe the altruistic personality and health benefits of volunteerism.
▼ Contrast the health effects of hope and hopelessness.

The philosopher Michel de Saint-Pierre observed, "An optimist may see a light where there is none, but why must the pessimist always run to blow it out?" The differences in attitudes between optimists and pessimists — the way we perceive ourselves, our circumstances, and our possibilities — have a profound effect on how well we are.

▼ EXPLANATORY STYLE AND HEALTH

Explanatory style is *the way people perceive the events in their lives*. It's the habitual manner in which people explain the bad things that happen to them. In reality, it's a habit, a way of thinking that people use when all other factors are equal and when there are no clear-cut right and wrong answers.

People with a pessimistic explanatory style interpret a negative event as an "omen," a sign as to how the rest of their life will turn out. People with an optimistic explanatory style see an isolated bad event as just that: isolated.

The pessimistic explanatory style can be identified readily by three thought patterns that give clues about what they're thinking in their conversation.

1. Assuming the problem is stable, or *never-ending*; being convinced it will never go away.
2. Believing the problem is *global,* that it affects a broad spectrum of activities instead of an isolated incident.
3. *Internalizing* everything ("It's my fault"), often placing the wrong blame at the wrong time.

Once you've developed an explanatory style, are you stuck with it forever? That's a matter of considerable controversy among leading researchers. Many believe we stick to one explanatory style throughout our lives, and some evidence exists to support that notion. University of Pennsylvania psychologist Martin Seligman believes, however, that explanatory style — which is basically a belief system — can be changed, a belief he supports through the results of his own work.[1]

Regardless of whether explanatory style can be changed, researchers agree on one thing: Explanatory style has an extremely powerful influence on health and wellness. Explanatory style, Seligman says, is like a self-fulfilling prophecy: The way a person "explains events in his life can predict and determine his future. Those who believe they are the master of their fate are more likely to succeed than those who attribute events to forces beyond their control."[2]

A negative explanatory style affects both emotional and physical well-being. In the emotional arena, it can lead to anxiety, eating disorders, and dysphoria, in the form of depression, guilt, anger, or hostility. In the physical realm a negative explanatory style can halt the healing process. From his work with cancer patients, Bernie Siegel points out, "If I said to patients, you have two choices if you want to get well — you can change your lifestyle or have an operation — the majority would say, 'Operate. It hurts less.'"[3] Siegel, who works with patients to help them change their explanatory style and to resolve stress and conflict in their lives, says remarkable changes occur in the course of disease.

Siegel maintains that an optimistic explanatory style and the positive emotions it embraces — such as love, acceptance, and forgiveness — stimulate the immune system and kick the body's own healing systems into gear. An optimistic explanatory style, he says, sends "live" messages to your body and helps promote the healing process.

A growing body of evidence suggests that explanatory style can be a potent predictor of physical health. Christopher Peterson, an associate professor of psychology at the University of Michigan, rated a group of students as either optimistic or pessimistic and then observed the students for 4 weeks. He found that the pessimists were sick twice as many days as the optimists were during the study period. He then monitored the students over the next year. The pessimistic students still fared the worst: During the year they visited a doctor four times as often as the optimistic students. Of the pessimistic students, 95% had colds, sore throats, or the flu during the year. Some of them also had ear infections, pneumonia, and mononucleosis. All the pessimists' illnesses were infectious — suggesting that "how we view things may directly affect our immune system."[4]

A pessimistic explanatory style can influence healing time and the course of the illness in several major diseases, such as cancer and coronary disease. In one pilot study of cancer patients with advanced melanoma, University of Rochester researcher

Sandra Levy reported that an optimistic explanatory style was the number-one psychological predictor of who would live the longest.[5] In another study, this one of women who had recurring breast cancer, Levy and her colleagues studied the similarities among women who had the longest cancer-free period between episodes of the disease. The most common denominator among women whose cancer was slow to return was an optimistic explanatory style.[6]

Attitude and explanatory style can impact the circulatory system and outlook for people with coronary heart disease. Sophisticated instruments and testing procedures have enabled researchers to watch the brain in action. Blood flow to the brain actually changes as thoughts, feelings, and attitudes change. Findings from a variety of studies show that people with a pessimistic explanatory style have higher risk for atherosclerosis, blockage of coronary arteries, and heart attack.

Studies of explanatory style conducted at Yale University and the University of Pennsylvania verify that a negative explanatory style compromises immunity. Blood samples taken from people with a negative explanatory style revealed suppressed immune function, a low ratio of helper/suppressor T-cells, and fewer lymphocytes, the cells responsible for waging war against disease or infection.[7]

An optimistic style tends to increase the strength of the immune system. Robert Good, former president and director of the Memorial Sloan-Kettering Cancer Hospital in New York, maintains that an optimistic explanatory style and the positive attitude it fosters can alter our ability to resist infections, allergies, autoimmunities, and even cancer.

Michael Lerner, founder of Commonweal and a MacArthur Foundation Genius Award winner, says the attitudes linked to an optimistic explanatory style can boost the immune system enough to help fight cancer, that attitudes themselves have a potent effect on the immune system. You become the person who developed the cancer, he says. Becoming a different personality may change the environment the cancer grew in; it may become so inhospitable that the cancer shrinks.[8]

Becoming more optimistic not only increases one's enjoyment in life, but apparently provides protection against illness and disease as well. To boost your own optimism:

▶ Before you start to change your attitudes, surround yourself with people who care about you and can help you. Ideally, they should be optimistic people. When you surround yourself with optimists, you begin to "catch" their attitude. Tell others you want to change, and solicit their help and suggestions.

▶ Learn to genuinely like other people. Look for their good qualities, and respect their differences.

The Life Orientation Test: Are You an Optimist?

In the following spaces, write how much you agree with each of the items, using the following scale:

4 = strongly agree
3 = agree
2 = neutral
1 = disagree
0 = strongly disagree

1. In uncertain times, I usually expect the best. _____
2. If something can go wrong for me, it will. _____
3. I always look on the bright side of things. _____
4. I'm always optimistic about my future. _____
5. I hardly ever expect things to go my way. _____
6. Things never work out the way I want them to. _____
7. I'm a believer in the idea that "every cloud has a silver lining." _____
8. I rarely count on good things happening to me. _____

How to Score

For items 2, 5, 6, and 8, you will need to reverse the numbers. For example, if you strongly agree with statement 8, "I rarely count on good things happening to me," change your score from 0 to 4. Now total up your score.

Interpreting Your Results

This test seems to demonstrate a relationship between an optimistic or a pessimistic outlook and physical well-being. When college students completed this test 4 weeks before final exams, the higher-scoring optimists (with 20 points and over) reported far fewer health problems. The pessimists complained of more dizziness, fatigue, sore muscles, and coughs.

Adapted from R. Ornstein and D. Sobel, *Healthy Pleasures* (Reading, MA: Addison-Wesley, 1989), pp. 162–163. © 1990 Robert Ornstein/David Sobel. Reprinted by permission of Addison-Wesley Publishing Co.

- Realize that changing your explanatory style is a big commitment. In essence, it's a change in lifestyle. You didn't develop an explanatory style overnight, and you won't be able to change it overnight, either. Be patient with yourself and expect some hard work.
- You'll undoubtedly suffer a few setbacks. Everybody does. Get past disappointments. Look at these as challenges to face and don't let them debilitate you.
- Look for evidence to support the way you want to feel. You'll be surprised to find it! Too often, we adopt pessimistic or negative attitudes based on faulty beliefs when the evidence really suggests otherwise.
- Set small, attainable goals, then reward yourself richly when you meet those goals. Celebrate your accomplishments.
- Look beyond yourself. The world does *not* revolve around you. Get involved in volunteerism or service to expand your horizons.
- Guard against exaggeration. An argument with a friend doesn't mean the friendship is collapsing; one poor exam score doesn't mean your college career is doomed. Work to develop a keen perspective on things — and relax!
- Gather all the facts before you form a conclusion. Take the time to research things; you'll probably develop a whole new set of ideas!
- Avoid overgeneralization. Just because you couldn't get a professor you wanted, don't believe that *nothing* ever turns out the way you want. Think of all the successes, all the good.
- Face your problems head-on. Develop strategies for solving them instead of trying to escape them.
- Above all, have fun. Learn to laugh at yourself, enjoy yourself, and respect yourself. That's what being optimistic is all about.

LOCUS OF CONTROL AND HEALTH

The concept of locus of control originated several years ago with the work of Julian Rotter. It involves the belief that our own actions are effective enough to master or control the environment. Control does not mean we need to control everything around us — other people, the environment, our circumstances, good or bad. Control *does* entail a deep-seated belief that we can impact a situation by how we look at the problem. We can choose how we react and respond. If we regard a loss with gloom and doom, we allow it to hurt us. If we view it as a chance for growth and opportunity, we minimize its ability to hurt us.

Researchers working in the field of psychoneuroimmunology theorize that, as far as a sense of control is concerned, a person is somewhere along a continuum. At one end of the continuum is the *external locus of control*. At the opposite end is the *internal locus of control*. Where a person is along the continuum relates to his or her health (see Figure 5.1).

People with an external locus of control believe that the things that happen to them are unrelated to their own behavior and, therefore, are beyond their control. At the opposite end of the spectrum are the people with an internal locus of control, who believe that negative events are a consequence of personal actions and, thus, *potentially* can be controlled.

Psychologists Suzanne Kobasa and Salvatore Maddi first conceived the now well-accepted theory that people who are able to stay healthy even while under stress have behaviors and personalities marked by hardiness,[9] a concept discussed in Chapter 3. One of the key components of hardiness, they say, is a sense of control. The control that characterizes hardiness is a belief that we can influence events, coupled with willingness to act on that belief rather than just be a victim of circumstances. As researcher Phillip Rice so aptly put it, "If the theme song of the external is *Cast Your Fate to the Winds*, the theme song of the internal is *I Did It My Way*."[10]

The results of a host of studies show the importance of control. As a whole, people with a greater sense of control are at less risk for illness. As new research is completed, scientists are realizing that an internal locus of control has an even more profound role in protecting health than we once thought.

Former *Saturday Review* editor Norman Cousins, renowned for his work linking attitudes and health, maintained that, in general, "Anything that restores a sense of control to a patient can be a profound aid to a physician in treating serious illness. That sense of control is more than a mere mood or attitude, and may well be a vital pathway between the brain, the endocrine system, and the immune system. The assumed possibility is that it may serve as the basis

LOCUS OF CONTROL

External ← CONTINUUM → Internal

FIGURE 5.1 ▼ A person's position along the continuum of the locus of control relates to his or her health.

for what may well be a profound advancement in the knowledge of how to confront serious illness."[11]

According to a study reported in *Clinical Psychiatry News*,[12] researchers at the University of Connecticut School of Medicine followed a group of more than 200 heart attack survivors for 8 years. The researchers noted that the patients who accepted the responsibility for their attacks had fewer second attacks than patients who blamed their genes, their mate, or other factors. According to study leader Glenn Affleck, the value in accepting responsibility for a heart attack may be in taking control. Passing the buck, on the other hand, could indicate the very sort of thinking that may contribute to heart attack in the first place — feeling a lack of control. This, in turn, could produce a feeling of helplessness in making adaptive lifestyle changes.

One reason control has such a profound influence over health is that a lack of control disturbs the biochemical balance in the brain and body. An internal locus of control has a significant influence over the body's release of hormones, which has been found to be a powerful determinant of health. Three of the hormones influenced by a lack of control are: serotonin, which regulates moods, relieves pain, and helps control the release of the pain-killing endorphines; dopamine, which is largely responsible for a sense of reward and pleasure; and norepinephrine, which, when depleted, causes depression.

When a person has little sense of control, the level of corticosteroids in the bloodstream soars. The corticosteroids, released by the body during stress, cause a variety of physical damage. They lower the body's resistance to disease and suppress the body's manufacture of the three hormones named, making lack of control a two-edged sword. A lack of control may have an even stronger influence over health than do high levels of stress.

Various studies among work populations have shown that lack of control can be deleterious to health. People with little control but high demands have more than three times the risk of heart disease and chronically escalated blood pressure than people with few demands but a high level of control. According to researchers with the Framingham Heart Study, female clerical workers and others with little control had twice the incidence of heart disease as women in occupations that allowed higher levels of control.[13]

A person in a stressful situation who believes he or she has some control over the situation has far less of the physiological damage normally associated with stress. And control acts as a buffer against stress when we *believe* we have control, even if we really don't.

One reason control has such a powerful impact on health lies with the immune system. According to research, control may have a significant effect on the body's immune defenses. People who feel powerless, helpless, and out of control generally have compromised immunity, whereas those who feel a sense of control have healthier immune systems.

When physicians tested women with early-stage breast cancer, those who felt some control over their lives and their disease were compared to women who felt a distressing lack of control. The women with control had a much higher level of natural killer cell activity, a much stronger immune system.[14]

A sense of control also seems to trigger the body's internal healing mechanisms. Several different studies with patients about to undergo surgery demonstrate that a sense of control can have a significant effect on the healing process. In one, psychologist Ellen Langer took a randomly selected group of surgical patients at Yale-New Haven Hospital and divided the patients into three groups. The people in the third group — those who were given coping information explaining how they could exercise control over their bodies — used half as many painkillers and sedatives and stayed in the hospital fewer days than the others.[15]

In a separate but similar study, patients about to undergo coronary bypass surgery were given a similar course on coping. According to the researchers at the University of Iowa School of Medicine who conducted the study, the patients who received enough information to gain a sense of control fared significantly better on all counts. They had less hypertension, anxiety, and pain. The researchers concluded that a greater sense of control proved to be the most powerful predictor of recovery without complication.[16]

▼ SELF-ESTEEM AND HEALTH

Self-esteem is *a sense of positive self-regard*. It's a way of viewing oneself as a good person who is well in all aspects. It's a sense of feeling good about one's capabilities, physical limitations, goals, place in the world, and relationship to others. Self-esteem is a powerful element as perceptions about self set the boundaries for what we can and cannot do. Self-esteem can be called the blueprint for behavior.

American humorist and author Samuel Clemens — the legendary Mark Twain — believed that being approving of ourselves is a hundred times more valuable than having the approval of others. A century after he penned that advice, it is proving to be true.

According to a growing body of evidence, healthy self-esteem is one of the best things a person can do for overall health, both mental and physical. A good, strong sense of self can boost the immune system, protect against disease, and aid in healing.

Whether people do or do not get sick — and how long they stay that way — may depend in part on the strength of their self-esteem. A growing body of evidence indicates that low self-esteem often is a factor in chronic pain, for example. And several studies show that recovery from infectious mononucleosis is related to "ego strength." The higher the self-esteem, the more rapid the recovery.

Self-esteem is so powerful an influence on health that it even impacts the way we react to life events. In their research, scientists have found that if we have strong self-esteem, the outlook is good. The more positive the life events, the better our health. If our self-esteem is poor, however, our health can decline in direct proportion as our life becomes peppered with more negative life events.

Results of various studies show that positive self-esteem helps protect health by boosting immunity. In one study, good self-esteem was shown to be related to the strongest natural killer cell activity.[17] In another, two victims of AIDS were compared for immune function and prognosis. The one whose self-esteem had been battered had a much poorer immune function than the one with good self-esteem, even though the second man had deleterious health habits that should have hurt his immunity.[18]

The way people regard their own health even serves as sort of a self-fulfilling prophecy, mostly because of its link to self-esteem. When Canadian researchers asked more than 3,500 elderly people to rate their own health and then followed those volunteers for 7 years, they found that actual health seven years later correlated to the self-ratings. Actually, the ratings the elderly people gave themselves were more accurate and predictive than the health measures provided by physicians who examined the patients.[19]

Belief in oneself is one of the most powerful weapons we have in protecting our health and living longer. It has a startling impact on wellness, and we are able to harness it to our advantage. As Madeline Gershwin said, "What wise people and grandmothers have always known is that the way you feel about yourself, your attitudes, beliefs, values, have a great deal to do with your health and well-being."[20]

To boost your self-esteem:

▶ Use *affirmations*, positive statements that help reinforce the most positive aspects of your personality and experience. Every day, you can

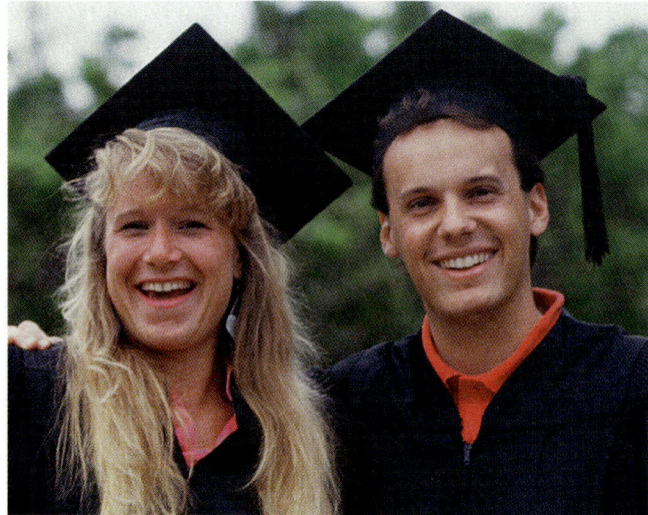

Self-eseteem can contribute to mental and physical health.

How Do You Feel About Yourself?

This scale is designed to assist you in understanding your self-image. Positive attitudes toward oneself are important components of maturation and emotional well-being.

Self-image aspect	Strongly agree	Agree	Disagree	Strongly disagree
1. I feel that I'm a person of worth, at least on an equal plane with others.	A	B	C	D
2. I feel that I have a number of good qualities.	A	B	C	D
3. All in all, I am inclined to feel that I am a failure.	A	B	C	D
4. I am able to do things as well as most other people.	A	B	C	D
5. I feel I do not have as much to be proud of as others.	A	B	C	D
6. I take a positive attitude toward myself.	A	B	C	D
7. On the whole, I am satisfied with myself.	A	B	C	D
8. I wish I could have more respect for myself.	A	B	C	D
9. I certainly feel useless at times.	A	B	C	D
10. At times I think I am no good at all.	A	B	C	D

How to Score

Use the following table to determine the number of points to assign to each of your answers. To determine your total score, add up all the numbers that match the letter (A, B, C, or D) you circled for each statement.

Statement	A	B	C	D
1.	4	3	2	1
2.	4	3	2	1
3.	1	2	3	4
4.	4	3	2	1
5.	1	2	3	4
6.	4	3	2	1
7.	4	3	2	1
8.	1	2	3	4
9.	1	2	3	4
10.	1	2	3	4

Total: _____ This is your self-esteem score.

Interpreting Your Score

Classify your score in the appropriate score range.

Score range	Current self-esteem level
Less than 20	Low self-esteem
20-29	Below-average self-esteem
30-34	Above-average self-esteem
35-39	High self-esteem
40	Highest self-esteem

The higher your score, the more positive your self-esteem.

High self-esteem means that individuals respect themselves, consider themselves worthy, but do not necessarily consider themselves better than others. They do not feel themselves to be the ultimate in perfection; on the contrary, they recognize their limitations and expect to grow and improve.

Self-esteem is the most important variable in regard to human development and maturation. It is the master key that can open the door to the actualization of an individual's human potential.

M. Rosenburg, *Society and the Adolescent Self-Image* (Hanover, NH: Wesleyan University Press, 1986).

boost your sense of esteem by saying positive things about you to yourself, such as, "I am honest and open in expressing my feelings." Write some affirmations of your own.

▶ List the things you would like to have or experience. Construct the statements as if you were already enjoying the situations you list, beginning each sentence with "I am." For example, "I am feeling great about doing well in my classes," or "I am enjoying the opportunity to meet new people." Visualize each situation, and get in the habit of repeating this process several times a day.

▶ When your internal critic — the negative inner voice we all have — starts putting you down, tune it out. Force yourself to think of a situation that you handled well or something about yourself that you're especially proud of.[21]

▼ PROTECTING HEALTH WITH A FIGHTING SPIRIT

A fighting spirit has been defined as *the open expression of emotions, whether they are negative or positive*. The opposite of a fighting spirit is hopelessness, a surrender to, rather than an open expression of, despair.

Physicians have found that fighting spirit can play a major role in recovery from disease. According to researchers, attitudes of patients faced with serious illness fall into one of four categories: a fighting spirit, denial, stoic acceptance, or helplessness and hopelessness. People with a fighting spirit fully accept the diagnosis, adopt an optimistic attitude filled with faith, seek information about how to help themselves, and are determined to fight the disease.

In one study, researchers followed a group of women with breast cancer that had not yet spread beyond the breast. Five years after surgery, those with a fighting spirit were most likely to be alive and free of recurrences.[22] Patients who express helplessness or hopelessness have the poorest prognosis, say the researchers.

A growing number of researchers believes that a fighting spirit may be the underlying factor in what is called *spontaneous remission*, the inexplicable recovery from incurable illness. More and more physicians believe that the patient is the key in spontaneous remission, and that the phenomenon is real. These researchers believe the patient's attitude, especially the presence of a fighting spirit, is responsible for victory over disease. "The forces exist in the body to arouse its natural disease-fighting abilities," says Dr. Lloyd Old of Memorial Sloan-Kettering Cancer Center in New York City. "The task ahead is to find ways to unleash them."

Fighters aren't stronger or better or more capable than the rest of the people. They simply don't give up easily. In study after study, they have been shown to enjoy better health and live longer, even when physicians and laboratory tests say they shouldn't.

According to author Steve Fishman, specific factors bolster a fighting spirit and promote survival.[23] A fighting spirit makes a person take charge. When illness or disease is present, that makes a big difference. As heart surgeon Dr. Wayne Eisom of New York Hospital-Cornell Medical Center points out, "A fighter gets out of bed earlier and walks, even with painful incisions. A non-fighter doesn't, and gets an infection in his lungs."[24] Fighters are intrinsically different from people who give up, the researchers say, and their health reflects those differences.

Probably the most remarkable studies involving the effect of a fighting spirit have dealt with cancer, a disease that, by its very name, evokes medical terror in many people. The spirit with which a patient accepts the diagnosis apparently is a major determinant in how the disease will progress. According to some researchers, an overall fighting spirit may even help stave off cancer.

A style of giving up, as contrasted with an active, fighting style, has been shown repeatedly to significantly affect prognosis in cancer cases. Siegel used the example of a patient with liver cancer, a financial advisor who invested people's life savings according to statistics. "His oncologist told him what statistics said about his chances, and from then on he refused to fight for his life," Siegel explains. "He said, 'I've spent my life making predictions based on statistics. Statistics tell me I'm supposed to die. If I don't die, my whole life doesn't make sense.' And he went home and died."[25]

The immune system may bear some of the greatest impact of a fighting spirit, and it may be the reason fighters do better in all kinds of disease situations. Convincing evidence from a host of studies indicates that a fighting spirit boosts immune function, mobilizing the body and empowering it to fight off disease and infection.

In discussing the power of a fighting spirit, psychoneuroimmunology pioneer Dr. George Solomon told the story of a Harvard professor who had been stricken with cancer; he had lesions in his head, lungs, and liver. Nonetheless, the professor continued teaching his classes, reassuring his friends and students. Solomon says of the professor, "It was thrilling to see how powerful the fighting spirit can be. For most of a year, he battled that cancer. And he won. The most important thing he had to teach us came not out of his medical lectures, but out of his own experience and example. He won against all the odds — against the predictions of the specialists and against the reports based on sophisticated technology." What the professor taught all around him was, in essence, that if we are willing to fight, we *can* win.

SPIRITUALITY AND HEALTH

In discussing the tremendous freedom spiritual health can bring, Yale surgeon and cancer specialist Bernie Siegel writes, "You always have a choice about how you feel. Listen to Jesse Jackson say that you may not have chosen to be down, but you have a choice as to whether you want to try to get up.... Listen to Mahatma Gandhi, who said, 'Let us not kill our enemies but kill their desire to kill.' And so you have a choice about how you behave, whether you are in prison, whether you are in a concentration camp, or whether you are sick. You have a choice."[26]

One researcher attempted to arrive at a definition of the spiritual dimension of health by questioning people in the health and medical fields. Combining all of the ideas with others she researched, she identified what she believes to be the four aspects of spiritual health: a *unifying force* that integrates the other dimensions of health; a force that creates or brings into focus a *meaning in life*; a *common bond* between individuals; and a dimension based on *individual perceptions and faith*.

Indications of spirituality include prayer, a sense of meaning in life, reading and contemplation, a sense of closeness to a higher being, interactions with others, and other experiences that reflect spiritual interaction or awareness. Using many of the same basic components, another researcher developed a slightly different definition of spiritual health. Optimum spiritual health, he says, is the ability to develop our spiritual nature to its fullest potential. Part and parcel of that is the ability to discover and articulate our own basic purpose in life and to learn how to experience love, joy, peace, and fulfillment. It's the experience of helping ourselves and others achieve full potential.[27] Through the spiritual dimension, we emphasize our connectedness to other members of the human family.

INFLUENCES OF SPIRITUALITY ON HEALTH

Spirituality and the cultivation of spiritual health — which is a process or journey, not an end point — can have a significant effect on physical, mental, and emotional health, sometimes in dramatic ways. Researchers are beginning to view spirituality with new interest, especially as it relates to physical health. One who is pioneering such research is Kenneth Pelletier — who, with his colleagues at the University of California at San Francisco, is investigating the link between spirituality and health.

Pelletier began his research by studying men and women he deemed to be "successful." He found, first, that most of the professionally successful men and women had strong spiritual values and beliefs. Further, virtually all of them had suffered a major psychological or physical trauma early in life but, perhaps because of their spirituality, had been able to weather the crisis and develop a more effective style of coping with life crises.[28] Preliminary findings from the study found the correlation between good spiritual health and good physical health "striking."

Similar findings have emerged from other studies over several decades of intense research. One of the reasons, say researchers, is that spirituality buffers stress; people with a deep sense of spirituality are not defeated by crisis. Spirituality helps people interpret crisis in a growth-producing way. As a result, they are able to use illness as a means of spiritual growth. Even when disease claims a life, spirituality can make the experience one of positive growth.

Not everyone is cured of disease, Siegel points out. At some time or another, everyone will die. Nevertheless, people who are busy living, who are trying to make changes in their lives, experience great growth even in the face of serious illness. People who meet disease with that attitude, Siegel says, "define their disease as a gift, a challenge, a wake-up call, a new beginning, and a beauty mark.

And they are not necessarily saying, 'I am cured.' The exceptional people accept their mortality. They have heard they're going to die, but they don't take it as a sentence. So they don't go home and die. They take it as an opportunity to live until they die."[29]

THE POWER OF PRAYER ON HEALTH

Prayer signals a commitment to a set of moral and ethical values. It is a signpost of our spirituality, at the core of most spiritual experiences. Research shows us that prayer also has powerful physiological effects on the body. In a nationwide poll asking doctors whether they feel patients benefit from prayer, half the doctors questioned said they believe prayer helps patients, and two-thirds of the doctors responding said they pray for their patients.

Dr. Herbert Benson, associate professor of medicine at the Harvard Medical School and chief of the Section on Behavioral Medicine at the New England Deaconess Hospital, has focused the last two decades of his clinical work on what he calls the "relaxation response," the body's ability to enter a "scientifically definable state" of relaxation[30] (see Chapter 2). According to Benson, the relaxation response, with all its physiological benefits, has most often and effectively been elicited through forms of prayer.

Prayer can have a powerful impact on people even when they don't know prayers are being offered in their behalf. One San Francisco cardiologist arranged for a group of people around the country to pray daily for 192 coronary care unit patients at San Francisco General Hospital, without telling the patients that anyone was praying for them. A second group of 201 control patients had no one praying for them. The praying continued for 10 months. Cardiologist Randy Byrd, who engineered the study, reported that the patients who were prayed for had significantly fewer complications while in the coronary care unit.[31]

THE HEALING POWER OF FORGIVENESS

Essential to a spiritual nature is forgiveness, *the ability to release from the mind all past hurts and failures, all sense of guilt and loss*. It is, as instructor of medicine Joan Borysenko put it, accepting the core of every human being the same as yourself and giving them the gift of not judging them.[32]

To understand the health benefits of forgiveness, we must understand what happens when we *don't* forgive: The body releases masses of "high-voltage" hormones that cause the heart to pound, blood pressure to skyrocket, muscles to contract, and abdominal pains to develop. If the situation continues unchecked, gastric ulcers, gastritis, or irritable bowel syndrome can result. With forgiveness, the anger and resentment dissolve. The body stops pouring high-voltage chemicals into the bloodstream, and the healing begins.

How can you learn to forgive? If you've been the victim of a major trespass — a parent sexually abused you, a mate deserted you — you may need the help of a professional counselor to complete the forgiveness process. But for day-to-day mishaps — a roommate offended you, you were served cold food in a restaurant — you *can* learn to forgive, and it may be easier than you think.

▶ Start out by practicing forgiveness of *very* minor infractions, things that are easy to forgive. Once you've learned the technique there, it's easier to transfer it to more major problems.

▶ Set aside a "forgiveness hour." For that hour, forgive *everything* that happens, even the things *you* do. Expand it to a "forgiveness day." Realize how great you feel to forgive someone instead of lugging around a burden of grudges and hard feelings.

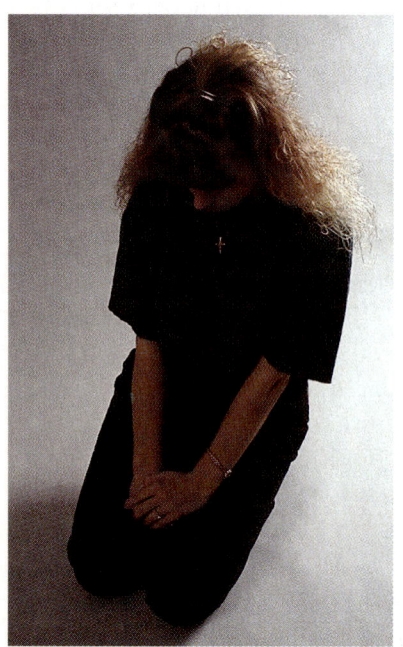

Sincere prayer can enhance health and buffer stress.

- Take a hard look at the way you judge others. Your own judgment, not the actions of someone else, often is what makes forgiveness difficult. Make it a policy to reserve judgment until you have all the facts. Better yet, make it a hard-and-fast rule to postpone all judgments for one year. (Chances are good that you will have forgotten the whole thing by then.)
- Don't say you've "forgiven" someone, then tell all your roommates what happened. Forgiving entails forgetting.
- Learn to forgive yourself, as you're often hardest on yourself. If you have to, say it aloud ("I forgive myself for cutting class and not being up front with the professor"). Learn from your mistakes, but turn them into positives instead of using them as ammunition against yourself forever.

CHURCH AFFILIATION AND HEALTH

According to an article published in *The Gerontologist*, religion is "the personal beliefs, values, and activities pertinent to that which is supernatural, mysterious, and awesome, which transcends immediate situations, and which pertains to questions of final causes and ultimate ends of man and the universe."[33] Basically, religion is a science in how to know God. Research has shown that people with active religious faith and people who are strongly affiliated with a church generally enjoy better health.

According to nationwide surveys, more than 90% of all Americans profess to a belief in God but, according to a recent Gallup poll, 78 million Americans either do not belong to a church or synagogue or they attend only infrequently, on special occasions. Even so, extensive research indicates that active participation in a church or synagogue boosts health, acts as a buffer against stress, and may even prolong life. People who attend a church or synagogue regularly have a much lower rate for a number of diseases than those who attend less frequently or do not attend at all. Churchgoers have especially low rates of heart disease, lung disease, cirrhosis of the liver, and some kinds of cancer.

Even though no one knows for certain how religious participation protects health, probable reasons have been advanced. Many churches prescribe behavior that prevents illness or assists in treating illness; many also discourage behavior that is harmful to health. Organized churches provide social support, reduce loneliness, and place people in support groups in times of need. Churches also promote more positive approaches toward illness, pain, or disability, which can influence the outcome of disease.

Regardless of *why* religion works to boost health, regular attendance or participation seems to be a key. Those who attend and participate regularly reap the greatest health benefits from religion. Regular participation has been shown to increase lifespan and decrease mortality, even after controlling for age and various other risk factors.

Regular church attendance apparently has an impact on a number of specific diseases, too, especially cardiovascular disease. Researchers have found that the more active in a religion a person is, the less chance that person has of incurring myocardial infarction. Regular church attenders also are at lower risk for myocardial degeneration, chronic endocarditis, arteriosclerotic heart disease, and degenerative heart disease. People with high conformity to religious belief have lower blood pressure; a slower, more steady heartbeat; and a healthier cardiovascular system.

Research also has found that regular participation in certain religious organizations can mean specific benefits in some areas. Seventh-Day Adventists have

How to Boost Church Affiliation

If you don't belong to a church now, consider joining. Investigate various religions until you find one that mirrors your general beliefs. If you already belong to a church, synagogue, temple, or mosque, try the following:

▼ Research the general beliefs and principles of the religion. Study. To really participate, you need to know what you're doing.

▼ Actively participate in what the church offers. Your church might offer a singles group or a Bible study; join, attend, and get the most out of what goes on.

▼ Cultivate friendships with the people you meet at church.

▼ Vow to attend meetings regularly. If your church encourages volunteers for various committees or projects, sign up.

a much lower risk of developing cancer, for example. Members of the Church of Jesus Christ of Latter-day Saints (the "Mormons") have lower mortality rates among all ages, lower risk of cancer and heart disease, and fewer fatal illnesses of all kinds. Active Christians in general have a significantly better margin of health than non-Christians or more passive Christians.

ALTRUISM AND HEALTH

One of the aspects of spirituality is altruism, the act of *giving of oneself out of a genuine concern for other people*. Physician and philosopher Albert Schweitzer proclaimed, during a selfless career, what he believed to be the prescription for happiness. True happiness, he said, is to be found only by serving others. New clinical research has verified that service not only is a prescription for happiness but is a prescription for improved health as well.

The ability to put another's needs above one's own seems to contribute to a longer and healthier life. Scientists are beginning to conclude that doing good for others is good for a person, especially for the nervous system and the immune system. The effects of genuine altruism may be so powerful that even *thinking* about altruistic action may boost your immune system.

Researchers at Harvard wanted to do a precise study, so they had volunteers watch three films. The first was a gentle film on gardening; the second a Nazi war commentary; and the third a documentary about Mother Teresa, the Nobel Prize-winning nun who has dedicated charitable works to the poor in India's most poverty-stricken regions. Researchers took saliva samples before and after volunteers watched each of the films. Saliva measurements did not change during the first two films. After viewing the third film, however, the amount of an immune agent — a germ-fighting substance — in the volunteer's saliva rose sharply, even among those who said they disliked Mother Teresa. Volunteers who merely *watched* altruistic service experienced an actual physical change, one that could possibly help them stay healthier.[34]

New evidence shows that the cumulative effects of altruism are positive. Whereas stress can undermine the immune system, the positive emotions related to altruism help stabilize the immune system against the normal immunosuppressing effects of stress. That effect may be so strong that altruism might even help slow down the inevitable deterioration of the immune system as a person ages.

In a landmark study of more than 2,700 people in Tecumseh, Michigan, spanning more than a decade, researchers discovered a powerful testimony for altruism. Those who did regular volunteer work had better health and longer lives. The researchers found that doing volunteer work, more than any other activity, dramatically increased life expectancy, and probably health as well.[35] Among the Michigan residents studied, the men who did no volunteer work were two and a half times more likely to die during the study as men who volunteered at least once a week.

THE ALTRUISTIC PERSONALITY

What makes a person altruistic? Some believe it's instinct, stemming from the time when people lived in small groups of hunters and gatherers. Growing numbers believe altruism is a capacity everyone shares to some extent. Some believe in an altruistic "personality," that altruistic people have certain personality traits that enable them to reach out to others.

Based on a study of rescuers who helped the Jews during Hitler's reign of terror, Samuel Oliner and Pearl Oliner summarized the traits they believe are common to all altruistic people. According to the Oliners, altruistic people never regard others as inferiors; value human relationships more than money; believe ethical values should be applied universally; believe in the right of innocent people to be free from persecution; have a healthy perspective about themselves; are "connected" to others; have a profound commitment to caring; and believe they can control events and shape their own destiny but are willing to risk failure.

University of Massachusetts psychologist Ervin Staub believes altruistic people share three general traits:

1. They have a positive view of people in general.
2. They are concerned about others' welfare.
3. They take personal responsibility for how other people are doing.

In studying outstanding altruists, researcher Christie Kiefer found that background and family values help determine the altruistic personality. The altruists she studied came from families that were warm and nurturing. The emotional self-acceptance they developed in that environment liberated them to be generative, creative, playful, and relaxed.[36]

THE HEALTH BENEFITS OF VOLUNTEERISM

Acts of volunteering, helping, and serving seem to bring important health benefits to the volunteer. According to the national director of the Retired Senior Volunteer Program, doctors claim that elderly people who engage in volunteer work have better health, visit the doctor less often, and have fewer complaints.[37]

Research conducted at Carnegie Mellon University shows that volunteerism causes a release of endorphines resulting in a "helper's high," similar to the "runner's high" experienced during exercising.[38] The "healthy-helper syndrome," as researchers Allan Luks and Howard Andrews dubbed it, starts with a physical high, reported by 95% of the volunteers surveyed. The second stage is a longer-lasting sense of calm and heightened emotional well-being. Together, the two stages are a powerful antidote to stress, a key to happiness and optimism, and a way to combat feelings of helplessness and depression.

According to Luks and Howard, the volunteers who experienced the healthy-helper syndrome noticed an improvement in their own ills, including arthritis, lupus symptoms, asthma attacks, migraine headaches, colds, and bouts of flu. Based on their study, the researchers also believe that volunteerism alleviates the stress and other physiological conditions that lead to heart attack.

The benefits of volunteer work depend on several factors, according to the researchers:

1. The helpers must actually *connect with people* (one-on-one contact with people).
2. The helpers must have a *desire* to help (the word "volunteer" is a key).
3. The helpers must *like* what they are doing.
4. The helpers must be fairly *consistent* (the greatest health benefits have been reaped by those who do consistent, regular volunteer work, at least once a week).

According to researchers, *motive* is important: People do not fare as well if they expect repayment for their altruism or if they expect something in return. The "repayment" some volunteers expect varies tremendously. Some expect monetary reward; others expect payment in the form of more status.

The motivation behind true altruism is also an emotion that protects health and longevity. Love, a projection of one's own good feelings onto other people, promotes health and is important in the healing process. Bernie Siegel claims that love is an important facet of all healing. Based on his own practice as a physician, spanning three decades, he reflects: "Someday we will understand the physiological and psychological workings of love well enough to turn on its full force more reliably. Once it is scientific, it will be accepted."[39]

Research conducted at several universities indicates that the expression of love improves immune function. Those who love others and enjoy intimate relationships have more vital white blood cells, more lymphocytes, a high ratio of helper and suppressor T-cells, and low levels of stress hormones. All of this translates into better immune function and increased ability to resist disease and infection.

Psychotherapist Harmon Bro, a former professor at Syracuse University, emphasizes the importance of early, affirming love. People, he says, who have never developed the capacity for loving find lovelessness reflected in their bodies — in poor health, muscular tension, shallow breathing, and other physical ills that reflect in real ways an illness of the spirit.

Would you like to try your hand at being a volunteer? The best volunteer opportunities:

▶ Provide a regular schedule and a specific description of what the volunteers are expected to do.

▶ Provide personal contact with the people the volunteers are going to help.

▶ Utilize skills the volunteers already have or train them for something they'd like to be able to do.

▶ Fall within volunteers' area of interest. It's easier to stick with the volunteer work if it's something they really enjoy doing.

▶ Expect a reasonable commitment; 2 hours a week is a good goal to shoot for.

Before making a commitment, the volunteer should check out what's available in the area, visit the facilities, watch what goes on, then narrow the choices. Before signing up for volunteer work, the volunteer should get as much information as possible and not be afraid to ask questions.

Volunteering to help others can bring tremendous health benefits, but, if people overextend themselves or get involved in the wrong kind of activity for them, they will get burned out and run the risk of getting sick instead of protecting their health. To guard against burnout, volunteers should:

▶ Not try to do too much. A good goal is roughly 2 hours of volunteer work a week. With a tight schedule, just an hour a week may be advisable.

▶ Do something they enjoy and something they feel comfortable doing. A suicide hotline may be begging for volunteers, but if that kind of work makes a person extremely uncomfortable, another volunteer option would be better.

▶ Realize that *any* line of work, volunteer or paid, has occasional setbacks or bad experiences, but that plenty of good happens in the meantime.

▶ Realize that they are not responsible for anyone else. They can't keep a person from committing suicide or an addict from returning to cocaine. They can provide help and support, but the responsibility is up to the person being helped.

▶ Get out of any situation that isn't right for them; look for something else. Just because the other volunteers seem to be doing well and enjoying themselves, it doesn't mean this specific situation is the best one for everybody.

▼ THE HEALING POWER OF FAITH

French authoress George Sand penned the sentiment that faith "is an excitement and an enthusiasm; it is a condition of intellectual magnificence to which we must cling as to a treasure, and not squander in the small coin of empty words." If the results of scientific studies are correct, faith is, as Sand stated, a treasure — not only in the spiritual sense of the word but also as a potent factor in good health and healing.

Medical and scientific research conducted over the past two decades or so has demonstrated clearly that what exists is not as important as what we *believe* to exist. Personal belief gives us an unseen power that enables us to do the impossible, to perform miracles, even to heal ourselves. Patients with faith become less concerned about their symptoms, have less severe symptoms, and have symptoms less frequently with longer periods of relief than patients who lack faith.

History is rich with examples of people who have been affected by faith's healing power. According to cardiologist Herbert Benson, medical and scientific research is demonstrating ever more clearly that the things we can touch, taste, and measure frequently have to take a back seat to what we *perceive* or *believe* to be real. If the mind is that powerful, what the mind believes can have tremendous influence over the body. Apparently, Benson says, just having a strong belief is enough to cause things to happen in our physiology.

According to Benson, countless studies have shown that faith has a powerful influence over the body. It has relieved headaches, reduced angina pains, controlled hypertension, overcome insomnia, prevented hyperventilation attacks, helped alleviate backaches, enhanced cancer treatment, controlled panic attacks, reduced cholesterol levels, lowered overall stress, and alleviated the symptoms of anxiety (including nausea, vomiting, diarrhea, and constipation).

A good example of faith's power over physiological processes is its influence over blood pressure. According to researchers in Virginia and Texas, devoutly faithful groups of people tend to have lower blood pressure.[40]

Faith also apparently increases the ability to resist stress, and it strengthens the body against the physical changes that accompany stress. One study measured the daily amounts of hydrocortisone (an adrenal hormone secreted in response to stress) in women for the 3 days before a group of women underwent biopsies for breast cancer. These women, who were in a literally life-threatening situation, were expected to have high levels of the hormone. Some did not, and they were the ones who reported their faith and prayer helped them cope with life's stressful events.[41]

The power of faith is probably apparent in the healing process more than any other aspect of medicine. Researcher Daniel Goleman maintains that faith is the hidden ingredient in Western medicine and every traditional system of healing. A large number of illnesses can be treated more successfully if the patient believes in a cure.[42]

One of the best-known healing shrines is Lourdes, a healing spring in the French countryside that attracts more than 2 million pilgrims each year, who travel to the site from all parts of the world in the hope of being healed. For most, the journey is a last resort. They have been told their condition has no cure. Many people are, indeed, healed, probably as a result of the expectant faith of the pilgrim who comes to be healed.

One of the most striking and profound examples of how faith influences even the course of medication is the well-known story of a patient treated by Dr. Bruno Klopfer in the late 1950s. The patient was suffering from a widespread lymphoma — a serious cancer of the immune system — that was in its late stages. At the time, a drug called Krebiozen was being touted as a cure for cancer. The patient demanded that Klopfer administer Krebiozen, and the doctor agreed. Within 2 days of receiving the Krebiozen, the patient had a remarkable turnaround. According to one account, the large tumors that covered his body began "melting like snowballs." After 10 days of treatment with Krebiozen, the patient was released from the hospital, apparently free of disease. Klopfer believed a medical miracle had occurred, but it was because of the patient's faith in the Krebiozen, not the drug itself. As fate would have it, that faith was short-lived. A few months after the patient was released from the hospital, newspapers around the country announced that Krebiozen was worthless. The patient's tumors promptly reappeared.

Klopfer was fascinated by this turn of events. Based on the patient's history, he strongly suspected the patient's *belief* was what had cured him and that the drug had nothing to do with it. Klopfer became convinced that he once again could harness the man's faith if the conditions were right. He called his patient in, reassured him, told him that the newspaper accounts were inaccurate, and that an extra-strength, improved, refined form of the drug had just been released to physicians. Klopfer offered this "refined" form of the drug to his eager patient. Klopfer didn't actually have any improved Krebiozen. What he gave his patient was actually distilled water. With distilled water coursing through his veins, the patient who believed he had a new super Krebiozen staged another remarkable recovery. Within days, his tumors again disappeared. He was released from the hospital a second time, apparently disease-free.

Unfortunately, that didn't last either. Three months after his recovery, the patient read a newspaper report published by the American Medical Association. Definitive tests had proven beyond a doubt, the report said, that Krebiozen was worthless. Top-ranking officials in the American Medical Association proclaimed the drug as useless in the fight against cancer. The patient, who had left the hospital 3 months earlier free of tumors, read the report. His faith was shattered. His tumors ballooned. Two days after he read the newspaper report, he literally laid down and died.

THE HEALING POWER OF HOPE

Hope — defined as *a wealth of optimism, a want of fear* — apparently is one of the strongest influences on health and the human body. Medical lore is replete with examples of "terminal" patients who, awash with hope, defied all medical odds. Some lived months or years longer than predicted. Some were able to remain symptom-free and enjoyed comfort for the last period of their lives. Some defied the odds in a total way: They lived, and they were healed. More and more, physicians are finding that hope is a powerful tool in their work with patients.

Psychologist Robert Ornstein and physician David Sobel define hope as "a special type of positive expectation. Unlike denial, which involves a negation of reality, hope is an active way of coping with threatening situations by focusing on the positive. No matter how dark or grim a situation may appear, certain people seem to be able to extract the positive aspects and concentrate on them. They fill their mind with hopeful scenarios, stories with happy endings, or lucky outcomes."[42]

Hope has a powerful influence on the physical health and well-being of all of us. It can bring not only enhanced health but a longer life as well. Dr. Elisabeth Kubler-Ross, whose work with dying patients revolutionized the medical profession, stressed the importance of hope, saying that dying patients insist on holding on to some hope. Even though they can't hope for a cure, she says, "they can hope for a few more days or hours of life, for contact with loved ones, for freedom from pain, or for peaceful death with dignity. . . . Hope is a satisfaction unto itself and need not be fulfilled to be appreciated."

Physicians and patients alike are beginning to speak out more frequently about the importance of hope. Hope sets in motion an entirely new set of expectations. It boosts belief about what can be achieved, and it makes possible the setting of new goals. Washington, DC journalist Natalie Davis Spingarn, who has lived with cancer for 10 years, claims that "hope is the essential ingredient. Without it, patients find no reason for struggling to survive; without it, we find it easy to give up and stay in bed."[44]

HOPELESSNESS VERSUS HOPE

If hope can profoundly influence health for the better, its opposite, hopelessness, can have the opposite effect.[45] According to a definition in the *Journal of Psychosocial Nursing*, hopelessness is marked by negative future expectations and the belief that the future holds nothing good or positive. It also is characterized by the inability to reach a desired goal, futility in planning for goals, and a lack of motivation for taking constructive action to gain control of life. Further, people who feel hopeless usually feel despondent, desperate, and despairing; they feel they have lost control and feel helpless about what the future holds.

In an editorial published in the *Western Journal of Medicine*,[46] Los Angeles physician Alexandra Levine gives a poignant example of what happens when hope is lost. She remembers a 55-year-old woman who was admitted to the hospital with a lesion in the upper lobe of her lung. Levine describes her as "a real dynamo, vigorous and friendly. She became the extra pair of hands on the ward, helping to pass the meal trays, running minor errands. We all came to love her."

When the woman underwent biopsy, it revealed a deadly cancer that already had invaded the nodes. The surgeons could not remove it, so they closed the incision. The next day a group of residents and interns surrounded her bed. One of them looked down and said, "Well, it's cancer, and we couldn't really resect it, so we just opened and closed."

The patient kept repeating the question, "Opened and closed?" As the intern nodded and repeatedly confirmed the procedure, she finally asked, "You mean you left the cancer in there?" "Yes," he replied. She closed her eyes and told the interns she was tired. They left the room.

The woman died that night. The autopsy indicated no specific cause of death, just the cancer, but it had been there for months. Levine wrote, "I have never been able to get her words out of my mind . . . I don't really know why she died, but to be honest, I will always believe that she died because all hope had been taken away from her. . . . The resident's words took away her hope, and I honestly believe, as crazy as it may seem, that those words took away some of her potential lifetime."

THE IMPACT OF HOPE ON HEALTH

Researchers in the field of psychoneuroimmunology have found that what happens in the brain — our thoughts and emotions, the attitudes with which we face the world — can have a definite effect on the body. An attitude such as hope is not just a mental state; it causes specific electrochemical changes in the body that influence not only the strength of the immune system but the workings of individual organs in the body as well.

Norman Cousins is perhaps best known for his work with what he calls "the biology of hope." As he explains it, hope is tremendous expectation, and expectation can have a powerful influence over the human body. One of his favorite examples of expectation occurred when a man collapsed on the Rancho Golf Course near Cousins's home. Paramedics were there, and from the monitor Cousins could see that the man was having premature contractions of the heart. The paramedics were not talking to the man. Cousins leaned over and assured the man that he was in good hands and would be just fine within a few minutes. Cousins kept his eye on the cardiac monitor. Within *30 seconds*, the cardiogram began to change. In just 2 minutes, the man's heartbeat had slowed, and his pulse was under 100 beats per minute.

Hope is so powerful and so real, say an increasing number of physicians, that it can influence the outcome of supposedly terminal and irreversible diseases, such as cancer. Siegel says, "If there is one thing I learned from my years of working with cancer patients, it's that there is no such thing as false hope. Hope is real and physiological. It's something I feel perfectly comfortable giving people — no matter what their situation. I know people are alive today because I said to them, 'You don't have to die'."[47]

In a variety of studies, hope has been shown to be a surprisingly accurate predictor of cancer. Two

Are Your Thoughts Helping or Hurting Your Longevity?

Does an extraordinary challenge make you freeze up with fear? Do you let yourself dwell on minor slights? If so, you're prone to destructive thinking patterns that can prevent you from doing your best, fostering successful relationships and, in general, coping well and living long. Pessimists are less likely to survive major surgery, for example. And anyone who's easily offended will have trouble enjoying the camaraderie that is a key to living a long life.

The antidote for destructive thoughts is cultivating constructive ones. To help you do that, Seymour Epstein, Ph.D., professor of psychology at the University of Massachusetts and author of *You're Smarter Than You Think*, adapted the following quiz from a psychological test he uses to help patients strengthen their coping skills. This exercise will tell how constructive a thinker you are overall and identify the areas that could stand some pumping up.

Rate each statement from 1 to 5 according to this scale:

 1 = completely false
 2 = mainly false
 3 = undecided
 4 = mainly true
 5 = completely true

Be honest. Don't answer according to how you think you should be but how you naturally are.

1. I don't worry about things I can do nothing about. _____
2. I am the kind of person who takes action, not just complains about things. _____
3. I don't let little things bother me. _____
4. If I have an unpleasant chore to do, I try to make the best of it by thinking in positive terms. _____
5. I don't feel I have to perform exceptionally well in order to consider myself a worthwhile person. _____
6. I look at challenges not as something to fear, but as opportunities to test myself and learn. _____
7. I tend to dwell more on pleasant than unpleasant incidents from the past. _____
8. When I have a difficult task, I think encouraging thoughts that help me do my best. _____
9. I tend not to take things personally. _____
10. When faced with upcoming unpleasant events, I usually think carefully how I will deal with them. _____

Total A _____

11. I feel that if people treat you badly, you should treat them in kind. _____
12. Talking about something I want to succeed at all but ensures failure. _____
13. I believe in astrology. _____
14. There are two kinds of people: good and bad. _____
15. When something good happens to me, I believe it will be balanced by something bad. _____
16. I have at least one good-luck charm. _____
17. There are many wrong ways to do something, but only one right way. _____
18. I believe in good and bad omens. _____
19. I believe in ghosts. _____
20. I tend to classify people as being either for or against me. _____
21. I sometimes think that if I want something to happen too badly, it probably won't. _____
22. I believe some people are able to read other people's thoughts. _____
23. I tend to be very judgmental. _____
24. I've learned not to hope for something too much — that usually means it won't happen. _____
25. I believe there are people who can literally see into the future. _____

Total B (90 minus total for 11-25) _____

Grand Total (A + B) _____

SCORING

Above 99 = VERY HIGH. You are a very constructive thinker. Keep up the good work.

89-99 = HIGH. You are a better-than-average constructive thinker. You usually expect good things to happen and they often do. But there's room for improvement.

74-88 = AVERAGE. Like most people, you're prone to some destructive thoughts. Go back through the exercise and try to identify a pattern. For example, statements 11, 14, 17, 20 and 23 represent categorical thinking — seeing situations and people as either good or bad; statements 12, 15, 18, 21 and 24 are examples of superstitious thinking; and 13, 16, 19, 22 and 25 show a kind of thinking that relies on belief in the paranormal. If you gave more than a 3 to these questions, try to catch yourself before lapsing into your usual assumptions. In addition, shore up your constructive thinking by reviewing the positive statements, 1 through 10, paying particular attention to those to which you gave less than a 3.

63-73 = LOW. Your habitual thinking is somewhat more destructive than most people's, and it interferes with your happiness and efficiency. Follow the advice given for average scorers. You have much to gain from working hard to improve your constructive thinking.

Below 63 = VERY LOW. Your destructive thinking is likely to be the source of serious problems. Work at identifying and correcting it. If you have trouble doing so, consider seeing a therapist. But regardless, don't expect your destructive thoughts to go away overnight.

researchers with the Carrier Foundation in New Jersey concluded from their studies that hope was as great a factor in predicting lung cancer as was cigarette smoking. Those who felt hopeless were dramatically more likely to develop lung cancer.

In another study, Dr. Arthur Schmale and Dr. Howard Iker interviewed a number of women who were coming to the hospital for a cervical biopsy. Each woman was rated according to the amount of hope she had. When the biopsy results came in, the findings were surprising: Of the 18 who lacked hope, 11 were diagnosed with cancer. Of the 33 who were brimming with hope, only 7 were diagnosed with cancer.[48]

In a separate but similar study, Schmale and Iker tried to predict which women would be diagnosed with cervical cancer based on their attitudes prior to their biopsies. They were able to predict with 68% accuracy which women had cancer, based only on their attitudes of hopelessness. And they were able to predict accurately 77% of the cancer-free women, based solely on their hopeful attitudes.[49]

Studies have shown that an attitude of hope contributes significantly to the healing process. In one study, physicians, social workers, and health professionals worked to transform a bleak Veterans Administration hospital into a place of hope, where patients could expect to be healed and eventually discharged from care. Results of the program were "impressive": Even though most patients had been hospitalized from 3 to 10 years, the discharge rate rose to 70% within 3 months. The discharge rate continued over the next 2½ years. Even more impressive, 40% of those who were released became self-supporting, which means they were not only physically healthier but also psychologically better adjusted.[50]

Hope can function as a survival factor. In a report published in *Medical World News*, the writers proclaimed that hope can play an important role in vulnerability to disease, the course of illness, and possibly in determining whether a patient lives or dies. University of Arkansas psychiatrist Fred Henker stated in the same report that "whether we acknowledge the influence of hope or not, it's real, and it may even determine the life or death outcome of a patient."[51]

DENIAL: MAKING ROOM FOR HOPE

At first thought, denial may seem to be a negative emotion. As we have learned through the work of countless researchers, negative emotions tend to have a negative effect on health. Denial can be positive, however, especially for health. Denial makes room for hope. In regard to serious illness, Norman Cousins remarked, "Don't deny the diagnosis. Try to defy the verdict."[52]

Researchers do point out the difference between total denial — the kind that does not leave room for hope — and "informed denial," which allows for and actually inspires hope. In one study conducted at Yale University, men who had suffered a heart attack or coronary bypass surgery (or both) were followed for a year after being discharged from the hospital. The deniers did better at first. They spent less time in the hospital and had fewer complications while they were there. Once they were discharged from the hospital, however, they didn't do as well. They were in total denial, which kept them from taking steps to improve their chances of recovery.[53]

Informed denial, on the other hand, allows for hope. According to psychologist Richard Lazarus of the University of California, Berkeley, "Illusion can sometimes allow hope, which is healthy. The critical determinant is whether you're denying facts or the implications. Let's say I get a biopsy that says I have a malignant tumor. I can face the facts, decide that this is a terrible illness, that I'm in trouble, will die very soon, and so give up hope. Or I can face the fact that this is a serious illness, but acknowledge the ambiguity; people sometimes recover; it's curable. I've got to be treated, but I don't have to give up."[54]

In summing up the importance of hope, Cousins leaves us with this thought:

> Hope, faith, love, and a strong will to live offer no promise of immortality, only proof of our uniqueness as human beings and the opportunity to experience full growth even under the grimmest circumstances. The clock provides only a technical measurement of how long we live. Far more real than the ticking of time is the way we open up the minutes and invest them with meaning. Death is not the ultimate tragedy in life. The ultimate tragedy is to die without discovering the possibilities of full growth."[55]

NOTES

1. Martin E. P. Seligman, *Learned Optimism* (New York: Alfred A. Knopf, 1991), p. 178.
2. Seligman.
3. "Mind Over Cancer: An Exclusive Interview with Yale Surgeon Dr. Bernie Siegel," *Prevention*, March 1988, pp. 59-64.
4. Carolyn Jabs, "New Reasons to be An Optimist," *Self*, September 1987, pp. 170-173.
5. Nan Silver, "Do Optimists Live Longer?" *American Health*, November 1986, pp. 50-53.
6. Silver.
7. Leslie Kamen-Siegel, Judith Rodin, Martin E. P. Seligman, and John Dwyer, "Explanatory Style and Cell-Mediated Immunity in Elderly Men and Women," *Health Psychology*, 10:4 (1991), pp. 229-235.
8. Daniel Goleman, "The Mind Over the Body," *New Realities*, March/April 1988, pp. 14-19.
9. Aaron Antonovsky, *Unraveling the Mystery of Health: How People Manage Stress and Stay Well* (San Francisco, CA: Jossey-Bass Publishers, 1987), pp. 36-37.
10. Phillip L. Rice, *Stress and Health* (Monterey, California: Brooks/Cole Publishing Company, 1987), p. 109.
11. Norman Cousins, *Head First: The Biology of Hope* (New York: E. P. Dutton, 1989), p. 120.
12. *Clinical Psychiatry News*, as reported in "Health Briefs," *Executive Fitness*, November 1987, p. 8.
13. S. G. Haynes, "Type A Behavior, Employment Status, and Coronary Heart Disease in Women," *Behavioral Medicine Update*, 6:4 (1984), pp. 11-15.
14. Sandra M. Levy, *Emotional Expression and Survival in Breast Cancer Patients: Immunological Correlates*, Paper Presented at the Meetings of the American Psychological Association, August 1983, Anaheim, California.
15. Case cited in Steven Locke and Douglas Colligan, *The Healer Within* (New York: E. P. Dutton, 1986), p. 96.
16. Blair Justice, *Who Gets Sick: Thinking and Health* (Houston, Texas: Peak Press, 1987), pp. 61-62.
17. "Research Strengthens Link Between Poor Mental and Physical Health," *Sexuality Today Newsletter*, November 24, 1986, p. 4.
18. Steven Locke and Douglas Colligan, *The Healer Within* (New York: E. P. Dutton, 1986), pp. 131-132.
19. Cited in Ornstein and Sobel, *The Healing Brain*, pp. 246-248.
20. Ornstein and Sobel, *The Healing Brain*, pp. 249-250.
21. Morris Rosenberg, *Society and The Adolescent Self-Image*.
22. Joan Borysenko, and Myrin Borysenko, "On Psychoneuroimmunology: How the Mind Influences Health and Disease ...and How to Make the Influence Beneficial," *Executive Health*, 19:10 (July 1983).
23. Steve Fishman, "Absolutely, Positively, Refusing to Die," *Longevity*, September 1990, p. 69.
24. Donald Robinson, "Mind Over Disease: Your Attitude Can Make You Well," *Reader's Digest*, April 1987, pp. 73-78.
25. Editors, *The Complete Book of Cancer Prevention*.
26. Florence Graves, "The High Priest of Healing," *New Age Journal*, May/June 1989, p. 34.
27. Larry S. Chapman, "Developing a Useful Perspective on Spiritual Health: Love, Joy, Peace, and Fulfillment," *American Journal of Health Promotion*, Fall, 1987, p. 12.
28. From "The Spirit of Health," *Advances: Journal of the Institute for the Advancement of Health*, 5:4 (1988), p. 4.
29. Graves.
30. Herbert Benson, *Your Maximum Mind* (New York: Times Books/Random House, Inc., 1987), p. 6.
31. "Does Prayer Help Patients?" *MD*, December 1986, p. 35; and Blair Justice, *Who Gets Sick: Thinking and Health* (Houston, Texas: Peak Press, 1987), p. 284.
32. Joan Borysenko, *Minding the Body, Mending the Mind* (Reading, Massachusetts: Addison-Wesley Publishing Company, Inc., 1987), p. 176.
33. Harold G. Koenig, James N. Kvale, and Carolyn Ferrel, "Religion and Well-Being in Later Life," *The Gerontologist*, 28:1 (1988), pp. 18-27.
34. Eileen Rockefeller Growald and Allan Luks, "Beyond Self," *American Health*, March 1988, pp. 51-53.
35. Growald and Luks, pp. 51-53.
36. "Research: Altruism and Transformation," *Noetic Sciences Review*, Autumn 1990, p. 33.
37. Allan Luks with Peggy Payne, "Helper's High," *New Age Journal*, September/October 1991, pp. 49, 121; from Allan Luks with Peggy Payne, *The Healing Power of Doing Good: The Health and Spiritual Benefits of Helping Others* (Ballantine Books, 1991).
38. Allan Luks, "Helper's High," *Psychology Today*, October 1988, p. 39.
39. Blair Justice, "Think Yourself Healthy," *Prevention*, June 1988, pp. 31-32, 105-108.
40. Sarah Lang, "Extend Your Hand, Extend Your Life," *Longevity*, March 1989, p. 18.
41. S. I. McMillen, *None of These Diseases*, revised (Old Tappan, New Jersey: Fleming H. Revell Company, 1984), pp. 188-189.
42. Tom Hurley, "Another Look at Altruism: Notes on an International Conference," *Noetic Sciences Building*, August/September 1989, p. 3.
43. Robert Ornstein and David Sobel, *The Healing Brain* (New York: Simon and Schuster, 1987), p. 243.
44. "Hope: That Sustainer of Man," *Executive Health*, Section II, 20:3 (December 1983), pp. 1-4.
45. *Journal of Psychosocial Nursing*, 25:2 (1987), p. 21.
46. Alexandra M. Levine, "The Importance of Hope," *Western Journal of Medicine*, 150 (May 1989), p. 609.

47. "Mind Over Cancer: An Exclusive Interview with Yale Surgeon Dr. Bernie Siegel," *Prevention*, March 1988, pp. 59-64.
48. Ornstein and Sobel.
49. Ornstein and Sobel, p. 245.
50. Jerome Frank, "The Medical Power of Faith," *Human Nature*, August 1978, pp. 40-47.
51. "Studies Show Hope Can Play Role in a Patient's Risk, Illness, Death," *Medical World News*, June 11, 1984, pp. 101-102.
52. Cousins.
53. Beryl Lieff Benderly, "Ill-Fated Denial," *Psychology Today*.
54. Ornstein and Sobel, p. 242.
55. Norman Cousins, *Head First: The Biology of Hope* (New York: E. P. Dutton, 1989), pp. 65-66.

Fitness Assessment For Wellness

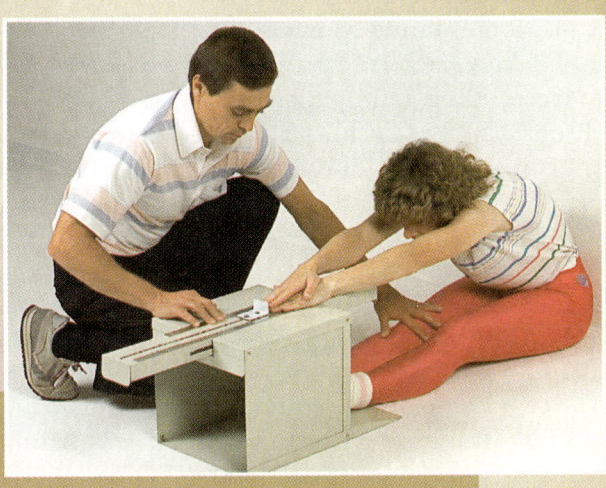

Objectives

▼ Define physical fitness.

▼ Identify the major health problems in the United States.

▼ Learn the difference between health standards and physical fitness standards.

▼ Understand the benefits and the significance of participating in a lifetime fitness program.

▼ Identify risk factors that may interfere with safe exercise participation.

▼ List the components of health-related and skill-related fitness.

▼ Learn to assess cardiovascular endurance, strength endurance, and flexibility.

▼ Be able to interpret health-related fitness test results.

Movement and physical activity are basic functions for which the human organism was created. Advances in modern technology, however, have almost completely eliminated the need for physical activity in the daily life of most people.

Physical activity is no longer a natural part of our existence. We live in an automated society, in which most of the activities that used to require strenuous physical exertion can be accomplished by machines with the simple pull of a handle or push of a button. The available scientific evidence shows that physical inactivity and a sedentary lifestyle pose a serious threat to our health and rapidly increase the deterioration rate of the human body.

At the beginning of the 20th century, the most common health problems in the United States were infectious diseases such as tuberculosis, diphtheria, influenza, kidney disease, polio, and other diseases of infancy. Progress in the field of medicine largely eliminated these diseases. Nevertheless, as the American people started to enjoy the "good life" (sedentary living, alcohol, fatty foods, excessive sweets, tobacco, drugs), a parallel increase was seen in chronic diseases such as hypertension, atherosclerosis, coronary heart disease, strokes, diabetes, cancer, emphysema, and cirrhosis of the liver.

▼ FITNESS AND HEALTH

The two leading causes of death in the United States are cardiovascular disease and cancer, accounting for approximately 70% of all deaths in 1991. During the late 1960s and in the 1970s, scientists began to realize that good fitness was important in the fight against chronic diseases, particularly those of the cardiovascular system. In the 1980s, research also pointed toward lower cancer incidence and death rates among exercise participants.

Consequently, a fitness and wellness trend gradually took hold over the last two and a half decades. People began to realize that good health is largely self-controlled and that the leading causes of premature death and illness in the United States could be prevented by adhering to a healthy lifestyle program.

Several significant research studies linking physical activity habits and mortality rates have shown a decrease in premature mortality rates among physically active people. Work conducted by Dr. Ralph Paffenbarger and colleagues,[1] published in the *Journal of the American Medical Association*, showed that as the amount of weekly physical activity increased, the risk of cardiovascular deaths decreased. The results of this study, conducted among 16,936 Harvard alumni, indicated that the greatest decrease in cardiovascular deaths was observed among alumni who used in excess of 2,000 calories per week through physical activity (see Figure 6.1).

Another major study, also published in the *Journal of the American Medical Association*, conducted by Dr. Steve Blair and associates,[2] upheld the findings of the Harvard alumni study. Based on data from 13,344 people who were followed over an average of 8 years, the results confirmed that the level of cardiovascular fitness is related to mortality from all causes.

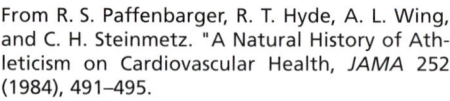
From R. S. Paffenbarger, R. T. Hyde, A. L. Wing, and C. H. Steinmetz. "A Natural History of Athleticism on Cardiovascular Health, *JAMA* 252 (1984), 491–495.

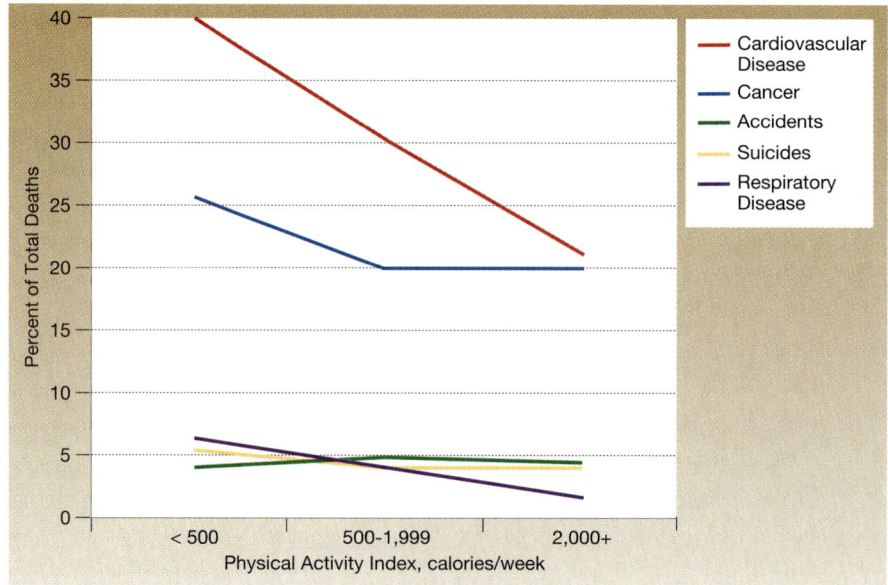

FIGURE 6.1 ▼ Cause-specific death rates per 10,000 man-years of observation among 16,936 Harvard alumni, 1962–1978, by physical activity index. Adjusted for differences in age, cigarette smoking, and hypertension.

The results of this research showed a graded and consistent inverse relationship between cardiovascular fitness and mortality, regardless of age and other risk factors. In essence, the higher the level of cardiovascular fitness, the longer the life (see Figure 6.2). Death-rate from all causes for the least fit (group 1) men was 3.4 times higher than it was for the most fit men. For the least fit women, the death rate was 4.6 times higher than it was for the most fit women.

The study also reported a much lower rate of premature deaths even at moderate fitness levels that most adults can achieve. Even greater protection was attained when a higher fitness level was combined with elimination of other risk factors such as hypertension, high cholesterol, cigarette smoking, and excessive body fat.

The importance of regular physical activity in preventing disease and enhancing quality of life was clearly pointed out in July of 1993 at a news briefing held at the National Press Club in Washington, D.C. At this briefing, the American College of Sports Medicine and the U.S. Centers for Disease Control and Prevention, in conjunction with the President's Council on Physical Fitness and Sports, provided the American public with a set of recommendations on the types and amounts of physical activity that are needed for maintenance and promotion of health.

In this summary statement, every American is encouraged to accumulate at least 30 minutes of moderate-intensity physical activity on an almost daily basis. Such daily routine has been labeled as an effective way to improve health. Some of the activities recommended include: walking part or all the way to and from work, walking up stairs, gardening, raking leaves, and dancing. The 30 minutes of physical activity also can be conducted during a planned exercise program (for example, jogging, cycling, or swimming). The entire contents of this statement on the benefits of physical activity are given in Figure 6.3.

▼ BENEFITS OF A LIFETIME PHYSICAL FITNESS PROGRAM

Many benefits accrue from participating in a regular fitness and wellness program, including a better chance to live longer. Most people exercise because it improves personal appearance and makes them feel good about themselves. The greatest benefit of all, however, is that physically fit individuals enjoy a better quality of life. These people live life to its

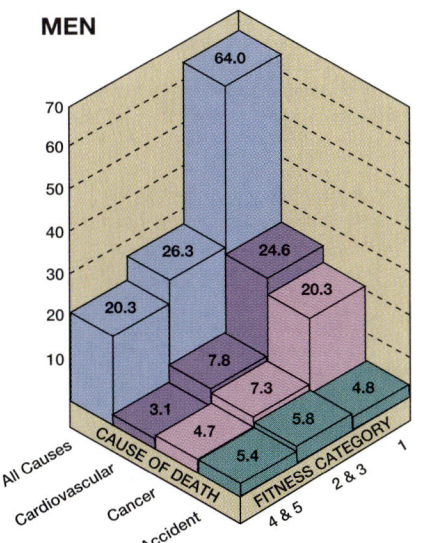
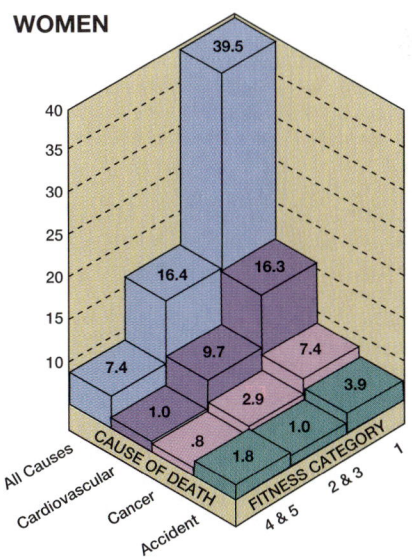

Least fit group = 1, most fit group = 5

Based on data from S. N. Blair, H. W. Kohl III, R. S. Paffenbarger, Jr., D. G. Clark, K. H. Cooper, and L. W. Gibbons, "Physical Fitness and All-Cause Mortality: A Prospective Study of Healthy Men and Women, *JAMA* 262 (1989), 2395–2401. Aerobics Center Longitudinal Study in Dallas, Texas.

FIGURE 6.2 ▼ Age-Adjusted Cause-Specific Death Rates per 10,000 Person-Years of Follow-up (1970–1985) by Physical Fitness Groups (one person-year indicates one person followed up 1 year later).

— SUMMARY STATEMENT —
Workshop On
Physical Activity and Public Health

Sponsored By:
U. S. Centers for Disease Control and Prevention
and
American College of Sports Medicine

In Cooperation with the President's Council on Physical Fitness and Sports

Regular physical activity is an important component of a healthy lifestyle — preventing disease and enhancing health and quality of life. A persuasive body of scientific evidence, which has accumulated over the past several decades, indicates that regular, moderate-intensity physical activity confers substantial health benefits. Because of this evidence, the U.S. Public Health Service has identified increased physical activity as a priority in Healthy People 2000, our national health objectives for the year 2000.

A primary benefit of regular physical activity is protection against coronary heart disease. In addition, physical activity appears to provide some protection against several other chronic diseases such as adult-onset diabetes, hypertension, certain cancers, osteoporosis, and depression. Furthermore, on average, physically active people outlive inactive people, even if they start their activity late in life. It is estimated that more than 250,000 deaths per year in the U.S. can be attributed to lack of regular physical activity, a number comparable to the deaths attributed to other chronic disease risk factors such as obesity, high blood pressure, and elevated blood cholesterol.

Despite the recognized value of physical activity, few Americans are regularly active. Only 22% of adults engage in leisure time physical activity at the level recommended for health benefits in Healthy People 2000. Fully 24% of adult Americans are completely sedentary and are badly in need of more physical activity. The remaining 54% are inadequately active and they too would benefit from more physical activity. Participation in regular physical activity appears to have gradually increased during the 1960s, 1970s, and early 1980s, but has plateaued in recent years. Among ethnic minority populations, older persons, and those with lower incomes or levels of education, participation in regular physical activity has remained consistently low.

Why are so few Americans physically active? Perhaps one answer is that previous public health efforts to promote physical activity have overemphasized the importance of high-intensity exercise. The current low rate of participation may be explained, in part, by the perception of many people that they must engage in vigorous, continuous exercise to reap health benefits. Actually the scientific evidence clearly demonstrates that regular, moderate-intensity physical activity provides substantial health benefits. A group of experts brought together by the U.S. Centers for Disease Control and Prevention (CDC) and the American College of Sports Medicine (ACSM) reviewed the pertinent scientific evidence and formulated the following recommendation:

Every American adult should accumulate 30 minutes or more of moderate-intensity physical activity over the course of most days of the week. Incorporating more activity into the daily routine is an effective way to improve health. Activities that can contribute to the 30-minute total include walking up stairs (instead of taking the elevator), gardening, raking leaves, dancing, and walking part or all of the way to or from work. The recommended 30 minutes of physical activity may also come from planned exercise or recreation such as jogging, playing tennis, swimming, and cycling. One specific way to meet the standard is to walk two miles briskly.

Because most adult Americans fail to meet this recommended level of moderate-intensity physical activity, almost all should strive to increase their participation in moderate or vigorous physical activity. Persons who currently do not engage in regular physical activity should begin by incorporating a few minutes of increased activity into their day, building up gradually to 30 minutes of additional physical activity. Those who are irregularly active should strive to adopt a more consistent pattern of activity. Regular participation in physical activities that develop and maintain muscular strength and joint flexibility is also recommended.

This recommendation has been developed to emphasize the important health benefits of moderate physical activity. But recognizing the benefits of physical activity is only part of the solution to this important public health problem. Today's high-tech society entices people to be inactive. Cars, television, and labor-saving devices have profoundly changed the way many people perform their jobs, take care of their homes, and use their leisure time. Furthermore, our surroundings often present significant barriers to participation in physical activity. Walking to the corner store proves difficult if there are no sidewalks; riding a bicycle to work is not an option unless safe bike lanes or paths are available.

Many Americans will not change their lifestyles until the environmental and social barriers to physical activity are reduced or eliminated. Individuals can help to overcome these barriers by modifying their own lifestyles and by encouraging family members and friends to become more active. In addition, local, state, and federal public health agencies; recreation boards; school groups; professional organizations; and fitness and sports organizations should work together to disseminate this critical public health message and to promote national, community, worksite, and school programs that help Americans become more physically active.

The American College of Sports Medicine and the U.S. Centers for Disease Control and Prevention, in cooperation with the President's Council on Physical Fitness and Sports, released this statement July 29, 1993, at the National Press Club in Washington, D.C.

From Summary Statement: Workshop On Physical Activity and Public Health, sponsored by U.S. Centers for Disease Control and Prevention and American College of Sports Medicine, *Sports Medicine Bulletin,* 28(4), 7. Reproduced by permission.

FIGURE 6.3 ▼ Summary Statement: Workshop On Physical Activity and Public Health.

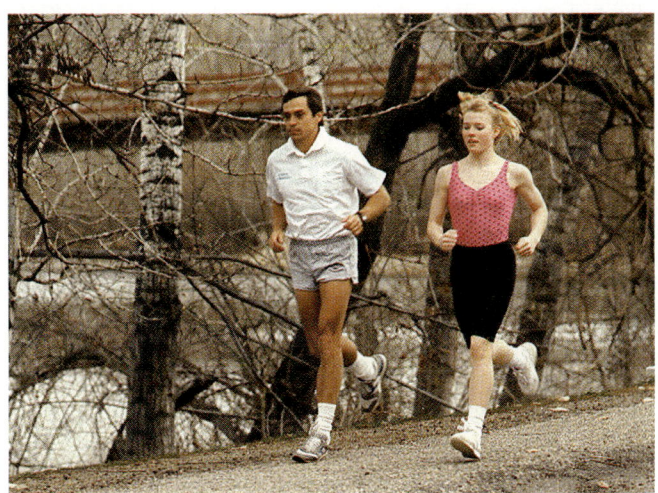

Regular participation in a lifetime exercise program increases quality of life and longevity.

fullest potential, with fewer health problems than inactive individuals who also may indulge in negative lifestyle patterns.

In addition to health benefits, the economic impact of sedentary living has left a strong impression on the nation's economy. As the need for physical exertion steadily decreased during the last century, the nation's health care expenditures dramatically increased. Health care costs in the United States have risen from $12 billion in 1950 to more than $800 billion in 1993.

If the rate of escalation continues, health care expenditures could double every five years. The 1993 figure represents more than 12% of the gross national product (GNP), and it is projected to reach 17% by the year 2000 and 37% by 2030. The 1989 average health care cost per person in the United States ($2,354) was almost twice as high as most other industrialized nations, including Great Britain ($836), (West) Germany ($1,232), France ($1,274), and Switzerland ($1,376).

As a result of the recent staggering rise in medical costs, many organizations are beginning to realize that it costs less to keep employees healthy than to treat them once they are sick. Consequently, health care cost containment, through fitness and wellness programs, has become a major issue for many organizations around the country.

The Prudential Insurance Company of Houston, Texas, released the findings of a study conducted on its 1,386 employees. Those who participated for at least a year in the company's fitness program averaged 3.5 days of disability, as compared to 8.6 days for nonparticipants. A further breakdown by level of fitness showed no disability days for those in the high fitness group, 1.6 days for the good fitness group, and 4.1 disability days for the fair fitness group.

Data analysis conducted by Tenneco Inc., Houston, Texas, showed a significant reduction in medical care costs for men and women who participated in an exercise program. Annual medical care costs for male and female exercisers were about 44% to 58% lower than for the nonexercising group. Sick leave also was lower among the men and women exercisers.

Furthermore, a survey of the more than 3,000 employees in the Tenneco study found that job productivity is related to fitness. The company reported that individuals with high job performance ratings also rated high in exercise participation.

Strong data also are coming in from Europe. Research in Germany (West Germany prior to reunification) reported 68.6% less absenteeism by workers with cardiovascular symptoms who participated in a fitness program. In Germany, the law mandates that corporations employing workers for sedentary jobs must provide an in-house facility for physical exercise. The Goodyear Company in Norrkoping, Sweden, indicated a 50% reduction in absenteeism following implementation of a fitness program. Studies in the former Soviet Union reported increased physical work capacity and motor coordination, lower incidence of disease, shorter duration of illness, and fewer relapses among individuals participating in industrial fitness programs.

▼ THE FITNESS CHALLENGE FOR THE 21st CENTURY

A better and healthier life is something every person should strive to attain. As we approach the 21st century, the biggest challenge is to teach people how to take control of their personal health habits by engaging in positive lifestyle activities. With impressive data available on the benefits of fitness and wellness programs, improving the quality and possible length of our lives is a matter of personal choice.

Because of current scientific data and the fitness and wellness movement of the past two decades, most Americans now see a need to participate in programs that will improve and maintain adequate health. Many people still are not taking part, however, because they are unaware of the basic principles of safe and effective exercise participation. Others are exercising incorrectly and, therefore, not reaping the full benefits of their program.

Although almost half of the adult population in the United States claims to participate in some sort of physical activity, a recent report by the U. S. Public Health Service indicated that less than 20% exercised vigorously enough to develop the cardiovascular system. Cardiovascular or aerobic activities are the most popular form of exercise, so perhaps even a lower percentage of the population participates in and derives benefits from strength and flexibility programs.

▼ PERSONALIZED FITNESS PROGRAMS

Fitness needs, interests, and objectives vary significantly from one individual to the other. Therefore, exercise prescriptions must be personalized for best results. The information provided in this and the next chapter provides the guidelines necessary to develop an individualized personal lifetime program to improve fitness and promote preventive health care and personal wellness.

As you work through this chapter and assess the various components of fitness, you will be able to develop a fitness profile. When you obtain the information pertaining to each component of fitness, you can enter your results on the profile found in Figure 6.6 at the end of this chapter.

Once the results for each component have been established, either with your instructor's help or using your own judgment, you can set the target goals to achieve over the next 10 to 14 weeks. You then may proceed with an exercise program as outlined in Chapter 7. Following 8 to 12 weeks of exercise training, you should retest each component to assess improvements in physical fitness.

▼ HEALTH SCREENING PRIOR TO EXERCISE PARTICIPATION

Even though exercise testing and participation are relatively safe for most apparently healthy individuals under age 40, the reaction of the cardiovascular system to more intense levels of physical activity cannot always be predicted. Consequently, people face a small but real risk of some bodily changes during exercise testing or participation. These changes may include abnormal blood pressure, irregular heart rhythm, fainting, and, rarely, a heart attack or cardiac arrest.

Before you start an exercise program or participate in any exercise testing, you should fill out the Physical Activity Readiness Questionnaire (PAR–Q) in Figure 6.3. This questionnaire was developed by the British Columbia Ministry of Health in Canada, and it is used widely in the United States and Canada as a screening instrument prior to fitness testing.

If your answer to any of the PAR-Q questions is positive, you should consult a physician before participating in fitness testing or a fitness program. Exercise testing or participation is not advised under some of the conditions listed in the questionnaire and may require a stress electrocardiogram (ECG) test (see Chapter 7). If you have any questions regarding your current health status, you should consult your doctor before initiating, continuing, or increasing your level of physical activity.

▼ PHYSICAL FITNESS

Physical fitness has been defined in several ways and has meant different things to different people. Perhaps the most comprehensive definition has been given by the American Medical Association, which defined physical fitness as the *general capacity to adapt and respond favorably to physical effort*. This implies that individuals are physically fit when they can meet the ordinary and the unusual demands of daily life safely and effectively, without being overly fatigued, and still have energy left for leisure and recreational activities.

As the fitness concept gained ground in the last two decades, it became clear that no single test was sufficient to assess overall fitness. Rather, a battery of tests was necessary because several specific components have to be established to determine an individual's overall level of fitness.

Most authorities agree that physical fitness can be classified into health-related and motor skill-related fitness. As illustrated in Figure 6.4, the four fitness

| NAME | Course: |

For most people, physical activity should not pose any problem or hazard. This questionnaire has been designed to identify the small number of adults for whom physical activity might be inappropriate or those who should have medical advice concerning the most suitable type of activity.

1. Has your doctor ever said you have heart trouble? Yes____ No____
2. Do you frequently suffer from chest pains? Yes____ No____
3. Do you often feel faint or have spells of severe dizziness? Yes____ No____
4. Has a doctor ever said your blood pressure was too high? Yes____ No____
5. Has a doctor ever told you that you have a bone or joint problem such as arthritis that has been aggravated by exercise, or might be made worse with exercise? Yes____ No____
6. Is there any other good physical reason why you should not follow an activity program even if you want to? Yes____ No____
7. Are you over 65 and not accustomed to vigorous exercise? Yes____ No____

If you answer "yes" to any question, vigorous exercise or exercise testing should be postponed. Medical clearance may be necessary. I have read this questionnaire, I understand it does not provide a medical assessment in lieu of a physical examination by a physician.

Student's Signature   Instructor's Signature   Date

Adapted from PAR-Q Validation Report, British Columbia Department of Health, June 1975.

FIGURE 6.3 ▼ Physical Activity Readiness Questionnaire (PAR-Q).

components, from a health point of view, are cardiovascular (aerobic) endurance, muscular strength and endurance, muscular flexibility, and body composition. The first three components of health-related fitness are discussed in this chapter. Body composition is discussed in Chapter 9.

The motor skill-related components of fitness are more important in athletics. Motor skill-related fitness includes agility, balance, coordination, power, reaction time, and speed. Although these components are important in achieving success in athletics, they are not crucial for developing better health.

In terms of health and wellness, the main emphasis of fitness programs should be placed on the health-related components. That is the focus of the fitness information provided in this book.

▼ FITNESS STANDARDS: HEALTH FITNESS VERSUS PHYSICAL FITNESS

A meaningful debate recently has arisen to determine recommended fitness standards for the nation. For instance, cardiovascular endurance is measured in terms of the maximal amount of oxygen (VO_{2max}) that each kilogram of body weight is able to utilize per minute of physical activity (ml/kg/min). Individual values can range from about 10 ml/kg/min in

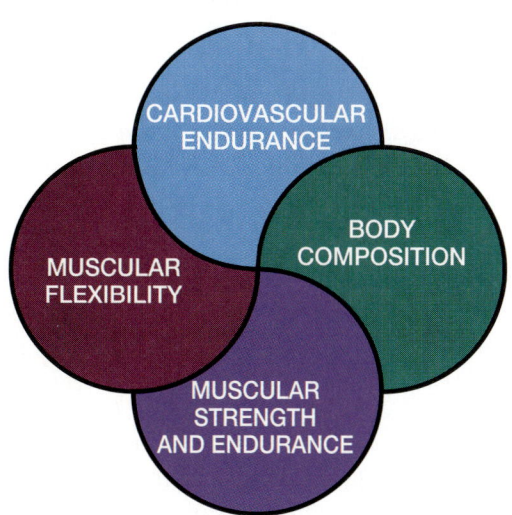

FIGURE 6.4 ▼ Health-related components of physical fitness.

cardiac patients to approximately 85 ml/kg/min in world-class runners and cross-country skiers. The debate now focuses on determining sound age- and gender-related fitness standards for the general population. Two standards have begun to develop in this regard: a health fitness standard and a physical fitness standard.

HEALTH FITNESS STANDARDS

The proposed health fitness standards are based on epidemiological* data linking minimum fitness values to health and disease prevention. According to the results of the research study presented in Figure 6.2, the data seem to indicate that VO_{2max} values of 35 and 32.5 ml/kg/min for men and women, respectively, may be sufficient to significantly decrease the risk for mortality from all causes. Although greater improvements in fitness yield a slightly lower risk of premature death, the largest drop in mortality risk is seen between the lowest fit (group 1) and the moderately fit groups (2 and 3). Therefore, the 35 and 32.5 ml/kg/min values could be selected as the health fitness standards.

PHYSICAL FITNESS STANDARDS

Physical fitness standards usually are set higher than the health fitness norms. Many experts believe that people who meet the criteria of "good" physical fitness should be able to perform moderate to vigorous amounts of physical activity without undue fatigue and to maintain this capability throughout life.

In this context, physically fit people of all ages will have the freedom to enjoy most of life's daily and recreational activities to their fullest potential. Current health fitness standards may not be enough to achieve these objectives. Sound physical fitness offers the individual a degree of independence throughout life that most people in the United States do not enjoy.

Though not with the same intensity, people should be able to carry out in their later years activities similar to those they conducted in their youth. A person does not have to be an elite athlete to climb several flights of stairs, play a vigorous game of basketball, go mountain biking, play soccer with grandchildren, walk several miles around a lake, hike through a national park, change a tire, and chop wood; yet these activities require more than the current "average fitness" level of American people.

WHICH STANDARD TO USE?

For purposes of this book, fitness standards for cardiovascular endurance, strength, flexibility, and body composition provide both a health fitness standard and a physical fitness standard. The individual has to decide his or her own objectives. If the main objective of a fitness program is to lower the risk of disease, attaining the health fitness standards may be enough to ensure better health. If an individual wants to participate in moderate to vigorous fitness activities, on the other hand, achieving a high physical fitness standard is recommended.

CARDIOVASCULAR ENDURANCE ASSESSMENT

Cardiovascular endurance has been defined as *the ability of the lungs, heart, and blood vessels to deliver adequate amounts of oxygen to the cells to meet the demands of prolonged physical activity*.

As a person breathes, part of the oxygen in the air is taken up in the lungs and transported in the blood to the heart. The heart then pumps the oxygenated blood through the circulatory system to all organs and tissues of the body. At the cellular level, oxygen is used to convert food substrates, primarily carbohydrates and fats, into energy necessary to conduct body functions and maintain a constant internal equilibrium.

During physical exertion, a greater amount of energy is needed to perform the activity. As a result, the heart, lungs, and blood vessels have to deliver more oxygen to the cells to supply the required energy. During prolonged exercise, an individual with a high level of cardiovascular endurance is able to deliver the required amount of oxygen to the tissues quite easily. The cardiovascular system of a person with a low level of endurance has to work much harder, because the heart has to pump more often to supply the same amount of oxygen to the tissues and, consequently, fatigues faster. A higher capacity to deliver and utilize oxygen (oxygen uptake), then, indicates a more efficient cardiovascular system.

---

*Epidemiology is the study of diseases that affect many individuals within a population.

A sound cardiovascular endurance program greatly enhances health. Of the four components of physical fitness, cardiovascular endurance is the single most important one. Certain amounts of muscular strength and flexibility are necessary in daily activities to lead a normal life. Even so, a person can get by without a lot of strength and flexibility but cannot do without a good cardiovascular system.

Again, the level of cardiovascular endurance, cardiovascular fitness, or aerobic capacity is determined by the maximal amount of oxygen the human body is able to utilize per minute of physical activity (usually expressed in ml/kg/min). Because all tissues and organs of the body require oxygen to function, a higher oxygen consumption indicates a more efficient cardiovascular system.

The most precise way to determine VO_{2max} is through direct gas analysis. This is done using a metabolic cart through which the amount of oxygen consumed by the body can be measured directly. This type of equipment is not available in most health/fitness centers, so several alternative methods of estimating VO_{2max} have been developed.

Even though most cardiovascular endurance tests probably are safe to administer to apparently healthy individuals (those with no major coronary risk factors or symptoms), the American College of Sports Medicine[3] recommends that a physician be present for all maximal exercise tests on apparently healthy men over age 40 and women over 50. A maximal test is any test that requires the participant's all-out or nearly all-out effort. For submaximal exercise tests a physician should be present when testing higher risk/symptomatic individuals or diseased people, regardless of the participant's current age.

Two exercise tests frequently used to assess cardiovascular fitness are the 1.5-Mile Run test and the 1.0-Mile Walk test. Depending on fitness level and personal preference, you may choose either or both of these tests. The running test is recommended for individuals who exercise regularly, whereas the walking test is preferred for those who have not yet initiated an exercise program. Because these are field tests to estimate VO_{2max}, each test will not necessarily yield exactly the same results. To make valid comparisons, the same test should be used for pre- and post-assessments.

THE 1.5-MILE RUN TEST

The 1.5-Mile Run Test is used most frequently to predict cardiovascular fitness according to the time it takes to run (or walk) a 1.5-mile course. VO_{2max} is estimated based on the time required to cover the distance (see Table 6.1).

The only equipment necessary to conduct this test is a stopwatch and a 440-yard track (6 laps to complete the 1.5 miles) or a premeasured 1.5-mile course. A person should be cautious prior to doing the 1.5-mile run. Because the objective of this test is to cover the distance in the shortest time, it is considered a maximal exercise test. Therefore, its use should be limited to conditioned individuals who have been cleared for exercise. The 1.5-Mile Run Test is not recommended for unconditioned beginners, men over 40, and women over 50, without proper medical clearance, symptomatic individuals, and those with known disease or coronary heart disease risk factors. Unconditioned individuals should participate in at least 6 weeks of aerobic training before taking this test.

Before the actual run, participants should warm up properly by doing some stretching exercises, walking, and slow jogging. Equally important, at the end of the 1.5-mile run, participants should cool down by slowly walking or jogging another 3 to 5 minutes. Participants should not sit or lie down after the test. If any unusual symptoms arise during the run, the test should be terminated immediately and the person should cool down through slow jogging or walking. The test may be retaken following 6 weeks of aerobic training.

According to the performance time, Table 6.1 can be consulted to find the estimated VO_{2max}. The corresponding fitness categories, based on VO_{2max} are found in Table 6.2.

THE 1.0-MILE WALK TEST*

For the walking test, either a 440-yard track (4 laps to a mile) or a premeasured 1.0-mile course can be used. Prior to the walk, participants have to know their body weight in pounds. A stopwatch is required to determine total walking time and exercise heart rate.

Participants should walk the 1.0-mile course at a brisk pace in such a way that the exercise heart rate at the end of the test is above 120 beats per minute. At the end of the 1.0-mile walk, walking time is

---
*Source: G. Kline et al., "Estimation of VO_{2max} from a One-Mile Track Walk, Gender, Age, and Body Weight," *Medicine and Science in Sports and Exercise* 19(3):253–259, 1987. © American College of Sports Medicine. Used by permission.

TABLE 6.1 ▼ Estimated Maximal Oxygen Uptake (VO$_{2max}$) in ml/kg/min for the 1.5-Mile Run Test

Time	VO$_2$ max	Time	VO$_2$ max	Time	VO$_2$ max	Time	VO$_2$ max
6:10	80.0	9:30	54.7	12:50	39.2	16:10	30.5
6:20	79.0	9:40	53.5	13:00	38.6	16:20	30.2
6:30	77.9	9:50	52.3	13:10	38.1	16:30	29.8
6:40	76.7	10:00	51.1	13:20	37.8	16:40	29.5
6:50	75.5	10:10	50.4	13:30	37.2	16:50	29.1
7:00	74.0	10:20	49.5	13:40	36.8	17:00	28.9
7:10	72.6	10:30	48.6	13:50	36.3	17:10	28.5
7:20	71.3	10:40	48.0	14:00	35.9	17:20	28.3
7:30	69.9	10:50	47.4	14:10	35.5	17:30	28.0
7:40	68.3	11:00	46.6	14:20	35.1	17:40	27.7
7:50	66.8	11:10	45.8	14:30	34.7	17:50	27.4
8:00	65.2	11:20	45.1	14:40	34.3	18:00	27.1
8:10	63.9	11:30	44.4	14:50	34.0	18:10	26.8
8:20	62.5	11:40	43.7	15:00	33.6	18:20	26.6
8:30	61.2	11:50	43.2	15:10	33.1	18:30	26.3
8:40	60.2	12:00	42.3	15:20	32.7	18:40	26.0
8:50	59.1	12:10	41.7	15:30	32.2	18:50	25.7
9:00	58.1	12:20	41.0	15:40	31.8	19:00	25.4
9:10	56.9	12:30	40.4	15:50	31.4		
9:20	55.9	12:40	39.8	16:00	30.9		

Adapted from Cooper, K. H. "A Means of Assessing Maximal Oxygen Intake." *JAMA* 203:201-204, 1968; Pollock, M. L. et. al. *Health and Fitness Through Physical Activity*. New York: John Wiley and Sons, 1978: Wilmore, J. H. *Training for Sport and Activity*. Boston: Allyn and Bacon, 1982.

TABLE 6.2 ▼ Cardiovascular Fitness Classification According to Maximal Oxygen Uptake (VO$_{2max}$) in ml/kg/min

Gender	Age	Fitness Classification				
		Poor	Fair	Average	Good	Excellent
Men	≤29	≤24.9	25–33.9	34–43.9	44–52.9	≥53
	30–39	≤22.9	23–30.9	31–41.9	42–49.9	≥50
	40–49	≤19.9	20–26.9	27–38.9	39–44.9	≥45
	50–59	≤17.9	18–24.9	25–37.9	38–42.9	≥43
	60–69	≤15.9	16–22.9	23–35.9	36–40.9	≥41
Women	≤29	≤23.9	24–30.9	31–38.9	39–48.9	≥49
	30–39	≤19.9	20–27.9	28–36.9	37–44.9	≥45
	40–49	≤16.9	17–24.9	25–34.9	35–41.9	≥42
	50–59	≤14.9	15–21.9	22–33.9	34–39.9	≥40
	60–69	≤12.9	13–20.9	21–32.9	33–36.9	≥37

High physical fitness standard
Health fitness standard

checked and the pulse is counted immediately for 10 seconds.

You can take your pulse on the wrist by placing two fingers over the radial artery (inside of the wrist on the side of the thumb) or over the carotid artery in the neck just below the jaw next to the voice box. Next, multiply the 10-second pulse count by 6 to obtain the exercise heart rate in beats per minute.

Now convert the walking time from minutes and seconds to minute units. Because each minute has 60 seconds, divide the seconds by 60 to obtain the fraction of a minute. For instance, a walking time of 12 minutes and 15 seconds equals $12 + (15 \div 60)$ or 12.25 minutes.

To obtain the estimated VO_{2max} in ml/kg/min for the 1.0-Mile Walk Test, plug your values into the following equation:

$VO_{2max} = 132.853 - (.0769 \times W) - (.3877 \times A) +$
$+ (6.315 \times G) - (3.2649 \times T) - (.1565 \times HR)$

Where:

- W = weight in pounds
- A = age in years
- G = gender (use 0 for women and 1 for men)
- T = total time for the mile walk in minutes
- HR = exercise heart rate in beats per minute at the end of the mile walk

For example, a 19-year-old female subject weighing 140 pounds completed the mile walk in 14 minutes and 39 seconds with an exercise heart rate of 148 beats per minute. The estimated VO_{2max} is:

- W = 140 lbs
- A = 19
- G = 0 (female gender = 0)
- T = 14:39 = $14 + (39 \div 60)$ = 14.65 min
- HR = 148 bpm

$VO_{2max} = 132.853 - (.0769 \times 140) - (.3877 \times 19) + (6.315 \times 0) - (3.2649 \times 14.65) - (.1565 \times 148)$

$VO_{2max} = 43.7$ ml/kg/min

As with the 1.5-Mile Run Test, the fitness categories, based on VO_{2max} are found in Table 6.2. The cardiovascular fitness test results are recorded on the fitness profile in Figure 6.5 at the end of this chapter.

▼ MUSCULAR STRENGTH ASSESSMENT

Strength, a basic component of fitness and wellness, is crucial for optimal performance in daily activities such as sitting, walking, running, lifting and carrying objects, doing housework, or even for enjoying recreational activities. Strength also is of great value in improving posture, personal appearance, self-image, in developing sports skills, and in meeting

Pulse taken at the radial artery.

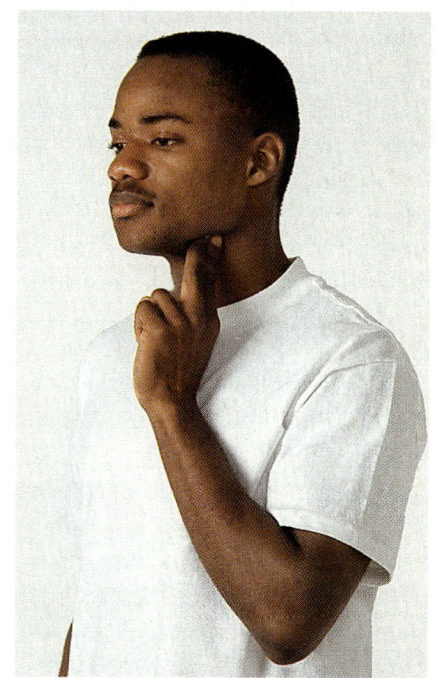

Pulse taken at the carotid artery.

certain emergencies in life in which strength is necessary to cope effectively.

From a health standpoint, strength helps to maintain muscle tissue and a higher resting metabolism (see Chapter 10), facilitates weight loss and weight control, decreases the risk for injury, and helps to prevent and correct chronic low back pain. Strength also is thought to help with childbearing and delivery.

STRENGTH VERSUS ENDURANCE

When discussing strength, the difference between muscular strength and muscular endurance has to be clarified. Although these components are interrelated, they have a basic difference. Strength is defined as *the ability to exert maximum force against resistance*. Endurance is *the ability of a muscle to exert submaximal force repeatedly over a period of time*.

Muscular endurance (also referred to as localized muscular endurance) depends to a large extent on muscular strength. Weak muscles cannot repeat an action several times or sustain it for a long time. Keeping these two principles in mind, strength tests and training programs have been designed to measure and develop absolute muscular strength, muscular endurance, or a combination of both.

Muscular strength usually is determined by the maximal amount of resistance (one repetition maximum, or 1 RM) that an individual is able to lift in a single effort. This assessment gives a good measure of absolute strength, but it does require a considerable amount of time, as the 1 RM is determined through trial and error.

For example, the strength of the chest muscles frequently is measured with the bench press exercise. If the individual has not trained with weights, he or she may try 100 pounds and lift this resistance quite easily. Then 50 pounds is added, but the person fails to lift the resistance. The resistance then is decreased by 10 or 20 pounds, and finally, after several trials, the 1 RM is established. Fatigue also becomes a factor, because by the time the 1 RM is established, several maximal, or near-maximal attempts have been performed already.

Muscular endurance is commonly established by the number of repetitions an individual can perform against a submaximal resistance such as lifting 80 pounds 20 times. It also can be determined by the length of time a given contraction is sustained — for example, how long the chin can be maintained above a bar while holding onto the bar with the hands, and the body freely suspended from the ground.

MUSCULAR ENDURANCE TEST

We live in a world in which muscular strength and endurance both are required. Because muscular endurance depends to a large extent on muscular strength, a muscular endurance test has been selected to determine strength.

Three exercises that assess the endurance of the upper body, lower body, and abdominal muscle groups have been selected for the muscular endurance test. A stopwatch, a metronome, a bench or gymnasium bleacher 16¼ inches high, and a partner are needed to administer the three test (exercise) items. The exercises conducted for this test are bench-jumps, modified-dips (men) or modified push-ups (women), and abdominal crunches.

Bench-jumps

Using a bench or gymnasium bleacher 16¼ inches high, attempt to jump up and down the bench as many times as possible in a 1-minute period. If you cannot jump the full minute, step up and down. A repetition is counted each time both feet return to the floor.

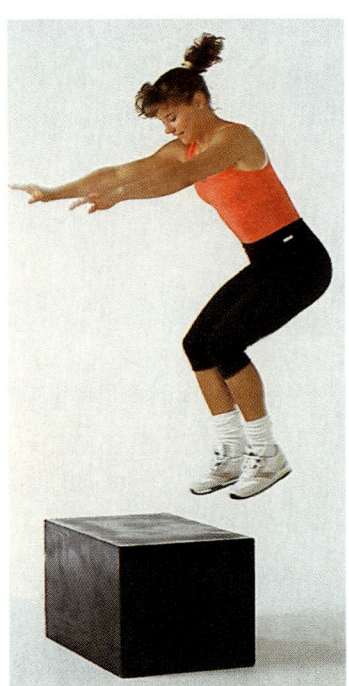

Bench-jumps.

Modified-dips

This upper-body exercise is performed by men only. Using the same bench or gymnasium bleacher 16¼ inches high, place the hands on the bench with the fingers pointing forward. Have a partner hold your feet in front of you. Your hips should be bent at approximately 90°. Lower your body by flexing your elbows until you reach a 90° angle at this joint, and then return to the starting position. (A repetition does not count if you do not reach 90°.) Perform the repetitions to a two-step cadence (down-up), regulated with a metronome set at 56 beats per minute. Perform as many continuous repetitions as possible. The test is also terminated if you fail to follow the metronome cadence.

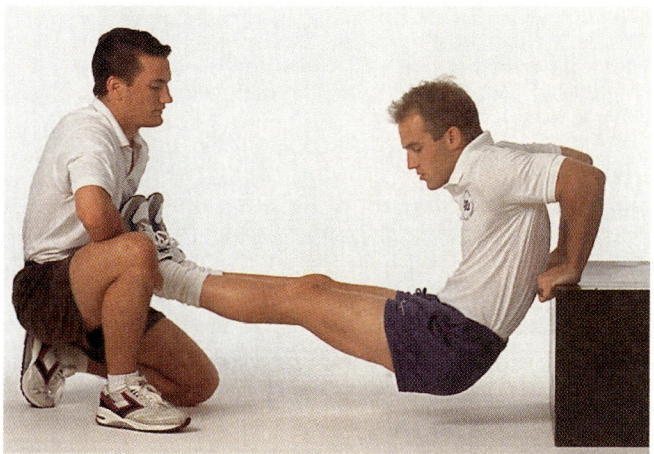

Modified-dips.

Modified push-ups

Women are to perform the modified push-up exercise instead of the modified-dip exercise. Lie down on the floor (face down), bend your knees (feet up in the air), and place your hands on the floor by the shoulders with your fingers pointing forward. The lower body will be supported at the knees (rather than the feet) throughout the test. The objective is to raise and lower the upper body by fully extending and flexing the elbows. The chest must touch the floor on each repetition.

As with the modified-dip exercise, the repetitions are performed to a two-step cadence (up-down) regulated with a metronome set at 56 beats per minute. Perform as many continuous repetitions as possible. The test is stopped when you can't do any more repetitions or you can no longer follow the metronome cadence.

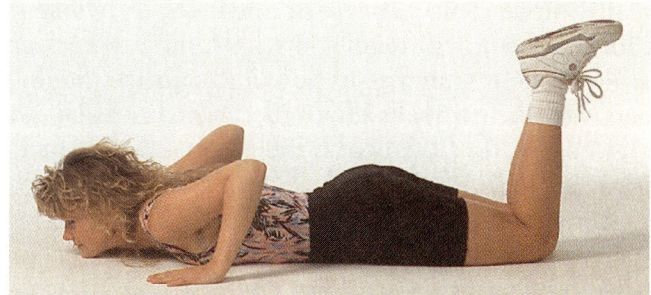

Modified push-ups.

Abdominal crunches

Tape a 3½ x 30" strip of cardboard onto the floor. Lie down on the floor in a supine position (face up) with the knees bent at approximately 100-degrees and the legs slightly apart. The feet should be on the floor and you must hold them in place yourself throughout the test. Straighten out your arms and place them on the floor alongside the trunk with the palms down and the fingers fully extended. The fingertips of both hands should barely touch the closest edge of the cardboard. Bring the head off the floor until the chin is 1 to 2" away from your chest. The head should remain in this position during the entire test (do not move the head by flexing or extending the neck). You are now ready to begin the test.

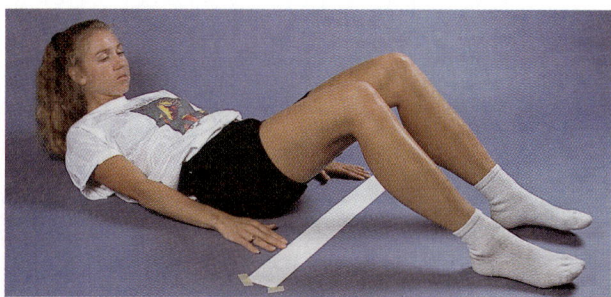

The fingertips of both hands should barely touch the closest edge of the cardboard.

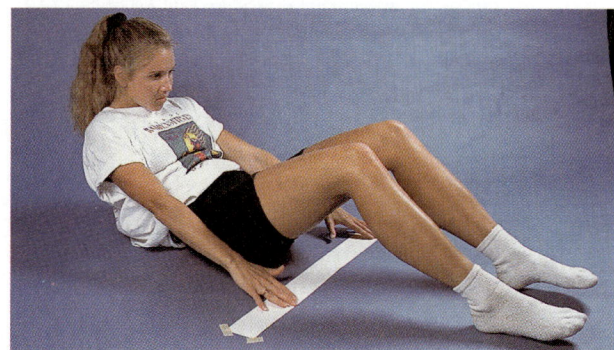

As you curl up, slide the fingers over the cardboard until the fingertips reach the far end of the board.

The repetitions are performed to a two-step cadence (up-down) regulated with a metronome set at 60 beats per minute. As you curl up, slide the fingers over the cardboard until the fingertips reach the far end (3½") of the board, then return to the starting position.

Allow a brief practice period of five to ten seconds to familiarize yourself with the cadence. The up movement is initiated with the first beat, and the down movement with the next beat. One repetition is accomplished every two beats of the metronome. Count as many repetitions as you are able to perform following the proper cadence. You may not count a repetition if the fingertips fail to reach the distant end of the cardboard.

The test is terminated if: (a) you fail to maintain the appropriate cadence, (b) the heels come off the floor, (c) the chin is not kept close to the chest, (d) you accomplish 100 repetitions, or (e) you can no longer perform the test. Have your partner check the angle at the knees throughout the test to make sure that the 100-degree angle is maintained as close as possible.

For this test you may also use a Crunch-Ster Curl-Up Tester available from Novel Products.*

*Novel Products Figure Finder Collection, P.O. Box 408, Rockton, IL 61072-0408, (800) 624-4888.

Photographs of the test performed with this equipment are shown below.

According to your results, look up the strength fitness category for each exercise in Table 6.3. Record this information in Figure 6.5.

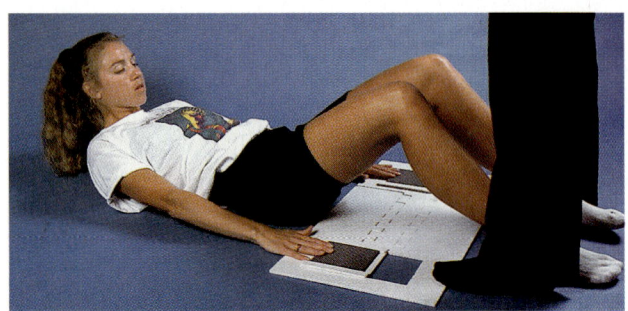
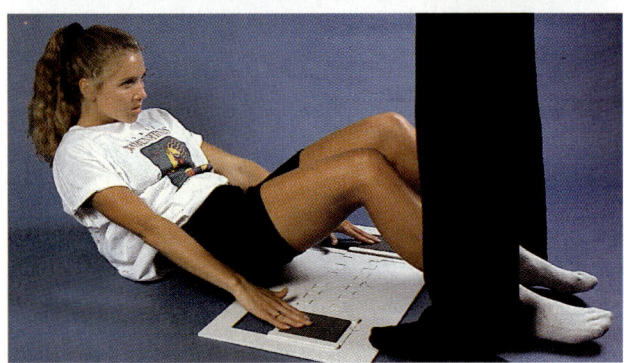

Abdominal crunches using a Crunch-Ster Curl-Up Tester.

TABLE 6.3 ▼ Percentile Ranks and Fitness Standards for the Muscular Endurance Test

Percentile Rank	MEN			WOMEN			Fitness Classification
	Bench Jumps	Modified Dips	Abdominal Crunches	Bench Jumps	Modified Push-ups	Abdominal Crunches	
99	66	54	100	58	95	100	
95	63	50	100	54	70	100	Excellent
90	62	38	100	52	50	69	
80	58	32	66	48	41	49	Good
70	57	30	45	44	38	37	
60	56	27	38	42	33	34	Average
50	54	26	33	39	30	31	
40	51	23	29	38	28	27	Fair
30	48	20	26	36	25	24	
20	47	17	22	32	21	21	
10	40	11	18	28	18	15	Poor
5	34	7	16	26	15	0	

■ High physical fitness standard
■ Health fitness standard

▼ MUSCULAR FLEXIBILITY ASSESSMENT

Flexibility is defined as *the ability of a joint to move freely through its full range of motion*. Sports medicine specialists believe that many muscular/skeletal problems and injuries, especially in adults, may be related to a lack of flexibility. Improving and maintaining good range of motion in the joints throughout life enhances the quality of life.

Because flexibility is joint-specific and good flexibility in one joint does not necessarily indicate the same is true in other joints, two tests are used to obtain an indication of current flexibility levels: the Modified Sit-and-Reach and the Total Body Rotation tests. Participants should properly warm up with a few stretching exercises before performing any flexibility testing. Assistance from another person is necessary to administer both tests.

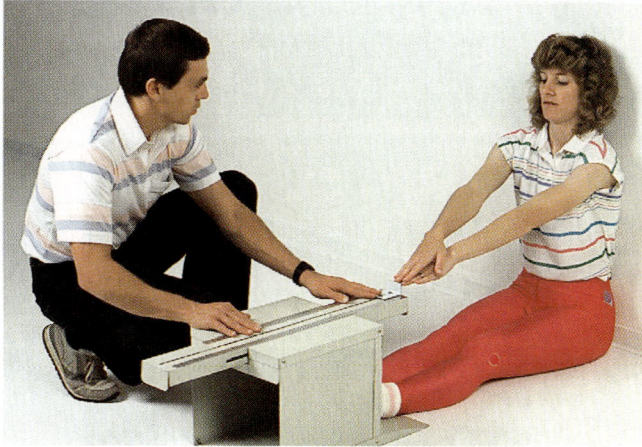

Determining the starting position for the modified sit-and-reach test.

MODIFIED SIT-AND-REACH TEST

To administer the modified Sit-and-Reach test, an Acuflex I* flexibility tester is needed, or you may design your own equipment by placing a yardstick on top of a box 12 inches high. To perform the test, remove your shoes and sit on the floor with your hips, back, and head against a wall. Your legs should be fully extended, with the bottom of your feet placed against the box.

Position one hand on top of the other, and reach forward as far as possible without letting your head or back come off the wall. The person assisting with the test then should slide the reach indicator (or yardstick) until the zero (end) point of the scale touches your fingers. He or she must then hold the indicator firmly in place throughout the rest of the test.

Your head and back now can come off the wall, and you should gradually reach forward as far as possible on the indicator, holding the final position at least 2 seconds. Be sure that, during the test, you keep the back of your knees flat against the floor.

Two trials are necessary and the average of the two scores, each recorded to the nearest half inch, is used as the final test score. Flexibility fitness categories for this test are provided in Table 6.4).

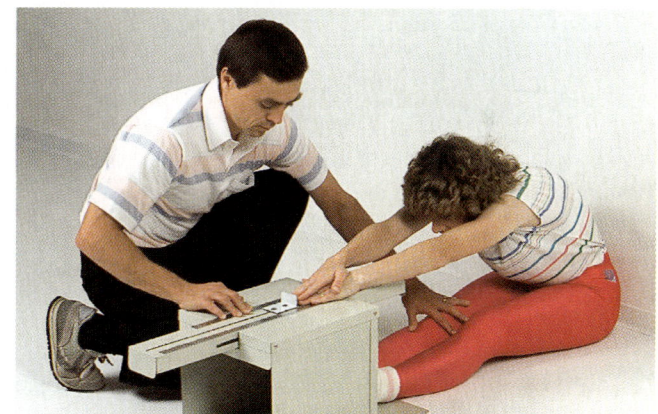

Sit-and-reach test.

TOTAL BODY ROTATION TEST

An Acuflex II flexibility tester or a measuring scale with a sliding panel is needed to administer this test. The Acuflex II or scale is placed on the wall at shoulder height and should be adjustable to accommodate individual differences in height.

If you need to build your own scale, use two measuring tapes, each at least 30 inches long, and

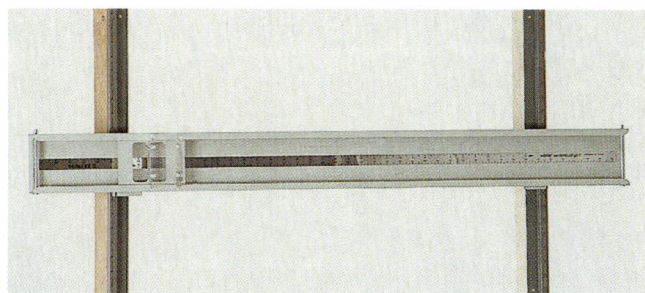

Acuflex II measuring device for the total body rotation test.

---

*Acuflex I and II flexibility equipment can be obtained from Novel Products Figure Finder Collection, P.O. Box 408, Rockton, IL 61072-0408, (800) 624-4888.

TABLE 6.4 ▼ Percentile Ranks and Fitness Standards for the Modified Sit-and-Reach Test

	MEN						WOMEN				
Percentile Rank	Age Category				Fitness Category	Percentile Rank	Age Category				Fitness Category
	<18	19–35	36–49	>50			<18	19–35	36–49	>50	
99	20.8	20.1	18.9	16.2		99	22.6	21.0	19.8	17.2	
95	19.6	18.9	18.2	15.8	Excellent	95	19.5	19.3	19.2	15.7	Excellent
90	18.2	17.2	16.1	15.0		90	18.7	17.9	17.4	15.0	
80	17.8	17.0	14.6	13.3	Good	80	17.8	16.7	16.2	14.2	Good
70	16.0	15.8	13.9	12.3		70	16.5	16.2	15.2	13.6	
60	15.2	15.0	13.4	11.5	Average	60	16.0	15.8	14.5	12.3	Average
50	14.5	14.4	12.6	10.2		50	15.2	14.8	13.5	11.1	
40	14.0	13.5	11.6	9.7	Fair	40	14.5	14.5	12.8	10.1	Fair
30	13.4	13.0	10.8	9.3		30	13.7	13.7	12.2	9.2	
20	11.8	11.6	9.9	8.8		20	12.6	12.6	11.0	8.3	
10	9.5	9.2	8.3	7.8	Poor	10	11.4	10.1	9.7	7.5	Poor
05	8.4	7.9	7.0	7.2		05	9.4	8.1	8.5	3.7	
01	7.2	7.0	5.1	4.0		01	6.5	2.6	2.0	1.5	

■ High physical fitness standard
■ Health fitness standard

---

glue them above and below the sliding panel, centered at the 15-inch mark. If no sliding panel is available, simply tape the measuring tapes onto a wall. Also, draw a line centered with the 15-inch mark on the floor.

Stand sideways, an arm's length away from the wall, your feet straight ahead, slightly separated, and your toes right up to the corresponding line drawn on the floor. Hold out the arm opposite to the wall horizontally from your body, making a fist with your hand. The Acuflex II, measuring scale, or tapes should be shoulder height at this time. Rotate your trunk, the extended arm going backward (always maintaining a horizontal plane) and making contact with the panel, gradually sliding it forward as far as possible. If no panel is available, slide your fist alongside the tapes as far as possible. Hold the final position for at least 2 seconds.

Your hand should be positioned with the little finger side forward during the entire sliding movement. It is crucial to have the proper hand position. Many

Homemade measuring device for the total body rotation test.

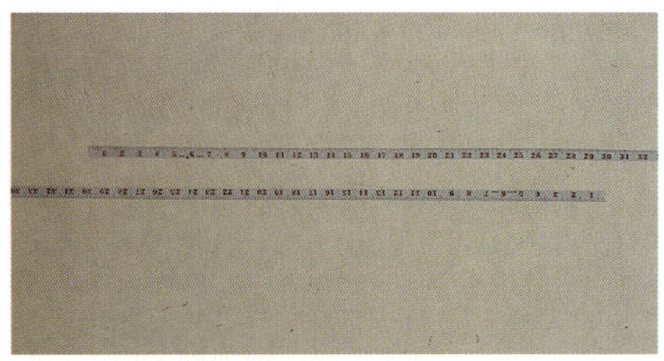

Measuring tapes for the total body rotation test.

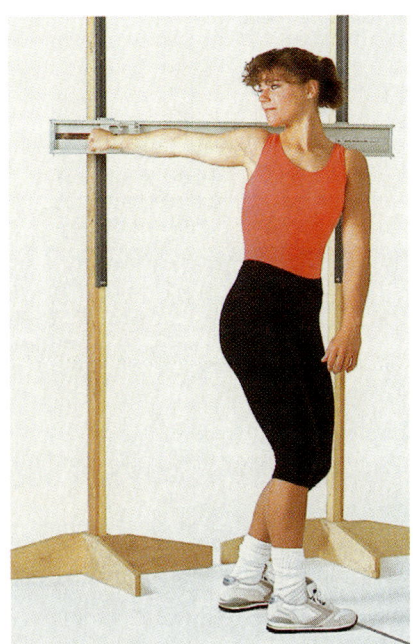

Total body rotation test.

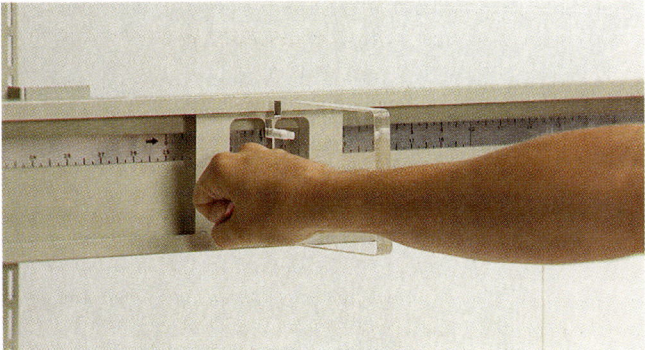

Proper hand position for total body rotation test.

After obtaining your flexibility scores and fitness categories, record the results in the fitness profile given at the end of the chapter (Figure 6.7).

▼ EXERCISE PRESCRIPTION

Upon completing the health-related fitness assessment, Chapter 7 will help you learn how to develop and implement your own exercise programs for cardiovascular endurance, muscular strength, and muscular flexibility. In Chapter 9 you also will learn how to assess your body composition (the fourth component of health-related fitness) and compute your recommended body weight based on your current percent body fat. Guidelines for a weight management program are provided in Chapter 10. Before advancing to the next chapter, however, record all of your fitness test results and categories in the fitness profile provided in Figure 6.5.

people attempt to open the hand or push with extended fingers or slide the panel with the knuckles, none of which is an acceptable test procedure. During the test, the knees can be slightly bent, but the feet cannot be moved; they always must point straight forward. The body must be kept as straight (vertical) as possible.

Conduct the test on either the right or the left side of the body. You are allowed two trials on the selected side. The farthest point reached, measured to the nearest half inch and held for at least 2 seconds, is recorded. The average of the two trials becomes the final test score. Flexibility fitness categories for the test are provided in Table 6.5.

▼ NOTES

1. Paffenbarger, R. S., Jr., R. T. Hyde, A. L. Wing, and C. H. Steinmetz. "A natural history of athleticism and cardiovascular health." *Journal of the American Medical Association* 252:491–495, 1984.

2. Blair, S. N., H. W. Kohl III, R. S. Paffenbarger, Jr, D. G. Clark, K. H. Cooper, and L. W. Gibbons. "Physical fitness and all-cause mortality: A prospective study of healthy men and women." *Journal of the American Medical Association* 262:2395–2401, 1989.

3. American College of Sports Medicine. *Guidelines for Exercise Testing and Prescription.* Philadelphia: Lea & Febiger, 1991.

TABLE 6.5 ▼ Percentile Ranks and Fitness Standards for the Total Body Rotation Test

	Percentile Rank	Left Rotation				Right Rotation				Fitness Category
		<18	19–35	36–49	>50	<18	19–35	36–49	>50	
Men	99	29.1	28.0	26.6	21.0	28.2	27.8	25.2	22.2	Excellent
	95	26.6	24.8	24.5	20.0	25.5	25.6	23.8	20.7	
	90	25.0	23.6	23.0	17.7	24.3	24.1	22.5	19.3	
	80	22.0	22.0	21.2	15.5	22.7	22.3	21.0	16.3	Good
	70	20.9	20.3	20.4	14.7	21.3	20.7	18.7	15.7	
	60	19.9	19.3	18.7	13.9	19.8	19.0	17.3	14.7	Average
	50	18.6	18.0	16.7	12.7	19.0	17.2	16.3	12.3	
	40	17.0	16.8	15.3	11.7	17.3	16.3	14.7	11.5	Fair
	30	14.9	15.0	14.8	10.3	15.1	15.0	13.3	10.7	
	20	13.8	13.3	13.7	9.5	12.9	13.3	11.2	8.7	Poor
	10	10.8	10.5	10.8	4.3	10.8	11.3	8.0	2.7	
	05	8.5	8.9	8.8	0.3	8.1	8.3	5.5	0.3	
	01	3.4	1.7	5.1	0.0	6.6	2.9	2.0	0.0	
Women	99	29.3	28.6	27.1	23.0	29.6	29.4	27.1	21.7	Excellent
	95	26.8	24.8	25.3	21.4	27.6	25.3	25.9	19.7	
	90	25.5	23.0	23.4	20.5	25.8	23.0	21.3	19.0	
	80	23.8	21.5	20.2	19.1	23.7	20.8	19.6	17.9	Good
	70	21.8	20.5	18.6	17.3	22.0	19.3	17.3	16.8	
	60	20.5	19.3	17.7	16.0	20.8	18.0	16.5	15.6	Average
	50	19.5	18.0	16.4	14.8	19.5	17.3	14.6	14.0	
	40	18.5	17.2	14.8	13.7	18.3	16.0	13.1	12.8	Fair
	30	17.1	15.7	13.6	10.0	16.3	15.2	11.7	8.5	
	20	16.0	15.2	11.6	6.3	14.5	14.0	9.8	3.9	Poor
	10	12.8	13.6	8.5	3.0	12.4	11.1	6.1	2.2	
	05	11.1	7.3	6.8	0.7	10.2	8.8	4.0	1.1	
	01	8.9	5.3	4.3	0.0	8.9	3.2	2.8	0.0	

■ High physical fitness standard
■ Health fitness standard

Date: _____ Course: _____ Section: _____
Name: _____ Age: _____ Male or Female: M / F
Body Weight: _____ . _____

Fitness Component	Test Data	Test Results	Fitness Classification
Cardiovascular Endurance	Time	VO$_2$ max.	
1.5-Mile Run	_____ : _____	_____ : _____	_____
	Time		
1.0-Mile Walk	_____ : _____		
	Heart Rate	VO$_2$ max.	
	_____	_____ : _____	_____
Muscular Strength / Endurance	Reps	Percentile	
Bench Jumps	_____	_____	_____
Chair Dips / Mod. Push-Ups	_____	_____	_____
Abdominal Curl-Ups	_____	_____	_____
Average Percentile		_____	_____
Muscular Flexibility	Inches	Percentile	
Modified Sit-and-Reach	_____	_____	_____
Body Rotation (R/L)	_____	_____	_____
Average Percentile		_____	_____
Body Composition			
Skinfolds			
Chest/Triceps	_____		
Abdominal/Suprailium	_____		
Thigh	_____		
Sum of Skinfolds	_____		
Girth Measurements			
Men			
Waist (inches)	_____		
Wrist (inches)	_____		
Women			
Upper Arm (cm)	_____		
Hip (cm)	_____		
Wrist (cm)	_____		
Percent Body Fat		_____	_____
Lean Body Mass (lbs)		_____	

FIGURE 6.5 ▼ Physical fitness profile.

Exercise Prescription For Wellness

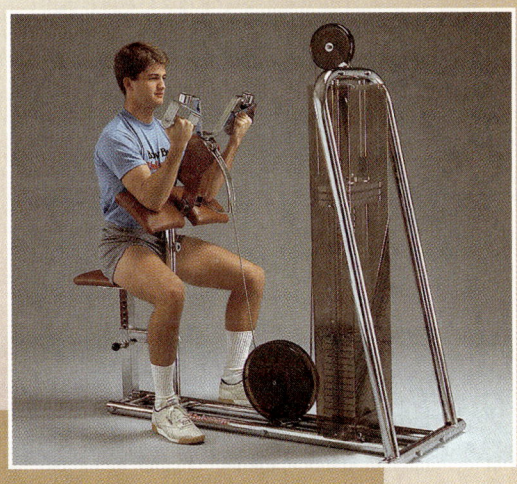

Objectives

▼ Understand the benefits of an active lifestyle.
▼ Define aerobic and anaerobic exercise.
▼ Learn the guidelines for cardiovascular, strength, and flexibility exercise prescription.
▼ Understand the overload principle for strength development.
▼ Clarify misconceptions related to exercise training programs.
▼ Become familiar with concepts for injury prevention and treatment.
▼ Learn basic skills to enhance exercise adherence.

A most inspiring story illustrating what fitness can do for a person's health and well-being is that of George Snell from Sandy, Utah. At age 45, Snell weighed approximately 400 pounds, his blood pressure was 220/180, he was blind because of diabetes he didn't know he had, and his blood glucose level was 487. Snell had determined to do something about his physical and medical condition, so he started a walking/jogging program.

After about 8 months of conditioning, Snell had lost almost 200 pounds, his eyesight had returned, his glucose level was down to 67, and he was taken off medication. Two months later, less than 10 months after initiating his personal exercise program, he completed his first marathon, a running course of 26.2 miles.

Results of epidemiological research have established that participating in a lifetime exercise program greatly contributes to good health (see Chapter 6). Nonetheless, too many individuals who exercise regularly find, when they take a battery of fitness tests, that they may not be as conditioned as they thought they were. Although these individuals may be exercising regularly, they most likely are not following the basic principles for exercise prescription and, therefore, are not reaping the full benefits of their exercise program.

A key principle in exercise prescription is that all programs must be individualized to obtain optimal results. Our bodies are not all alike, and fitness levels and needs vary among individuals. The information presented in this chapter provides the necessary guidelines to write a personalized cardiovascular, strength, and flexibility exercise program that promotes and maintains physical fitness. Information on weight control to achieve and maintain ideal body composition, a key component of good physical fitness, is given in Chapter 10.

▼ CARDIOVASCULAR ENDURANCE

Cardiovascular endurance refers to the ability of the lungs, heart, and blood vessels to deliver adequate amounts of oxygen to the cells to meet the demands of prolonged physical activity. Because the body uses oxygen to convert food (carbohydrates and fats) into energy, a greater capacity to deliver and utilize oxygen (referred to as oxygen uptake or VO_2) indicates a more efficient cardiovascular system.

Cardiovascular endurance activities also are called aerobic exercise. The word *aerobic* means

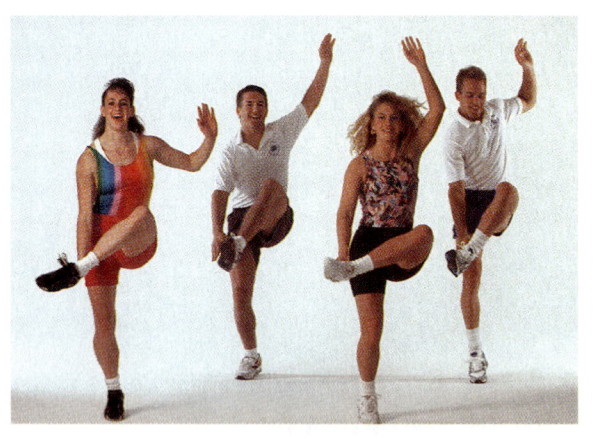
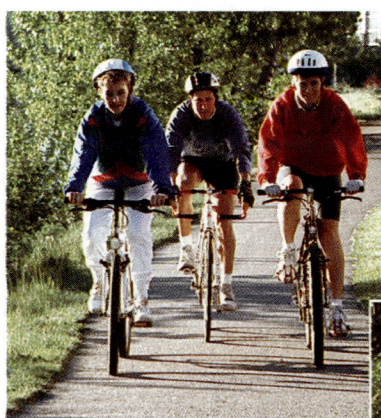
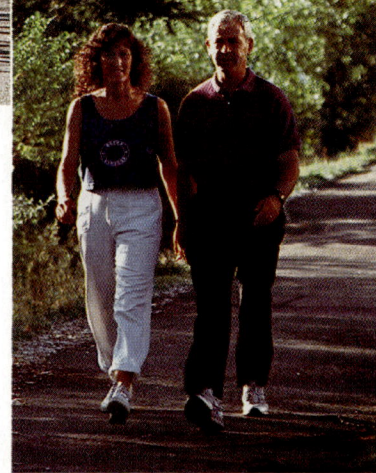
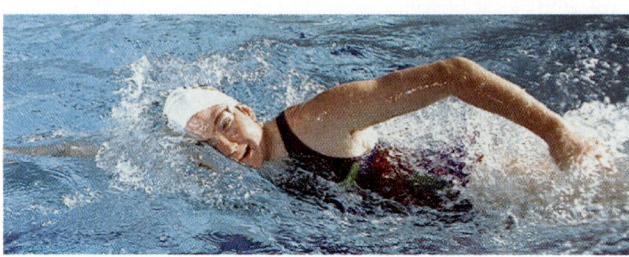

Aerobic exercise requires oxygen to supply the energy needed to carry out the activity.

"with oxygen." Whenever an activity requires oxygen to produce energy, it is considered an aerobic exercise. Examples of cardiovascular or aerobic exercise are walking, jogging, swimming, cycling, cross-country skiing, water aerobics, rope skipping, and aerobics.

Anaerobic activities, on the other hand, are carried out "without oxygen." The intensity of anaerobic exercise is so high that oxygen is not utilized to produce energy. Because energy production is limited without oxygen, these activities can be carried out for only short periods (2 to 3 minutes). The higher the intensity of the activity, the shorter the duration.

Activities such as the 100, 200, and 400 meters in track and field, the 100 meters in swimming, gymnastics routines, and weight training are good examples of anaerobic activities. Anaerobic activities will not contribute much to development of the cardiovascular system. Only aerobic activities will enhance cardiovascular endurance.

SIGNIFICANCE OF CARDIOVASCULAR ENDURANCE

Physical activity is no longer a natural part of our existence. If we need to go to a store only a couple of blocks away, most people drive their cars and then spend a couple of minutes driving around the parking lot to find a spot 10 yards closer to the store's entrance. We do not even have to carry out the groceries any more. A youngster working at the store usually takes them out in a cart and places them in your vehicle. During a normal visit to a multilevel shopping mall, almost everyone chooses to ride the escalators instead of taking the stairs. Automobiles, elevators, escalators, telephones, intercoms, remote controls, and electric garage door openers — all are modern-day commodities that minimize body movement and effort.

One of the most detrimental effects of modern-day technology has been an increase in chronic conditions related to a lack of physical activity. Some examples are hypertension, heart disease, chronic low back pain, and obesity. These conditions also are called *hypokinetic diseases*. "Hypo" means low or little, and "kinetic" denotes motion.

Lack of adequate physical activity is a reality of modern life that most people no longer can avoid, but to enjoy modern-day commodities and still expect to live life to its fullest, a personalized

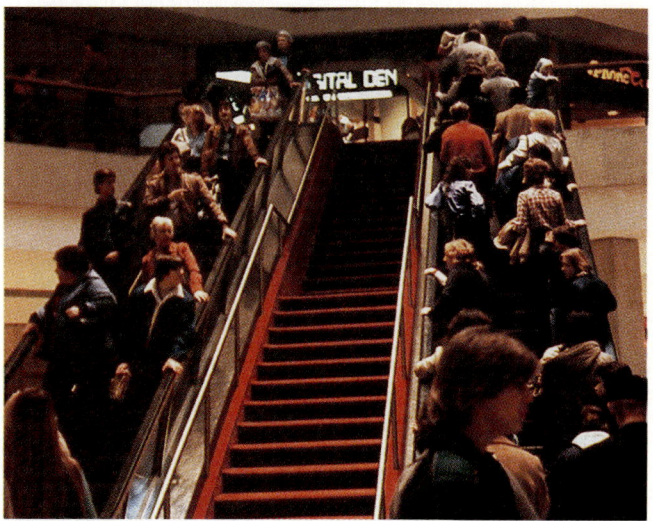

Advances in modern technology have almost completely eliminated the need for physical activity, significantly enhancing the deterioration rate of the human body.

lifetime exercise program must become part of daily living. Based on current estimates by the Centers for Disease Control in Atlanta, Georgia, only about 20% of the adult population exercises vigorously enough to develop the cardiovascular system.

Aerobic exercise is especially important in preventing coronary heart disease. A poorly conditioned heart that has to pump more often just to keep a person alive is subject to more wear-and-tear than a well-conditioned heart. In situations that place strenuous demands on the heart, such as doing yard work, lifting heavy objects or weights, or running to catch a train, the unconditioned heart may not be able to sustain the strain.

In addition, regular participation in cardiovascular endurance activities helps achieve and maintain recommended body weight, the fourth component of health-related physical fitness. Weight management is the topic of Chapter 10.

Everyone who initiates a cardiovascular or aerobic exercise program can expect a number of physiological adaptations from training. Among the most significant adaptations are:

1. *A higher maximal oxygen uptake* (VO_{2max}). The amount of oxygen the body is able to use during physical activity significantly increases. This allows the individual to exercise longer and at a higher rate before becoming fatigued.

    Small increases in VO_{2max} can be observed in as few as 2 to 3 weeks of aerobic training. Depending on the initial fitness level, VO_{2max} may

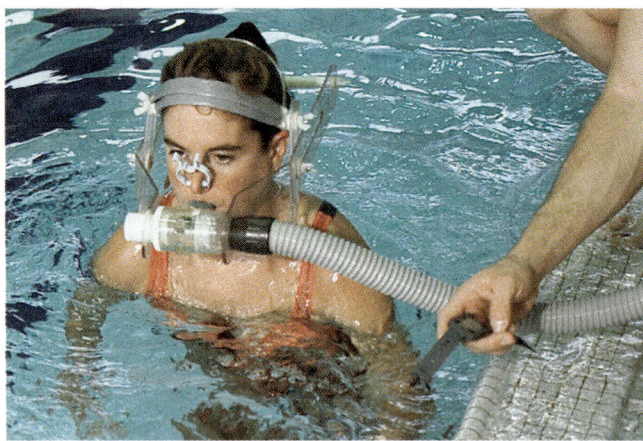

Physical work capacity, measured through a maximal oxygen uptake (VO$_{2max}$) test, increases with aerobic training.

rise as much as 30%, although higher increases have been reported in people with very low initial levels of fitness.

2. *A decrease in resting heart rate and an increase in cardiac muscle strength.* During resting conditions, the heart ejects between 5 and 6 liters of blood per minute (a liter is slightly larger than a quart). This amount of blood, also referred to as *cardiac output,* meets the energy demands in the resting state.

   Like any other muscle, the heart responds to training by gaining strength and size. As the heart gets stronger, the muscle can produce a more forceful contraction. A stronger contraction causes a greater ejection of blood with each beat (stroke volume), yielding a lower heart rate. This reduction in heart rate also allows the heart to rest longer between beats.

   Resting heart rates frequently decrease 10 to 20 beats per minute (bpm) after only 6 to 8 weeks of training. A reduction of 20 bpm saves the heart about 10,483,200 beats per year. The average heart beats between 70 and 80 bpm. Resting heart rates in highly trained athletes frequently are around 45 bpm.

3. *A lower heart rate at given workloads.* When compared with untrained individuals, a trained person has a lower heart rate response to a given task, because of higher efficiency of the cardiovascular system. Following several weeks of training, a given workload (let's say a 10-minute mile) elicits a much lower heart rate response as compared to the response when training first started.

4. *An increase in the number and size of the mitochondria.* All energy necessary for cell function is produced in the mitochondria. As the size and number increase, so does the potential to produce energy for muscular work.

5. *An increase in the number of functional capillaries.* These smaller vessels allow for the exchange of oxygen and carbon dioxide between the blood and the cells. As more vessels open up, more gas exchange can take place, thereby decreasing the onset of fatigue during prolonged exercise. This increase in capillaries also speeds up the rate at which waste products of cell metabolism can be removed. Increased capillarization also is seen in the heart, which enhances the oxygen delivery capacity to the heart muscle itself.

6. *A decrease in recovery time.* Trained individuals have a faster recovery time following exercise. A fit system is able to more rapidly restore any internal equilibrium disrupted during exercise.

7. *A decrease in blood pressure and blood lipids.* A regular aerobic exercise program will result in lower blood pressure and fats such as cholesterol and triglycerides, linked to the formation of the atherosclerotic plaque, which obstructs the arteries. This reduction lowers the risk for coronary heart disease (see Chapter 11). High blood pressure also is a leading risk factor for strokes.

8. *An increase in fat-burning enzymes.* Fat is lost primarily by burning it in muscle. As the concentration of the enzymes increases, so does the ability to burn fat.

GUIDELINES FOR CARDIOVASCULAR EXERCISE PRESCRIPTION

To develop the cardiovascular system, the heart muscle has to be overloaded like any other muscle in the human body. Just as the biceps muscle in the upper arm is developed through strength-training exercises, the heart muscle also has to be exercised to increase in size, strength, and efficiency. To better understand how the cardiovascular system can be developed, we have to be familiar with the four basic principles of intensity, mode, duration, and frequency of exercise. These principles are discussed separately in this section, and Figure 7.1 summarizes the cardiovascular exercise prescription guidelines according to the American College of Sports Medicine.[1]

Activity:	Aerobic (examples: walking, jogging, cycling, swimming, aerobics, racquetball, soccer, stair climbing)
Intensity:	60–90% of Maximal Heart Rate
Duration:	20–60 minutes of continuous aerobic activity
Frequency:	3 to 5 days per week

The recommended quantity and quality of exercise for developing and maintaining cardiorespiratory and muscular fitness in healthy adults by the American College of Sports Medicine. *Medical Science Sports Exercise.* 22(1990):265–274.

FIGURE 7.1 ▼ Cardiovascular exercise prescription guidelines.

The American College of Sports Medicine, the leading sports medicine organization in the world, recommends that a medical exam and a diagnostic exercise stress test or stress ECG be administered prior to vigorous exercise by apparently healthy men over age 40 and women over 50. The American College of Sports Medicine has defined vigorous exercise as an exercise intensity above 60% of VO_{2max}. This intensity is the equivalent of exercise that provides a "substantial challenge" to the participant or one that cannot be maintained for 20 continuous minutes.

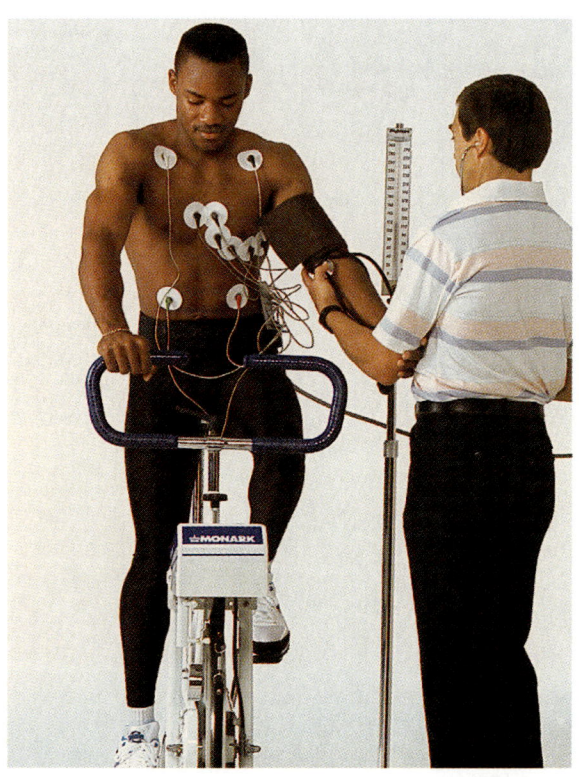

Exercise stress electrocardiogram test (stress ECG).

INTENSITY OF EXERCISE

When trying to develop the cardiovascular system, the intensity of exercise perhaps is the most commonly ignored factor. This principle refers to how hard a person has to exercise to improve cardiovascular endurance.

Muscles have to be overloaded to a given point for them to develop. While the training stimulus to develop the biceps muscle can be accomplished with curl-up exercises, the stimulus for the cardiovascular system is provided by making the heart pump at a faster rate for a certain period of time. Research has shown that cardiovascular development occurs when working between 60% and 90% of maximal heart rate. Faster development can be obtained by working closer to the higher end of the range. For this reason, many experts prescribe exercise between 70% and 90% for young people.

Exercise intensity can be calculated easily and training can be monitored by checking your pulse. To determine the intensity of exercise or cardiovascular training zone:

1. Estimate your maximal heart rate (MHR). The maximal heart rate depends on the person's age and can be estimated according to the following formula: MHR = 220 minus age (220 – age)

2. Calculate the training intensities (TI) at 60%, 70%, and 90%. Multiply MHR by the respective 60%, 70%, and 90%. For example, the 60%, 70%, and 90% training intensities for a 20-year-old person are:

   MHR: 220 – 20 = 200 beats per minute (bpm)
   60% TI = (200 × .60) = 120 bpm
   70% TI = (200 × .70) = 140 bpm
   90% TI = (200 × .90) = 180 bpm

Cardiovascular training zone: 120 to 180 bpm

According to your present age, you also may look up your cardiovascular training zone in Table 7.1. The training zone indicates that whenever you exercise to improve the cardiovascular system, you should maintain the heart rate between the 60% and 90% training intensities to obtain adequate development.

If you have been physically inactive, you should train around 60% intensity during the first 4 to 6 weeks of the exercise program. After the first few weeks, you should exercise between 70% and 90% training intensity.

TABLE 7.1 ▼ Recommended Cardiovascular Exercise Intensities

Age	Estimated Max HR*	60% HR* Intensity	70% HR* Intensity	90% HR* Intensity
15	205	123	144	185
20	200	120	140	180
25	195	117	137	176
30	190	114	133	171
35	185	111	130	167
40	180	108	126	162
45	175	105	123	158
50	170	102	119	153
55	165	99	116	149
60	160	96	112	144
65	155	93	109	140
70	150	90	105	135
75	145	87	102	131

*HR = Heart Rate

Monitor your exercise heart rate regularly during exercise to make sure you are training in the respective zone. Wait until you are about 5 minutes into the exercise session before taking your first rate. When checking exercise heart rate, count your pulse for 10 seconds. Next, multiply the 10-second count by 6 to obtain the rate in beats per minute. Exercise heart rate will remain at the same level for about 15 seconds following exercise. After 15 seconds, heart rate will drop rapidly. Do not hesitate to stop during your exercise bout to check your pulse. If the rate is too low, increase the intensity of exercise. If the rate is too high, slow down.

Health Versus Fitness Intensities

To develop the cardiovascular system, you do not have to exercise above the 90% rate. From a fitness standpoint, training above this percentage will not yield extra benefits and actually may be unsafe for some people.

For unconditioned people and older adults, cardiovascular training should be conducted at about the 60% rate. This lower rate is recommended to reduce potential problems associated with high-intensity exercise.

Training benefits obtained by exercising at the 60% training intensity may place a person only in an average or "moderately fit" category (see Table 6.2 in Chapter 6). Even though it is not an excellent fitness rating, exercising at this lower intensity does significantly decrease the risk for cardiovascular mortality (health fitness) and other chronic diseases. An excellent fitness rating is obtained by exercising closer to the 90% threshold.

Rate of Perceived Exertion

Many people do not check their heart rate during exercise, so an alternative method of prescribing intensity of exercise has become more popular recently. This method uses a rate of perceived exertion (RPE) scale developed by Gunnar Borg. Using the scale in Figure 7.2, a person subjectively rates the perceived exertion or difficulty of exercise when training in the appropriate target zone. The exercise heart rate then is associated with the corresponding RPE value.

If the training intensity requires a heart rate zone between 150 and 170 bpm, for example, this is associated with training between "hard" and "very hard" (15 and 17 on the scale). Some individuals, however, may perceive less exertion than others when training in the correct zone. Therefore, you should associate your own inner perception of the task with the phrases given on the scale. You then may proceed to exercise at that rate of perceived exertion.

Whether you monitor the intensity of exercise by checking your pulse or through rate of perceived

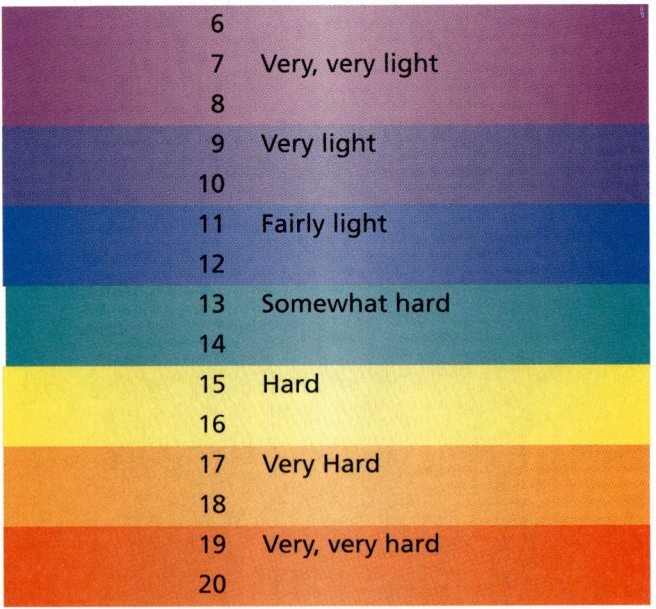

From G. Borg, "Perceived Exertion: A Note on History and Methods." *Medicine and Science in Sports and Exercise* 5:90–93, 1983.

FIGURE 7.2 ▼ Rate of perceived exertion scale.

exertion, changes in normal exercise conditions affect the training zone. For example, exercising on a hot or humid day or at high altitude increases the heart rate response to a given task. Therefore, the intensity of your exercise may have to be adjusted.

MODE OF EXERCISE

The type of exercise that develops the cardiovascular system has to be aerobic in nature. Once you have established your cardiovascular training zone, any activity or combination of activities that will get your heart rate up to that training zone and keep it there for as long as you exercise will produce adequate development. Examples of these activities are walking, jogging, aerobics, swimming, water aerobics, cross-country skiing, rope skipping, cycling, racquetball, stair climbing, and stationary running or cycling.

The activity you choose should be based on your personal preferences, what you enjoy doing most, and your physical limitations. Different activities may affect the amount of strength or flexibility developed, but as far as the cardiovascular system is concerned, the heart doesn't know whether you are walking, swimming, or cycling. All the heart knows is that it has to pump at a certain rate, and as long as that rate is in the desired range, cardiovascular development will take place.

DURATION OF EXERCISE

The general recommendation is that a person should train between 20 and 60 minutes per session. Duration is based on how intensely a person trains. If the training is done around 90%, 20 minutes are sufficient. At 60% intensity, a person should train at least 30 minutes. As mentioned, unconditioned people and older adults should train at lower percentages; therefore, the activity should be carried out over a longer period of time.

Although most experts recommend 20 to 30 minutes of aerobic exercise per session, 1990 research published in the *American Journal of Cardiology* by Dr. Robert DeBusk and co-workers[2] indicates that three 10-minute exercise sessions per day (separated by at least 4 hours), at approximately 70% of maximal heart rate, also produce training benefits. Increases in VO_{2max} with this program were not as large (only 57%) as those in a group performing a continuous 30-minute bout of exercise per day, but the researchers concluded that moderate-intensity exercise training, conducted for 10 minutes three times per day, benefits the cardiovascular system. The results of this study are meaningful because people often mention lack of time as the reason for not taking part in an exercise program. Many think they must exercise at least 20 minutes to get any benefits at all. Even though 20 to 30 minutes are ideal, short, intermittent bouts of exercise also are beneficial to the cardiovascular system.

The training session always should include a 5-minute warm-up and a 5-minute cool-down period (see Figure 7.3). The warm-up should consist of general calisthenics, stretching exercises, or exercising at a lower intensity level than the actual target zone. To cool down, the intensity of exercise is gradually decreased. Abruptly stopping causes blood to pool in the exercised body parts, diminishing the return of blood to the heart. A decreased blood return can cause dizziness and faintness or even bring on cardiac abnormalities.

FREQUENCY OF EXERCISE

Ideally, a person should engage in aerobic exercise three to five times per week. Research indicates that, when starting an exercise program, three to five 20- to 30-minute training sessions per week improves VO_{2max}. When training is conducted more than 5 days per week, further improvements are minimal.

For people on a weight loss program, 45- to 60-minute exercise sessions of low to moderate intensity, conducted 5 or 6 days a week, are recommended. Longer exercise sessions increase caloric expenditure for faster weight reduction (see Chapter 10).

MAINTAINING CARDIOVASCULAR FITNESS

A decrease in cardiovascular fitness has been observed in as little as 2 weeks of nontraining. Depending on the length of participation in the aerobic program, complete loss of training benefits is seen between 3 and 8 months after discontinuing the program. Following an aerobic conditioning program, a person must continue a regular training program to maintain cardiovascular fitness.

The key to maintaining fitness seems to be the intensity of training. Research indicates that, though duration and frequency of training can be reduced,

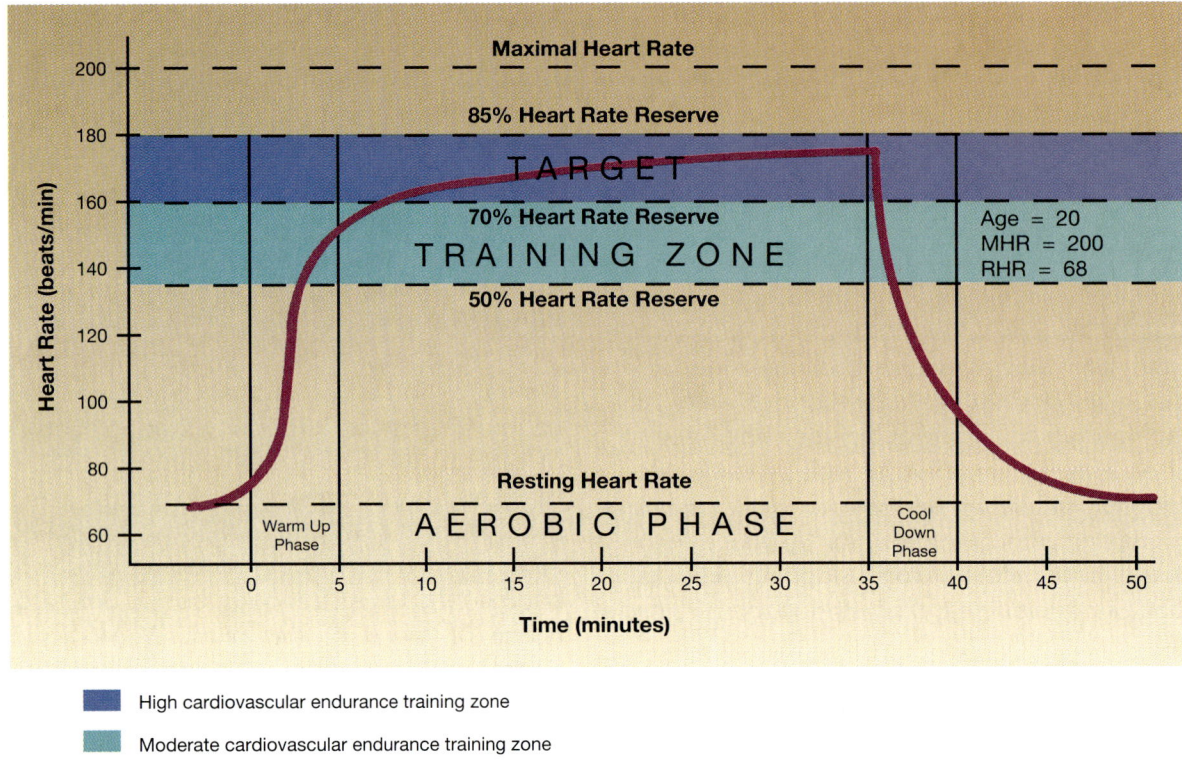

FIGURE 7.3 ▼ Typical aerobic training pattern.

VO_{2max} does not decline as long as the proper intensity is maintained. Three 20-minute training sessions per week, on nonconsecutive days, maintains cardiovascular fitness as long as the heart rate is in the appropriate target zone.

MUSCULAR STRENGTH

An adequate level of strength is an important component of good physical fitness. The two forms of strength, as defined in Chapter 6, are muscular strength and muscular endurance. Muscular strength is the ability to exert maximum force against resistance; muscular endurance is the ability of a muscle to exert submaximal force repeatedly over a period of time. For example, a person may have the muscular strength to lift 180 pounds once but may not have the muscular endurance to lift 140 pounds 12 times.

Over the years it has been well-documented that the capacity of muscle cells to exert force increases and decreases according to the demands placed upon the muscular system. If muscle cells are overloaded beyond their normal use, such as in strength-training programs, the cells increase in size (hypertrophy) and strength. If the demands placed on the muscle cells decrease, such as in sedentary living or required rest because of illness or injury, the cells decrease in size (atrophy) and lose strength.

SIGNIFICANCE OF STRENGTH

Strength is important for optimal performance in daily tasks and recreational activities, to improve personal appearance and self-image, to lessen the risk of injury, and to cope with emergency situations in life. Adequate strength levels also contribute to weight control and enhanced overall health and well-being.

Perhaps one of the most significant benefits of maintaining a good strength level is its relationship to human metabolism. Metabolism is defined as *all energy and material transformations that occur within living cells.*

A primary result of a strength-training program is an increase in muscle mass or size (lean body mass), known as *muscle hypertrophy.* Muscle tissue uses energy even at rest, whereas fatty tissue uses very little energy and may be considered metabolically inert from the point of view of caloric use.

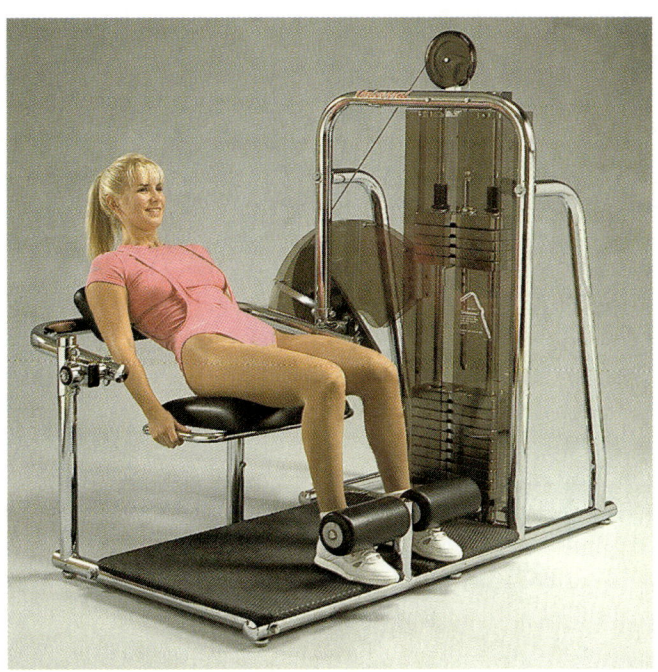

A regular strength-training program facilitates weight loss and lifetime weight management.

As muscle size increases, so does the resting metabolism or the amount of energy (expressed in calories) an individual requires during resting conditions to sustain proper cell function. Even small increases in muscle mass may affect resting metabolism.

Each additional pound of muscle tissue is estimated to increase resting metabolism by 30 to 50 calories per day. All other factors being equal, if two individuals at 150 pounds have different amounts of muscle mass — let's say 5 pounds — the one with the greater muscle mass will have a higher resting metabolic rate. A higher metabolic rate indicates that this person can afford to eat more calories to maintain the additional muscle tissue.

Loss of lean tissue is thought to be the main reason for the decrease in metabolism as people grow older. Contrary to some beliefs, metabolism does not slow down with aging. We slow down.

Lean body mass declines with sedentary living, which, in turn, slows down the resting metabolic rate. If people continue eating at the same rate, body fat increases. The average decrease in resting metabolism for a 60-year-old individual is about 300 to 400 calories per day, as compared to a 25-year-old person. Hence, participating in a strength-training program is a means of preventing and reducing obesity.

One of the most common misconceptions about physical fitness relates to women and strength training. Because of the increase in muscle mass commonly seen in men, some women think strength-training programs are counterproductive because they, too, will develop large muscles. Although the quality of muscle in men and women is the same, endocrinological differences will not allow women to achieve the same amount of muscle hypertrophy (size) as men. Men also have more muscle fibers, and because of the male sex-specific hormones, each fiber has a greater potential for hypertrophy.

As the number of women who participate in sports has increased steadily in the last few years, the myth that strength training for women leads to larger muscle size has waned. In recent years, better body appearance has become the rule rather than the exception for women who participate in strength-training programs. Some of the most attractive women movie stars and many beauty pageant participants train with weights to further improve their personal image.

Another benefit of strength training, accentuated even more when combined with aerobic exercise, is a decrease in adipose (fatty) tissue. Research has shown that the decrease in fatty tissue often is greater than the amount of muscle hypertrophy gained through strength training. Therefore, losing inches but not body weight is a typical outcome.

Because muscle tissue is more dense than fatty tissue, and despite the fact that inches are being lost, people, especially women, often become discouraged because they cannot readily see the results on the scale. This discouragement can be offset easily by regularly determining body composition to monitor changes in percent body fat rather than simply measuring total body weight changes.

GUIDELINES FOR STRENGTH DEVELOPMENT

Because muscular strength and endurance are important in developing and maintaining overall fitness and well-being, the principles necessary to develop a strength-training program have to be followed, as in the prescription of cardiovascular exercise. These principles are built around mode, resistance, sets, and frequency of training. Before discussing these principles, the concepts of *overload* and *specificity of training* are explained.

OVERLOAD PRINCIPLE

Strength gains are achieved in two ways: (a) through greater ability of individual muscle fibers to get a stronger contraction, and (b) by recruiting a greater proportion of the total available fibers for each contraction. These two factors combine in the overload principle. This principle states that, for strength to improve, the demands placed on the muscle must be increased systematically and progressively over a period of time, and the resistance must be of a magnitude significant enough to cause physiologic adaptation. In simpler terms, just like all other organs and systems of the human body, muscles have to be taxed beyond their accustomed loads to increase in physical capacity.

SPECIFICITY OF TRAINING

The principle of specificity of training states that, for a muscle to increase in strength or endurance, the training program must be specific to obtain the desired effects. In like manner, to increase static (isometric) versus dynamic (isotonic) strength, an individual must use static against dynamic training procedures to achieve the desired results.

MODE OF TRAINING

Two basic types of training methods are used to improve strength: *isometric* (static) and *isotonic* (dynamic). Isometric training refers to a muscle contraction producing little or no movement, such as pushing or pulling against immovable objects. Isotonic training refers to a muscle contraction with movement, such as lifting an object over the head.

Isometric training does not require much equipment. It was commonly used several years ago, but its popularity has waned. As strength gains with isometric training are specific to the angle of muscle contraction, this type of training is beneficial in a sport such as gymnastics, which requires regular static contractions during routines.

Isotonic training programs can be conducted without weights or with free weights (barbells and dumbbells), fixed resistance machines, variable resistance machines, and isokinetic equipment. When performing isotonic exercises without weights (for example, pull-ups, push-ups), with free weights, or with fixed resistance machines, a constant resistance (weight) is moved through a joint's full range of motion.

A limitation of isotonic training is that the greatest resistance that can be lifted equals the maximum weight that can be moved at the weakest angle of the joint. This is because of changes in muscle length and angle of pull as the joint moves through its range of motion.

As strength training became more popular, new strength-training machines were developed. This technology brought about isokinetic and variable resistance training. These training programs require special machines equipped with mechanical devices that provide varying amounts of resistance, with the intent of overloading the muscle group maximally through the entire range of motion.

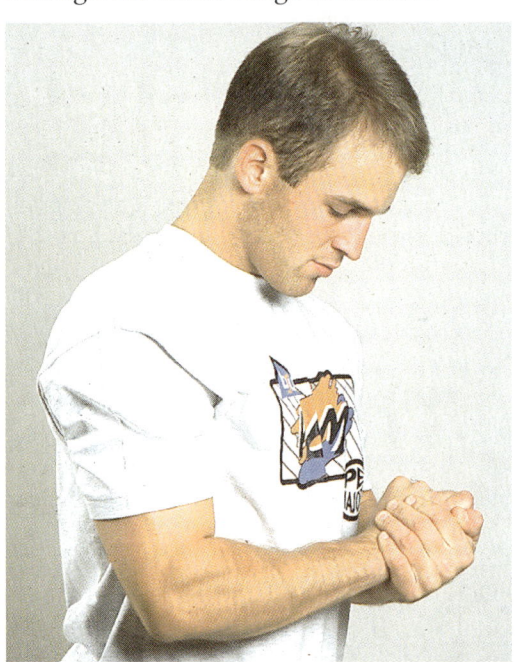

Isometric training.

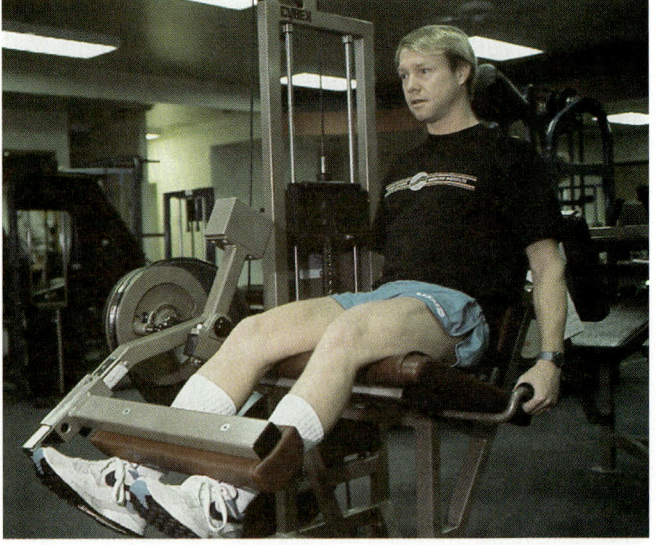

Isotonic training.

A distinction of isokinetic training is that the speed of the muscle contraction is kept constant because the machine provides resistance to match the user's force through the range of motion. The mode of training an individual uses depends mainly on the type of equipment available and the specific objective the training program is attempting to accomplish.

Isotonic training is the most popular mode for strength training. The main advantage is that strength is gained through the full range of motion. Most daily activities are isotonic in nature. We are constantly lifting, pushing, and pulling objects, and strength is needed through a complete range of motion. Another advantage is that improvements are easily measured by the amount lifted.

The benefits of isokinetic and variable resistance training are similar to the other isotonic training methods. Theoretically, strength gains should be better because maximum resistance is applied at all angles. Research, however, has not shown this type of training to be more effective than other modes of isotonic training.

A possible advantage of isokinetic training is that specific speeds used in various sport skills can be duplicated more closely with this type of training, which may enhance performance (specificity of training). A disadvantage is that the equipment is not readily available to many people.

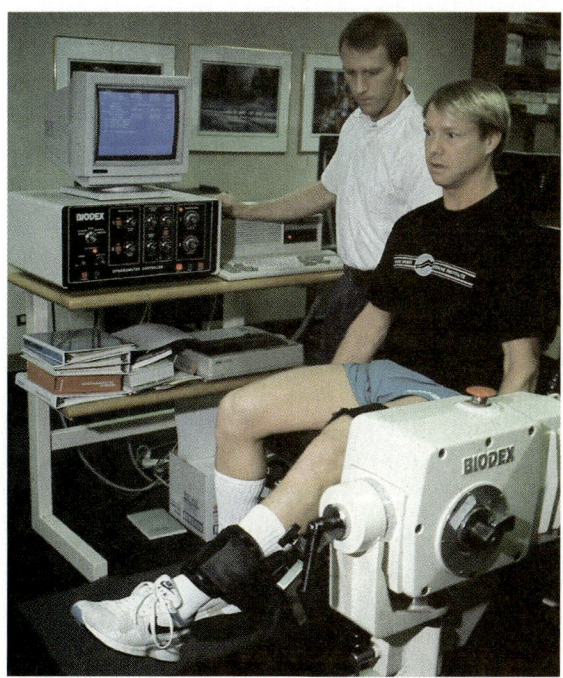

Isokinetic training.

RESISTANCE

Resistance in strength training is the equivalent of intensity in cardiovascular exercise prescription. The amount of resistance, or weight lifted, depends on whether the individual is trying to develop muscular strength or muscular endurance.

To stimulate strength development, a resistance of approximately 80% of the maximum capacity (1 RM) is recommended. For example, a person who can press 150 pounds should work with at least 120 pounds (150 × .80). Using less than 80% will increase muscular endurance rather than strength. Because of the time factor involved in constantly determining the 1 RM on each lift to ensure that the person is indeed working above 80%, a rule of thumb that many authors and coaches accept is that individuals should perform between 3 and 12 repetitions maximum (3 to 12 RM) for adequate strength gains.

For example, if a person is training with a resistance of 120 pounds and cannot lift it more than 12 times, the training stimulus is adequate for strength development. Once the person can lift the weight more than 12 times, the resistance should be increased by 5 to 10 pounds and the person again should build up to 12 repetitions. If training is conducted with more than 12 repetitions, primarily muscular endurance will be developed.

Research on strength indicates that the closer a person trains to the 1 RM, the greater are the strength gains. A disadvantage of constantly working at or near the 1 RM is that it increases the risk for injury.

Highly trained athletes seeking maximum strength development often use 3 to 6 repetitions maximum. Working around 10 repetitions maximum seems to produce the best results in terms of muscular hypertrophy. From a health-fitness point of view, 8 to 12 repetitions maximum are ideal for adequate development. We live in an "isotonic world" in which muscular strength and endurance both are required to lead an enjoyable life. Therefore, working near a 10-repetition threshold seems best to improve overall performance.

SETS

In strength training, a set has been defined as the number of repetitions performed for a given exercise. For example, a person lifting 120 pounds 8 times has performed 1 set of 8 repetitions (1 × 8 × 120). The number of sets recommended for optimum development is 3 sets per exercise.

Because of the characteristics of muscle fiber, the number of sets that can be done is limited. As the number of sets increases, so does muscle fatigue and subsequent recovery time. Therefore, if too many sets are performed, strength gains may be lessened. A recommended program for beginners in their first year of training is 3 heavy sets, up to the maximum number of repetitions, preceded by 1 or 2 light warm-up sets using about 50% of the 1 RM.

To make the exercise program more time-effective, two or three exercises that require different muscle groups may be alternated. In this way, an individual will not have to wait too long before proceeding to a new set on a different exercise. For example, bench press, leg extensions, and abdominal crunches may be combined so the person can go almost directly from one set to the next.

To avoid muscle soreness and stiffness, new participants ought to build up gradually to the 3 sets of maximal repetitions. This can be done by doing only 1 set of each exercise with a lighter resistance on the first day. During the second session, 2 sets of each exercise can be performed, one light and the second with the regular resistance. On the third session, 3 sets could be performed, one light and two heavy. After that, a person should be able to do all 3 heavy sets.

FREQUENCY OF TRAINING

Strength training should be done either with a total body workout three times per week, or more frequently if using a split-body routine (upper body one day, lower body the next). After a maximum strength workout, the muscles should be rested for about 48 hours to allow adequate recovery.

People who are not completely recovered in 2 or 3 days most likely are overtraining and, therefore, not reaping the full benefits of their program. In that case, decreasing the total number of sets or exercises performed during the previous workout is recommended.

To achieve significant strength gains, a minimum of 8 weeks of consecutive training is needed. Once an ideal level of strength is achieved, one training session per week will be sufficient to maintain the new strength level.

DESIGNING A STRENGTH-TRAINING PROGRAM

Two strength-training programs are illustrated at the end of this chapter. Only a minimum of equipment is required for the first program, "Strength-Training Exercises Without Weights." (Exercises 1 through 10). This program can be done within the walls of your own home. Your body weight is used as the primary resistance for most exercises. A few exercises call for a friend's help or some basic implements from around the house to provide more resistance.

"Strength-Training Exercises With Weights" (Exercises 11 through 17) requires machines such as those shown in the photographs. Some of these machines use fixed resistance; others use variable resistance. Many of these exercises also can be done with free weights.

Depending on the facilities available to you, you should be able to choose one of the two training programs outlined in this chapter. The resistance and the number of repetitions you use should be based on whether you want to increase your muscular strength or your muscular endurance. Do up to 10–12 repetitions maximum for strength gains and muscle hypertrophy, and more than 12 for muscular endurance.

As pointed out, three training sessions per week on nonconsecutive days is an ideal arrangement for proper development. Because both strength and endurance are required in daily activities, 3 sets of about 8 to 12 repetitions maximum for each exercise are enough. In doing this, you will obtain good strength gains and yet be close to the endurance threshold.

Perhaps the only exercises that call for more repetitions are abdominal exercises. The abdominal muscles are considered primarily antigravity or postural muscles. Hence, a little more endurance may be required. When doing abdominal work, most people do about 20 repetitions.

If time is a concern in completing a strength-training exercise program, the American College of Sports Medicine recommends as a minimum: (a) 1 set of 8 to 12 repetitions performed to near fatigue, and (b) 8 to 10 exercises involving the major muscle groups of the body, conducted twice a week (see Figure 7.4). This recommendation is based on research showing that this training generates 70% to 80% of the improvements reported in other programs using 3 sets of about 10 RM.

Mode:	8 to 10 isotonic strength-training exercises involving the body's major muscle groups.
Resistance:	Enough resistance to perform 8 to 12 repetitions to near fatigue
Sets:	A minimum of 1 set
Frequency:	At least two times per week

Source: The recommended quantity and quality of exercise for developing and maintaining cardiorespiratory and muscular fitness in healthy adults by the American College of Sports Medicine. *Medical Science Sports Exercise* 22, (1990):265–274.

FIGURE 7.4 ▼ Strength-training guidelines.

MUSCULAR FLEXIBILITY

Flexibility is defined as the ability of a joint to move freely through its full range of motion. Health care professionals and practitioners generally have underestimated and overlooked the contribution of good muscular flexibility to overall fitness and preventive health care.

SIGNIFICANCE OF FLEXIBILITY

Approximately 80% of all low back problems in the United States are attributable to improper alignment of the vertebral column and pelvic girdle, a direct result of inflexible and weak muscles. This backache syndrome costs American industry more than $1 billion each year in lost productivity and services alone, and an extra $225 million in Worker's Compensation. In daily life we often have to make rapid or strenuous movements we are not accustomed to making, which may cause injury. And physical therapists have indicated that improper body mechanics are often the result of poor flexibility.

Participating in a regular flexibility program helps a person maintain good joint mobility, increases resistance to muscle injury and soreness, prevents low-back and other spinal column problems, improves and maintains good postural alignment, promotes proper and graceful body movement, improves personal appearance and self-image, and helps to develop and maintain motor skills throughout life. In addition, flexibility exercises have been prescribed successfully to treat dysmenorrhea (painful menstruation) and general neuromuscular tension (stress).

Furthermore, stretching exercises in conjunction with calisthenics are helpful in warm-up routines to prepare the human body for more vigorous aerobic or strength-training exercises, as well as cool-down routines following exercise to help the person return to a normal resting state. Fatigued muscles tend to contract to a shorter than average resting length, and stretching exercises help fatigued muscles re-establish their normal resting length.

Total range of motion around a joint is highly specific and varies from one joint to the other (hip, trunk, shoulder), as well as from one individual to the next. The amount of muscular flexibility relates primarily to genetic factors and index of physical activity. Other factors that influence range of motion about a joint include joint structure, ligaments, tendons, muscles, skin, tissue injury, adipose tissue (fat), body temperature, age, and gender.

Because of the specificity of flexibility, to indicate what constitutes an ideal level of flexibility is difficult. Nevertheless, flexibility is important to everyone's health, and even more so during the aging process.

GUIDELINES FOR FLEXIBILITY DEVELOPMENT

Although genetics play a crucial role in body flexibility, range of joint mobility can be increased and maintained through a regular flexibility exercise program. Because range of motion is highly specific to each body part (ankle, trunk, shoulder), a comprehensive stretching program, which includes all body parts and adheres to the basic guidelines for flexibility development, should be followed to obtain optimal results.

The overload and specificity of training principles discussed in conjunction with strength development also apply to the development of muscular flexibility. To increase the total range of motion of a joint, the specific muscles surrounding that joint have to be stretched progressively beyond their accustomed length. Principles of mode, intensity, repetitions, and frequency of exercise also can be applied to flexibility programs.

MODE OF EXERCISE

Three modes of stretching exercises can be used to increase flexibility: (a) ballistic stretching, (b) slow-sustained stretching, and (c) proprioceptive neuromuscular facilitation stretching. Although research has indicated that all three types of stretching are effective in developing better flexibility, each technique has certain advantages.

Ballistic (or *dynamic*) *stretching* exercises are performed using jerky, rapid, and bouncy movements that provide the necessary force to lengthen the muscles. Studies have shown that this type of stretching helps to develop flexibility, but the ballistic actions may cause muscle soreness and injury because of small tears to the soft tissue.

Precautions must be taken not to overstretch ligaments, as they undergo plastic or permanent elongation. If the stretching force cannot be controlled, as in fast, jerky movements, ligaments can be easily overstretched. This, in turn, leads to excessively loose joints, heightening the risk for injuries, including joint dislocation and sublaxation (partial dislocation). Most authorities, therefore, do not recommend ballistic exercises for flexibility development.

With *slow-sustained stretching* technique, muscles are lengthened gradually through a joint's complete range of motion, and the final position is held for a few seconds. Using a slow-sustained stretch causes the muscles to relax so greater length can be achieved. This type of stretch causes little pain and has a low risk for injury. Slow-sustained stretching exercises are used most frequently and are recommended for flexibility development programs.

Proprioceptive neuromuscular facilitation (PNF) stretching has become more popular in the last few years. This technique is based on a "contract and relax" method and requires the assistance of another person. The procedure is as follows:

1. The person assisting with the exercise provides an initial force by slowly pushing in the direction of the desired stretch. The initial stretch does not cover the entire range of motion.

2. The person being stretched then applies force in the opposite direction of the stretch, against the assistant, who tries to hold the initial degree of stretch as closely as possible. An isometric contraction is being performed at that angle.

3. After 4 or 5 seconds of isometric contraction, the muscle(s) being stretched are relaxed completely. The assistant then slowly increases the degree of stretch to a greater angle.

4. The isometric contraction is then repeated for another 4 or 5 seconds, after which the muscle is relaxed again. The assistant then can slowly increase the degree of stretch one more time. This procedure is repeated two to five times, until the exerciser feels mild discomfort. On the last trial, the final stretched position should be held for several seconds.

Theoretically, with the PNF technique, the isometric contraction helps relax the muscle(s) being stretched, which results in greater muscle length. Although some fitness leaders believe that PNF is more effective than slow-sustained stretching, the disadvantages are more pain with PNF, a second person is required to assist, and more time is needed to conduct each session.

INTENSITY OF EXERCISE

Before starting any flexibility exercises, the muscles always should be warmed up using some calisthenic exercises. A good time to do flexibility exercises is after aerobic workouts. Higher body temperature can increase joint range of motion significantly. Failing to do a proper warm-up increases the risk for muscle pulls and tears.

When doing flexibility exercises, the intensity or degree of stretch should be only to a point of mild discomfort. Pain does not have to be a part of the stretching routine.

Excessive pain is an indication that the load is too high and may lead to injury. Stretching should be done to slightly below the pain threshold. As participants reach this point, they should try to relax the muscle or muscles being stretched as much as

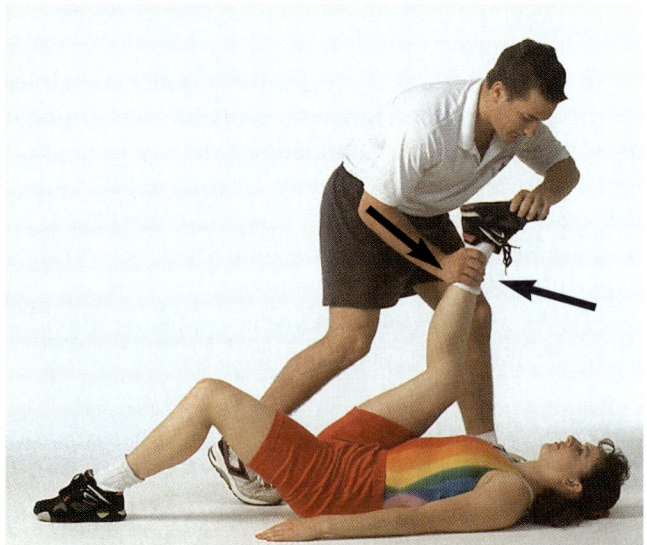

Proprioceptive Neuromuscular Facilitation (PNF) stretching technique.

possible. After completing the stretch, the body part is brought back gradually to the starting point.

REPETITIONS

In an exercise session, the time required for flexibility development is based on the number of repetitions performed and the length of time each repetition (final stretched position) is held. The general recommendation is that each exercise be done four or five times, holding the final position each time for about 10 seconds. As flexibility increases, the individual can gradually increase the time each repetition is held, to a maximum of a minute.

FREQUENCY OF TRAINING

Flexibility exercises should be conducted five to six times a week in the initial stages of the program. After a minimum of 6 to 8 weeks of almost daily stretching, flexibility levels can be maintained with only two or three sessions per week, using about 3 repetitions of 10 to 15 seconds each. Figure 7.5 provides a summary of flexibility development guidelines.

DESIGNING A FLEXIBILITY PROGRAM

To improve body flexibility, each major muscle group should be subjected to at least one stretching exercise. A complete set of exercises for developing muscular flexibility is presented at the end of this chapter. With some of the exercises, you may not be able to hold a final stretched position (examples are lateral head tilts and arm circles), but you still should perform the exercise through the joint's full range of motion. Depending on the number and the length of the repetitions, a complete workout will last between 15 and 30 minutes.

Mode:	Static stretching or proprioceptive neuromuscular facilitation (PNF)
Intensity:	Stretch to the point of mild discomfort
Repetitions:	Repeat each exercise 4 to 5 times and hold the final stretched position for 10 to 60 seconds
Frequency:	2 to 6 days per week

FIGURE 7.5 ▼ Flexibility development guidelines.

PREVENTING AND REHABILITATING LOW BACK PAIN

Few people make it through life without having low back pain at some point. An estimated 75 million Americans currently have chronic low back pain each year. About 80% of the time, backache syndrome is preventable and is caused by: (a) physical inactivity, (b) poor postural habits and body mechanics, and (c) excessive body weight.

Lack of physical activity is the most common contributor to chronic low back pain. Deterioration or weakening of the abdominal and gluteal muscles, along with tightening of the lower back (erector spine) muscles, brings about an unnatural forward tilt of the pelvis. This tilt puts extra pressure on the spinal vertebrae, causing pain in the lower back. Accumulation of fat around the midsection of the body contributes to the forward tilt of the pelvis, which further aggravates the condition.

Low back pain frequently is associated with faulty posture and improper body mechanics (body positions in all of life's daily activities, including sleeping, sitting, standing, walking, driving, working, and exercising). Incorrect posture and poor mechanics, as explained in Figure 7.6, increase strain not only on the lower back but on many other bones, joints, muscles, and ligaments as well.

The incidence and frequency of low back pain episodes can be reduced greatly by including some specific stretching and strengthening exercises in the regular fitness program. In most cases, back pain is present only with movement and physical activity.

If the pain is severe and persists even at rest, the first step is to consult a physician, who can rule out any disc damage and most likely will prescribe proper bed rest using several pillows under the knees for leg support. This position helps release muscle spasms by stretching the muscles involved.

The physician also may prescribe a muscle relaxant or anti-inflammatory medication (or both) and some type of physical therapy. Once the individual is pain-free in the resting state, he or she needs to start correcting the muscular imbalance by stretching the tight muscles and strengthening the weak ones. Stretching exercises always are performed first.

Several exercises for preventing and rehabilitating the back are given at the end of this chapter. These exercises can be done twice or more daily when a person has back pain. Under normal circumstances,

Your Back and How to Care For It

HOW TO STAY ON YOUR FEET WITHOUT TIRING YOUR BACK

To prevent strain and pain in everyday activities, it is restful to change from one task to another before fatigue sets in. Housewives can lie down between chores; others should check body position frequently, drawing in the abdomen, flattening the back, bending the knees slightly.

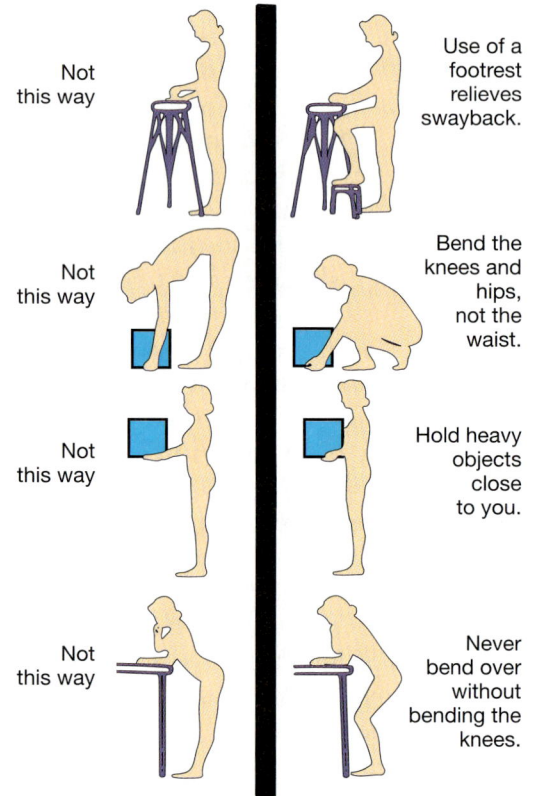

- Not this way / Use of a footrest relieves swayback.
- Not this way / Bend the knees and hips, not the waist.
- Not this way / Hold heavy objects close to you.
- Not this way / Never bend over without bending the knees.

HOW TO PUT YOUR BACK TO BED

For proper bed posture, a firm mattress is essential. Bedboards, sold commercially, or devised at home, may be used with soft mattresses. Bedboards, preferably, should be made of 3/4 inch plywood. Faulty sleeping positions intensify swayback and result not only in backache but in numbness, tingling, and pain in arms and legs.

Incorrect:

Lying flat on back makes swayback worse.

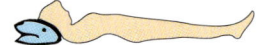
Use of high pillow strains neck, arms, shoulders.

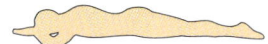
Sleeping face down exaggerates swayback, strains neck and shoulders.

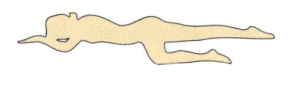
Bending one hip and knee does not relieve swayback.

Correct:

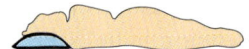
Lying on side with knees bent effectively flattens the back. Flat pillow may be used to support neck, especially when shoulders are broad.

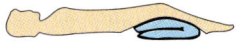
Sleeping on back is restful and correct when knees are properly supported.

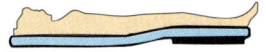
Raise the foot of the mattress eight inches to discourage sleeping on the abdomen.

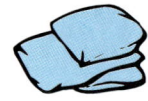
Proper arrangement of pillows for resting or reading in bed.

HOW TO SIT CORRECTLY

A back's best friend is a straight, hard chair. If you can't get the chair you prefer, learn to sit properly on whatever chair you get. To correct sitting position from forward slump: Throw head well back, then bend it forward to pull in the chin. This will straighten the back. Now tighten abdominal muscles to raise the chest. Check position frequently.

Relieve strain by sitting well forward, flatten back by tightening abdominal muscles, and cross knees.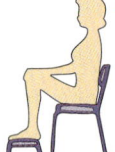

TV slump leads to "dowager's hump," strains neck and shoulders.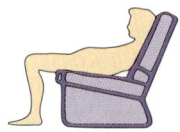

Driver's seat too far from pedals emphasizes curve in lower back.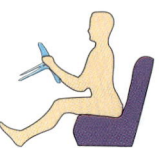

Use of footrest relieves swayback. Aim is to have knees higher than hips.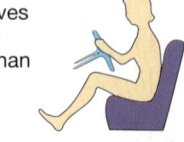

If chair is too high, swayback is increased.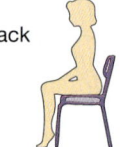

Strained reading position. Forward thrusting strains muscles of neck and head.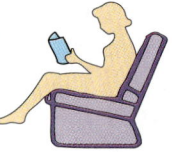

Correct way to sit while driving, close to pedals. Use seat belt or hard backrest, available commercially.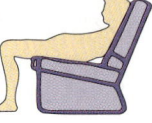

Keep neck and back in as straight a line as possible with the spine. Bend forward from hips.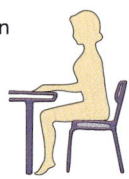

Reproduced with permission of Schering Corporation. Copyright Schering Corporation, Kenilworth, NJ

FIGURE 7.6 ▼ Your back and how to care for it.

three to four times a week is sufficient to prevent the syndrome.

MANAGEMENT OF EXERCISE-RELATED INJURIES

To enjoy and maintain physical fitness, preventing injury during a conditioning program is essential. Exercise-related injuries, nonetheless, are common in individuals who participate in exercise programs. Surveys show that more than half of all new exercise participants will incur injuries during the first 6 months of the conditioning program. The three most common causes of injuries are: (a) rapid conditioning programs — doing too much too quick, (b) improper shoes or training surfaces, and (c) anatomical predisposition (body propensity). Substantial increases in quantity, intensity, and duration of activities comprise the most common cause of injuries, by far. The body requires time to adapt to more intense activities. Most of these injuries could be prevented through a more gradual and proper conditioning program.

The best treatment always has been prevention itself. If an activity is causing unusual discomfort or chronic irritation, you need to treat the cause by decreasing the intensity, switching activities, or using better equipment such as proper-fitting shoes.

In the case of acute injury, the standard method of treatment is cold application, compression or splinting, and elevation of the affected body part. Cold should be applied three to five times a day for 15 to 20 minutes at a time during the first 36 to 48 hours. Cold can be applied by submerging the injured area in cold water, using an ice bag, or applying ice massage to the affected part. Compression can be applied with an elastic bandage or wrap. Elevating the body part, whenever possible, will decrease blood flow to it. The purpose of this treatment is to minimize swelling in the area, which greatly increases recovery time. After the first 36 to 48 hours, heat can be applied in the absence of further swelling or inflammation. If you have doubts regarding the nature or seriousness of the injury (such as suspected fracture), however, you should seek a medical evaluation.

Whenever an obvious deformity (such as in fractures, dislocations, or partial dislocations) is present, splinting, cold application with an ice bag, and medical attention are required. No one other than medical personnel should attempt to correct these conditions, as muscles, ligaments, and nerves could be further damaged. A quick reference guide for the signs or symptoms and treatment of exercise-related problems is provided in Table 7.2.

EXERCISE INTOLERANCE

As you start your exercise program, be sure to stay within the safe limits for exercise participation. The best method to determine whether you are exercising too strenuously is to check your heart rate and make sure it does not exceed the limits of your target zone. Exercising above this target zone may not be safe for unconditioned or high-risk individuals. You do not need to exercise beyond your target zone to gain the desired benefits for the cardiovascular system.

In addition, several physical signs will tell you when you are exceeding functional limitations. These include a rapid or irregular heart rate, difficult breathing, nausea, vomiting, lightheadedness, headaches, dizziness, pale skin, flushness, extreme weakness, lack of energy, shakiness, sore muscles, cramps, and tightness in the chest. If you notice any of these symptoms, you should seek medical attention before continuing your exercise program. One of the basic things you will need to learn with exercise is to listen to your body.

Your recovery heart rate also can be an indicator of overexertion. To a certain extent, recovery heart rate is related to fitness level. The higher your cardiovascular fitness level, the faster your heart rate will decrease following exercise. As a rule of thumb, heart rate should be below 120 beats per minute 5 minutes into recovery. If your heart rate is above 120, you have most likely overexerted yourself or could possibly have some other cardiac abnormality. If you decrease the intensity or duration of exercise and you still have a fast heart rate 5 minutes into recovery, consult your physician.

LEISURE-TIME PHYSICAL ACTIVITY

Although individuals have notable differences, the average person in developed countries has about 3.5 hours of "free" or leisure-time daily. Unfortunately,

TABLE 7.2 ▼ Reference Guide For Exercise-Related Problems

Injury	Signs/Symptoms	Treatment*
Bruise (contusion)	Pain, swelling, discoloration	Cold application, compression, rest
Dislocations Fractures	Pain, swelling, deformity	Splinting, cold application, seek medical attention
Heat cramps	Cramps, spasms and muscle twitching in the legs, arms, and abdomen	Stop activity, get out of the heat, stretch, massage the painful area, drink plenty of fluids
Heat exhaustion	Fainting, profuse sweating, cold/clammy skin, weak/rapid pulse, weakness, headache	Stop activity, rest in a cool place, loosen clothing, rub body with cool/wet towel, drink plenty of fluids, stay out of heat for 2–3 days
Heat stroke	Hot/dry skin, no sweating, serious disorientation, rapid/full pulse, vomiting, diarrhea, unconsciousness, high body temperature	*Seek immediate medical attention*, request help and get out of the sun, bathe in cold water / spray with cold water / rub body with cold towels, drink plenty of cold fluids
Joint sprains	Pain, tenderness, swelling, loss of use, discoloration	Cold application, compression, elevation, rest, heat after 36 to 48 hours (if no further swelling)
Muscle cramps	Pain, spasm	Stretch muscle(s), use mild exercises for involved area
Muscle soreness and stiffness	Tenderness, pain	Mild stretching, low-intensity exercise, warm bath
Muscle strains	Pain, tenderness, swelling, loss of use	Cold application, compression, elevation, rest, heat after 36 to 48 hours (if no further swelling)
Shin splints	Pain, tenderness	Cold application prior to and following any physical activity, rest, heat (if no activity is carried out)
Side stitch	Pain on the side of the abdomen below the rib cage	Decrease level of physical activity or stop altogether, gradually increase level of fitness
Tendonitis	Pain, tenderness, loss of use	Rest, cold application, heat after 48 hours

* Cold should be applied 3 to 4 times a day for 15 minutes
  Heat can be applied 3 times a day for 15 to 20 minutes

in the current automated society, most of this time is spent in sedentary living.

Leisure-time physical activity usually is viewed as any activity undertaken during an individual's discretionary time that helps to increase resting energy or caloric expenditure. These activities are selected based on personal interests. Motivational factors for participation include health, aesthetics, weight control, competition and challenge, fun, social interaction, mental arousal, relaxation, and stress management.

Frequently, leisure-time physical activity does not include exercise performed during a regular exercise program. It consists of activities such as walking, hiking, gardening, yard work, occupational work and chores, and moderate sports such as tennis, table tennis, badminton, golf, and croquet.

Every small increase in daily physical activity contributes to the development of health and wellness. Small increases in physical activity have a large impact in decreasing early risk for disease and premature death. Therefore, a new, concerted effort must be made to spend leisure-time in activities that promote energy expenditure, provide a break from daily tasks, and contribute to health-related fitness.

▼ TIPS TO ENHANCE EXERCISE ADHERENCE

Different things motivate different people to join and remain in a fitness program. Regardless of the initial reason for beginning an exercise program, you now need to plan for ways to make your workout fun. The psychology behind it is simple. If you enjoy an activity, you will continue to do it. If you don't, you will quit. Some of the following suggestions may help:

1. Start your exercise program slowly. Adhering to new behaviors takes time. Don't be discouraged if you can exercise only a few minutes or if you miss one or more exercise sessions. The key to success is perseverance.
2. Select aerobic activities you enjoy doing. Picking an activity you don't enjoy makes you less likely to keep exercising. Don't be afraid to try out a new activity, even if that means learning new skills.
3. Combine different activities. You can train by doing two or three different activities the same week. Some people find that this counteracts the monotony of repeating the same activity every day. Try lifetime sports. Many endurance sports such as racquetball, basketball, soccer, badminton, in-line skating, cross-country skiing, and surfing (paddling the board) provide a nice break from regular workouts.
4. Set aside a regular time for exercise. If you don't plan ahead, exercise is a lot easier to skip. Holding your exercise hour "sacred" helps you adhere to the program.
5. Obtain the proper equipment for exercise. A poor pair of shoes, for example, can increase the risk for injury, discouraging you right from the beginning.
6. Find a friend or a group of friends to exercise with. Social interaction makes exercise more fulfilling. Besides, exercise is harder to skip if someone else is waiting for you.
7. Set goals and share them with others. Quitting is tougher when someone else knows what you are trying to accomplish. When you reach a specific goal, reward yourself with a new pair of shoes or a jogging suit.
8. Don't become a chronic exerciser. Learn to listen to your body. Overexercising can lead to chronic fatigue and injuries. Exercise should be enjoyable, and in the process you will need to "stop and smell the roses."
9. Exercise in different places and facilities. This practice adds variety to your workouts.
10. Keep a regular record of your activities. Keeping a record allows you to monitor your progress and compare it with previous months and years.
11. Conduct periodic assessments. Improving to a higher fitness category is a reward in itself.
12. If health problems arise, see a physician. When in doubt, "better safe than sorry."

To stay fit, you need to maintain a regular exercise program, even during vacations. If you have to interrupt your program for reasons beyond your control, do not attempt to resume your training at the same level you left off. Rather, build up gradually again.

NOTES

1. American College of Sports Medicine. *Guidelines for Exercise Testing and Prescription.* Philadelphia: Lea & Febiger, 1991.

2. DeBusk, R. F., U. Stenestrand, M. Sheehan, and W. L. Haskell. Training effects of long versus short bouts of exercise in healthy subjects." *The American Journal of Cardiology* 65:1010–1013, 1990.

SEVEN ▼ *Exercise Prescription For Wellness*   153

STRENGTH-TRAINING EXERCISES

EXERCISE 1

Step-Up

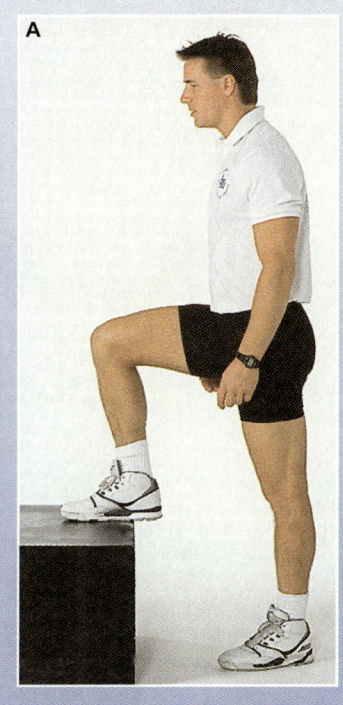 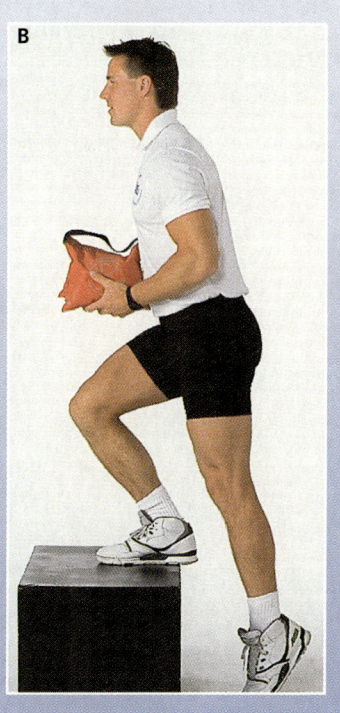

Action: Step up and down using a box or chair approximately twelve to fifteen inches high. Conduct one set using the same leg each time you go up and then conduct a second set using the other leg. You could also alternate legs on each step-up cycle. You may increase the resistance by holding a child or some other object in your arms (hold the child or object close to the body to avoid increased strain in the lower back).

Muscles Developed: Gluteal muscles, quadriceps, gastrocnemius, and soleus.

EXERCISE 2

High-Jumper

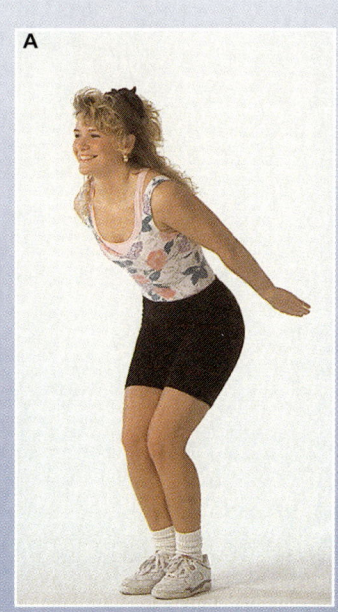 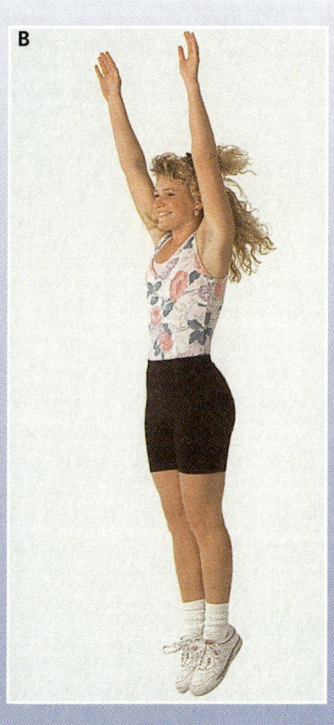

Action: Start with the knees bent at approximately 150° and jump as high as you can, raising both arms simultaneously.

Muscles Developed: Gluteal muscles, quadriceps, gastrocnemius, and soleus.

EXERCISE 3

Push-Up

Action: Maintaining your body as straight as possible, flex the elbows, lowering the body until you almost touch the floor, then raise yourself back up to the starting position. If you are unable to perform the push-up as indicated, you can decrease the resistance by supporting the lower body with the knees rather than the feet (see illustration c) or using an incline plane and supporting your hands at a higher point than the floor (see illustration d). If you wish to increase the resistance, have someone else add resistance to your shoulders as you are coming back up (see illustration e).

Muscles Developed: Triceps, deltoid, pectoralis major, erector spinae, and abdominals.

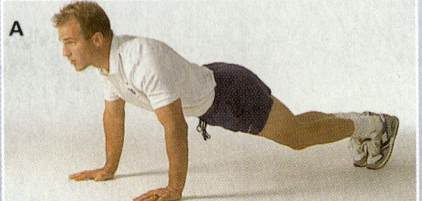
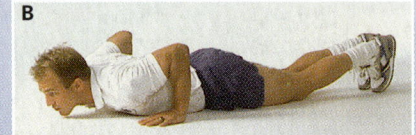
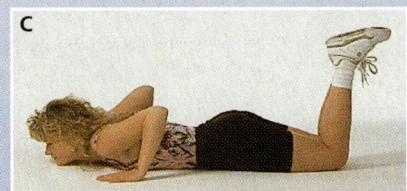
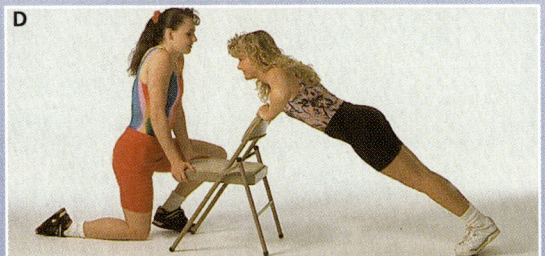
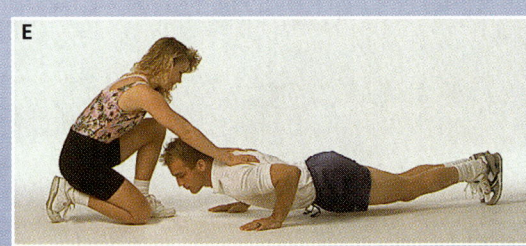

EXERCISE 4

Abdominal Crunch and Abdominal Curl-Up

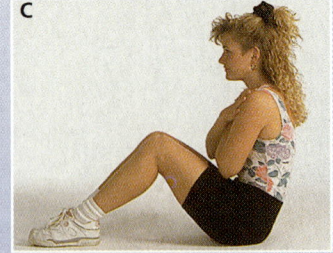
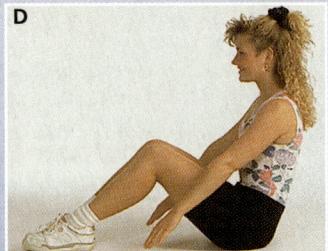

Action: Start with your head and shoulders off the floor, arms crossed on your chest, and knees slightly bent (the greater the flexion of the knee, the more difficult the curl-up). Now curl up to about 30° (abdominal crunch — see illustration b) or curl all the way up (abdominal curl-up), then return to the starting position without letting the head or shoulders touch the floor, or allowing the hips to come off the floor. If you allow the hips to raise off the floor and the head and shoulders to touch the floor, you will most likely "swing up" on the next repetition, which minimizes the work of the abdominal muscles. If you cannot curl up with the arms on the chest, place the hands by the side of the hips or even help yourself up by holding on to your thighs (illustrations d and e). Do not perform the sit-up exercise with your legs completely extended, as this will cause strain on the lower back.

Muscles Developed: Abdominal muscles and hip flexors.

EXERCISE 5

Leg Curl

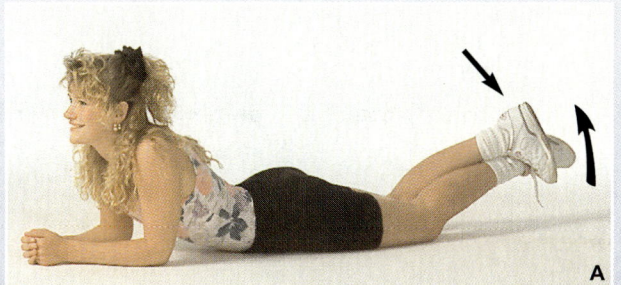

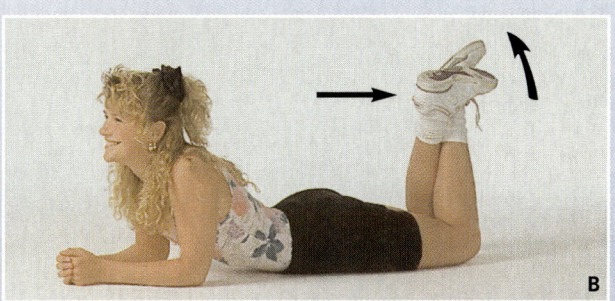

Action: Lie on the floor face down. Cross the right ankle over the left heel. Apply resistance with your right foot, while you bring the left foot up to 90° at the knee joint. (Apply enough resistance so that the left foot can only be brought up slowly.) Repeat the exercise, crossing the left ankle over the right heel.

Muscles Developed: Hamstrings (and quadriceps).

EXERCISE 6

Modified Dip

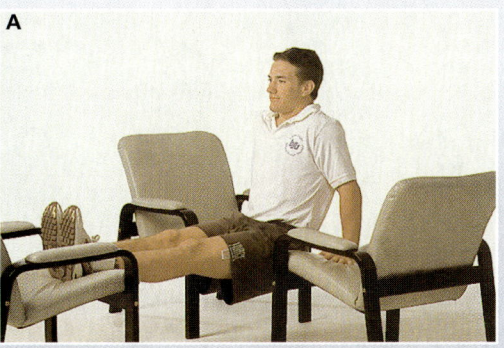

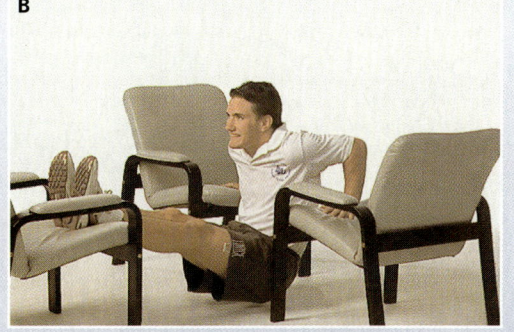

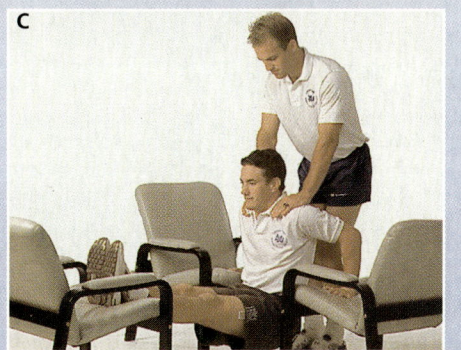

Action: Place your hands and feet on opposite chairs with knees slightly bent (make sure that the chairs are well stabilized). Dip down at least to a 90° angle at the elbow joint, then return to the initial position. To increase the resistance, have someone else hold you down by the shoulders on the way up (see illustration c).

Muscles Developed: Triceps, deltoid, and pectoralis major.

EXERCISE 7

Pull-Up

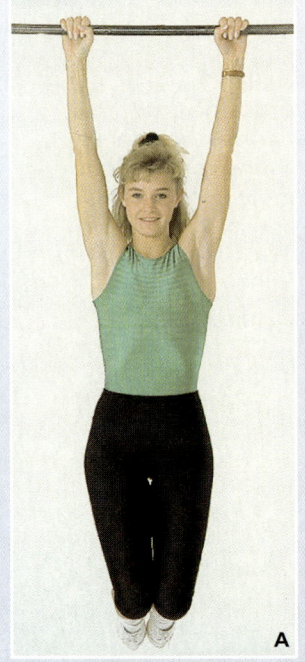
A

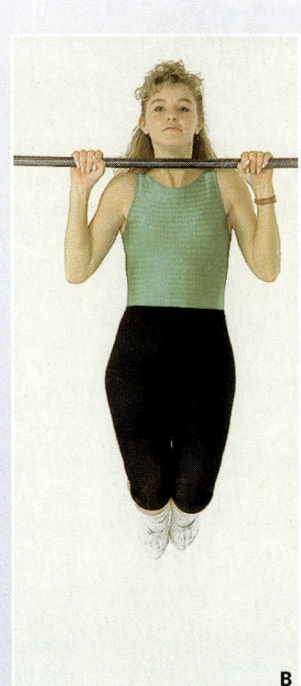
B

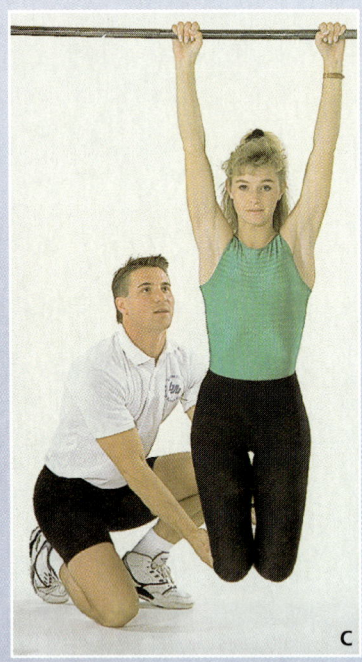
C

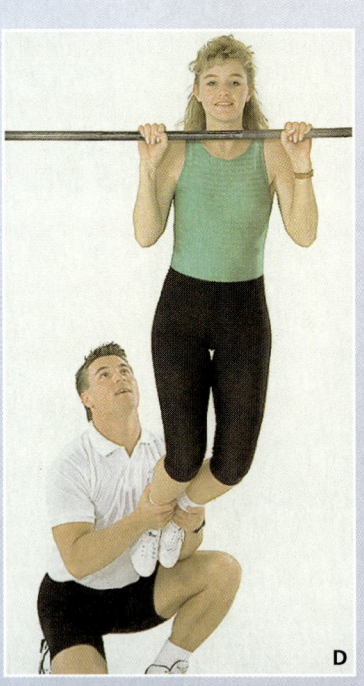
D

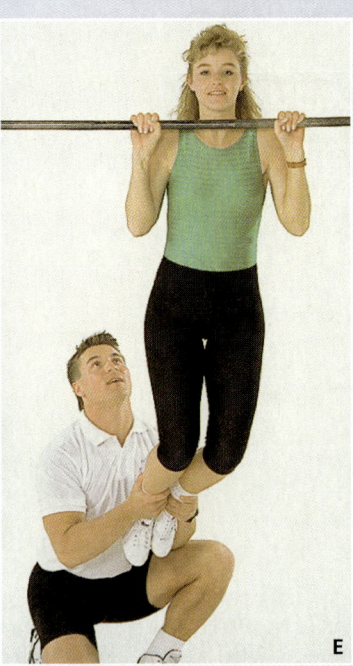
E

Action: Suspend yourself from a bar with a pronated grip (thumbs in). Pull your body up until your chin is above the bar, then lower the body slowly to the starting position. If you are unable to perform the pull-up as described, either have a partner hold your feet to push off and facilitate the movement upward (illustrations c and d) or use a lower bar and support your feet on the floor (illustration e).

Muscles Developed: Biceps, brachioradialis, brachialis, trapezius, and latissimus dorsi.

EXERCISE 8

Arm Curl

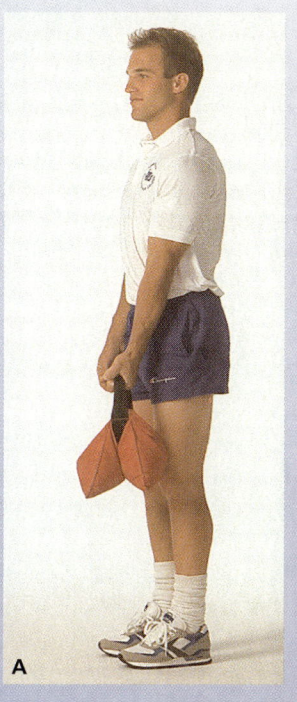
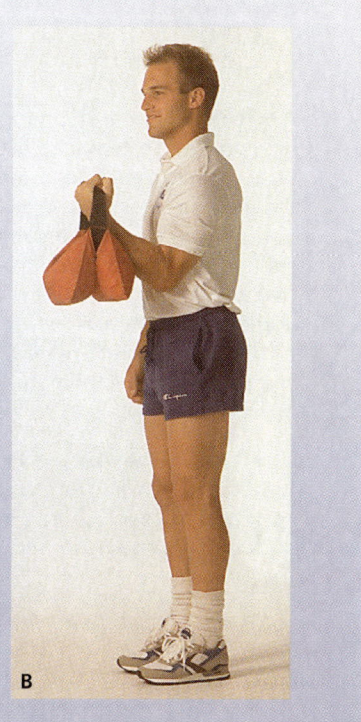

Action: Using a palms-up grip, start with the arm completely extended, and with the aid of a sandbag or bucket filled (as needed) with sand or rocks, curl up as far as possible, then return to the initial position. Repeat the exercise with the other arm.

Muscles Developed: Biceps, brachioradialis, and brachialis.

EXERCISE 9

Heel Raise

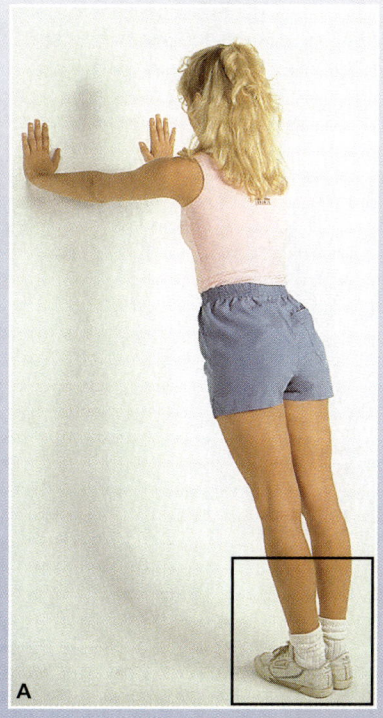
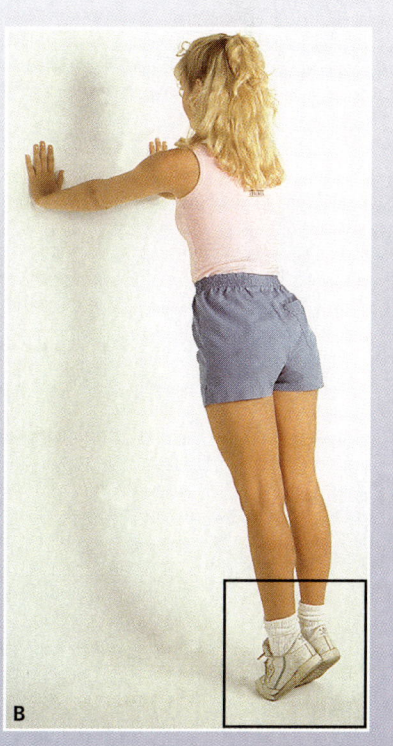

Action: From a standing position with feet flat on the floor, raise and lower your body weight by moving at the ankle joint only (for added resistance, have someone else hold your shoulders down as you perform the exercise).

Muscles Developed: Gastrocnemius and soleus.

EXERCISE 10

Leg Abduction and Adduction

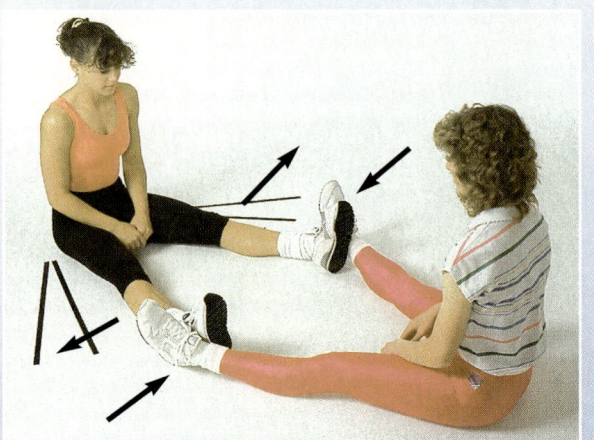

Action: Both participants sit on the floor. The subject on the left places the feet on the inside of the other participant's feet. Simultaneously, the subject on the left presses the legs laterally (to the outside — abduction), while the subject on the right presses the legs medially (adduction). Hold the contraction for five to ten seconds. Repeat the exercise at all three angles, and then reverse the pressing sequence. The subject on the left places the feet on the outside and presses inward, while the subject on the right presses outward.

Muscles Developed: Hip abductors (rectus femoris, sartori, gluteus medius and minimus), and adductors (pectineus, gracilis, adductor magnus, adductor longus, and adductor brevis).

STRENGTH-TRAINING EXERCISES WITH WEIGHTS

EXERCISE 11

Arm Curl

Action: Use a supinated or palms-up grip, and start with the arms almost completely extended. Now curl up as far as possible, then return to the starting position.

Muscles Developed: Biceps, brachioradialis, and brachialis.

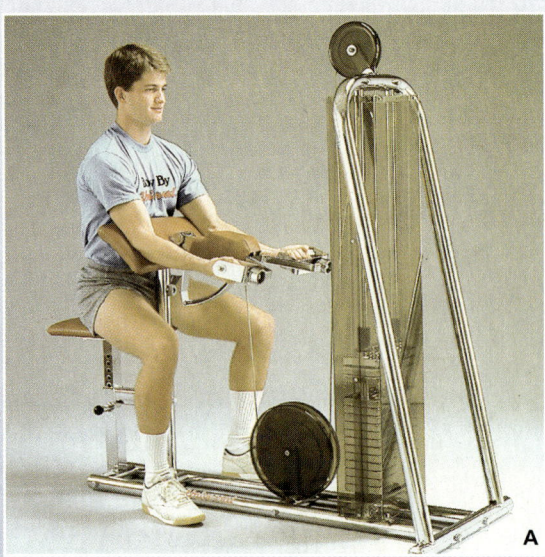
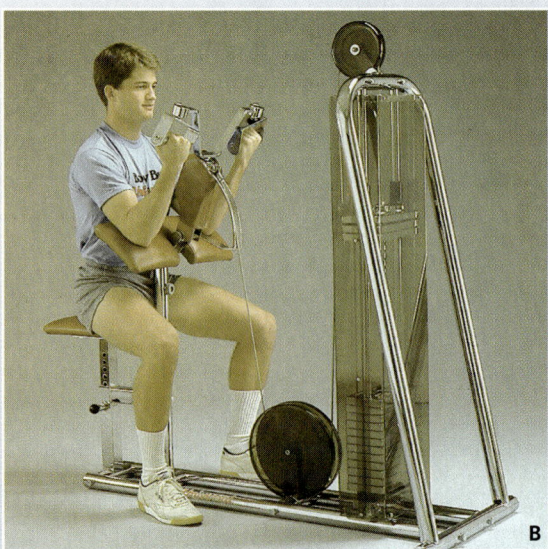

A   B

EXERCISE 12

Bench Press

Action: Lie down on the bench with the head by the weight stack, the bench press bar above the chest, and keep the feet on the floor. Grasp the bar handles and press upward until the arms are completely extended, then return to the original position. Do not arch the back during this exercise. CAUTION: If you are susceptible to low back pain, place your feet on the bench.

Muscles Developed: Pectoralis major, triceps, and deltoid.

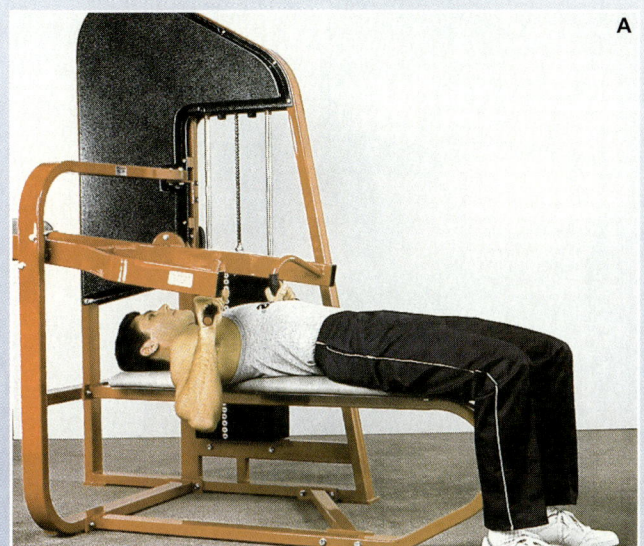
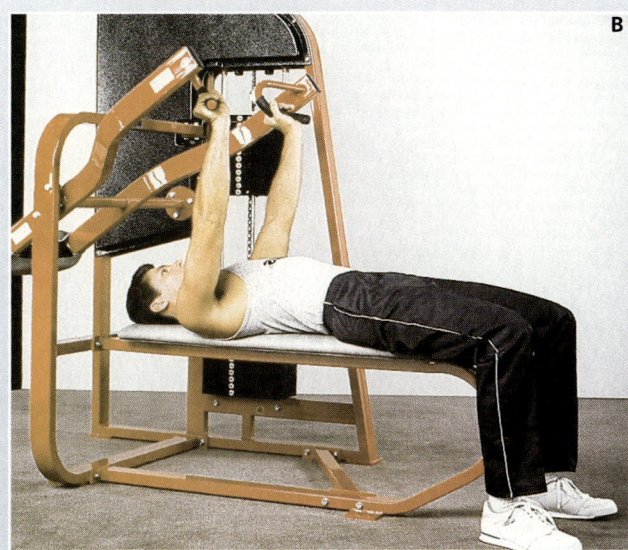

EXERCISE 13

Abdominal Crunch and Abdominal Curl-up

See exercise 4 in this chapter.

EXERCISE 14

Leg Extension

Action: Sit in an upright position with the feet under the padded bar and grasp the handles at the sides. Extend the legs until they are completely straight, then return to the starting position.

Muscles Developed: Quadriceps.

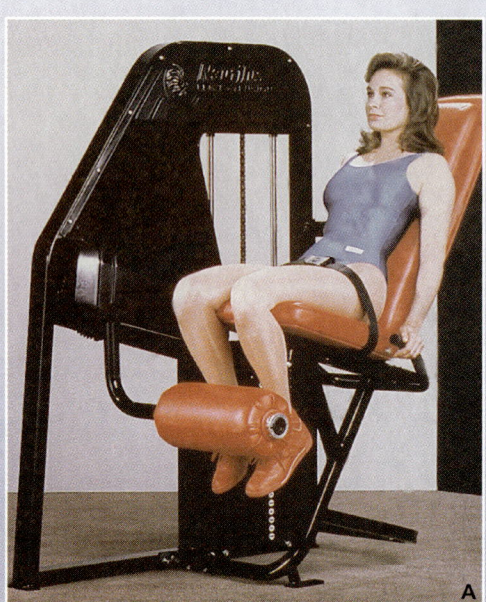
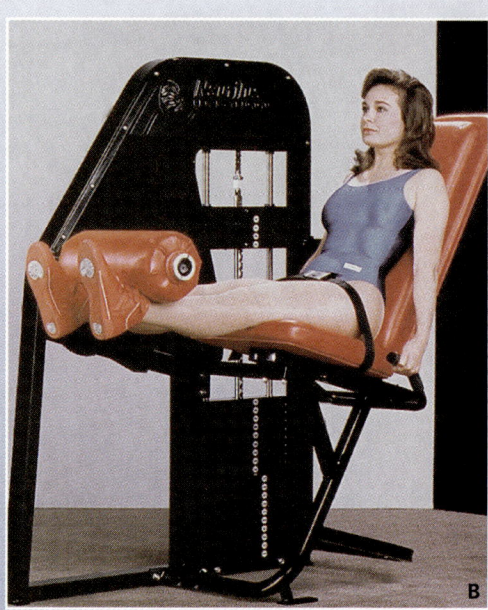

EXERCISE 15

Leg Curl

Action: Lie with the face down on the bench, legs straight, and place the back of the feet under the padded bar. Curl up to at least 90°, and return to the original position.

Muscles Developed: Hamstrings.

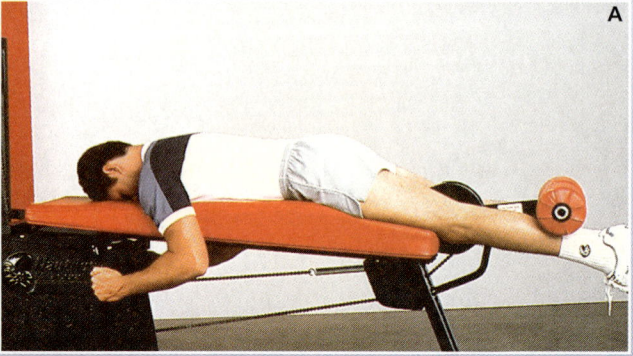
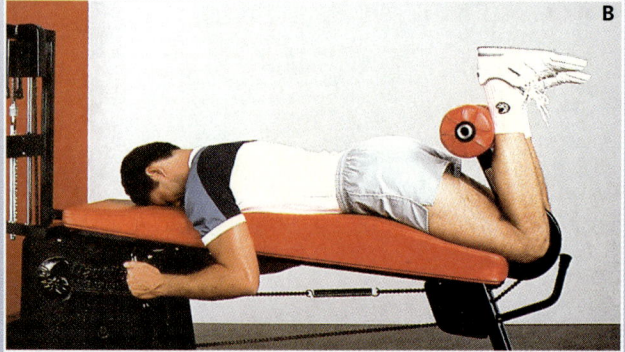

EXERCISE 16

Lat Pull-Down

Action: Start from a sitting position, and hold the exercise bar with a wide grip. Pull the bar down until it touches the base of the neck, then return to the starting position (if a heavy resistance is used, stabilization of the body may be required by either using equipment as shown or by having someone else hold you down by the waist or shoulders).

Muscles Developed: Latissimus dorsi, pectoralis major, and biceps.

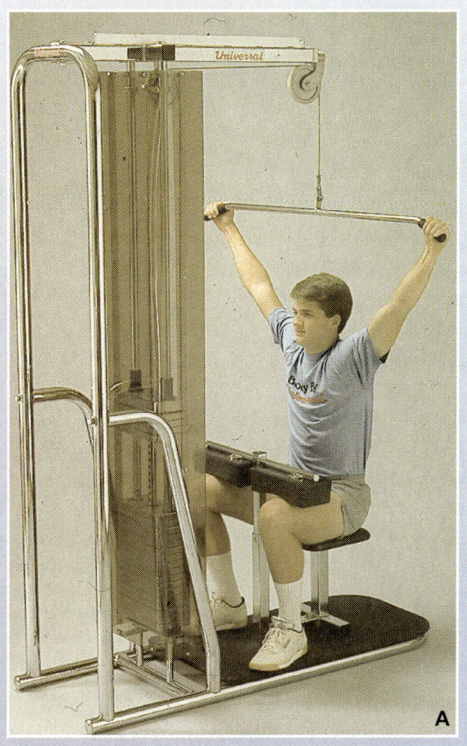
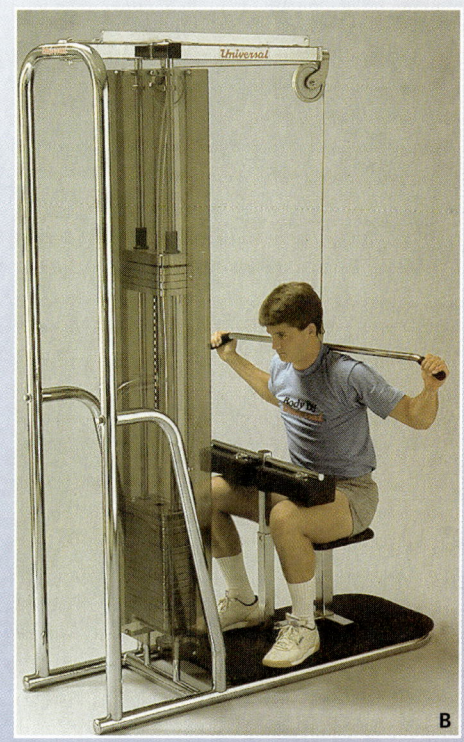

EXERCISE 17

Heel Raise

Action: Start with your feet either flat on the floor or the front of the feet on an elevated block, then raise and lower yourself by moving at the ankle joint only. If additional resistance is needed, you can use a squat strength-training machine.

Muscles Developed: Gastrocnemius and soleus.

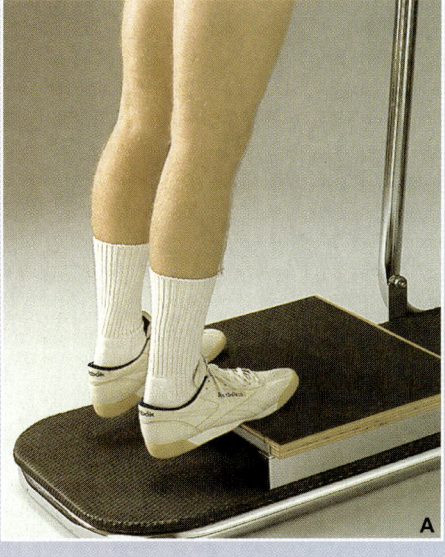
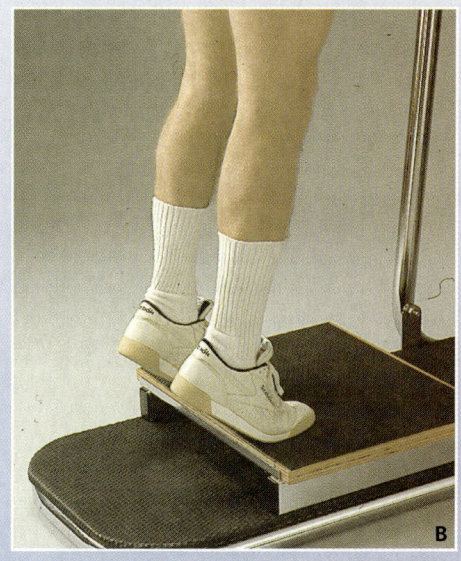

FLEXIBILITY EXERCISES

EXERCISE 18

Lateral Head Tilt

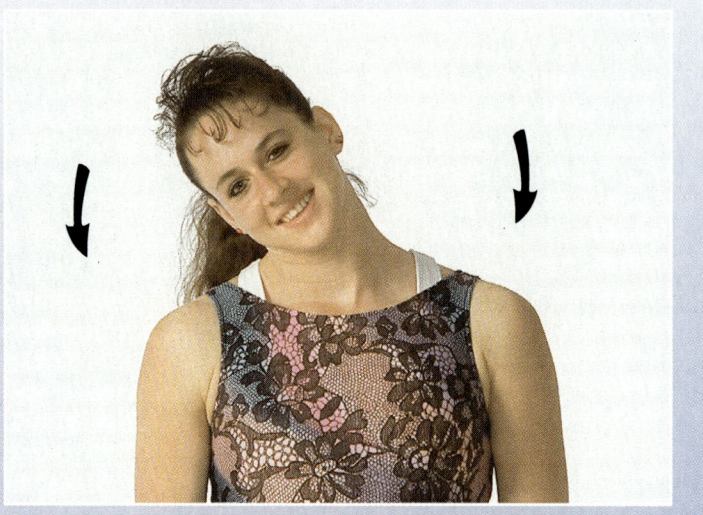

Action: Slowly and gently tilt the head laterally. Repeat several times to each side.

Areas Stretched: neck flexors and extensors and ligaments of the cervical spine.

EXERCISE 19

Arm Circles

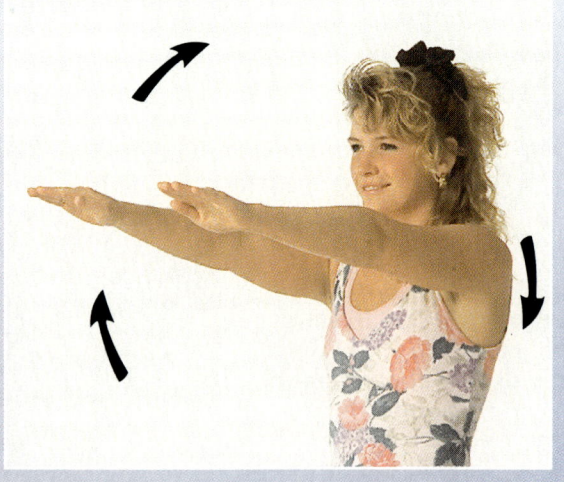

Action: Gently circle your arms all the way around. conduct the exercise in both directions.

Areas Stretched: Shoulder muscles and ligaments.

EXERCISE 20

Side Stretch

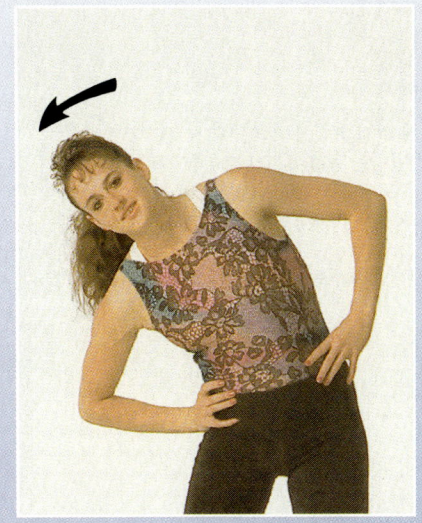

Action: Stand straight up, feet separated to shoulder width, and place your hands on your waist. Now move the upper body to one side and hold the final stretch for a few seconds. Repeat on the other side.

Areas Stretched: Muscles and ligaments in the pelvic region.

EXERCISE 21

Body Rotation

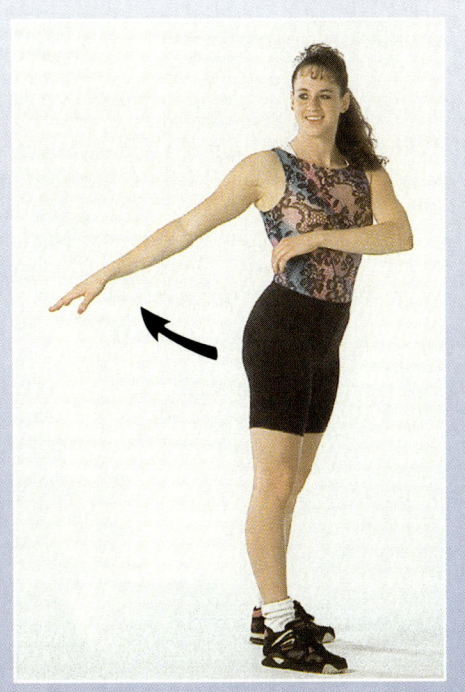

Action: Place your arms slightly away from your body and rotate the trunk as far as possible, holding the final position for several seconds. Conduct the exercise for both the right and left sides of the body. You can also perform this exercise by standing about two feet away from the wall (back toward the wall), and then rotate the trunk, placing the hands against the wall.

Areas Stretched: Hip, abdominal, chest, back, neck, and shoulder muscles; hip and spinal ligaments.

Chest Stretch

Action: Kneel down behind a chair and place both hands on the back of the chair. Gradually push your chest downward and hold for a few seconds.

Areas Stretched: Chest (pectoral) muscles and shoulder ligaments.

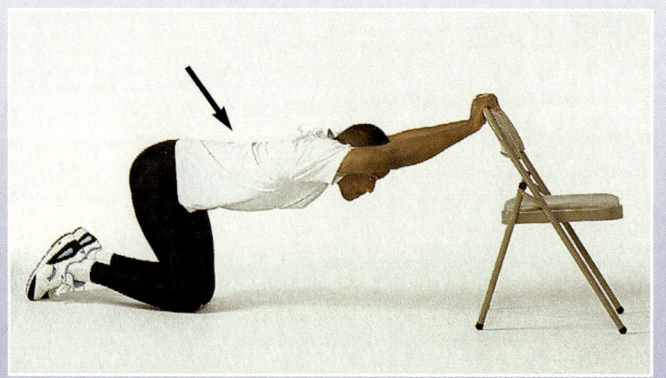

Shoulder Hyperextension Stretch

Action: Have a partner grasp your arms from behind by the wrists and slowly push them upward. Hold the final position for a few seconds.

Areas Stretched: Deltoid and pectoral muscles, and ligaments of the shoulder joint.

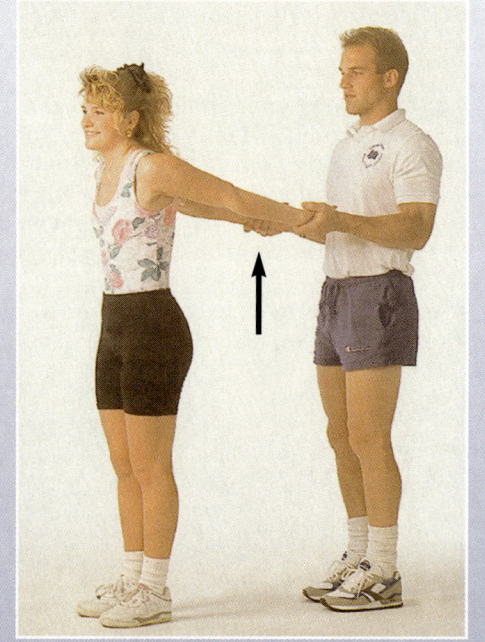

Shoulder Rotation Stretch

Action: With the aid of surgical tubing or an aluminum or wood stick, place the tubing or stick behind your back and grasp the two ends using a reverse (thumbs-out) grip. Slowly bring the tubing or stick over your head, keeping the elbows straight. Repeat several times (bring the hands closer together for additional stretch).

Areas Stretched: Deltoid, latissimus dorsi, and pectoral muscles; shoulder ligaments.

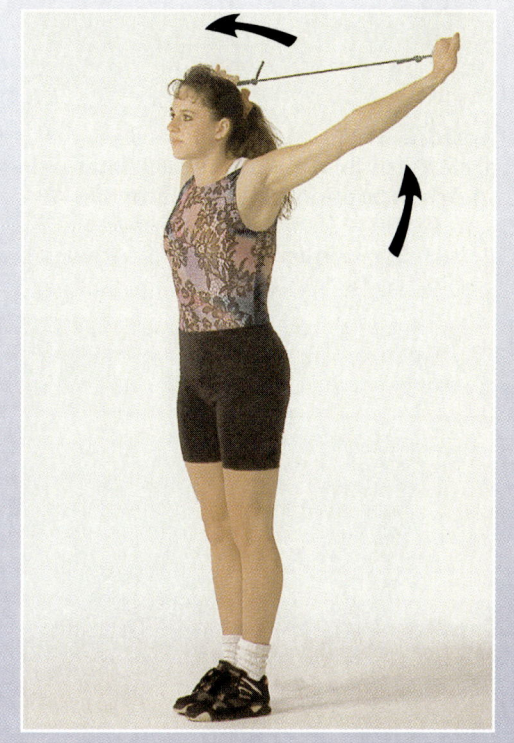

Quad Stretch

Action: Lie on your side and move one foot back by flexing the knee. Grasp the front of the ankle and pull the ankle toward the gluteal region. Hold for several seconds. Repeat with the other leg.

Areas Stretched: Quadriceps muscle, and knee and ankle ligaments.

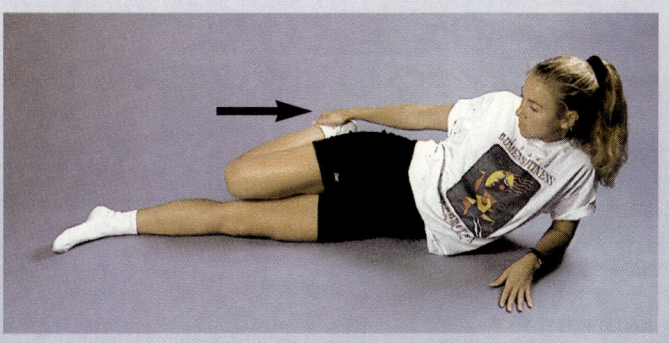

EXERCISE 26

Heel Cord Stretch

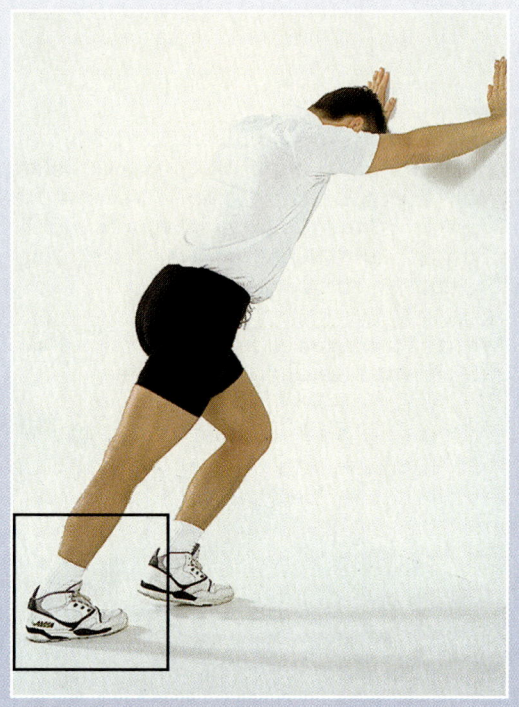

Action: Stand against the wall or at the edge of a step and stretch the heel downward, alternating legs. Hold the stretched position for a few seconds.

Areas Stretched: Heel cord (Achilles tendon), gastrocnemius, and soleus muscles.

EXERCISE 27

Adductor Stretch

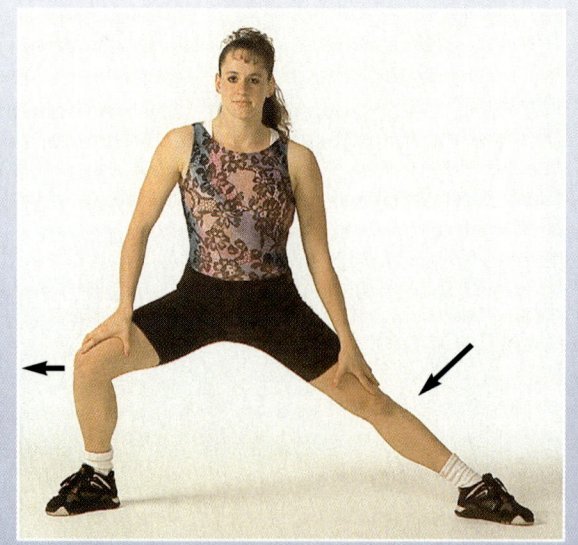

Action: Stand with your feet about twice shoulder width and place your hands slightly above the knee. Flex one knee and slowly go down as far as possible, holding the final position for a few seconds. Repeat with the other leg.

Areas Stretched: Hip adductor muscles.

EXERCISE 28

Sitting Adductor Stretch

Action: Sit on the floor and bring your feet in close to you, allowing the soles of the feet to touch each other. Now place your forearms (or elbows) on the inner part of the thigh and push the legs downward, holding the final stretch for several seconds.

Areas Stretched: Hip adductor muscles.

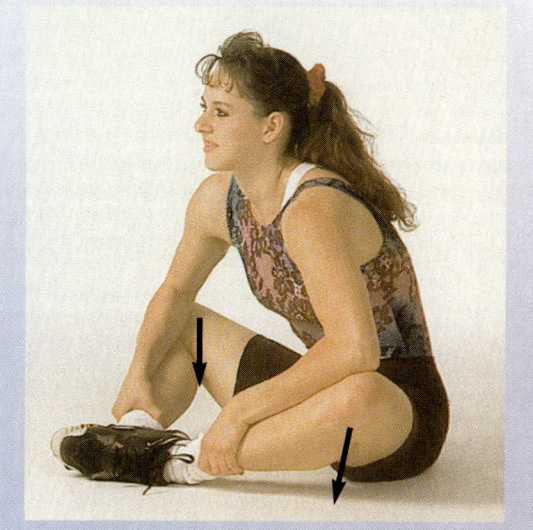

EXERCISE 29

Sit-and-Reach Stretch

Action: Sit on the floor with legs together and gradually reach forward as far as possible. Hold the final position for a few seconds. This exercise may also be performed with the legs separated, reaching to each side as well as to the middle.

Areas Stretched: Hamstrings and lower back muscles, and lumbar spine ligaments.

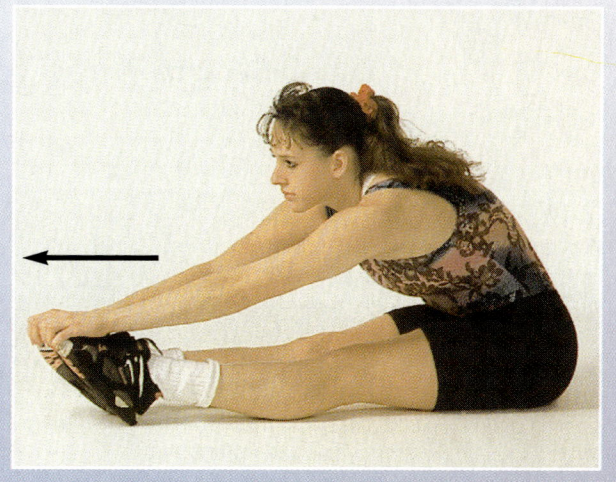

EXERCISE 30

Triceps Stretch

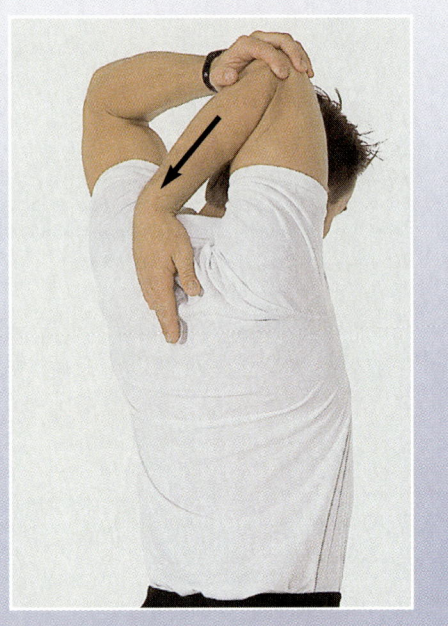

Action: Place the right hand behind your neck. Grasp the right arm above the elbow with the left hand. Gently pull the elbow backward. Repeat the exercise with the opposite arm.

Areas Stretched: Back of upper arm (triceps muscle) and shoulder joint.

EXERCISES FOR THE PREVENTION AND REHABILITATION OF LOW BACK PAIN

EXERCISE 31

Single-Knee to Chest Stretch

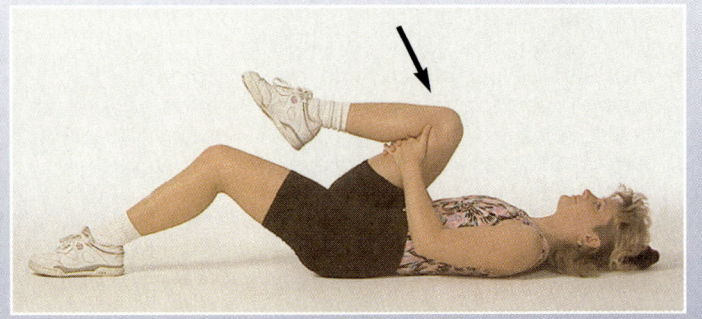

Action: Lie down flat on the floor. Bend one leg at approximately 100° and gradually pull the opposite leg toward your chest. Hold the final stretch for a few seconds. Switch legs and repeat the exercise.

Areas Stretched: Lower back and hamstring muscles, and lumbar spine ligaments.

SEVEN ▼ *Exercise Prescription For Wellness*

EXERCISE 32

Double-Knee to Chest Stretch

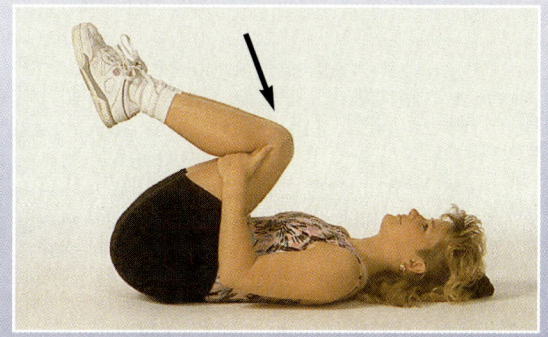

Action: Lie flat on the floor and then slowly curl up into a fetal position. Hold for a few seconds.

Areas Stretched: Upper and lower back and hamstring muscles; spinal ligaments.

EXERCISE 33

Upper and Lower Back Stretch

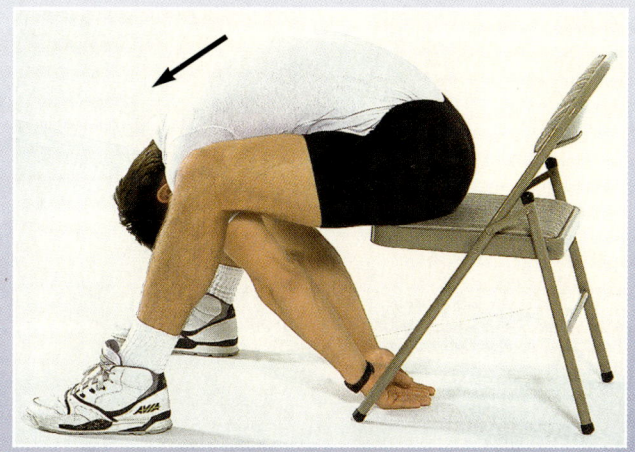

Action: Sit in a chair with feet separated greater than shoulder width. Place your arms to the inside of the thighs and bring your chest down toward the floor. At the same time, attempt to reach back as far as you can with your arms.

Areas Stretched: Upper and lower back muscles and ligaments.

EXERCISE 34

Sit-and-Reach Stretch

See exercise 29 in this chapter.

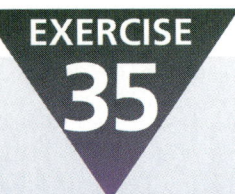

Exercise 35: Back Extension

Action: Lie face down on the floor with the elbows by the chest, forearms on the floor, and the hands beneath the chin. Gently raise the trunk by extending the elbows until you reach an approximate 90° angle at the elbow joint. Be sure that the forearms remain in contact with the floor at all times. DO NOT extend the back beyond this point. Hyperextension of the lower back may lead to or aggravate an already existing back problem. Hold the stretched position for about 10 seconds.

Areas Stretched: Abdominal region.

Additional Benefit: Restoration of lower back curvature.

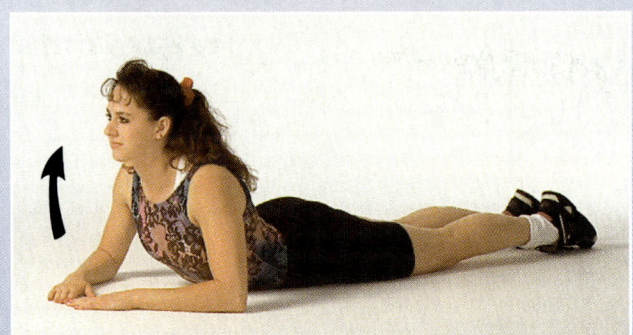

Exercise 36: Gluteal Stretch

Action: Sit on the floor, bend the right leg and place your right ankle slightly above the left knee. Grasp the left thigh with both hands and gently pull the leg toward your chest. Repeat the exercise with the opposite leg.

Areas Stretched: Buttock area (gluteal muscles).

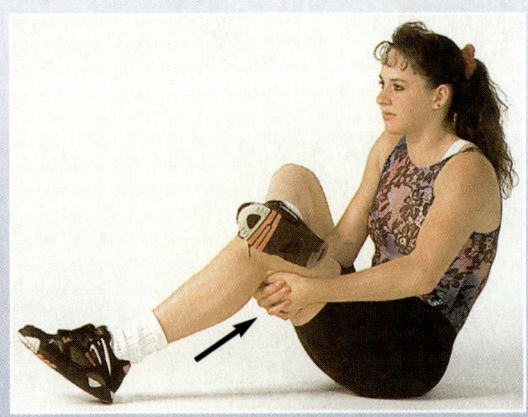

EXERCISE 37

Trunk Rotation and Lower Back Stretch

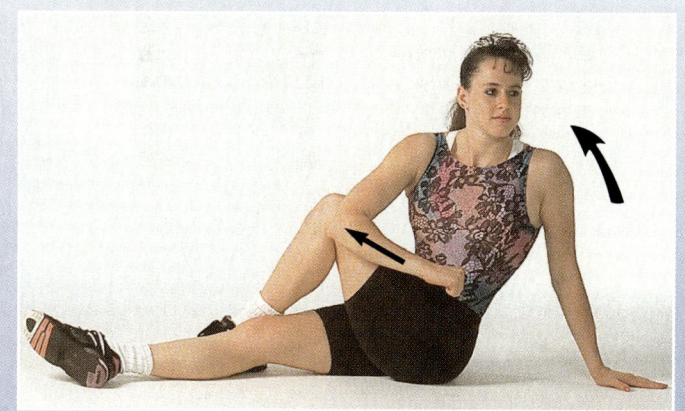

Action: Sit on the floor and bend the left leg, placing the left foot on the outside of the right knee. Place the right elbow on the left knee and push against it. At the same time, try to rotate the trunk to the left (counterclockwise). Hold the final position for a few seconds. Repeat the exercise with the other side.

Areas Stretched: Lateral side of the hip and thigh; trunk, and lower back.

EXERCISE 38

Pelvic Tilt

Action: Lie flat on the floor with the knees bent at about a 70° angle. Tilt the pelvis by tightening the abdominal muscles, flattening your back against the floor, and raising the lower gluteal area ever so slightly off the floor (see photo b). Hold the final position for several seconds. The exercise can also be performed against a wall (as shown in photo c).

Areas Stretched: Low back muscles and ligaments.

Areas Strengthened: Abdominal and gluteal muscles.

Note: This is perhaps the most important exercise for the care of the lower back. It should be included as a part of your daily exercise routine and should be performed several times throughout the day when pain in the lower back is present as a result of muscle imbalance.

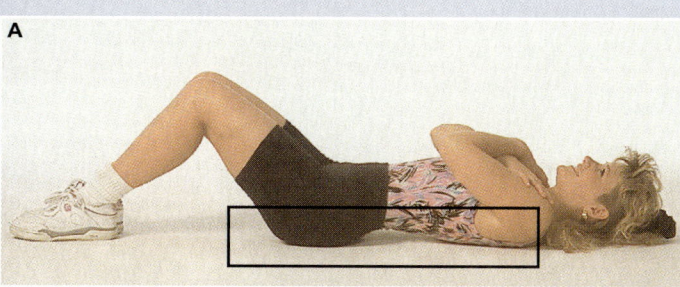
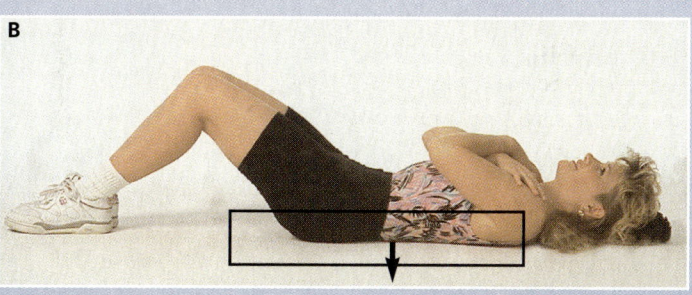
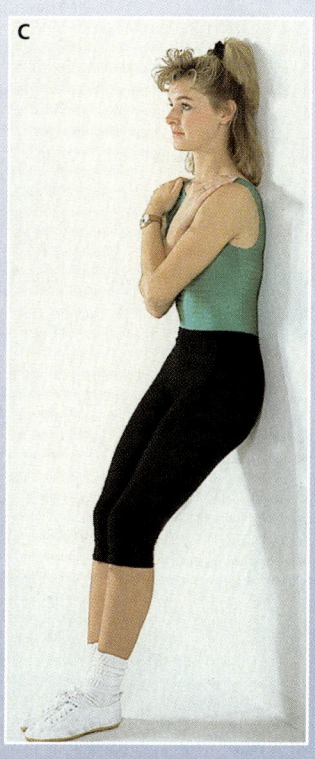

Abdominal Crunch and Abdominal Curl-Up

See exercise 4 in this chapter.

It is important that you do not stabilize your feet when performing either of these exercises, because doing so decreases the work of the abdominal muscles. Also, remember not to "swing up" but rather to curl up as you perform these exercises.

Nutrition and Wellness

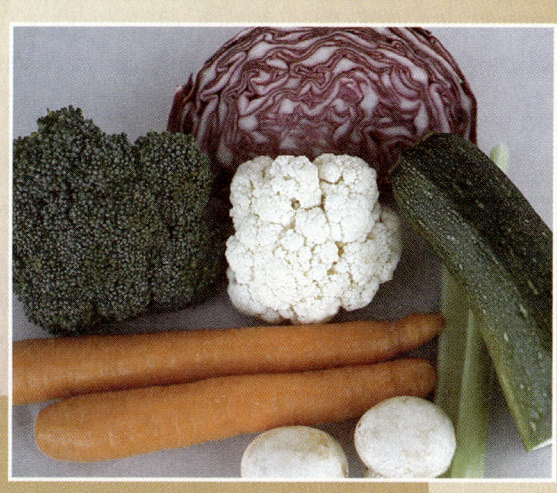

Objectives

- ▼ Identify the trends and eating habits of the average American.
- ▼ Enumerate the six basic elements of nutrition, their functions and sources.
- ▼ Learn the types of fat and what each does in the body.
- ▼ Understand cholesterol and its functions.
- ▼ Differentiate the types of carbohydrates and the role of fiber.
- ▼ List the types of vitamins, their sources and functions.
- ▼ Identify the minerals the body needs, their sources and functions.
- ▼ Become acquainted with the recommended dietary guidelines.
- ▼ Learn how to read food labels on packaged products.
- ▼ Develop personalized guidelines for a nutritional wellness plan.

The typical American family of five decades ago was a classic Norman Rockwell vision: Dad in his shirt and tie sat at the head of the table while Mom, complete with a ruffled apron, hurried to bring dinner to her smiling family. It was the age of two-parent, one-career families who sat down to a solid, home-cooked meal three times a day.

As a nation, our eating habits have changed dramatically since then: Dinner is more likely to be a frozen entree popped into the microwave or a hamburger and fries grabbed on the run from a fast-food drive-through. The U.S. Restaurant Association estimates that approximately 45.8 million people — one-fifth of the U.S. population — eat at a fast-food restaurant every day.

The growing trends away from agricultural populations and toward single-person households, single-parent families, and women in the workforce have had a marked influence on the way we as a nation eat. Fifty or 60 years ago, large numbers of Americans grew their own food and ate diets rich in grains, vegetables and fruits. The average diet was significantly lower in fats and refined sugars than our diets are today. Table 8.1 compares the typical American diet to the recommended one in three of the basic nutrients.

Perhaps America's changing eating habits are mirrored most in the trend toward fast-food eating. In the single decade between 1970 and 1980, the number of fast-food restaurants in this country more than quadrupled. Today, the United States has more than 175,000 fast-food outlets, including those on college campuses and military bases. Today, few people sit down to breakfast or lunch at home, and as many as a fourth of all Americans eat dinner at a fast-food restaurant, too. Some estimate that America's fast-food restaurants serve up approximately 200 hamburgers *every second*.

Fare from a fast-food restaurant doesn't have to be nutritionally bankrupt. Neither do frozen dinners — or snacks, for that matter. In a position statement on fast food and the American diet, the American Council on Science and Health reported that, contrary to common belief, fast food has substantial nutritional value. Its potential nutritional contribution to the diet is limited only by the variety of menu items available and the choices individual consumers make. People who want to eat healthfully can incorporate fast food into a balanced diet by varying their selections, choosing menu items that contribute to nutrient needs, and choosing meals of appropriate calorie content.

THE SIX BASIC ELEMENTS OF NUTRITION

The six basic elements of nutrition — proteins, fats, carbohydrates, vitamins, minerals, and water — provide what the body needs to maintain itself. The process of converting these nutrients into body tissue and functions (such as muscle contraction) is called *metabolism*. The six basic nutrients fuel metabolism to help the body with:

▶ Growth and the formation of new tissue.
▶ Repair of damaged tissue.

TABLE 8.1 ▼ Typical American Diet Compared to Recommended Diet

Current Diet	Dietary Goals
Fat: 42% total	*Fat:* 30% total
16% saturated	10% saturated
19% monounsaturated	10% monounsaturated
7% polyunsaturated	10% polyunsaturated
Protein: 12%	*Protein:* 12%
Carbohydrates: 46% total	*Carbohydrates:* 58% total
22% complex carbohydrates	48% complex carbohydrates and
6% naturally occurring sugars	naturally occurring sugars
(not processed or refined)	10% refined and processed sugars
18% refined and processed sugars	

▼

Eating Healthy At Fast-Food Restaurants

If much of your fare comes from fast-food restaurants or cafeterias, that's okay, as long as you make food choices like these:

▼ Look for chains that offer healthy alternatives such as whole-grain buns, salads, or baked potatoes.

▼ For breakfast, choose English muffins or pancakes. Avoid fried hash browns, eggs, bacon, sausage, croissants, butter, and Danish rolls.

▼ If you can, choose a salad bar; lightly sprinkle on cheese and dressing.

▼ Skip the milk shake or soda; drink juice, low-fat milk, or water instead.

▼ **Baked potatoes:** A good option, but get a vegetable topping (such as broccoli) if you can instead of butter, sour cream, or cheese.

▼ **Hamburgers:** Get a single, plain burger; condiments, bacon, and cheese are all high in fat. Better yet, choose roast beef.

▼ **Chicken:** Order skinless, or take the skin off yourself. Avoid "extra crispy," as the crispness comes from added fat. Avoid chicken nuggets; they usually contain ground-up chicken skin, which is high in fat.

▼ **Mexican:** Choose chicken tacos or burritos instead of beef; order soft flour tortillas instead of corn tortillas; choose dishes with lots of beans and vegetables and little cheese.

▼ **Pizza:** Choose vegetable toppings and go light on cheese. Steer away from sausage, pepperoni, olives, extra cheese.

▶ Production of energy.
▶ Conduction of nerve impulses.
▶ Reproduction.

PROTEINS

With their specialized chemical structure, proteins are the body's "building blocks," providing the basic materials for cell growth and repair. Protein helps build skin, blood, muscles, and bone; aids in the formation of hormones; regulates the body's chemical processes; forms enzymes; carries nutrients to all body cells; and is a major constituent of the immune system.

Protein is composed of carbon, oxygen, hydrogen, and nitrogen. The nitrogen in protein is what gives it the ability to maintain and regulate the body tissues and functions. Good animal sources of protein include milk and milk products, eggs, meat, poultry, and fish. Good plant sources of protein include whole grains, rice, pastas, legumes (peas and beans), and seeds.

Proteins derived from both plant and animal sources are made up of about 20 *amino acids*, the chemical structures that form protein's ability to build and repair tissue, regulate the formation of hormones and enzymes, and maintain the body's chemical balance. Of these 20 amino acids, 11 can be manufactured by the body itself. Nine of them, called *essential amino acids*, cannot be produced by the body and must be obtained from the foods we eat.

A *complete protein* (such as chicken or cheddar cheese) contains all nine essential amino acids. An *incomplete protein* (such as pinto beans or brown rice) contains only some of the essential amino acids. Before an incomplete protein source can be converted to a complete protein, it has to be combined with another food that supplies the missing essential amino acids. The best complete protein source is the egg.

Only about 12% of your total calories for the day should come from protein, and most Americans eat far too much protein. An American woman, for example, needs only about 46 to 48 grams of protein a day, the equivalent of a cup of low-fat yogurt, a cup of low-fat milk, and 4 ounces of chicken. Of course, the proper amount of protein is essential for the body's growth and repair, but too much protein can wreak havoc on the body. Excess protein is stored as fat. Evidence also suggests that too much protein accelerates growth of tumors and contributes to heart disease, cancer, and osteoporosis. It causes the body to excrete calcium (needed for strengthening bones and teeth). If you eat too much protein, the extra nitrogen is excreted in your urine, which can strain the kidneys.

Commenting on the reality that we eat too much protein, nutritionist and author Jane Brody said, "Americans excrete the most expensive urine in the world. If it were economical to collect and dry it, tons of nitrogen could be harvested from the nation's toilet bowls each day."

FATS

The most concentrated form of food energy, fat provides 9 calories per gram, more than twice the calories in a gram of carbohydrates or proteins. Fats transport fat-soluble vitamins in the body, insulate and protect body organs, regulate hormones, contribute to growth, provide a concentrated source of energy, and are essential for healthy skin. Although the right amount of fat is essential to growth and functioning of the body, too much fat is harmful. Excess dietary fat can lead to high blood pressure, stroke, heart disease, diabetes, and other diseases. Excessive body fat is the leading factor in heart disease. It also has been linked to cancers of the colon, breast, uterus, and prostate.

The average American eats six to eight times as much fat as is recommended or healthy. According to estimates, in any single year the average American eats more than 55 pounds of visible fat (salad oil, butter, shortening, for example) and more than 130 pounds of invisible fat (such as fat in eggs, dairy products, meats, and nuts).

The greatest single source of dietary fat in Americans of all ages other than infants is thought to be ground beef. According to the National Research Council, more than half the total fat, including all the cholesterol and more than three-fourths of the saturated fats, in the typical American diet comes from milk and milk products, eggs, red meats (beef, pork, veal, and lamb), fish and shellfish, and separated animal fats (such as lard).

The American Heart Association and the U.S. Department of Health and Human Services recommend that no more than 30% of the total calories in the diet comes from fat and the percentage should be less if you are overweight or have a high cholesterol level. (Interestingly, your cholesterol level is not affected as much by the cholesterol you eat as by the overall percentage of fat in your diet.) Of that 30%, less than one-third should come from saturated fats, less than one-third from polyunsaturated fats, and the rest from monounsaturated fats. All fats are chains of carbon atoms. The *kind* of fat depends on how many hydrogen atoms are linked to the carbon atoms. Because chemical analysis isn't practical for most of us, you can identify, in some simple ways, the kinds of fat you're eating. Table 8.2 lists some common foods according to their percent-fat categories.

A useful guideline when figuring out the fat content of individual foods is: As shown in Figure 8.1, all you have to do is multiply the grams of fat by 9 and divide by the total calories in that particular food. You then multiply that number by 100 to get the percentage. For example, if a food label lists a total of 100 calories and 7 grams of fat, the fat content is 63% of total calories. This simple guideline can help you decrease the fat in your diet. The fat content of selected foods, given in grams and as a percent of total calories, is presented in Figure 8.2.

Beware also of products labeled 97% fat-free. These products use weight and not percent of total calories as a measure of fat. As illustrated in Figure 8.1, many of these foods are still in the range of 30% fat calories.

Caloric Value of Food

Sources of Calories
1 gram of carbohydrate .... 4 calories
1 gram of protein .... 4 calories
1 gram of fat .... 9 calories
1 gram of alcohol .... 7 calories

Computation For Fat Content in Food

Example:
Caloric Distribution for Turkey Breast, 97% Fat Free

Portion size .... 1 slice (1 oz)
Calories 29
Protein .... 4 grams × 4 calories = 16 calories
Carbohydrate .... 1 gram × 4 calories = 4 calories
Fat .... 1 gram × 9 calories = 9 calories
                        Total calories   = 29 calories

Percent Fat Calories =
  (grams of fat × 9) divided by total calories × 100

Percent fat calories in 97% fat free turkey =
  [(1 × 9) ÷ 29] × 100 = 31%

FIGURE 8.1 ▼ How to determine fat calories in food.

Saturated Fats

In pure form these fats, the ones with the highest number of hydrogen atoms, are solid at room temperature (see Figure 8.3). The only exceptions are coconut oil, palm oil, and palm kernel oil (the "tropical oils"), which are highly saturated but liquid at room temperature. Saturated fats raise the cholesterol level in the bloodstream and have been linked the most strongly to heart disease and other degenerative diseases. Examples of foods high in saturated fats are butter, cheese, milk, cream, nondairy cream substitutes, lard, pork, bacon, beef, veal, lamb, poultry skin, hot dogs, luncheon meats, chocolate, cocoa, coconut oil, and palm oil.

TABLE 8.2 ▼ Percentage of Fat Calories in Common Foods

Type of Food	Less Than 15% of Calories from Fat	15%-30% of Calories from Fat	30%-50% of Calories from Fat	More Than 50% of Calories from Fat
Fruits and Vegetables	Fruits, plain vegetables, juices, pickles, sauerkraut		French fries, hash browns	Avocados, coconuts, olives
Bread and Cereals	Grains and flours, most breads, most cereals, corn tortillas, pita, matzoh, bagels, noodles and pasta	Corn bread, flour tortillas, oatmeal, soft rolls and buns, wheat germ	Breakfast bars, biscuits and muffins, granola, pancakes and waffles, donuts, taco shells, pastries, croissants	
Dairy Products	Nonfat milk, dry curd cottage cheese, nonfat cottage cheese, nonfat yogurt	Buttermilk, low-fat yogurt, 1% milk, low-fat cottage cheese	Whole milk, 2% milk, creamed cottage cheese	Butter, cream, sour cream, half & half, most cheeses (including part-skim and "lite" cheeses)
Meats		Beef round; veal loin, round, and shoulder; pork tenderloin	Beef and veal, lamb, fresh and picnic hams	All ground beef, spareribs, cold cuts, bacon, sausages, corned beef, hot dogs, pastrami
Poultry Products	Egg whites	Chicken and turkey (light meat without skin)	Chicken and turkey (light meat with skin, dark meat without skin), duck and goose (without skin)	Chicken/turkey (dark meat with skin), chicken/turkey hot dogs and bologna, egg yolks, whole eggs
Seafood	Clams, cod, crab, crawfish, flounder, haddock, lobster, perch, sole, scallops, shrimp, tuna (in water)	Bass and sea bass, halibut, mussels, oyster, tuna (fresh)	Anchovies, catfish, salmon, sturgeon, trout, tuna (in oil, drained)	Herring, mackerel, sardines
Beans and Nuts	Dried beans and peas, chestnuts, water chestnuts		Soybeans	Tofu, most nuts and seeds, peanut butter
Fats and Oils	Oil-free and some "lite" salad dressings			Butter, margarine, all mayonnaise (including reduced-calorie), most salad dressings, all oils
Soups	Bouillons, broths, consomme	Most soups	Cream soups, bean soups, "just add water" noodle soups	Cheddar cheese soup, New England clam chowder
Desserts	Angel food cake, gelatin, some new fat-free cakes	Pudding, tapioca	Most cakes, most pies	
Frozen Desserts	Sherbet, low-fat frozen yogurt, sorbet, fruit ices	Ice milk	Frozen yogurt	All ice cream
Snack Foods	Popcorn (air-popped), pretzels, rye crackers, rice cakes, fig bars, raisin biscuit cookies, marshmallows, most hard candy, fruit rolls	"Lite" microwave popcorn, Scandinavian "crisps," plain crackers, caramels, fudge, gingersnaps, graham crackers	Snack crackers, popcorn (popped in oil), cookies, candy bars, granola bars	Most microwave popcorn, corn and potato chips, chocolate, buttery crackers

American Heart Association/USDA.

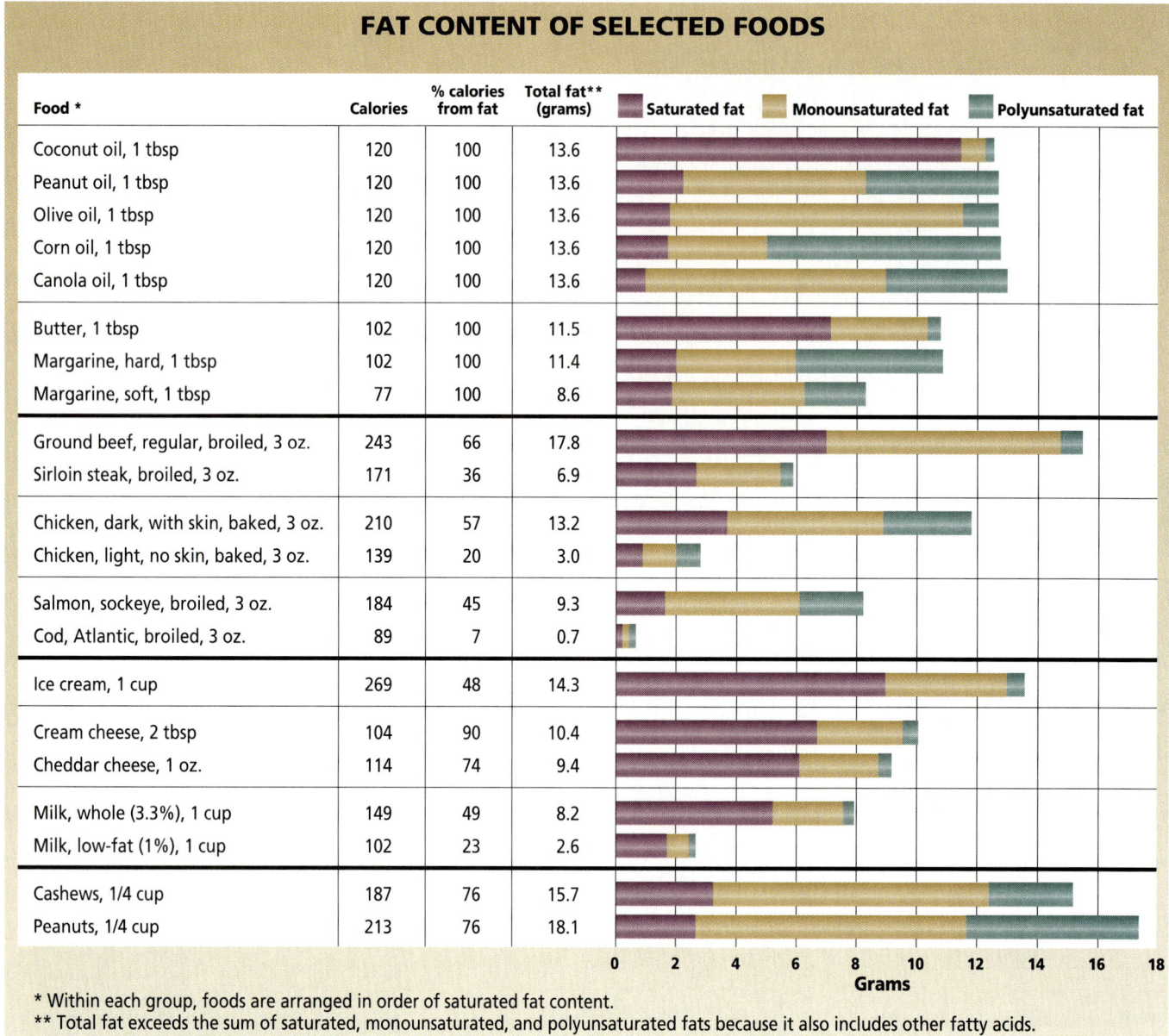

FIGURE 8.2 ▼ Saturated fat, monounsaturated fat, and polyunsaturated fat content of selected foods.

Monounsaturated fats

These fats, which can accept two more hydrogen atoms, seem to help lower the cholesterol level in the bloodstream. They are found in peanuts, cashews, olives, and avocados, as well as olive oil, peanut oil, cottonseed oil, and canola oil.

Polyunsaturated fats

Fats that can accept four more hydrogen atoms, polyunsaturated fats lower the level of cholesterol in the bloodstream. They come from foods such as fish, margarine, mayonnaise, walnuts, almonds, pecans, corn oil, safflower oil, sunflower oil, sesame oil, and soybean oil.

Where fat is concerned, reading labels is important. Some mono- or polyunsaturated fats are *hydrogenated* during manufacturing. During the process, hydrogen is added to the fat to increase shelf life and to make it harder or more spreadable. Eating a vegetable oil that has been hydrogenated may carry as many health risks as eating a saturated fat.

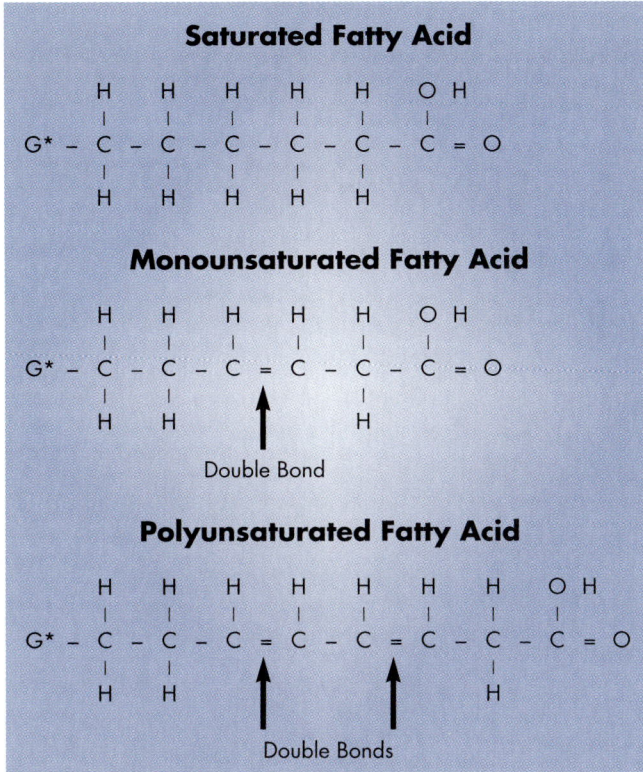

*Glyceride component

FIGURE 8.3 ▼ Chemical structure of saturated and unsaturated fats.

negative publicity given to cholesterol, you might not realize it has a beneficial role in the body. It aids in digestion, is a major component of the membranes that protect nerve fibers, aids in production of vitamin D, and helps the body produce the sex hormones estrogen, progesterone, and androgen. But that's in moderation. If you have too much cholesterol in your bloodstream, you run a significantly higher risk of developing heart disease.

Your liver produces most of the cholesterol you need to stay healthy. Additional cholesterol from the foods you eat, if eaten in excess, can lead to heart disease. The American Heart Association recommends that cholesterol intake be limited to 300 mg a day. Plant foods contain no cholesterol, and you need to limit the amount of milk, cheese, dairy products, egg yolks, and meat you eat to keep cholesterol at a healthy level. Additional information on cholesterol is given in Chapter 11. One of the best ways to reduce the production of cholesterol in the body is to reduce the intake of saturated fat.

Fish oil. A study of traditional Eskimo diets turned up an amazing discovery about fat: Even though the traditional Eskimo diet is about 40% fat, Eskimos have the lowest rate of heart disease in the world. Research shows that the reason seems to be fish. Fish are rich in polyunsaturated fats called *omega-3 oils*, which have been shown to reduce cholesterol levels and prevent the buildup of plaque in coronary arteries. In one study, the death rate from heart disease was 50% lower in people who ate at least an ounce of fish every day than those who didn't eat fish.

Research also shows that taking fish-oil capsules every day isn't as effective as eating fish even once a week. Instead, the diet should include fish rich in omega-3 oils. Tuna, sardines, salmon, mackerel, and herring are best.

Cholesterol. Any discussion of dietary fat would not be complete without attention to cholesterol, a yellow, waxy, fatlike substance produced by the liver and found in animal tissue. Cholesterol isn't actually a fat but technically is a steroid alcohol. With all the

Tips on Cutting Fat From Your Diet

▼ Drink fortified skim milk, and choose dairy products (such as cheeses) made from skim or low-fat milk.

▼ Eat meatless or low-meat main dishes at least several times a week.

▼ Eat more fish; bake, broil, or stew it.

▼ Eat no more than 5 to 7 ounces of meat, poultry, and seafood a day.

▼ Avoid fatty meats, such as corned beef, sausage, hot dogs, luncheon meats, spareribs, regular ground beef, and heavily marbled meat.

▼ Eat red meat only a few times a week. Choose lean cuts, such as round, rump, or flank. Trim all visible fat before you cook, and cook the meat so the fat can drain away from it.

▼ Remove skin from chicken and turkey before you cook it.

▼ Cook stews, soups, and gravies a day ahead; refrigerate and lift off congealed fat.

▼ Bake, broil, roast, barbecue, or stew foods instead of frying them.

▼ Limit nuts, peanuts, and peanut butter.

▼ Eat no more than four egg yolks a week, including the ones you use in cooking.

Test for Fats

True/False

1. Egg yolks contain the "bad" cholesterol called LDL.

2. Mayonnaise made from canola oil has less fat than regular mayonnaise, which is generally made from soybean oil.

3. The more unsaturated fat a food has, the more it will raise blood-cholesterol levels.

4. Polyunsaturated fats are converted to saturated fats when heated, such as in deep-fat frying.

5. A jar of peanut butter labeled as "cholesterol free" is better than regular brands.

6. A label that reads "95% fat free" means the food contains only 5% of its calories from fat.

7. The best way to decrease blood-cholesterol levels is to eat less cholesterol.

8. A third of the average U.S. woman's fat intake comes from salad dressing, margarine, cheese, and beef.

9. A label that reads "low cholesterol" means the food has fewer calories than regular brands and no saturated fat.

10. Veggie burgers are always a low-fat alternative to hamburgers.

Multiple-Choice

Select the best answer to the following questions.

11. A product is labeled as containing only vegetable oils. It would be:
    a. high in only saturated fat
    b. high in only unsaturated fat
    c. high in either saturated fat or unsaturated fat
    d. high in unsaturated fat and might contain some cholesterol

12. A woman has a total blood-cholesterol level of 220 mg/dl and an HDL level of 60 mg/dl. What is this person's ratio of total cholesterol to HDL cholesterol? Is she at high or low risk for heart disease?
    a. 3:7 ratio and low risk
    b. 2:7 ratio and low risk
    c. 7:2 ratio and low risk
    d. 4:5 ratio and high risk

13. A 5-ounce serving of ground beef has how much more fat than the same size serving of skinless chicken breast?
    a. 50%   c. 75%
    b. 65%   d. 95%

14. There are 30 grams of fat and 309 calories in an avocado. What is the percentage of fat calories?
    a. 42%   c. 87%
    b. 62%   d. 97%

15. A food is considered low-fat if it has how many grams of fat per 100 calories?
    a. 3   c. 10
    b. 5   d. 30

16. According to the American Heart Association, people ideally should adopt a low-fat diet that contains no more than 30% fat calories:
    a. starting at birth
    b. at 2 years of age
    c. at puberty
    d. in early adulthood

17. An olive-oil label states that the product is "extra light." This means
    a. it has a lighter color and taste than other olive oils
    b. it weighs less
    c. it has fewer calories
    d. it is lower in saturated fats

18. Whole milk gets 48% of its calories from fat. What percentage of calories come from fat in 2% low-fat milk?
    a. 2%   c. 25%
    b. 15%   d. 30%

19. Experts recommend limiting your saturated-fat intake to no more than 10% of total calorie intake. If you eat 2,000 calories per day, your saturated-fat allowance would be
    a. 10 grams   c. 27 grams
    b. 22 grams   d. 36 grams

20. A Taco Bell taco salad contains how many teaspoons of fat?
    a. 9   c. 15
    b. 12   d. 25

Answers:

1. False. LDL is a carrier of cholesterol in the blood. It is not found in food.

2. False. They contain similar amounts of fat and calories.

3. False. The more *saturated* fat in your diet, the more your blood-cholesterol level will be raised.

4. False. However, frying does expose these fats to oxygen, and once oxidized, they can increase heart-disease risk.

5. False. Cholesterol is found only in animal products.

6. False. The label refers only to fat content by weight. The percentage of calories from fat would be much higher. For instance, a 95% fat-free Janet Lee Chopped Ham contains 60% fat calories (2 grams of fat per 30-calorie slice).

7. False. Reducing your saturated fat intake is the most important dietary factor for lowering blood cholesterol.

8. True. The average woman in the United States gets 9% of her fat from salad dressing, 8% from margarine, 8% from cheese and 7% from beef, for a total of one-third.

9. False. A food can be cholesterol-free and still be high in calories and/or saturated fat.

10. False. Commercial veggie burgers get anywhere from 6% of 66% of their calories from fat.

11. c. Most vegetable oils are high in unsaturated fats. However, manufacturers also use tropical oils, such as palm or coconut oils, which are as saturated as lard.

12. a.
13. d.
14. c.
15. a. There are 9 calories per gram of fat, so a food that has 3 grams of fat per 100 calories is 27% fat; a food that is less than 30% fat is considered low-fat.
16. b.
17. a.
18. d.
19. b.
20. c.

To find your score, total your correct answers.

18 or more: All of that label reading has paid off! You are a bona fide fat sleuth.

15 to 17: You put the average American to shame. If you practice what you know, your diet is probably within the low-fat zone.

12 to 14: You keep company with the majority of Americans and may be confused when it comes to fat. Review the answers and see if you can improve your score.

Less than 12: Oops. It's time to take the fat issue more seriously.

From Facing Fats by Elizabeth Somer in SHAPE, January, 1994.

CARBOHYDRATES

Two different kinds of carbohydrates are available in the foods you eat: simple carbohydrates (sugars) and complex carbohydrates (starches).

Simple Carbohydrates

Simple carbohydrates, which include refined and processed sugars, have given carbohydrates the reputation of being "fattening." Simple carbohydrates include refined white sugar, honey, sucrose, corn syrup, fructose, dextrose, sorghum, and maltose, among others. Those that have been refined or extracted from their natural sources contain many calories but little, if any, nutritional value — earning them the popular nickname of "empty calories." A diet high in simple carbohydrates can lead to obesity and give you dental cavities, as well as health problems such as heart disease, diabetes, and hypoglycemia.

Simple carbohydrates are divided into monosaccharides and disaccharides. These carbohydrates — with *-ose* endings — often take the place of more nutritive foods in the diet.

Monosaccharides, the simplest sugars, are formed by five- or six-carbon skeletons. The three most common monosaccharides are glucose, fructose, and galactose.

1. *Glucose* is a natural sugar found in food, but it also is produced in the body from other simple and complex carbohydrates.
2. *Fructose*, or fruit sugar, occurs naturally in fruits and honey.
3. *Galactose* is produced from milk sugar in the mammary glands of lactating animals.

Both fructose and galactose are readily converted to glucose in the body. Glucose is used as a source of energy, or it may be stored in the muscles and liver in the form of *glycogen* (a long chain of glucose molecules hooked together). Excess glucose in the blood is converted to fat and stored in adipose (fat) tissue. Some of it is eliminated by the kidneys through the urine.

Disaccharides are formed by the linkage of two monosaccharide units, one of which is glucose. The three major disaccharides are:

1. *Sucrose* or table sugar (glucose + fructose).
2. *Lactose* (glucose + galactose).
3. *Maltose* (glucose + glucose).

Most Americans eat about 130 pounds of refined sugars a year, or about 20% of their total caloric intake. The dietary guidelines for Americans recommend that no more than 10% of your total calories come from sugar — cutting the amount of sugar you eat in half if you're typical.

A key to cutting sugar is learning to read labels. The word *sugar* doesn't always appear. Instead, manufacturers may list the various kinds of sweeteners they use separately, so the label may have a long list of ingredients such as corn syrup, corn starch, sucrose, and honey. These hidden sugars can be deceptive. Jell-O is 83% sugar, and a single 8-ounce can of Coke has approximately 10 teaspoons of sugar.

Artificial sweeteners — some of which are 220 times sweeter than sucrose, or table sugar — can actually increase your cravings for sweets. Whereas sugar produces a feeling of fullness or satisfaction, studies show that artificial sweeteners do nothing to ease hunger pangs or appease the appetite. Some studies show they may have a physical effect that boosts the desire for sweets. Even worse, other studies show that people who use artificial sweeteners tend to increase the amount of fats they eat as well.

▼ Tips For Cutting the Amount of Sugar You Eat

- ▼ Substitute water and unsweetened fruit juices for sodas, which is the number-one source of sugar in the typical American diet.
- ▼ Cut back on the number-two source: processed baked goods, such as doughnuts, cookies, cakes, and pies.
- ▼ Buy fruit that is canned in its own juice instead of packed in sweetened juices.
- ▼ Buy cereals that are low in sugar or contain no sugar.
- ▼ Gradually reduce the amount of sugar you add to foods such as tea, coffee, or cereal.
- ▼ Cut back on desserts and sweetened snacks; instead, try fresh fruits.
- ▼ Cut back on the amount of sugar you use in recipes. Sometimes it can be cut in *half* without affecting flavor or texture. Experiment.
- ▼ Above all, *read labels*, and cut back on foods that list any type of sugar as one of the first three ingredients.

Complex Carbohydrates

Diets high in complex carbohydrates (often called starches) tend to be lower in fat, lower in calories, and higher in dietary fiber. These factors combine to keep the blood sugar at a steady level, stave off malnutrition, and reduce the risks of heart disease, cancer, and other degenerative diseases.

Because they are nutritionally dense, most complex carbohydrate foods are rich in vitamins and minerals. Many contain a significant amount of protein. Complex carbohydrates provide a steady source of energy, making them an excellent choice for physically active people (especially those competing in marathon events). Dietary guidelines recommend that nearly half of daily calories come from carbohydrates, at least 80% of which are complex carbohydrates. The best sources of complex carbohydrates are grains, such as wheat, rice, oats, corn, rye, barley, and millet; potatoes, sweet potatoes, and yams; fruits; vegetables; and legumes, such as soybeans, garbanzo beans, black-eyed peas, kidney beans, butter beans, and peanuts.

One of the "non-nutrients" in complex carbohydrates is *fiber* — formerly called "roughage" — the part of the plant that is not digested in the small intestine and provides the bulk needed to keep the digestive system running smoothly. *Soluble fiber*, such as gels and pectins, dissolves in water and forms a thick, gel-like substance when mixed with water. It isn't digested in the small intestine, but it is absorbed in the large intestine. It helps lower blood cholesterol level, slows emptying of the stomach (prolonging a sense of fullness), and slows the absorption of sugars from the small intestine. Good sources of soluble fiber are oats, oat bran, corn bran, apples, pears, prunes, oranges, sweet potatoes, dried beans, and a variety of grains, fruits, and vegetables.

Insoluble fiber, which can't be dissolved in water, is not digested at all and comes mostly from the skins of fruits and vegetables, the seeds of fruits (such as strawberries and raspberries), and the outer tough bran of grains (such as wheat and rice). Insoluble fiber has a number of important health benefits. It speeds the transit time of materials through the intestines, stimulates muscles tone in the intestinal walls, softens stools, helps prevent constipation, helps the colon produce more mucus, and has been shown to help prevent cancer of the colon. A diet

▼ Are You Meeting Your Fiber Quota?

To find out how close you come to meeting your daily fiber quota, keep track of everything you eat for 3 days. Then, take the quiz below and add up your points. This quiz was developed with assistance from nutrition lecturer Liz Applegate, and nutrition professor Judith Stern, both at the University of California, Davis.

1. What type of bread (including rolls and muffins) did you usually eat?
    a. whole-wheat or whole-grain   +4
    b. white or partial whole-wheat   +2

2. How many servings of oat products did you average daily? (1 serving = 1 cup cooked oatmeal or oat bran.)
    a. 2 or more   +4
    b. 1   +3
    c. 1/2   +2
    d. none   0

3. How many times during the last 3 days did you eat beans (legumes), such as kidney beans, pintos, garbanzos, soybeans, lentils, and split peas?
    a. 3 or more   +4
    b. 2   +3
    c. 1   +2
    d. none   0

4. How many times during the 3-day period did you eat high-fiber breakfast cereals?
    a. 3 or more   +4
    b. 2   +3
    c. 1   +2
    d. none   0

5. How many times during the 3-day period did you eat cooked whole-grain side dishes, such as brown rice or barley?
    a. 3 or more   +4
    b. 2   +3
    c. 1   +2
    d. none   0

6. Approximately how many servings of canned or fresh fruits and vegetables did you eat daily? (Use an average from the previous 3 days. 1 serving = 1/2 cup cooked or 1 cup or 1 piece raw.)
    a. 7 or more   +5
    b. 5-6   +4
    c. 3-4   +2
    d. 1-2   +1
    e. none   −2

Scoring: If your overall score is over 20, your fiber intake is probably adequate. If it is lower, try to increase your fiber intake using the foods mentioned above.

high in insoluble fiber also has been shown to help prevent diverticulosis and diverticulitis, disease conditions that occur when the intestine bulges out into "pockets" that can become infected or rupture.

The best source of insoluble fiber is wheat bran. Other good sources are dried beans and peas, fresh fruits and vegetables eaten with their skins, and most whole grains. Table 8.3 compares some sources of fiber in common foods.

Most Americans eat about 15 grams of fiber a day. The National Cancer Institute recommends doubling that

Boosting The Fiber Content of Your Diet

If your diet is low in fiber, introduce it gradually over a period of 4 to 6 weeks, with these suggestions:

▼ Substitute brown rice for white rice.
▼ Substitute whole wheat products for those made with white wheat. Start by trying those made partially of whole wheat.
▼ Add brown rice, millet, bulgur, or barley to soups, stews, and casseroles.
▼ Cook with recipes that include bran and other good sources of fiber.
▼ Don't overcook vegetables. Steaming and stir-frying are two good methods to prevent the breakdown of fiber.
▼ Sprinkle wheat germ or bran on applesauce, pudding, yogurt, cottage cheese, custard, ice cream.
▼ Whenever you can, eat unpeeled fresh fruits and vegetables (scrubbed well).
▼ Choose high-fiber snacks such as popcorn, fruits, and raw vegetables.
▼ Read labels. Look for whole-grain breads, macaroni, egg noodles, and cereals.
▼ When buying bread, look for "stone-ground wheat" or "whole wheat" as the first ingredient. Other breads usually are made from refined flour (with the bran removed) that has been colored brown.

TABLE 8.3 ▼ Fiber Content of Selected Foods (in grams)

		Serving Size	Dietary Fiber
Grains	Bread, white	1 slice	0.6
	Bread, whole wheat	1 slice	1.5
	Oat bran, dry	⅓ cup	4.0
	Oatmeal, dry	⅓ cup	2.7
	Rice, brown, cooked	½ cup	2.4
	Rice, white, cooked	½ cup	0.8
Fruits	Apple, with skin	1 small	2.8
	Apricots, with skin	4 fruit	3.5
	Banana	1 small	2.2
	Blueberries	¾ cup	1.4
	Figs, dried	3 fruit	4.6
	Grapefruit	½ fruit	1.6
	Pear, with skin	1 large	5.8
	Prunes, dried	3 medium	1.7
Vegetables	Asparagus, cooked	½ cup	1.8
	Broccoli, cooked	½ cup	2.4
	Carrots, cooked, sliced	½ cup	2.0
	Peas, green, frozen, cooked	½ cup	4.3
	Tomatoes, raw	1 medium	1.0
Legumes	Kidney beans, cooked	½ cup	6.9
	Lima beans, canned	½ cup	4.3
	Pinto beans, cooked	½ cup	5.9
	Beans, white, cooked	½ cup	5.0
	Lentils, cooked	½ cup	5.2
	Peas, blackeyed, canned	½ cup	4.7

From James W. Anderson, *Plant Fiber in Foods, 2d Edition,* University of Kentucky, College of Medicine, HCF Nutrition Foundation, P.O. Box 22124, Lexington, KY 40522.

amount, or aiming for about 30 grams of fiber a day. Don't worry about the ratio of insoluble to soluble fibers. Both kinds are beneficial, and you should eat a good variety of foods that provide fiber. Because meat is extremely low in fiber, it makes sense to substitute plenty of complex carbohydrates.

VITAMINS

Vitamins fuel the chemical reactions in the body and enable metabolism to take place. They promote good vision, help form normal blood cells, create strong bones and teeth, and enable proper functioning of the heart and the nervous system.

The 13 vitamins fall into two categories. *Fat-soluble vitamins*, including vitamins A, D, E, and K, are stored in the body's fat cells. They are not excreted in the urine and are accumulated in the fat tissues of the body. If you get too many, they can be toxic. *Water-soluble vitamins*, including vitamin C and the B-complex vitamins, readily dissolve in water and are excreted in the urine. Good sources and important functions of vitamins are given in Table 8.4.

Vitamins C, E, beta-carotene (a precursor to vitamin A) and the mineral selenium serve as antioxidants, preventing oxygen from combining with other substances that it may damage. During metabolism oxygen changes carbohydrates and fats into energy. In this process oxygen is transformed into stable forms of water and carbon dioxide. A small amount of oxygen, however, ends up in an unstable form, referred to as *oxygen free radicals*. Solar radiation, cigarette smoke, radiation, and other environmental factors also seem to encourage the formation of free radicals.

A free radical molecule has a normal proton nucleus with a single unpaired electron. Having only one electron makes the free radical extremely reactive, and it constantly looks to pair the electron up with one from another molecule. When it steals the second electron from another molecule, that other molecule in turn becomes a free radical. This chain reaction goes on until two free radicals meet to form a stable molecule. Antioxidants help stabilize free radicals so they will not be as reactive until a match can be found.

Free radicals attack and damage proteins and lipids, in particular the cell membrane and DNA. This damage is thought to play a key role in the development of conditions such as heart disease, cancer, and emphysema.

Researchers believe that antioxidants offer protection by absorbing free radicals before they can cause damage and also by interrupting the sequence of reactions once damage has begun, thwarting certain chronic diseases.

MINERALS

Minerals are inorganic substances found in all living cells. They are used in the metabolic process and help form enzymes, hormones, and other chemicals essential to metabolism. Some minerals resemble fat-soluble vitamins: They are not excreted easily by the body, are stored in body cells, and can become toxic if excessive. Other minerals resemble water-soluble vitamins: They don't accumulate in the tissues and are excreted easily by the body.

Of the approximately 31 nutritional minerals, 24 are considered essential for sustaining life. The nutritional minerals fall into two basic categories: macrominerals and trace minerals.

The *macrominerals*, or "major" minerals, are those the body needs in relatively large amounts. These major minerals constitute as much as 80% of all inorganic material in the human body. Because they are found in so many different foods, deficiencies are not common if people eat even a moderate variety of foods. The one exception is calcium. According to the National Academy of Sciences, 80% of the women over age 18 who were surveyed consumed too little calcium, a deficiency that may cause osteoporosis later in life. The macrominerals, in order of importance to the human body, are: calcium, phosphorus, potassium, sulfur, sodium, chloride, and magnesium.

Trace minerals are those the body needs in very small amounts; 14 trace minerals are essential to good health. The most abundant, and probably the most important, are iron, zinc, and iodine. Table 8.5 lists selected minerals of both types, along with their safe intake levels.

Three minerals are especially essential to health and sustaining life. These are calcium, iron, and sodium.

Calcium

Among its other functions, calcium aids in the formation of bones, and that's an important factor not

TABLE 8.4 ▼ Major Functions of Vitamins

Nutrient	Good Sources	Major Functions	Deficiency Symptoms
Vitamin A	Milk, cheese, eggs, liver, and yellow/dark green fruits and vegetables	Required for healthy bones, teeth, skin, gums, and hair. Maintenance of inner mucous membranes, thus increasing resistance to infection. Adequate vision in dim light.	Night blindness, decreased growth, decreased resistance to infection, rough-dry skin.
Vitamin D	Fortified milk, cod liver oil, for salmon, tuna, egg yolk	Necessary for bones and teeth. Needed calcium and phosphorus absorption	Rickets (bone softening), fractures, and muscle spasms
Vitamin E	Vegetable oils, yellow and green leafy vegetables, margarine, wheat germ, whole grain breads and cereals	Related to oxidation and normal muscle and red blood cell chemistry	Leg cramps, red blood cell breakdown
Vitamin K	Green leafy vegetables, cauliflower, cabbage, eggs, peas, and potatoes	Essential for normal blood clotting	Hemorrhaging
Vitamin B_1 (Thiamine)	Whole grain or enriched bread, lean meats and poultry, organ fish, liver, pork, poultry, organ meats, legumes, nuts, and dried yeast	Assists in proper use of carbohydrates. Normal functioning of nervous system. Maintenance of good appetite.	Loss of appetite, nausea, confusion, cardiac abnormalities, muscle spasms
Vitamin B_2 (Riboflavin)	Eggs, milk, leafy green vegetables, whole grains, lean meats, dried beans and peas	Contributes to energy release from carbohydrates, fats, and proteins. Needed for normal growth and development, good vision, and healthy skin	Cracking of the corners of the mouth, inflammation of the skin, impaired vision.
Vitamin B_6 (Pyridoxine)	Vegetables, meats, whole grain cereals, soybeans, peanuts, and potatoes	Necessary for protein and fatty acids metabolism, and normal red blood cell formation	Depression, irritability, muscle spasms, nausea
Vitamin B_{12}	Meat, poultry, fish, liver, organ meats, eggs, shellfish, milk, and cheese	Required for normal growth, red blood cell formation, nervous system and digestive tract functioning	Impaired balance, weakness, drop in red blood cell count
Niacin	Liver and organ meats, meat, fish, poultry, whole grains, enriched breads, nuts, green leafy vegetables, and dried beans and peas	Contributes to energy release from carbohydrates, fats, and proteins. Normal growth and development, and formation of hormones and nerve-regulating substances	Confusion, depression, weakness, weight loss
Biotin	Liver, kidney, eggs, yeast, legumes, milk, nuts, dark green vegetables	Essential for carbohydrate metabolism and fatty acid synthesis	Inflamed skin, muscle pain, depression, weight loss
Folic Acid	Leafy green vegetables, organ meats, whole grains and cereals, and dried beans	Needed for cell growth and reproduction and red blood cell formation	Decreased resistance to infection
Pantothenic Acid	All natural foods, especially liver, kidney, eggs, nuts, yeast, milk, dried peas and beans, and green leafy vegetables	Related to carbohydrate and fat metabolism	Depression, low blood sugar, leg cramps, nausea, headaches
Vitamin C (Ascorbic Acid)	Fruits and vegetables	Helps protect against infection; formation of collagenous tissue. Normal blood vessels, teeth, and bones	Slow healing wounds, loose teeth, hemorrhaging, rough-scaly skin, irritability

Reprinted from *Principles & Labs for Physical Fitness & Wellness*. 2d Ed. Werner W. K. Hoeger, & Sharon Hoeger, Morton Publishing Co, 1994.

TABLE 8.5 ▼ Major Functions of Minerals

Nutrient	Good Sources	Major Functions	Deficiency Symptoms
Calcium	Milk, yogurt, cheese, green leafy vegetables, dried beans, sardines, and salmon	Required for strong teeth and bone formation. Maintenance of good muscle tone, heart beat, and nerve function	Bone pain and fractures, periodontal disease, muscle cramps
Iron	Organ meats, lean meats, seafoods, eggs, dried peas and beans, nuts, whole and enriched grains, and green leafy vegetables	Major component of hemoglobin. Aids in energy utilization	Nutritional anemia, and overall weakness
Phosphorus	Meats, fish, milk, eggs, dried beans and peas, whole grains, and processed foods	Required for bone and teeth formation. Energy release regulation.	Bone pain and fracture, weight loss, and weakness
Zinc	Milk, meat, seafood, whole grains, nuts, eggs, and dried beans	Essential component of hormones, insulin, and enzymes. Used in normal growth and development	Loss of appetite, slow healing wounds, and skin problems
Magnesium	Green leafy vegetables, whole grains, nuts, soybeans, seafood, and legumes	Needed for bone growth and maintenance. Carbohydrate and protein utilization. Nerve function. Temperature regulation	Irregular heartbeat, weakness, muscle spasms, and sleeplessness
Sodium	Table salt, processed foods, and meat	Body fluid regulation. Transmission of nerve impulse. Heart action	Rarely seen
Potassium	Legumes, whole grains, bananas, orange juice, dried fruits, and potatoes	Heart action. Bone formation and maintenance. Regulation of energy release. Acid-base regulation	Irregular heartbeat, nausea, weakness
Selenium	Seafood, meat, whole grains	Component of enzyme; functions in close association with vitamin E	Muscle pain, possible heart muscle deterioration; possible hair and nail loss

just for children and teenagers. Healthy adults replace about one-fifth of their bone tissue *every year*. This means you need plenty of calcium to help your bones keep pace with what you lose each year. Women have smaller, less dense bones than men and are about eight times more likely to develop brittle, porous bones, termed osteoporosis.

Young adulthood or even the teen years are the right time to form the health habits that help prevent osteoporosis. Still, it's never too late to begin. Bones, like skin, deserve special care.

Bones respond to physical activity by becoming denser and stronger. If you walk a lot, for example, your leg bones will respond by increasing their mass. If you regularly use your arms to lift weights or swing a tennis racket, the bones in your arms will grow stronger. To make sure you get enough calcium and maintain strong bones:

▶ Do weight-bearing exercise daily — walking, running, cycling, dancing, or weight-lifting — or activities such as housework or mowing the grass.

▶ Consume enough calcium. The daily recommended dietary allowance, (RDA) is 800 milligrams daily, except for adolescents and young adults and pregnant or lactating women, who are advised to consume 1,200 milligrams daily. A cup of milk provides 300 milligrams of calcium; 8 ounces of yogurt, 300 to 450 milligrams.

▶ If you smoke, stop.

Check Your Calcium Intake

If you are not a fan of dairy products, you may be coming up far short of your calcium needs. But even if you are a milk lover, how much calcium your body actually absorbs depends upon your genetic makeup. And how much you retain depends upon your intake of salt and protein. This duo increases the elimination of calcium, causing your body to steal calcium it needs from your bones.

The following quiz was developed with the assistance of Robert P. Heaney, professor of medicine at Creighton University School of Medicine, Omaha, Nebraska. It can tell you how close your diet comes to providing the appropriate amount of bone food. Just check the answer that applies to you.

1. I eat a serving of yogurt (8 ounces), milk (1 cup), or cheese (1 ounce) at least once a day.
   ____ True   +3
   ____ False   −1

2. Dairy products give me gas and bloating, so I avoid them.
   ____ True   −1
   ____ False   +1

3. I make sure I eat one or more of the following nondairy sources of calcium at least 3 times a week: leafy green vegetables (kale, bok choy, or broccoli), shellfish (oysters or clams), or canned fish with bones (salmon or sardines).
   ____ True   +1
   ____ False   0

4. I make an effort to slip dairy foods into my diet whenever I can (grating cheese over salads, for example).
   ____ True   +1
   ____ False   0

5. I eat calcium-enriched forms of products (such as breakfast cereal or fruit juice) whenever possible.
   ____ True   +1
   ____ False   −1

6. When given a choice, I drink carbonated soft drinks over low-fat dairy drinks or water.
   ____ True   −1
   ____ False   0

7. I tend to get my protein from meats.
   ____ True   −1
   ____ False   +1

8. I usually salt food automatically without tasting them.
   ____ True   −1
   ____ False   +1

Scoring: If you scored between 7 and 9, you are laying the dietary foundation for a rock-solid skeleton. (Remember, though, that even if you scored a perfect 9, you may still have a bone deficit if you are inactive, underweight or postmenopausal, have a family history of osteoporosis, or take aluminum-based antacids or other calcium-robbing drugs.) If you scored between 4 and 6, try to include more low-fat dairy products and go easy on the calcium bandits. If you scored below 4, your skeleton may be becoming perilously porous. Learn to love low-fat yogurt and make friends with skim milk. Ask your doctor about taking a calcium supplement.

- Eat foods rich in vitamins A and D; they help your body absorb calcium. Primary sources are milk (preferably nonfat) and dark leafy vegetables.
- Avoid too much meat or other protein-rich foods; they make your body excrete calcium.
- Cut down on alcohol, caffeine, and phosphates (found in soda); they also leach calcium from your body.

Iron

A deficiency of iron in the diet means too few red blood cells in the bloodstream. This can cause a condition called *iron deficiency anemia*, characterized by weakness, pallor, shortness of breath, susceptibility to infection, shortened attention span, impaired learning abilities, loss of vision, and other serious physical problems. Up to 15% of American women of childbearing age may have an iron deficiency, because of blood loss during menstruation.

A balance must be present, though, as too much iron can cause infections, tissue damage, and severe liver damage. Because the proper balance is so important, you should consult with your doctor before taking any iron supplement.

To make sure your body keeps and utilizes the iron you get in your diet:

- Eat foods rich in vitamin C, along with iron-rich foods; vitamin C triples iron absorption.
- Use cast-iron cookware to prepare your food; the body readily uses the iron the food picks up.

Is Osteoporosis in Your Future?

Risk factors you CANNOT control:

		YES	NO
1.	Are you female?	☐	☐
2.	Do you have a family history of osteoporosis?	☐	☐
3.	Are your ancestors from the British Isles, northern Europe, China, or Japan?	☐	☐
4.	Are you very fair-skinned?	☐	☐
5.	Are you small-boned?	☐	☐
6.	Are you over age 35?	☐	☐
7.	Have you had your ovaries removed, or did you have an early menopause?	☐	☐
8.	Did you breast-feed your baby?	☐	☐
9.	Are you allergic to milk and milk products?	☐	☐
10.	Have you never been pregnant?	☐	☐
11.	Do you have cancer or kidney disease?	☐	☐
12.	Do you have to take chemotherapy, steroids, anticonvulsants, or anticoagulants?	☐	☐

Risk factors you CAN control:

		YES	NO
13.	Is your daily routine stressful?	☐	☐
14.	Do you smoke?	☐	☐
15.	Do you drink alcohol?	☐	☐
16.	Do you avoid milk and cheese in your diet?	☐	☐
17.	Do you get very little exercise?	☐	☐
18.	Do you drink a lot of soft drinks?	☐	☐
19.	Is your diet high in protein?	☐	☐
20.	Do you consume a lot of caffeine (five or more cups of coffee per day or equivalent)?	☐	☐
21.	Are you amenorrhic (without a monthly period)?	☐	☐
22.	Do you get less than 1,000 mg. of calcium a day?	☐	☐
23.	Is your body weight very low?	☐	☐
24.	Do you crash diet?	☐	☐
25.	Do you have a high sodium (salt) intake?	☐	☐

If you answered "yes" to three (3) of the above questions, you are at risk for osteoporosis and may want to ask your doctor to give you a bone density screening test. The more questions you answered "yes" to, the higher your risk of developing osteoporosis in the future.

Many clinical studies suggest that osteoporosis is a preventable disease. As you can see from the quiz, you can do several things right now to help prevent osteoporosis in your future.

Adapted from Marion Laboratories, Inc.

▶ Avoid too much caffeine; it reduces your body's ability to absorb iron. Drink no more than three cups of tea or coffee a day.

Sodium

Sodium, commonly known as salt, is essential to life, but, according to the National Academy of Sciences, most Americans get as much as 10 times the amount they should. The average American consumes two to three times as much salt as is generally recommended. An estimated 5% to 10% of all people are sensitive to sodium. Their blood pressure rises, increasing the risk for stroke, kidney disease and heart disease.

Sodium is added to almost all processed foods during processing, and many restaurants add vast amounts of sodium to fast foods such as hamburgers, French fries, and even milk shakes. One fast-food meal of a quarter-pound cheeseburger, fries, and a chocolate shake provides almost 1000 mg more sodium than you should have in an *entire day*. A single apple pie from McDonald's contains more than 1,000 mg of sodium, almost as much as you need all day.

These hidden sources of sodium are what cause problems. One significant source of sodium is common condiments, such as ketchup, mustard, barbecue sauce, soy sauce, and MSG. You can overload on sodium even if you take certain medications, such as antacids.

Can You Find the Hidden Salt?

If you've already banned the saltshaker from the table and sworn off salty snacks — good for you! But to keep your intake at the recommended one-teaspoon-a-day limit takes a bit more vigilance. Three-fourths of your dietary sodium is hidden in already-prepared foods, experts say. And many salt-laced foods, such as cereal, diet soda and instant pudding don't taste a bit salty.

Just how good are you at avoiding this hidden salt? If you're eating more potassium-rich fresh fruits and vegetables than packaged convenience foods, for example, you're probably doing great. (Potassium helps rid your body of excess sodium.)

Take this quiz to find out where you stand on the hidden salt scale.

1. When barbecuing meat or fish, I'm more likely to brush on herbs or homemade marinara sauce than commercial ketchup, barbecue sauce, or soy sauce.
   ____ True   +1
   ____ False   −1

2. The fresh fruits and vegetables and lean meats in my grocery cart usually crowd out the canned, frozen, and processed food.
   ____ True   +1
   ____ False   −1

3. I buy only the low-salt type of margarine.
   ____ True   +1
   ____ False   −1

4. I usually have dehydrated, instant versions of soups, sauces, salad dressings, oatmeal, or other foods on hand.
   ____ True   −1
   ____ False   +1

5. I steam, microwave, broil, or stir-fry vegetables rather than boil them.
   ____ True   +1
   ____ False   −1

6. Processed cheese never passes my lips.
   ____ True   +1
   ____ False   −1

7. I rinse canned foods such as tuna, ham, and beans before preparing them.
   ____ True   +1
   ____ False   −1

8. I'm a sucker for deli food — cold cuts, prepared salads, pastrami, ham, smoked fish, and so on.
   ____ True   −1
   ____ False   +1

9. I usually order my hamburger with the works — cheese, pickles, ketchup, mustard and special sauce.
   ____ True   −1
   ____ False   +1

10. When dining out, I usually order oil and vinegar dressing for my salad, and ask for gravies and sauces on the side.
    ____ True   +1
    ____ False   −1

Scoring: 8-10: You're a top-notch salt sleuth. 5-7: There's room for improvement. Scan food labels closely for the key phrases "sodium-free" or "very low sodium." Below 5: You're probably relying on too many prepared condiments and packaged convenience foods. Try to cut down on these.

> ### Tips For Reducing Salt in Your Diet
>
> About a third of the salt in your diet comes from natural, unprocessed foods you eat. That's probably all you need. The rest comes from processed foods and the salt shaker, which you can safely eliminate. Try these tips:
>
> ▼ Taste food before you salt it. You might even try taking the salt shaker off the table.
>
> ▼ Cut back on the salt you use when cooking. Try other spices instead.
>
> ▼ Avoid salty processed foods, such as bacon, lunch meats, sausage, and ham.
>
> ▼ Remember that "hidden" salt in processed foods — gelatin, instant potatoes, American cheese, and canned fish — are some of the worst offenders.
>
> ▼ Learn to read labels. You should be getting 1100 to 3300 mg of sodium a day, and you can get all, if not most, in unprocessed fruits, vegetables, and meats.

WATER

You might not think of water as a nutrient, but, next to air, it is the element most necessary for survival and is the most important nutrient. Water helps your body use the other nutrients in your diet, helps your body get rid of wastes, helps you digest foods, carries oxygen and nutrients throughout the body, lubricates your joints, and regulates your body temperature — to name just a few functions.

Approximately 60% of your body is made up of water. Some of the denser tissues, such as bones, have less (approximately 20% for bones). Others have more (brain tissue, for example, is 75% water).

You get some water from the foods you eat. Fruits, for example, are as much as 80% water. Especially good choices are melons and apples. Even foods you don't typically think of as "wet," such as bread and meat, can be anywhere from 33% to 50% water. In addition to the foods you eat, you should drink eight to ten 8-ounce glasses of water a day — more if you are physically active, live in a hot climate, or perspire a lot.

You can't always rely on thirst to indicate a water deficit, according to Dr. Barbara Rolls of Johns Hopkins University School of Medicine. A rough indicator is the color of your urine. If it is dark amber or has a strong odor, you are not drinking enough water. Passing a full bladder of colorless or pale yellow urine at least four times a day means you're getting enough water.

In addition to drinking plenty of water:

▶ Avoid caffeine. It increases the body's need for water while it increases the amount of water the body puts out.

▶ Avoid alcohol. You need 8 ounces of water to metabolize a single ounce of alcohol.

▶ Cut down on the amount of sugar you eat. It increases your body's need for water.

▶ Cut back on protein to a healthy level. The wastes produced from proteins build up in the kidneys, and you need extra water to flush them out.

▶ Drink a steady amount of water throughout the day to keep your body supplied.

ENERGY (ATP) PRODUCTION

The energy derived from food is not used directly by the cells. It is transferred to form an energy-rich compound called **adenosine triphosphate**, or **ATP**. The subsequent breakdown of this compound provides the energy used by all energy-requiring processes of the body. ATP must be recycled continually to sustain life and work.

ATP can be resynthesized in three ways:

1. **ATP and ATP-CP system.** The body stores small amounts of ATP and creatine phosphate (CP). These stores are used during all-out activities up to 10 seconds in duration, such as sprinting, long jumping, and power (weight) lifting. The amount of stored ATP provides energy for just a few seconds. With all-out efforts, ATP is resynthesized from CP, another high-energy phosphate compound. This is referred to as the ATP-CP or phosphagen system.

   Depending on the amount of physical training, the concentration of CP stored in cells is sufficient to allow maximal exertion for up to 10 seconds. Once the CP stores are depleted, the person is forced to slow down or rest to allow ATP to form through anaerobic and aerobic pathways.

2. **Anaerobic or lactic acid system.** During high intensity (anaerobic) exercise that is sustained between 10 and 180 seconds maximum, ATP is replenished from the breakdown of glucose through a series of chemical reactions that do not require oxygen. In the process, though, lactic acid is produced, which causes muscular fatigue.

    Because of the accumulation of lactic acid with high intensity exercise, the formation of ATP is limited to about 3 minutes. A recovery period then is necessary to allow for the elimination of lactic acid. Formation of ATP through the anaerobic system is possible from glucose (carbohydrates) only.

3. **Aerobic system.** The production of energy during slow-sustained exercise is derived primarily through aerobic metabolism. Both glucose (carbohydrates) and fatty acids (fat) are used in this process. Oxygen is required to form ATP, and under steady state exercise conditions lactic acid accumulation is minimal.

    Because oxygen is required, a person's capacity to utilize oxygen (maximal oxygen uptake, or Max VO_2 (see Chapter 6) is critical for successful athletic performance in aerobic events. The higher the Max VO_2, the greater is the capacity to generate ATP through the aerobic system.

▼ NUTRIENT SUPPLEMENTATION

According to the Food and Drug Administration, four of every 10 adults in the United States take nutrient supplements daily, and one in every seven has a nutrient intake almost eight times the RDA. In reality, vitamin and mineral requirements for the body can be met by consuming as few as 1,200 calories per day, as long as the diet contains the recommended servings from the five food groups.

Water-soluble vitamins cannot be stored as long as fat-soluble vitamins. The body readily excretes excessive intakes. Small amounts, however, can be retained for weeks or months in various organs and tissues of the body. Fat-soluble vitamins, on the other hand, are stored in fatty tissue. Therefore, daily intake of these vitamins is not as crucial. Too much vitamin A and vitamin D actually can be detrimental to health.

People should not take megadoses of vitamins. For most vitamins, a megadose is 10 times the RDA or more. For vitamins A and D, it is respectively five and two times the RDA. Mineral doses should not exceed three times the RDA.

No standard percentage above the RDA is present to guide us in determining the level at which a high dose of a given nutrient may cause health problems. For some nutrients, a dose of five times the RDA taken over several months may create problems. For others, it may not pose any threat to human health.

Iron supplementation frequently is recommended for women who have heavy menstrual flow. Iron deficiency (determined through blood testing) is common in these women. Some pregnant and lactating women also may require supplements. According to 1990 guidelines by the National Academy of Science, the average pregnant woman who eats an adequate amount of a variety of foods needs only to take a low dose of daily iron supplement. Women who are pregnant with more than one baby may need additional supplements. In the above instances, supplements should be taken under a physician's supervision.

Other people who may benefit from supplementation are alcoholics and street-drug users who do not have a balanced diet, smokers, strict vegetarians, individuals on extremely low-calorie diets, elderly people who don't eat balanced meals regularly, and newborn infants (usually given a single dose of vitamin K to prevent abnormal bleeding).

For healthy people with a balanced diet, most supplements do not seem to provide additional benefits. They do not help people run faster, jump higher, relieve stress, improve sexual prowess, cure a common cold, or boost energy levels.

Much research currently is being done to study the effects of antioxidant supplements (vitamins C, E, beta-carotene, and the mineral selenium) in thwarting several chronic diseases (see the discussion earlier in this chapter on vitamins). Antioxidants are believed to offer protection, but the effects of supplements have not yet been clearly established.

The benefits of antioxidants have been researched primarily through diet alone, by studying people who eat foods high in antioxidants and not through supplements. Researchers do not know if the protective effects are caused by the antioxidants themselves, in combination with other nutrients, or actually by some other nutrients in food that have not yet been investigated. In the case of selenium, excessive amounts may be toxic. A diet with substantial fruits, vegetables, and grains is the best means to obtain ample amounts of antioxidants.

Many people who regularly eat fast foods high in fat content or too many sweets think they need vitamin and mineral supplementation to balance their diet. This is another fallacy about nutrition. The problem in these cases is not a lack of vitamins and minerals but, instead, a diet too high in calories, fat, and sodium. Supplementation will not offset these poor eating habits.

If you think your diet is not balanced, you first need to determine which nutrients are missing (see nutrient analysis). Then use the Healthy Eating Pyramid and the vitamin and mineral charts in this chapter, and eat more of the foods high in antioxidants and those with nutrients that are deficient in your diet.

▼ RECOMMENDED DIETARY GUIDELINES FOR AMERICANS

The U. S. Department of Agriculture (USDA) and the U. S. Department of Health and Human Services have issued a set of dietary guidelines for Americans. Based on an earlier U. S. Senate report called *Dietary Goals for the United States*, the guidelines consist of seven general practices geared toward good health:

- *Eat a variety of foods* to get the energy (calories), protein, vitamins, minerals, and fiber you need for good health.
- *Maintain a healthy weight* to reduce your chances of having high blood pressure, heart disease, a stroke, certain cancers, and the most common kind of diabetes.
- *Choose a diet low in fat, saturated fat, and cholesterol* to reduce your risk of heart disease and certain types of cancer. Because fat contains more than twice the calories of an equal amount of carbohydrates or protein, a diet low in fat can help you maintain a healthy weight.
- *Choose a diet with plenty of vegetables, fruits, and grain products* that provide needed vitamins, minerals, fiber, and complex carbohydrates. They are generally lower in fat.
- *Use sugars only in moderation* A diet with lots of sugars has too many calories and too few nutrients for most people and can contribute to tooth decay.
- *Use salt and other forms of sodium only in moderation* to help reduce your risk of high blood pressure.
- *If you drink alcoholic beverages, do so in moderation.* Alcoholic beverages supply calories but few or no nutrients. Drinking alcohol is also the cause of many health problems and accidents and can lead to addiction.

In addition to the seven guidelines issued by the USDA, the National Research Council, a division of the National Academy of Sciences, has issued the following specific suggestions:

- *Reduce total fat intake to no more than 30% of your daily calories.* Less than one-third of that should be saturated fat.
- *Reduce cholesterol intake to less than 300 mg per day.*
- *Eat plenty of vegetables and fruits.* You should have five or more servings a day of fruits and vegetables combined. Concentrate on citrus fruits and green and yellow vegetables.
- *Eat six or more servings of complex carbohydrates a day,* such as whole-grain breads, whole-grain cereals, fruits, vegetables, and dried beans or peas.
- *Eat a moderate amount of protein.*
- *Maintain an appropriate weight* by balancing what you eat with your level of physical activity.
- *Limit alcohol to an equivalent of less than 1 ounce per day.* That translates to two average cocktails, two glasses of wine, or two cans of beer. If you're pregnant, avoid alcohol completely.
- *Eat fewer than 6 grams of sodium a day.*
- *Get adequate calcium* through low-fat or nonfat dairy products, dark green vegetables, and other sources of calcium.
- *Avoid taking dietary supplements* that provide more than the recommended daily allowance of any vitamins, minerals, amino acids, proteins, fibers, or lecithin unless your physician or nutritionist instructs you to do so.

If you're an average American, following either set of guidelines probably represents some significant dietary changes for you. According to the U.S.

Senate select committee that issued the original set of dietary goals, the recommended changes stack up as shown in Figure 8.6, the Food Guide Pyramid.

The pyramid conveys three essential elements of a healthy diet:

▶ *Proportion.* Eat different amounts every day from the basic food groups. The shape of the pyramid tells you at a glance that grains, vegetables, and fruits should make up the bulk of your diet.

▶ *Moderation.* Use fats and sugars sparingly.

▶ *Variety.* Choose different foods from each major food group every day. The pyramid doesn't claim that any food is better or worse than another.

As you look at the pyramid, keep in mind that the USDA groups foods according to the most important nutrients they contain and how they're used. That's why you see legumes grouped with meat, poultry, fish, eggs, and nuts.

Legumes contain protein in amounts comparable to these other protein-rich foods, but they also provide fiber with virtually no fat — healthful qualities none of the other foods in this group have.

Don't worry about where legumes are grouped — with meats or with fruits and vegetables. Just remember to eat them.

FOOD LABELS: READING YOUR WAY TO BETTER HEALTH

Every ten years or so, the National Academy of Sciences issues a new RDA based on a review of the most current research on nutrient needs for healthy people. The RDA provides daily nutrient intake recommendations, usually set high enough to encompass 97.5% of the healthy population in the United States. Stated another way, the RDA recommendation for any nutrient is well above almost everyone's actual requirement.

Between the late 1960s and the early 1990s, nutrient information on labels was expressed in terms of the U. S. RDA — a set of standard values for the average consumer — derived from the 1968 edition of the RDA. In 1993, the Food and Drug Administration (FDA) revised food labeling regulations and has replaced the U. S. RDA with *Daily Values* (see Figure 8.7). These daily values are based on a 2,000 calorie diet and may require adjustments by the individual depending on daily caloric needs.

In setting the Daily Values, the FDA first created two sets of standards: Reference Daily Intakes (RDI) and Daily Reference Values (DRV). For FDA purposes, these two sets of standards serve different functions. To avoid consumer confusion in food

Food Guide Pyramid
A Guide to Daily Food Choices

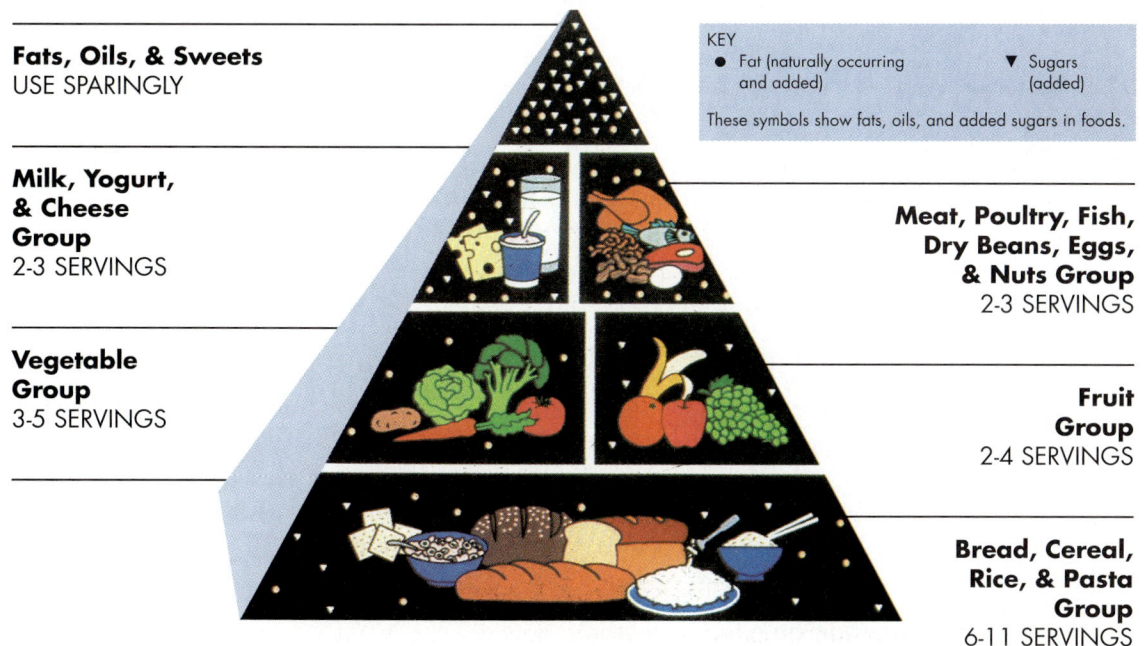

FIGURE 8.6

Nutrition Facts Title

The new title "Nutrition Facts" signals the new label.

Serving Size

Similar food products now have similar serving sizes. This makes it easier to compare foods. Serving sizes are based on amounts people actually eat.

New Label Information

Some label information may be new to you. The new nutrient list covers those most important to your health. You may have seen this information on some old labels, but it is now required.

Vitamins and Minerals

Only two vitamins, A and C, and two minerals, calcium and iron, are required on the food label. A food company can voluntarily list other vitamins and minerals in the food.

Label Numbers

Numbers on the nutrition label may be rounded for labeling.

Nutrition Facts
Serving Size 1 cup (228g)
Servings Per Container 2

Amount Per Serving
Calories 90   Calories from Fat 30

	% Daily Value*
Total Fat 3g	5%
Saturated Fat 0g	0%
Cholesterol 0mg	0%
Sodium 300mg	13%
Total Carbohydrate 13g	4%
Dietary Fiber 3g	12%
Sugars 3g	
Protein 3g	

Vitamin A	80%	•	Vitamin C	60%
Calcium	4%	•	Iron	4%

*% Daily Values are based on a 2000 calorie diet. Your daily values may be higher or lower depending on your calorie needs:

	Calories	2000	2500
Total Fat	Less than	65g	80g
Sat Fat	Less than	20g	25g
Cholesterol	Less than	300mg	300mg
Sodium	Less than	2400mg	2400mg
Total Carbohydrate		300g	375g
Dietary Fiber		25g	30g

Calories per gram:
Fat 9 • Carbohydrates 4 • Protein 4

Foods that have only a few of the nutrients required on the standard label can use a short label format. What's on the label depends on what's in the food. Small- and medium-sized packages with very little label space also can use a short label.

% Daily Value

% Daily Value shows how a food fits into a 2000-calorie reference diet.

You can use % Daily Value to compare foods and see how the amount of a nutrient in a serving of food fits in a 2000-calorie reference diet.

Daily Values Footnote

Daily Values are the new label reference numbers. These numbers are set by the government and are based on current nutrition recommendations.

Some labels list the daily values for a daily diet of 2000 and 2500 calories. Your own nutrient needs may be less than or more than the Daily Values on the label.

Calories Per Gram Footnote

Some labels tell the approximate number of calories in a gram of fat, carbohydrate, and protein.

Some food packages make claims such as "light," "low fat," and "cholesterol free." These claims can be used only if a food meets strict government definitions. Here are some of the meanings.

Label claim	Definition*
Calorie-Free	Less than 5 calories
Light or Lite	1/3 fewer calories or 50% less fat; if more than half the calories are from fat, fat content must be reduced by 50% or more
Light in Sodium	50% less sodium
Fat-Free	Less than 1/2 gram fat
Low-Fat	3 grams or less fat**
Cholesterol-Free	Less than 2 milligrams cholesterol and 2 grams or less saturated fat**
Low Cholesterol	20 milligrams or less cholesterol and 2 grams or less saturated fat**
Sodium-Free	Less than 5 milligrams sodium**
Very Low Sodium	35 milligrams or less sodium**
Low-Sodium	140 milligrams or less sodium**
High Fiber	5 grams or more fiber

*Per Reference Amount (standard serving size). Some claims have higher nutrient levels for main dish products and meal products, such as frozen entrees and dinners.

**Also per 50 g for products with small serving sizes (reference amount is 30 g or less or 2 tbsp or less).

Some food packages may now carry health claims. A health claim is a label statement that describes the relationship between a nutrient and a disease or health-related condition. A food must meet certain nutrient levels to make a health claim. Seven types of health claims are allowed. These nutrient-disease relationships include:

A diet:	And:
High in calcium	Osteoporosis (brittle bone disease)
High in fiber-containing grain products, fruits, and vegetables	Cancer
High in fruits or vegetables (high in dietary fiber or vitamins A or C)	Cancer
High in fiber from fruits, vegetables, and grain products	Heart disease
Low in fat	Cancer
Low in saturated fat and cholesterol	Heart disease
Low in sodium	High blood pressure

FIGURE 8.7 ▼ Information on new food label.

labeling, however, the FDA combined the RDI and DRV into the Daily Values.

The RDI are reference values for protein, vitamins, and minerals. These are similar in purpose to the old U. S. RDA, but reflecting average allowances based on the 1989 RDA.

The DRV are standards for nutrients and food components that do not have an established RDA. The DRV include carbohydrate, fat, saturated fat, fiber, cholesterol, and sodium. These standards (computed in grams and milligrams based on a 2,000 calorie diet) represent dietary intakes to attain or restrict based on a consensus of critical values that are associated with health. For example, carbohydrate intake should be 60% of total daily calories (300 grams), while fat intake should be limited to less than 30% (65 grams).

Both the RDA and the Daily Values apply only to healthy people. They are not intended for people who are ill and may require additional nutrients.

Using the food label can help you make healthful food choices in the supermarket, at the dinner table, and on the road. You can use the food label to compare foods and plan healthful meals. The label also gives the information to make wise food choices that may help reduce your chances for diseases such as heart disease, high blood pressure, stroke, obesity, diabetes, and some forms of cancer.

▼ DESIGNING A NUTRITIONAL PLAN FOR WELLNESS

The best nutritional plan for you is one that is *personalized* for your situation. The food choices you make depend on how much time you have, where you eat (a dormitory cafeteria? a fast-food restaurant? your own kitchen?), and what kinds of foods you *like*. To design a food plan that includes Brussels sprouts, turnip greens, and tuna casserole is senseless if you really dislike those things.

Designing a nutritional plan involves two fairly simple steps:

1. Identify the things you need to change.
2. Make some *gradual* changes. You'll be much more successful if you plan to change things bit-by-bit, allowing yourself time to adjust your habits and tastes.

In general, aim for a good variety of foods from all four food groups. Eat lots of complex carbohydrates (fruits, vegetables, whole grains) and only a little protein (meats). Steer away from foods that are high in fats or refined sugars. Make some alternative selections for snacks and desserts — air-popped popcorn, fresh fruits and vegetables, low-fat crackers. Drink soda, tea, coffee, and alcohol in moderation. Drink plenty of water.

GUIDELINES

▶ Keep a written list for a week or two, and note the foods you eat regularly that don't provide much nutrition. Note the foods, too, that actually might be bad for you — foods high in saturated fats, refined sugars, salt. The list can serve as a basic blueprint of the things you need to change.

▶ Little by little, start to substitute nutritious and healthy foods for the things on the list you'd be better off without. (See Figure 8.8). If you're eating regular yogurt with fruit and flavorings, opt for nonfat yogurt topped with fresh fruit instead; you'll eliminate a lot of fat and sugar. Or try a halibut steak, broiled, in place of beef steak. Or a sweet glass of orange juice in place of the cola you normally have between classes.

▶ Eat a good variety of foods; you're more likely to get the recommended daily allowances of all the essential nutrients that way.

▶ Whenever you can, eat "natural" or fresh foods. A carrot you slice and steam is the best source of nutrients; frozen is second best; and canned is a poor substitute (it generally is loaded with sodium and stripped of many nutrients).

▶ Start out the day with a good breakfast that provides approximately a third of your daily requirements. You'll have more energy, will feel better, and won't suffer that traditional sugar crash midmorning, when you're tempted to snack on high-fat or sugar-laden foods.

▶ Make good breakfast choices, including low-fat or skim milk, whole-grain breads or cereals, bagels, bran muffins, nonfat yogurt topped with fresh fruit or sprinkled with wheat germ, fresh fruit, or fruit juice. If you make pancakes, use whole-wheat flour and top them with a low-fat, low-sugar topping, such as unsweetened applesauce. If you make French toast, use whole-grain

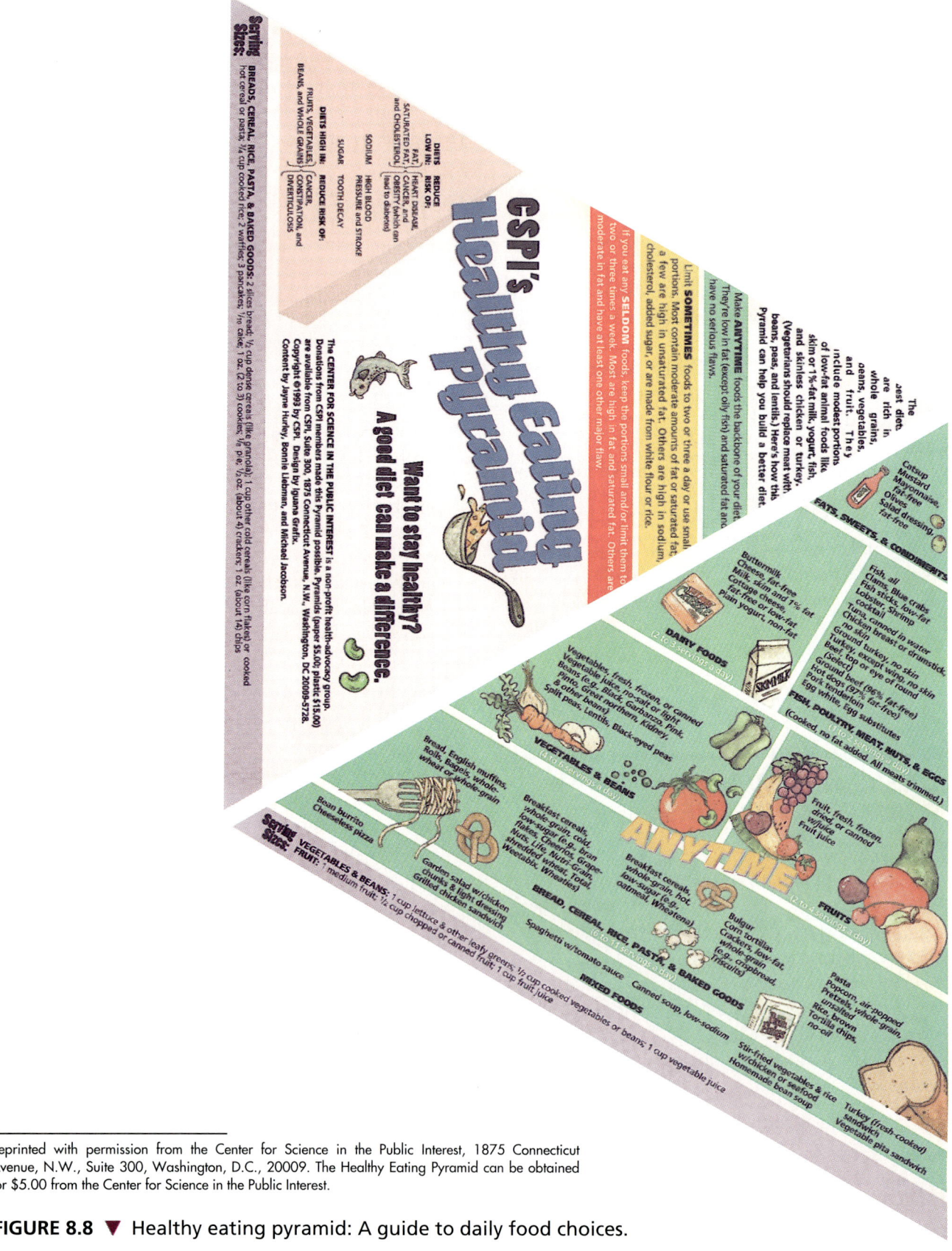

Reprinted with permission from the Center for Science in the Public Interest, 1875 Connecticut Avenue, N.W., Suite 300, Washington, D.C., 20009. The Healthy Eating Pyramid can be obtained for $5.00 from the Center for Science in the Public Interest.

FIGURE 8.8 ▼ Healthy eating pyramid: A guide to daily food choices.

EIGHT ▼ Nutrition and Wellness

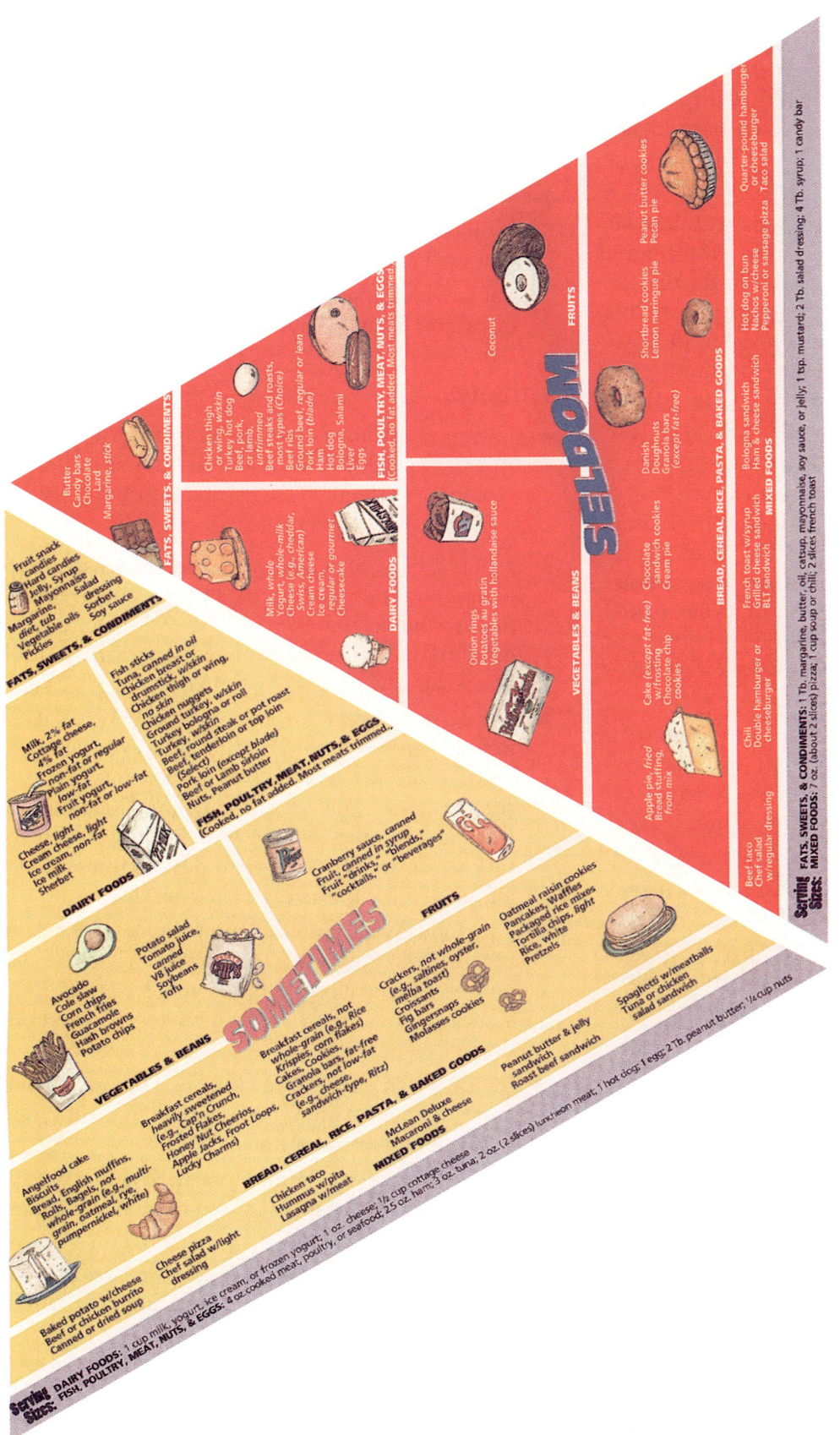

bread, egg whites, and low-fat or skim milk. Steer away from egg yolks, butter, and cream cheese.

▶ Eat at regular intervals throughout the day: breakfast in the morning, lunch at mid-day, and dinner in the early evening, with healthy snacks in between if you need them. You'll have higher energy levels and a better chance of keeping your blood sugar at a constant level.

▶ Make good lunch choices of salads with low-fat dressing; sandwiches made with whole-grain bread, low-fat spreads, and sliced roasted chicken or turkey; vegetable soups; vegetable pizza. At the salad bar, load up on fresh vegetables, legumes, and fruits. For the most part, avoid cream soups, predressed pasta salads, cheese, mayonnaise, fried foods, and processed lunch meats.

▶ Include healthy dinner choices such as skinless baked chicken breast; stir-fry foods (these normally emphasize vegetables and use meat only as an accompaniment); pasta; brown rice; whole-grain rolls; steamed vegetables. Top your baked potato with nonfat yogurt instead of butter and sour cream. Use lemon pepper on your vegetables instead of salt and butter.

▶ When cooking, use less fats. Cook in a nonstick skillet; poach, bake, broil, or roast instead of frying whenever you can; steam or microwave vegetables instead of cooking them in butter.

▶ If you're eating in a restaurant, find out if you can make substitutions. Ask for skinless chicken, a baked potato instead of French fries, sauces and dressings on the side. Look over the menu, and select items that are baked, roasted, broiled, or poached instead of fried; avoid creams, cheeses, and butter.

▶ Order several appetizers instead of one main course. A tomato or vegetable soup, a raw vegetable platter, rolls or bread sticks (without butter), or an artichoke (without sauce) are good possible choices.

SPECIAL CONCERNS

Vegetarians

If you are a vegetarian, consider these suggestions to help avoid nutritional deficiencies:

▶ Combine *complementary proteins* to make sure you get complete proteins. In essence, you should combine vegetables with grains — beans and corn (common in Mexican foods), beans and rice, tofu and rice, black bean and rice soup.

▶ Because vegetarian diets usually are low in fat, make sure you get at least 1 gram of fat a day so your body can absorb fat-soluble vitamins.

▶ Eat at least one cup of dark green vegetables a day to boost your iron intake.

▶ If you don't drink milk, eat at least two cups of legumes (dried beans and peas) a day to provide you with adequate calcium.

▶ Eat a wide range of foods to better your chance of getting balanced nutrients.

Athletes

If you are physically active, participate in sports, or compete as an athlete, you don't need a special diet, but you do need to increase certain nutrients in your diet. Follow these suggestions:

▶ Drink plenty of water. You need at least a cup before you start to exercise and one cup every 15 minutes while you exercise. Don't wait until you get thirsty. You probably won't feel thirsty until you're already quite dehydrated.

▶ Eat extra complex carbohydrates for 3 to 4 days before you compete. Pasta, fruit, rice, potatoes, and breads are good sources. Recent research recommends against "carbohydrate loading," a method of eating a high-protein, high-fat, low-carbohydrate diet for several days before switching to a high-carbohydrate, low-fat diet.

▶ Eat foods rich in potassium for several days before you compete, as potassium helps you retain essential electrolytes. If you decide to use a commercial electrolyte drink while you exercise, dilute it with water.

▶ If you're an endurance athlete, you may have more iron depletion and should consult your physician about supplementation.

▶ Resist the urge to eat more meat. You don't need more protein. Steer away from protein supplements, too.

▶ Consider that you might need more calories — generally, about 5% more than sedentary people of your same age and weight.

Maximizing Your Minerals

SELECTED MINERALS	ADULT RDA OR RESTIMATED SAFE & ADEQUATE INTAKE	MAJOR FOOD SOURCES	WHAT IT DOES; COMMENTS
Boron	None	Fruits and vegetables, especially apples, pears, broccoli, carrots.	May help regulate the body's use of calcium, phosphorus, and magnesium.
Calcium	1,200 milligrams (mg), age 11–24 and during pregnancy; 800 mg, age 25 and over (1,500 mg for women over 50, according to an NIH consensus panel).	Milk and milk products (one quart of milk has about 1,200 mg); dark green leafy vegetables; broccoli; sardines and salmon eaten with bones; some tofu; some fortified cereals; small amount in grain products.	Builds bone and teeth; maintains bone density and strength. Helps regulate heartbeat, muscle contractions, nerve function, and blood clotting. May help prevent hypertension. Adequate calcium intake (from pills or, preferably, foods) can help prevent or minimize osteoporosis. Vitamin D (from fortified milk and sun exposure) and lactose (milk sugar) help improve calcium absorption. Oxalic acid, found in spinach and some other greens, may reduce absorption.
Chlorine (chloride)	None.	Table salt (sodium chloride), fish.	Helps maintain fluid and acid-base balance; component of gastric juice.
Chromium	50–200 micrograms.*	Meat, whole grains, broccoli, brewer's yeast, fortified cereals.	Important in the metabolism of carbohydrates and fats. Many Americans don't consume enough chromium. Deficiency may impair action of insulin and the regulation of glucose in blood.
Copper	1.5–3 mg.*	Shellfish (especially oysters), beans, nuts, seeds, organ meats, whole grains, potatoes.	Helps in formation of red blood cells. Helps keep bones, blood vessels, nerves, and immune system healthy. Research into its role in heart disease has been inconclusive.
Fluorine (fluoride)	1.5–4 mg.*	Fluoridated water and foods grown or cooked in it, marine fish (with bones), tea.	Helps form bone and teeth. Some studies suggest it may help prevent osteoporosis.
Iodine	150 micrograms; 175 during pregnancy.	Primarily iodized salt; also seafood, seaweed, dairy products, crops from iodine-rich areas.	Necessary for function of the thyroid gland and thus normal cell metabolism. Prevents goiter (enlargement of thyroid). Widely dispersed in the food supply, so even if you eat little iodized salt, you probably get enough iodine.
Iron	15 mg, women age 11–50; 10 mg, women over age 50; 10 mg, men; 30 mg during pregnancy.	Meat, poultry, fish, eggs, liver, kidneys, peas, beans, nuts, dried fruits, leafy green vegetables, enriched pasta and bread, fortified cereals. Cooking in iron pots adds iron, especially to acidic food.	Essential to the formation of hemoglobin (which carries oxygen in blood) and myoglobin (in muscle). Part of several enzymes and proteins in the body. Heme iron, found in animal products, is better absorbed by the body than nonheme iron, found in plant products. To enhance absorption of nonheme iron, consume vitamin-C-rich foods or a small amount of meat.
Magnesium	280 mg, women; 350 mg, men; 320 mg during pregnancy.	Wheat bran, whole grains, leafy green vegetables, meat, milk, nuts, beans, bananas, apricots.	Aids in bone growth, basic metabolic functions, and the functioning of nerves and muscles, including the regulation of normal heart rhythm. Low intake has been linked to high blood pressure, heart-rhythm abnormalities, and heart attack.
Manganese	2–5 mg.*	Whole grains, nuts, vegetables, fruits, instant coffee, tea, cocoa powder, beans.	Needed for energy production and reproduction. May also be essential for building bones. Excess may interfere with iron absorption.
Molybdenum	75–250 micrograms.*	Whole grains, liver, beans, leafy vegetables.	Needed to activate certain enzymes in the body.
Phosphorus	1,200 mg, age 11–24 and during pregnancy; 800 mg, age 25 and over.	Almost all foods: especially fish, meat, poultry, dairy products, eggs, peas, beans, soft drinks, nuts.	Helps build bones and teeth and form cell membranes and genetic material. Vital for energy production. So plentiful in American diet that deficiencies are virtually unknown.
Potassium	1,600–2000 mg minimum.*	Most foods, especially oranges, orange juice, bananas, potatoes (with skin), dried fruits, yogurt, meat, poultry, milk.	Vital for muscle contraction, nerve impulses, and function of heart and kidneys. Helps regulate water balance in cells and blood pressure. There's some evidence that diets high in potassium (fruits and vegetables) reduce the risk of hypertension and stroke. Supplements, however, can supply dangerous amounts — take them only under a doctor's supervision.
Selenium	55 micrograms, women; 70 micrograms, men; 65 micrograms during pregnancy.	Fish, shellfish, red meat, grains, eggs, chicken, garlic, organ meats; amount in vegetables depends on soil.	Part of enzymes that act as antioxidants — that is, that help fight cell damage by oxygen-derived compounds and thus may protect against cancer. Needed for proper immune response. However, large doses, as supplied by some supplements, can be extremely toxic.
Sodium	2,400 mg maximum.*	Table salt and salt added to prepared foods, especially cheese, smoked meats, prepared soups, salty snacks, fast food.	Helps regulate blood pressure and water balance in the body.
Zinc	12 mg, women; 15 mg, men and during pregnancy.	Meat, seafood (especially oysters), liver, eggs, brewer's yeast, milk, beans, wheat germ.	Important in activity of enzymes needed for cell division, growth, and repair (wound healing), as well as proper functioning of immune system. Also plays a role in acuity of taste and smell. Large doses from pills can cause nausea, impaired immunity, and increased LDL ("bad") cholesterol.

* No RDA established. Instead, because less is known about many of these nutrients, the National Academy of Sciences has proposed ranges of Estimated Safe and Adequate Daily Dietary Intake. Recommendations for sodium and potassium are also from the National Academy of Sciences.

Recommended Dietary Allowances[a]

Category	Age	Weight[b] (lb)	Height[b] (in)	Protein (g)	Vitamin A (mcg RE)[c]	Vitamin D (mcg)[d]	Vitamin E (mg α-TE)[e]	Vitamin K (mcg)	Vitamin C (mg)	Thiamine (mg)
Infants	0-6 months	13	24	13	375	7.5	3	5	30	0.3
	6-12 months	20	28	14	375	10	4	10	35	0.4
Children	1-3	29	35	16	400	10	6	15	40	0.7
	4-6	44	44	24	500	10	7	20	45	0.9
	7-10	62	52	28	700	10	7	30	45	1.0
Males	11-14	99	62	45	1000	10	10	45	50	1.3
	15-18	145	69	59	1000	10	10	65	60	1.5
	19-24	160	70	58	1000	10	10	70	60	1.5
	25-50	174	70	63	1000	5	10	80	60	1.5
	51 plus	170	68	63	1000	5	10	80	60	1.2
Females	11-14	101	62	46	800	10	8	45	50	1.1
	15-18	120	64	44	800	10	8	55	60	1.1
	19-24	128	65	46	800	10	8	60	60	1.1
	25-50	138	64	50	800	5	8	65	60	1.1
	51 plus	143	63	50	800	5	8	65	60	1.0
Pregnant women				60	800	10	10	65	70	1.5
Lactating women	1st 6 months			65	1300	10	12	65	95	1.6
	2nd 6 months			62	1200	10	11	65	90	1.6

[a] The allowances, expressed as average daily intakes over time, are intended to provide for individual variations among most normal persons as they live in the United States under usual environmental stresses. Diets should be based on a variety of common foods in order to provide other nutrients for which human requirements have been less well defined.

[b] Weights and heights of Reference Adults are actual medians for the U.S. population of the designated age. The use of these figures does not imply that the height-to-weight ratios are ideal.

[c] Retinol equivalents. 1 retinol equivalent = 1 mcg retinol or 6 mcg beta carotene. To calculate IU value: for fruits and vegetables, multiply the RE value by ten; for animal-source foods, multiply the RE value by 3.3.

Other Recommended Intakes

The following nutrients have no RDA or Estimated Safe and Adequate Daily Dietary Intake. Instead the daily recommendations listed below are based on guidelines established by various health organizations and experts.

Beta Carotene	5 to 6 milligrams
Cholesterol	no more than 300 milligrams
Dietary Fiber	20 to 30 grams
Potassium	3000 milligrams
Sodium	no more than 2400 milligrams

Excerpted from The Wellness Encyclopedia of Food and Nutrition, © Health Letter Associates, 1992

Ribo-flavin (mg)	Niacin (mg NE)[f]	Vita-min B$_6$ (mg)	Folate[g] (mcg)	Vita-min B$_{12}$ (mcg)	Cal-cium (mg)	Phos-phorus (mg)	Mag-nesium (mg)	Iron (mg)	Zinc (mg)	Iodine (mcg)	Selen-ium (mcg)
0.4	5	0.3	25	0.3	400	300	40	6	5	40	10
0.5	6	0.6	35	0.5	600	500	60	10	5	50	15
0.8	9	1.0	50	0.7	800	800	80	10	10	70	20
1.1	12	1.1	75	1.0	800	800	120	10	10	90	20
1.2	13	1.4	100	1.4	800	800	170	10	10	120	30
1.5	17	1.7	150	2.0	1200	1200	270	12	15	150	40
1.8	20	2.0	200	2.0	1200	1200	400	12	15	150	50
1.7	19	2.0	200	2.0	1200	1200	350	10	15	150	70
1.7	19	2.0	200	2.0	800	800	350	10	15	150	70
1.4	15	2.0	200	2.0	800	800	350	10	15	150	70
1.3	15	1.4	150	2.0	1200	1200	280	15	12	150	45
1.3	15	1.5	180	2.0	1200	1200	300	15	12	150	50
1.3	15	1.6	180	2.0	1200	1200	280	15	12	150	55
1.3	15	1.6	180	2.0	800	800	280	15	12	150	55
1.2	13	1.6	180	2.0	800	800	280	10	12	150	55
1.6	17	2.2	400	2.2	1200	1200	320	30	15	175	65
1.8	20	2.1	280	2.6	1200	1200	355	15	19	200	75
1.7	20	2.1	260	2.6	1200	1200	340	15	16	200	75

[d] As cholecalciferol. 10 mcg cholecalciferol = 400 IU of vitamin D.

[e] α-tocopherol equivalents. 1 mg d-α tocopherol = 1 α-TE.

[f] t NE (niacin equivalent) is equal to 1 mg of niacin or 60 mg of dietary tryptophan.

[g] Felacin

Estimated Safe and Adequate Daily Dietary Intakes of Selected Vitamins and Minerals[a]

Category	Age	Vitamins		Trace Minerals[b]				
		Biotin (mcg)	Pantothenic acid (mg)	Copper (mg)	Manganese (mg)	Fluoride (mg)	Chromium (mcg)	Molybdenum (mcg)
Infants	0-6 months	10	2	0.4-0.6	0.3-0.6	0.1-0.5	10-40	15-30
	6-12 months	15	3	0.6-0.7	0.6-1.0	0.2-1.0	20-60	20-40
Children and adolescents	1-3	20	3	0.7-1.0	1.0-1.5	0.5-1.5	20-80	25-50
	4-6	25	3-4	1.0-1.5	1.5-2.0	1.0-2.5	30-120	30-75
	7-10	30	4-5	1.0-2.0	2.0-3.0	1.5-2.5	50-200	50-150
	11 plus	30-100	4-7	1.5-2.5	2.0-5.0	1.5-2.5	50-200	75-250
Adults		30-100	4-7	1.5-3.0	2.0-5.0	1.5-4.0	50-200	75-250

[a] Because there is less information on which to base allowances, these figures are not given in the main table of RDAs and are provided here in the form of ranges of recommended intakes.

[b] Since the toxic levels for many trace elements may be only several times usual intakes, the upper levels for the trace elements given in this table should not be habitually exceeded.

How's Your Diet?

The 40 questions below will help you focus on the key features of your diet. The (+) or (–) numbers under each set of answers instantly pat you on the back for good habits or alert you to problems you may not even realize you have.

The Grand Total rates your overall diet, on a scale from "Great" to "Arghh!"

The quiz focuses on fat, cholesterol, sodium, sugar, fiber, and vitamins A and C. It doesn't attempt to cover everything in your diet. Also, it doesn't try to measure precisely how much of these key nutrients you eat. What the quiz will do is give you a rough sketch of your current eating habits and, implicitly, suggest what you can do to improve them.

Don't despair over a less-than-perfect score. A healthy diet isn't built overnight.

INSTRUCTIONS

Under each answer is a number with a + or – sign in front of it. Circle the number that is directly beneath the answer you choose. That's your score for the question. (If you use a pencil, you can erase your answers and give the quiz to someone else.)

Circle only one number for each question, unless the instructions tell you to "average two or more scores if necessary."

How to average: In answering question 18, for example, if you drink club soda (+3) and coffee (–1) on a typical day, add the two scores (which gives you +2) and then divide by 2. That gives you a score of +1 for the question. If averaging gives you a fraction, round it to the nearest whole number.

If a question doesn't apply to you, skip it.

Pay attention to serving sizes. For example, a serving of vegetables is 1/2 cup. If you usually eat one cup of vegetables at a time, count it as two servings.

Add up all your + scores and your – scores.

Subtract your – scores from your + scores. That's your GRAND TOTAL.

QUIZ

1. How many times per week do you eat unprocessed red meat (steak, roast beef, lamb or pork chops, burgers, etc.)?
   (a) never (b) 1 or less (c) 2-3 (d) 4-5 (e) 6 or more
   +3   +2   0   –1   –3

2. After cooking, how large is the serving of red meat you usually eat? (To convert from raw to cooked, reduce by 25%. For example, 4 oz. of raw meat shrinks to 3 oz. after cooking. There are 16 oz. in a pound.)
   (a) 8 oz. or more (b) 6-7 oz. (c) 4-5 oz. (d) 3 oz. or less
   –3   –2   –1   0
   (e) don't eat red meat
   +3

3. Do you trim the visible fat when you cook or eat red meat?
   (a) yes (b) no (c) don't eat red meat
   +1   –3   0

4. How many times per week do you eat processed meats (hot dogs, bacon, sausage, bologna, luncheon meats, etc.)? (OMIT products that contain 1 gram of fat or less per serving.)
   (a) none (b) less than 1 (c) 1-2 (d) 3-4 (e) 5 or more
   +3   +2   0   –1   –3

5. What kind of ground meat or poultry do you usually eat?
   (a) regular ground beef (b) lean ground beef
   –3   –2
   (c) ground round (d) ground turkey
   0   +1
   (e) Healthy Choice™ (f) don't eat ground meat
   +2   +3

6. What type of bread do you usually eat?
   (a) whole wheat or other whole grain (b) rye
   +3   +2
   (c) pumpernickel (d) white, "wheat," French, or Italian
   +2   –2

7. How many times per week do you eat deep-fried foods (fish, chicken, vegetables, potatoes, etc.)?
   (a) none (b) 1-2 (c) 3-4 (d) 5 or more
   +3   0   –1   –3

8. How many servings of non-fried vegetables do you usually eat per day? (One serving = 1/2 cup. INCLUDE potatoes.)
   (a) none (b) 1 (c) 2 (d) 3 (e) 4 or more
   –3   0   +1   +2   +3

9. How many servings of cruciferous vegetables do you usually eat per week? (ONLY count kale, broccoli, cauliflower, cabbage, Brussels sprouts, greens, bok choy, kohlrabi, turnip, and rutabaga. One serving = 1/2 cup.)
   (a) none (b) 1-3 (c) 4-6 (d) 7 or more
   –3   +1   +2   +3

10. How many servings of vitamin-A-rich fruits or vegetables do you usually eat per week? (ONLY count carrots, pumpkin, sweet potatoes, cantaloupe, spinach, winter squash, greens, and apricots. One serving = 1/2 cup.)
    (a) none (b) 1-3 (c) 4-6 (d) 7 or more
    –3   +1   +2   +3

11. How many times per week do you eat at a fast-food restaurant? (INCLUDE burgers, fried fish or chicken, croissant or biscuit sandwiches, topped potatoes, and other main dishes. OMIT meals of just plain baked potato, broiled chicken, or salad.)
    (a) never (b) less than 1 (c) 1 (d) 2 (e) 3
    +3   +1   0   –1   –2
    (f) 4 or more
    –3

(continued)

From *Nutrition Action Healthletter*, March 1992.

12. How many servings of grains rich in complex carbohydrates do you eat per day? *(One serving = 1 slice of bread, 1 large pancake, 1 cup whole grain cold cereal, or 1/2 cup cooked cereal, rice, pasta, bulgur, wheat berries, kasha, or millet. OMIT heavily-sweetened cold cereals.)*
    (a) none   (b) 1-3   (c) 4-5   (d) 6-8   (e) 9 or more
       −3   0   +1   +2   +3

13. How many times per week do you eat fish or shellfish? *(OMIT deep-fried items, tuna packed in oil, shrimp, squid, and mayonnaise-laden tuna salad — a little mayo is okay.)*
    (a) never   (b) 1-2   (c) 3-4   (d) 5 or more
       −2   +1   +2   +3

14. How many times per week do you eat cheese? *(INCLUDE pizza, cheeseburgers, veal or eggplant parmigiana, cream cheese, etc. OMIT low-fat or fat-free cheeses.)*
    (a) 1 or less   (b) 2-3   (c) 4-5   (d) 6 or more
       +3   +2   −1   −3

15. How many servings of fresh fruit do you eat per day?
    (a) none   (b) 1   (c) 2   (d) 3   (e) 4 or more
       −3   0   +1   +2   +3

16. Do you remove the skin before eating poultry?
    (a) yes   (b) no   (c) don't eat poultry
      +3   −3   0

17. What do you usually put on your bread or toast? *(AVERAGE two or more scores if necessary.)*
    (a) butter or cream cheese   (b) margarine or peanut butter
              −3   −2
    (c) diet margarine   (d) jam or honey
           −1   0
    (e) fruit butter   (f) nothing
          +1   +3

18. Which of these beverages do you drink on a typical day? *(AVERAGE two or more scores if necessary.)*
    (a) water or club soda   (b) fruit juice   (c) diet soda
           +3   +1   −1
    (d) coffee or tea   (e) soda, fruit "drink," or fruit "ade"
          −1   −3

19. Which flavorings do you add to your foods most frequently? *(AVERAGE two or more scores if necessary.)*
    (a) garlic or lemon juice   (b) herbs or spices
          +3   +3
    (c) salt or soy sauce   (d) margarine   (e) butter   (f) nothing
          −2   −2   −3   +3

20. What do you eat most frequently as a snack? *(AVERAGE two or more scores if necessary.)*
    (a) fruits or vegetables   (b) sweetened yogurt   (c) nuts
          +3   +2   −1
    (d) cookies or fried chips   (e) granola bar
           −2   −2
    (f) candy bar or pastry   (g) nothing
          −3   0

21. What is your most typical breakfast? *(SUBTRACT an extra 3 points if you also eat bacon or sausage.)*
    (a) croissant, danish, or doughnut   (b) eggs
                  −3   −3
    (c) pancakes or waffles   (d) cereal or toast
            −2   +3
    (e) low-fat yogurt or cottage cheese   (f) don't eat breakfast
                  +3   0

22. What do you usually eat for dessert?
    (a) pie, pastry, or cake   (b) ice cream
            −3   −3
    (c) fat-free cookies or cakes   (d) frozen yogurt or ice milk
               −1   +1
    (e) nonfat ice cream or sorbet   (f) fruit
                +1   +3
    (g) don't eat dessert
          +3

23. How many times per week do you eat beans, split peas, or lentils?
    (a) none   (b) 1   (c) 2   (d) 3 or more
       −2   +1   +2   +3

24. What kind of milk do you drink?
    (a) whole   (b) 2% low-fat   (c) 1% low-fat
        −3   −1   +2
    (d) 1/2% or skim   (e) none
            +3   0

25. What dressings or toppings do you usually add to your salads? *(ADD two or more scores if necessary.)*
    (a) nothing, lemon, or vinegar   (b) fat-free dressing
                +3   +2
    (c) low- or reduced-calorie dressing   (d) regular dressing
                   +1   −1
    (e) croutons or bacon bits
           −1
    (f) cole slaw, pasta salad, or potato salad
                  −1

26. What sandwich fillings do you eat most frequently? *(AVERAGE two or more scores if necessary.)*
    (a) luncheon meat   (b) cheese or roast beef
            −3   −1
    (c) peanut butter   (d) low-fat luncheon meat
            0   +1
    (e) tuna, salmon, chicken, or turkey
            +3
    (f) don't eat sandwiches
           0

27. What do you usually spread on your sandwiches? *(AVERAGE two or more scores if necessary.)*
    (a) mayonnaise   (b) light mayonnaise
          −2   −1
    (c) ketchup, mustard, or fat-free mayonnaise   (d) nothing
                        0   +2

28. How many egg yolks do you eat per week? *(ADD 1 yolk for every slice of quiche you eat.)*
    (a) 2 or less   (b) 3-4   (c) 5-6   (d) 7 or more
         +3   0   −1   −3

(continued)

29. How many times per week do you eat canned or dried soups? *(OMIT low-sodium, low-fat soups.)*
    (a) none (b) 1-2 (c) 3-4 (d) 5 or more
      +3   0   −2   −3

30. How many servings of a rich source of calcium do you eat per day? *(One serving = 2/3 cup milk or yogurt, 1 oz. cheese, 1½ oz. sardines, 3½ oz. salmon, 5 oz. tofu made with calcium sulfate, 1 cup greens or broccoli, or 200 mg of a calcium supplement.)*
    (a) none (b) 1 (c) 2 (d) 3 or more
      −3   +1   +2   +3

31. What do you usually order on your pizza? *(Vegetable toppings include green pepper, mushrooms, onions, and other vegetables. SUBTRACT 1 point from your score if you order extra cheese.)*
    (a) no cheese with vegetables   (b) cheese with vegetables
         +3   +1
    (c) cheese   (d) cheese with meat toppings
         0   −3
    (e) don't eat pizza
         +2

32. What kind of cookies do you usually eat?
    (a) graham crackers or ginger snaps   (b) oatmeal
         +1   −1
    (c) sandwich cookies (like Oreos)
         −2
    (d) chocolate coated, chocolate chip, or peanut butter
         −3
    (e) don't eat cookies
         +3

33. What kind of frozen dessert do you usually eat? *(SUBTRACT 1 point from your score for each topping you use — whipped cream, hot fudge, nuts, etc.)*
    (a) gourmet ice cream   (b) regular ice cream
         −3   −1
    (c) sorbet, sherbet, or ices
         +1
    (d) frozen yogurt, fat-free ice cream, or ice milk
         +1
    (e) don't eat frozen desserts
         +3

34. What kind of cake or pastry do you usually eat?
    (a) cheesecake, pie, or any microwave cake
         −3
    (b) cake with frosting or filling   (c) cake without frosting
         −2   −1
    (d) unfrosted muffin, banana bread, or carrot cake
         0
    (e) angelfood or fat-free cake
         +1
    (f) don't eat cakes or pastries
         +3

35. How many times per week does your dinner contain grains, vegetables, or beans, but little or no animal protein (meat, poultry, fish, eggs, milk, or cheese)?
    (a) none (b) 1-2 (c) 3-4 (d) 5 or more
      −1   +1   +2   +3

36. Which of the following salty snacks do you typically eat? *(AVERAGE two or more scores if necessary.)*
    (a) potato chips, corn chips, or packaged popcorn
         −3
    (b) reduced-fat potato or tortilla chips   (c) salted pretzels
         −2   −1
    (d) unsalted pretzels or baked corn or tortilla chips
         +1
    (e) homemade air-popped popcorn
         +3
    (f) don't eat salty snacks
         +3

37. What do you usually use to saute vegetables or other foods? *(Vegetable oil includes safflower, corn, canola, olive, sunflower, and soybean.)*
    (a) butter or lard
         −3
    (b) more than one tablespoon of margarine or vegetable oil
         −1
    (c) no more than one tablespoon or margarine or vegetable oil
         0
    (d) no more than one tablespoon of olive oil
         +1
    (e) water or broth
         +2

38. What kind of cereal do you usually eat?
    (a) whole grain (like oatmeal or shredded wheat)
         +3
    (b) low-fiber (like cream of wheat or corn flakes)
         0
    (c) sugary low-fiber (like frosted flakes)   (d) granola
         −1   −2

39. With what do you make tuna salad, pasta salad, chicken salad, etc.?
    (a) mayonnaise   (b) light mayonnaise
         −2   −1
    (c) nonfat mayonnaise   (d) low-fat yogurt
         0   +2
    (e) nonfat yogurt
         +3

40. What do you typically put on your pasta? *(ADD one point if you also add sauteed vegetables. AVERAGE two or more scores if necessary.)*
    (a) tomato sauce   (b) tomato sauce with a little parmesan
         +3   +3
    (c) white clam sauce   (d) meat sauce or meat balls
         +1   −2
    (e) Alfredo, pesto, or other creamy sauce
         −3

YOUR GRAND TOTAL

+59 to +116	GREAT!	You're a nutrition superstar. Give yourself a big (non-butter) pat on the back.
0 to +58	GOOD	Pin your quiz on the nearest wall.
−58 to −1	FAIR	Hang in there
−117 to −59	ARGHH!	Empty your refrigerator and cupboard. It's time to start over.

9

Body Composition Assessment

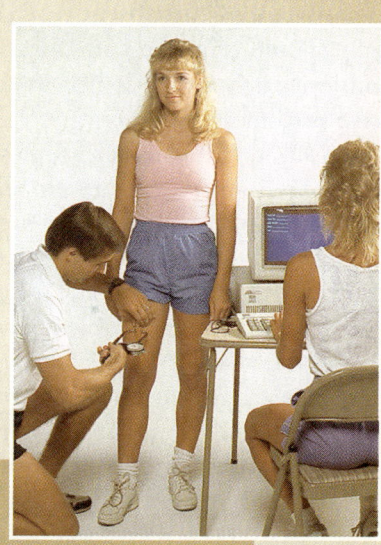

Objectives

▼ Define body composition and its relationship to recommended body weight assessment.

▼ Learn the difference between essential fat and storage fat.

▼ Understand the methodology used to assess body composition according to skinfold thickness and girth measurements.

▼ Be able to determine recommended weight according to recommended percent body fat values.

▼ Understand the importance of waist-to-hip ratio and body mass index.

Body composition is used in reference to the fat and nonfat components of the human body. The fat component usually is called fat mass or percent body fat. The nonfat component is termed lean body mass.

For many years people relied on height/weight charts to determine recommended body weight. We now know, however, that these tables can be highly inaccurate for many people and they fail to identify critical fat values associated with higher risk for disease. The proper way to determine **recommended weight** is through body composition by finding out what percent of total body weight is fat and what amount is lean tissue.

Once the fat percentage is known, recommended body weight can be calculated from recommended body fat. Recommended body weight, also called "healthy weight," is defined as the *body weight at which there seems to be no harm to human health*. This includes the absence of any medical condition that would improve with weight loss and a fat distribution pattern that is not associated with increased risk for illness.

Although various techniques for determining percent body fat were developed several years ago, many people still are unaware of these procedures and continue to depend on height/weight charts to find out their recommended body weight. The standard height/weight tables were first published in 1912. They were based on average weights (including shoes and clothing) for men and women who obtained life insurance policies between 1888 and 1905. The recommended body weight on these tables is obtained according to gender, height, and frame size. Because no scientific guidelines are given to determine frame size, most people choose their frame size based on the column in which the weight comes closest to their own!

To determine whether people are truly obese or falsely at recommended body weight, body composition must be established. Obesity is related to an excess of body fat. If body weight is the only criterion, an individual easily can be overweight, according to height/weight charts, yet not have any excess body fat. Football players, body builders, weight lifters, and other athletes with large muscle size are typical examples. Some of these athletes who appear to be 20 or 30 pounds overweight really have little body fat.

The inaccuracy of height/weight charts was illustrated clearly when a young man who weighed about 225 pounds applied to join a city police force but was turned down without having been granted an interview. The reason? He was "too fat," according to the height/weight charts. When this young man's body composition later was assessed at a preventive medicine clinic, he was shocked to find out that only 5% of his total body weight was in the form of fat — considerably lower than the recommended standard. In the words of the technical director of the clinic, "The only way this fellow could come down to the chart's target weight would have been through surgical removal of a large amount of his muscle tissue."

At the other end of the spectrum, some people who weigh very little and are viewed by many as skinny or underweight actually can be classified as obese because of their high body fat content. People who weigh as little as 100 pounds but are more than 30% fat (about one-third of their total body weight) are not uncommon. These cases are found more readily in sedentary people and those who are always dieting. Physical inactivity and constant negative caloric balance both lead to a loss in lean body mass (see Chapter 10). From these examples, body weight alone clearly does not always tell the true story.

▼ ESSENTIAL AND STORAGE FAT

Total fat in the human body is classified into two types: essential fat and storage fat. Essential fat is needed for normal physiological functions, and without it, human health deteriorates. This essential fat constitutes about 3% of the total fat in men and 12% in women. The percentage is higher in women because it includes sex-specific fat, such as that found in the breast tissue, the uterus, and other sex-related fat deposits.

Storage fat is the fat stored in adipose tissue, mostly beneath the skin (subcutaneous fat) and around major organs in the body. This fat serves three basic functions:

1. As an insulator to retain body heat.
2. As energy substrate for metabolism.
3. As padding against physical trauma to the body.

The amount of storage fat does not differ between men and women, except that men tend to store fat around the waist and women more so around the hips and thighs.

TECHNIQUES FOR ASSESSING BODY COMPOSITION

Body composition can be determined through several different procedures. The most common techniques are: (a) hydrostatic or underwater weighing, (b) skinfold thickness, (c) girth measurements, and (d) bioelectrical impedance.

When using the different techniques, slightly different values are obtained. Therefore, when assessing body composition, the same technique should be used for pre- and post-test comparisons.

HYDROSTATIC WEIGHING

Hydrostatic weighing has been called the "gold standard" of body composition. Almost all other techniques to determine body composition are validated against hydrostatic weighing. It is the most accurate technique available if it is administered properly and if the individual is able to perform the test adequately. The psychological factor of being weighed while submerged underwater makes hydrostatic weighing difficult to administer to the aqua-phobic.

The person's residual lung volume (the amount of air left in the lungs following complete forceful exhalation) must be measured to accurately determine percent body fat according to hydrostatic weighing. If the residual volume cannot be measured, as is the case in many health/fitness centers, the volume is estimated using predicting equations, which may sacrifice the accuracy of the assessment.

Because of the cost, time, and complexity of hydrostatic weighing, most health and fitness

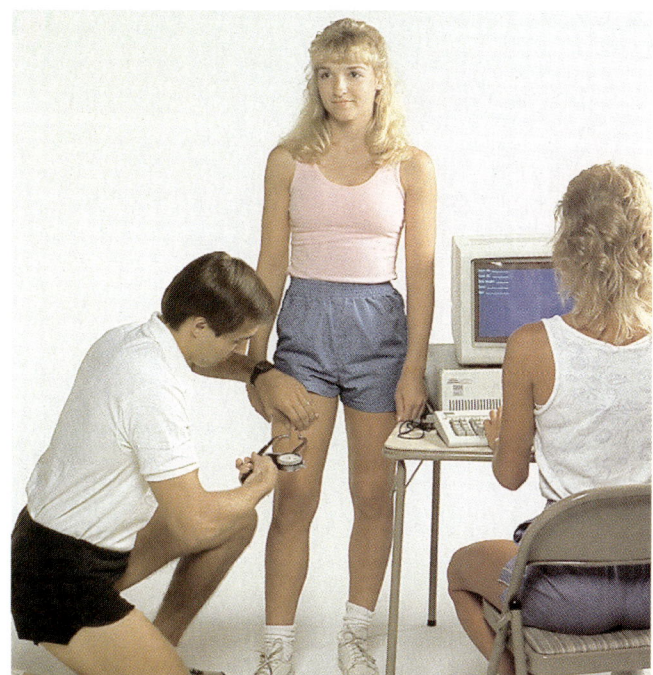

Skinfold thickness technique for body composition assessment.

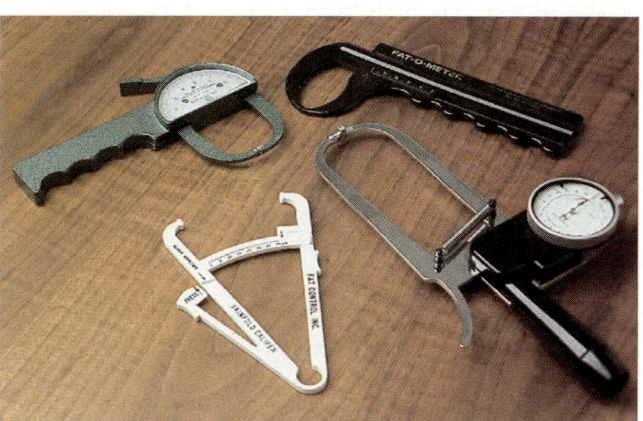

Various types of skinfold calipers used to assess skinfold thickness.

programs prefer anthropometric measurement techniques, which correlate quite well with hydrostatic weighing. These techniques, primarily skinfold thickness and girth measurements, allow a quick, simple, and inexpensive estimate of body composition.

SKINFOLD THICKNESS

Assessing body composition using skinfold thickness is based on the principle that approximately half of the body's fatty tissue is directly beneath the skin. Valid and reliable estimates of this tissue give a good indication of percent body fat.

The skinfold test is done with the aid of pressure calipers. Several sites must be measured to reflect the

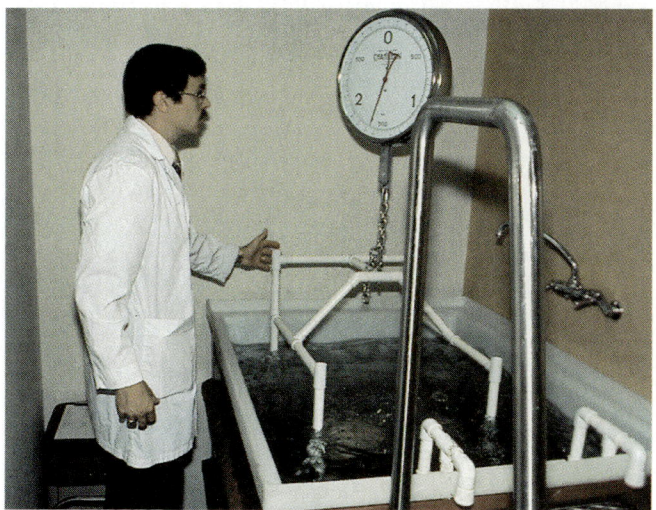

Hydrostatic weighing technique for body composition assessment.

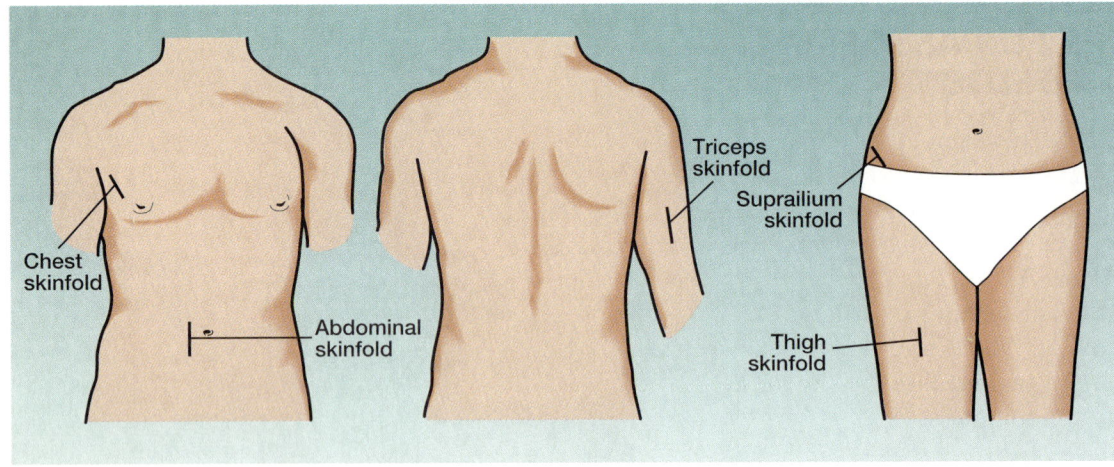

FIGURE 9.1 ▼ Anatomical landmarks for skinfold measurements.

total percentage of fat: triceps, suprailium, and thigh skinfolds for women; and chest, abdomen, and thigh for men (Figure 9.1). All measurements should be taken on the right side of the body.

Even with the skinfold technique, some training is necessary to obtain accurate measurements. Also, different technicians may produce slightly different measurements from the same person. Therefore, the same technician should take pre- and post-measurements.

Measurements should be done at the same time of the day, preferably in the morning, as changes in water hydration from activity and exercise can increase skinfold girth. The procedure for assessing percent body fat using skinfold thickness is given in Figure 9.2. If skinfold calipers* are available to you, you may proceed to assess your percent body fat with the help of your instructor or an experienced technician.

---

*This instrument is available at most colleges and universities. If unavailable, you can purchase an inexpensive, yet reliable skinfold caliper from: Fat Control Inc., P.O. Box 10117, Towson, MD 21204, Phone 301/296-1993.

Body Fat Assessment According to Skinfold Thickness Technique

1. Select the proper anatomical sites. For men, chest, abdomen, and thigh skinfolds are used. For women, use triceps, suprailium, and thigh skinfolds (see Figure 9.1). Take all measurements on the right side of the body with the person standing. The correct anatomical landmarks for skinfolds are:

   Chest: a diagonal fold halfway between the shoulder crease and the nipple.
   Abdomen: a vertical fold taken about one inch to the right of the umbilicus.
   Triceps: a vertical fold on the back of the upper arm, halfway between the shoulder and the elbow.
   Thigh: a vertical fold on the front of the thigh, midway between the knee and hip.
   Suprailium: a diagonal fold above the crest of the ilium (on the side of the hip).

2. Measure each site by grasping a double thickness of skin firmly with the thumb and forefinger, pulling the fold slightly away from the muscular tissue. The calipers are held perpendicular to the fold, and the measurement is taken one-half inch below the finger hold. Each site is measured three times and the values are read to the nearest .1 to .5 mm. The average of the two closest readings is recorded as the final value. The readings should be taken without delay to avoid excessive compression of the skinfold. Releasing and refolding the skinfold is required between readings.

3. When doing pre- and post-assessments, the measurement should be conducted at the same time of day. The best time is early in the morning to avoid water hydration changes resulting from activity or exercise.

4. Percent fat is obtained by adding the three skinfold measurements and looking up the respective values on Tables 9.1 for women, 9.2 for men under age 40, and 9.3 for men over 40.

For example, if the skinfold measurements for an 18-year-old female are: (a) triceps = 16, (b) suprailium = 4, and (c) thigh = 30 (total = 50), the percent body fat is 20.6%

FIGURE 9.2 ▼ Procedure for body fat assessment according to skinfold thickness technique.

TABLE 9.1 ▼ Percent Fat Estimates for Women Calculated From Triceps, Suprailium, and Thigh Skinfold Thickness

Sum of 3 Skinfolds	Under 22	23 to 27	28 to 32	33 to 37	38 to 42	43 to 47	48 to 52	53 to 57	Over 58
23- 25	9.7	9.9	10.2	10.4	10.7	10.9	11.2	11.4	11.7
26- 28	11.0	11.2	11.5	11.7	12.0	12.3	12.5	12.7	13.0
29- 31	12.3	12.5	12.8	13.0	13.3	13.5	13.8	14.0	14.3
32- 34	13.6	13.8	14.0	14.3	14.5	14.8	15.0	15.3	15.5
35- 37	14.8	15.0	15.3	15.5	15.8	16.0	16.3	16.5	16.8
38- 40	16.0	16.3	16.5	16.7	17.0	17.2	17.5	17.7	18.0
41- 43	17.2	17.4	17.7	17.9	18.2	18.4	18.7	18.9	19.2
44- 46	18.3	18.6	18.8	19.1	19.3	19.6	19.8	20.1	20.3
47- 49	19.5	19.7	20.0	20.2	20.5	20.7	21.0	21.2	21.5
50- 52	20.6	20.8	21.1	21.3	21.6	21.8	22.1	22.3	22.6
53- 55	21.7	21.9	22.1	22.4	22.6	22.9	23.1	23.4	23.6
56- 58	22.7	23.0	23.2	23.4	23.7	23.9	24.2	24.4	24.7
59- 61	23.7	24.0	24.2	24.5	24.7	25.0	25.2	25.5	25.7
62- 64	24.7	25.0	25.2	25.5	25.7	26.0	26.2	26.4	26.7
65- 67	25.7	25.9	26.2	26.4	26.7	26.9	27.2	27.4	27.7
68- 70	26.6	26.9	27.1	27.4	27.6	27.9	28.1	28.4	28.6
71- 73	27.5	27.8	28.0	28.3	28.5	28.8	29.0	29.3	29.5
74- 76	28.4	28.7	28.9	29.2	29.4	29.7	29.9	30.2	30.4
77- 79	29.3	29.5	29.8	30.0	30.3	30.5	30.8	31.0	31.3
80- 82	30.1	30.4	30.6	30.9	31.1	31.4	31.6	31.9	32.1
83- 85	30.9	31.2	31.4	31.7	31.9	32.2	32.4	32.7	32.9
86- 88	31.7	32.0	32.2	32.5	32.7	32.9	33.2	33.4	33.7
89- 91	32.5	32.7	33.0	33.2	33.5	33.7	33.9	34.2	34.4
92- 94	33.2	33.4	33.7	33.9	34.2	34.4	34.7	34.9	35.2
95- 97	33.9	34.1	34.4	34.6	34.9	35.1	35.4	35.6	35.9
98-100	34.6	34.8	35.1	35.3	35.5	35.8	36.0	36.3	36.5
101-103	35.2	35.4	35.7	35.9	36.2	36.4	36.7	36.9	37.2
104-106	35.8	36.1	36.3	36.6	36.8	37.1	37.3	37.5	37.8
107-109	36.4	36.7	36.9	37.1	37.4	37.6	37.9	38.1	38.4
110-112	37.0	37.2	37.5	37.7	38.0	38.2	38.5	38.7	38.9
113-115	37.5	37.8	38.0	38.2	38.5	38.7	39.0	39.2	39.5
116-118	38.0	38.3	38.5	38.8	39.0	39.3	39.5	39.7	40.0
119-121	38.5	38.7	39.0	39.2	39.5	39.7	40.0	40.2	40.5
122-124	39.0	39.2	39.4	39.7	39.9	40.2	40.4	40.7	40.9
125-127	39.4	39.6	39.9	40.1	40.4	40.6	40.9	41.1	41.4
128-130	39.8	40.0	40.3	40.5	40.8	41.0	41.3	41.5	41.8

Body density is calculated based on the generalized equation for predicting body density of women developed by A. S. Jackson, M. L. Pollock, and A. Ward. *Medicine and Science in Sports and Exercise* 12, (1980), 175–182. Percent body fat is determined from the calculated body density using the Siri formula.

TABLE 9.2 ▼ Percent Fat Estimates for Men 40 and Under Calculated from Chest, Abdomen, and Thigh Skinfold Thickness

Sum of 3 Skinfolds	Age to the Last Year							
	Under 19	20 to 22	23 to 25	26 to 28	29 to 31	32 to 34	35 to 37	38 to 40
8- 10	.9	1.3	1.6	2.0	2.3	2.7	3.0	3.3
11- 13	1.9	2.3	2.6	3.0	3.3	3.7	4.0	4.3
14- 16	2.9	3.3	3.6	3.9	4.3	4.6	5.0	5.3
17- 19	3.9	4.2	4.6	4.9	5.3	5.6	6.0	6.3
20- 22	4.8	5.2	5.5	5.9	6.2	6.6	6.9	7.3
23- 25	5.8	6.2	6.5	6.8	7.2	7.5	7.9	8.2
26- 28	6.8	7.1	7.5	7.8	8.1	8.5	8.8	9.2
29- 31	7.7	8.0	8.4	8.7	9.1	9.4	9.8	10.1
32- 34	8.6	9.0	9.3	9.7	10.0	10.4	10.7	11.1
35- 37	9.5	9.9	10.2	10.6	10.9	11.3	11.6	12.0
38- 40	10.5	10.8	11.2	11.5	11.8	12.2	12.5	12.9
41- 43	11.4	11.7	12.1	12.4	12.7	13.1	13.4	13.8
44- 46	12.2	12.6	12.9	13.3	13.6	14.0	14.3	14.7
47- 49	13.1	13.5	13.8	14.2	14.5	14.9	15.2	15.5
50- 52	14.0	14.3	14.7	15.0	15.4	15.7	16.1	16.4
53- 55	14.8	15.2	15.5	15.9	16.2	16.6	16.9	17.3
56- 58	15.7	16.0	16.4	16.7	17.1	17.4	17.8	18.1
59- 61	16.5	16.9	17.2	17.6	17.9	18.3	18.6	19.0
62- 64	17.4	17.7	18.1	18.4	18.8	19.1	19.4	19.8
65- 67	18.2	18.5	18.9	19.2	19.6	19.9	20.3	20.6
68- 70	19.0	19.3	19.7	20.0	20.4	20.7	21.1	21.4
71- 73	19.8	20.1	20.5	20.8	21.2	21.5	21.9	22.2
74- 76	20.6	20.9	21.3	21.6	22.0	22.2	22.7	23.0
77- 79	21.4	21.7	22.1	22.4	22.8	23.1	23.4	23.8
80- 82	22.1	22.5	22.8	23.2	23.5	23.9	24.2	24.6
83- 85	22.9	23.2	23.6	23.9	24.3	24.6	25.0	25.3
86- 88	23.6	24.0	24.3	24.7	25.0	25.4	25.7	26.1
89- 91	24.4	24.7	25.1	25.4	25.8	26.1	26.5	26.8
92- 94	25.1	25.5	25.8	26.2	26.5	26.9	27.2	27.5
95- 97	25.8	26.2	26.5	26.9	27.2	27.6	27.9	28.3
98-100	26.6	26.9	27.3	27.6	27.9	28.3	28.6	29.0
101-103	27.3	27.6	28.0	28.3	28.6	29.0	29.3	29.7
104-106	27.9	28.3	28.6	29.0	29.3	29.7	30.0	30.4
107-109	28.6	29.0	29.3	29.7	30.0	30.4	30.7	31.1
110-112	29.3	29.6	30.0	30.3	30.7	31.0	31.4	31.7
113-115	30.0	30.3	30.7	31.0	31.3	31.7	32.0	32.4
116-118	30.6	31.0	31.3	31.6	32.0	32.3	32.7	33.0
119-121	31.3	31.6	32.0	32.3	32.6	33.0	33.3	33.7
122-124	31.9	32.2	32.6	32.9	33.3	33.6	34.0	34.3
125-127	32.5	32.9	33.2	33.5	33.9	34.2	34.6	34.9
128-130	33.1	33.5	33.8	34.2	34.5	34.9	35.2	35.5

Body density is calculated based on the generalized equation for predicting body density of men developed by A. S. Jackson and M. L. Pollock, *British Journal of Nutrition* 40, (1978) 497–504. Percent body fat is determined from the calculated body density using the Siri formula.

TABLE 9.3 ▼ Percent Fat Estimates for Men Over 40 Calculated from Chest, Abdomen, and Thigh Skinfold Thickness

Sum of 3 Skinfolds	Age to the Last Year							
	41 to 43	44 to 46	47 to 49	50 to 52	53 to 55	56 to 58	59 to 61	Over 62
8- 10	3.7	4.0	4.4	4.7	5.1	5.4	5.8	6.1
11- 13	4.7	5.0	5.4	5.7	6.1	6.4	6.8	7.1
14- 16	5.7	6.0	6.4	6.7	7.1	7.4	7.8	8.1
17- 19	6.7	7.0	7.4	7.7	8.1	8.4	8.7	9.1
20- 22	7.6	8.0	8.3	8.7	9.0	9.4	9.7	10.1
23- 25	8.6	8.9	9.3	9.6	10.0	10.3	10.7	11.0
26- 28	9.5	9.9	10.2	10.6	10.9	11.3	11.6	12.0
29- 31	10.5	10.8	11.2	11.5	11.9	12.2	12.6	12.9
32- 34	11.4	11.8	12.1	12.4	12.8	13.1	13.5	13.8
35- 37	12.3	12.7	13.0	13.4	13.7	14.1	14.4	14.8
38- 40	13.2	13.6	13.9	14.3	14.6	15.0	15.3	15.7
41- 43	14.1	14.5	14.8	15.2	15.5	15.9	16.2	16.6
44- 46	15.0	15.4	15.7	16.1	16.4	16.8	17.1	17.5
47- 49	15.9	16.2	16.6	16.9	17.3	17.6	18.0	18.3
50- 52	16.8	17.1	17.5	17.8	18.2	18.5	18.8	19.2
53- 55	17.6	18.0	18.3	18.7	19.0	19.4	19.7	20.1
56- 58	18.5	18.8	19.2	19.5	19.9	20.2	20.6	20.9
59- 61	19.3	19.7	20.0	20.4	20.7	21.0	21.4	21.7
62- 64	20.1	20.5	20.8	21.2	21.5	21.9	22.2	22.6
65- 67	21.0	21.3	21.7	22.0	22.4	22.7	23.0	23.4
68- 70	21.8	22.1	22.5	22.8	23.2	23.5	23.9	24.2
71- 73	22.6	22.9	23.3	23.6	24.0	24.3	24.7	25.0
74- 76	23.4	23.7	24.1	24.4	24.8	25.1	25.4	25.8
77- 79	24.1	24.5	24.8	25.2	25.5	25.9	26.2	26.6
80- 82	24.9	25.3	25.6	26.0	26.3	26.6	27.0	27.3
83- 85	25.7	26.0	26.4	26.7	27.1	27.4	27.8	28.1
86- 88	26.4	26.8	27.1	27.5	27.8	28.2	28.5	28.9
89- 91	27.2	27.5	27.9	28.2	28.6	28.9	29.2	29.6
92- 94	27.9	28.2	28.6	28.9	29.3	29.6	30.0	30.3
95- 97	28.6	29.0	29.3	29.7	30.0	30.4	30.7	31.1
98-100	29.3	29.7	30.0	30.4	30.7	31.1	31.4	31.8
101-103	30.0	30.4	30.7	31.1	31.4	31.8	32.1	32.5
104-106	30.7	31.1	31.4	31.8	32.1	32.5	32.8	33.2
107-109	31.4	31.8	32.1	32.4	32.8	33.1	33.5	33.8
110-112	32.1	32.4	32.8	33.1	33.5	33.8	34.2	34.5
113-115	32.7	33.1	33.4	33.8	34.1	34.5	34.8	35.2
116-118	33.4	33.7	34.1	34.4	34.8	35.1	35.5	35.8
119-121	34.0	34.4	34.7	35.1	35.4	35.8	36.1	36.5
122-124	34.7	35.0	35.4	35.7	36.1	36.4	36.7	37.1
125-127	35.3	35.6	36.0	36.3	36.7	37.0	37.4	37.7
128-130	35.9	36.2	36.6	36.9	37.3	37.6	38.0	38.5

Body density is calculated based on the generalized equation for predicting body density of men developed by A. S. Jackson and M. L. Pollock, *British Journal of Nutrition* 40 (1978), 497–504. Percent body fat is determined from the calculated body density using the Siri formula.

GIRTH MEASUREMENTS

A simpler method to determine body fat is by measuring circumferences at various body sites. All this technique requires is a standard measuring tape, and good accuracy can be achieved with little practice. The limitation is that it may not be valid for athletic individuals (men or women) who actively participate in strenuous physical activity or people who can be classified visually as thin or obese.

The required procedure for girth measurements is given in Figure 9.3. Measurements for women include the upper arm, hip, and wrist; for men, the waist and wrist.

BIOELECTRICAL IMPEDANCE

The bioelectrical impedance technique is much simpler to administer, but it does require costly equipment. In this technique, the individual is hooked up to a machine and a weak electrical current (totally painless) is run through the body to analyze body composition (body fat, lean body mass, and body water). The technique is based on the principle that fat tissue is not as good a conductor of an electrical current as lean tissue is. The easier the conductance, the leaner the individual.

The accuracy of current equations used in estimating percent body fat with this technique is still questionable. More research is required before the

Body Fat Assessment According to Girth Measurements

Girth Measurements for Women*

1. Using a regular tape measure, determine the following girth measurements in centimeters (cm):

   Upper Arm: take the measure halfway between the shoulder and the elbow.
   Hip: measure at the point of largest circumference.
   Wrist: take the girth in front of the bones where the wrist bends.

2. Obtain the person's age.
3. Using Table 9.4, find the girth measurement for each site and age in the lefthand columns. Look up the constant values in the righthand columns. These values will allow you to derive body density (BD) by substituting the constants in the following formula:
   BD = A − B − C + D
4. Using the derived body density, calculate percent body fat (%F) according to the following equation:

   %F = (495 ÷ BD) − 450**

   Example: Jane is 20 years old, and the following girth measurements were taken: biceps = 27 cm, hip = 99.5 cm, wrist = 15.4 cm.

Data	Constant
Upper Arm = 27 cm	A = 1.0813
Age = 20	B = .0102
Hip = 99.5 cm	C = .1206
Wrist = 15.4 cm	D = .0971

BD = A − B − C + D
BD = 1.0813 − .0102 − .1206 + .0971 = 1.0476
%F = (495 ÷ BD) − 450
%F = (495 ÷ 1.0476) − 450 = 22.5

Girth Measurements for Men**

1. Using a regular tape measure, determine the following girth measurements in inches (the men's measurements are taken in inches as contrasted with centimeters for women):

   Waist: measure at the umbilicus (belly button)
   Wrist: measure in front of the bones where the wrist bends.

2. Subtract the wrist from the waist measurement.
3. Obtain the person's weight in pounds.
4. Look up the percent body fat (%F) in Table 9.5 by using the difference obtained in step 2 above and the person's body weight.

Example: John weighs 160 pounds, and his waist and wrist girth measurements are 36.5 and 7.5 inches, respectively.

Waist girth = 36.5 inches
Wrist girth = 7.5 inches
Difference = 29.0 inches
Body weight = 160.0 lbs.
%F = 22

* Reproduced by permission from R. B. Lambson, "Generalized Body Density Prediction Equations for Women Using Simple Anthropometric Measurements." Unpublished doctoral dissertation, Brigham Young University, August 1987.

** From W. E. Siri, *Body Composition From Fluid Spaces and Density*, (Berkeley: University of California, Donner Laboratory of Medical Physics, 1956).

*** Table 3.5 reproduced by permission from A. G. Fisher, and P. E. Allsen, *Jogging* (Dubuque, IA: Wm. C. Brown, 1987). This table was developed according to the generalized body composition equation for men using simple measurement techniques by K. W. Penrouse, A. G Nelson, and A G. Fisher, *Medicine and Science in Sports and Exercise* 17(2):189, 1985. © American College of Sports Medicine 1985.

FIGURE 9.3 ▼ Procedure for body fat assessment according to girth measurements.

TABLE 9.4 ▼ Conversion Constants from Girth Measurements (Centimeters) to Calculate Body Density for Women

Upper Arm (cm)	Constant A	Age	Constant B	Hip (cm)	Constant C	Hip (cm)	Constant C	Wrist (cm)	Constant D
20.5	1.0966	17	.0086	79	.0957	114.5	.1388	13.0	.0819
21	1.0954	18	.0091	79.5	.0963	115	.1394	13.2	.0832
21.5	1.0942	19	.0096	80	.0970	115.5	.1400	13.4	.0845
22	1.0930	20	.0102	80.5	.0976	116	.1406	13.6	.0857
22.5	1.0919	21	.0107	81	.0982	116.5	.1412	13.8	.0807
23	1.0907	22	.0112	81.5	.0988	117	.1418	14.0	.0882
23.5	1.0895	23	.0117	82	.0994	117.5	.1424	14.2	.0895
24	1.0883	24	.0122	82.5	.1000	118	.1430	14.4	.0908
24.5	1.0871	25	.0127	83	.1006	118.5	.1436	14.6	.0920
25	1.0860	26	.0132	83.5	.1012	119	.1442	14.8	.0933
25.5	1.0848	27	.0137	84	.1018	119.5	.1448	15.0	.0946
26	1.0836	28	.0142	84.5	.1024	120	.1454	15.2	.0958
26.5	1.0824	29	.0147	85	.1030	120.5	.1460	15.4	.0971
27	1.0813	30	.0152	85.5	.1036	121	.1466	15.6	.0983
27.5	1.0801	31	.0157	86	.1042	121.5	.1472	15.8	.0996
28	1.0789	32	.0162	86.5	.1048	122	.1479	16.0	.1009
28.5	1.0777	33	.0168	87	.1054	122.5	.1485	16.2	.1021
29	1.0775	34	.0173	87.5	.1060	123	.1491	16.4	.1034
29.5	1.0754	35	.0178	88	.1066	123.5	.1497	16.6	.1046
30	1.0742	36	.0183	88.5	.1072	124	.1503	16.8	.1059
30.5	1.0730	37	.0188	89	.1079	124.5	.1509	17.0	.1072
31	1.0718	38	.0193	89.5	.1085	125	.1515	17.2	.1084
31.5	1.0707	39	.0198	90	.1091	125.5	.1521	17.4	.1097
32	1.0695	40	.0203	90.5	.1097	126	.1527	17.6	.1109
32.5	1.0683	41	.0208	91	.1103	126.5	.1533	17.8	.1122
33	1.0671	42	.0213	91.5	.1109	127	.1539	18.0	.1135
33.5	1.0666	43	.0218	92	.1115	127.5	.1545	18.2	.1147
34	1.0648	44	.0223	92.5	.1121	128	.1551	18.4	.1160
34.5	1.0636	45	.0228	93	.1127	128.5	.1558	18.6	.1172
35	1.0624	46	.0234	93.5	.1133	129	.1563		
35.5	1.0612	47	.0239	94	.1139	129.5	.1569		
36	1.0601	48	.0244	94.5	.1145	130	.1575		
36.5	1.0589	49	.0249	95	.1151	130.5	.1581		
37	1.0577	50	.0254	95.5	.1157	131	.1587		
37.5	1.0565	51	.0259	96	.1163	131.5	.1593		
38	1.0554	52	.0264	96.5	.1169	132	.1600		
38.5	1.0542	53	.0269	97	.1176	132.5	.1606		
39	1.0530	54	.0274	97.5	.1182	133	.1612		
39.5	1.0518	55	.0279	98	.1188	133.5	.1618		
40	1.0506	56	.0284	98.5	.1194	134	.1624		
40.5	1.0495	57	.0289	99	.1200	134.5	.1630		
41	1.0483	58	.0294	99.5	.1206	135	.1636		
41.5	1.0471	59	.0300	100	.1212	135.5	.1642		
42	1.0459	60	.0305	100.5	.1218	136	.1648		
42.5	1.0448	61	.0310	101	.1224	136.5	.1654		
43	1.0434	62	.0315	101.5	.1230	137	.1660		

(Continued)

TABLE 9.4 ▼ Conversion Constants from Girth Measurements (Centimeters) to Calculate Body Density for Women *(continued)*

Upper Arm (cm)	Constant A	Age	Constant B	Hip (cm)	Constant C	Hip (cm)	Constant C	Wrist (cm)	Constant D
43.5	1.0424	63	.0320	102	.1236	137.5	.1666		
44	1.0412	64	.0325	102.5	.1242	138	.1672		
		65	.0330	103	.1248	138.5	.1678		
		66	.0335	103.5	.1254	139	.1685		
		67	.0340	104	.1260	139.5	.1691		
		68	.0345	104.5	.1266	140	.1697		
		69	.0350	105	.1272	140.5	.1703		
		70	.0355	105.5	.1278	141	.1709		
		71	.0360	106	.1285	141.5	.1715		
		72	.0366	106.5	.1291	142	.1721		
		73	.0371	107	.1297	142.5	.1728		
		74	.0376	107.5	.1303	143	.1733		
		75	.0381	108	.1309	143.5	.1739		
				108.5	.1315	144	.1745		
				109	.1321	144.5	.1751		
				109.5	.1327	145	.1757		
				110	.1333	145.5	.1763		
				110.5	.1339	146	.1769		
				111	.1345	146.5	.1775		
				111.5	.1351	147	.1781		
				112	.1357	147.5	.1787		
				112.5	.1363	148	.1794		
				113	.1369	148.5	.1800		
				113.5	.1375	149	.1806		
				114	.1382	149.5	.1812		
						150	.1818		

TABLE 9.5 ▼ Estimated Percent Body Fat for Men Obtained from Waist Minus Wrist Girth Measurements (Inches) and Body Weight

Body Weight	22	22.5	23	23.5	24	24.5	25	25.5	26	26.5	27	27.5	28	28.5	29	29.5	30	30.5	31	31.5	32	32.5	33	33.5	34	34.5	35	35.5	36	36.5	37	37.5	38	38.5	39	39.5	40	40.5	41	41.5	42	42.5	43	43.5	44	44.5	45	45.5	46	46.5	47	47.5	48	48.5	49	49.5	50
120	4	6	8	10	12	14	16	18	20	21	23	25	27	29	31	33	35	37	39	41	43	45	47	49	50	52	54	56	58																												
125	4	6	7	9	11	13	15	17	19	20	22	24	26	28	30	31	33	35	37	39	41	43	45	46	48	50	52	54	56	58																												
130	3	5	7	9	11	12	14	16	18	20	21	23	25	27	28	30	32	34	36	37	39	41	43	44	46	48	50	52	53	55	57																										
135	3	5	7	8	10	12	13	15	17	19	20	22	24	26	27	29	31	32	34	36	38	39	41	43	44	46	48	50	51	53	55	56																									
140	3	5	6	8	10	11	13	15	16	18	20	21	23	25	26	28	30	31	33	35	36	38	39	41	43	44	46	48	49	51	53	54	56																								
145	3	4	6	7	9	11	12	14	16	17	19	20	22	24	25	27	28	30	32	33	35	36	38	39	41	43	44	46	47	49	51	52	54	55																							
150	2	4	6	7	9	10	12	13	15	17	18	20	21	23	24	26	27	29	30	32	33	35	36	38	40	41	43	44	46	47	49	50	52	53	55																						
155	2	4	5	7	8	10	11	13	14	16	17	19	20	22	23	25	26	28	29	31	32	34	35	37	38	40	41	43	44	46	47	49	50	52	53	55																					
160	2	4	5	6	8	9	11	12	14	15	17	18	20	21	23	24	25	27	28	30	31	33	34	35	37	38	40	41	43	44	46	47	48	50	51	53	54																				
165	2	3	5	6	8	9	10	12	13	15	16	17	19	20	22	23	24	26	27	29	30	31	33	34	35	37	38	40	41	43	44	45	47	48	50	51	52	54																			
170	2	3	5	6	7	9	10	11	13	14	15	17	18	20	21	22	24	25	26	28	29	30	32	33	34	36	37	38	40	41	43	44	45	47	48	49	51	52	54																		
175	2	3	4	6	7	8	10	11	12	14	15	16	18	19	20	22	23	24	26	27	28	30	31	32	34	35	36	38	39	40	41	43	44	45	47	48	49	51	52	53																	
180		3	4	5	7	8	9	11	12	13	15	16	17	19	20	21	22	24	25	26	28	29	30	31	33	34	35	36	38	39	40	41	43	44	45	46	48	49	50	52	53																
185		3	4	5	6	8	9	10	12	13	14	15	17	18	19	20	22	23	24	25	27	28	29	30	32	33	34	35	37	38	39	40	41	43	44	45	46	48	49	50	51	53															
190		2	4	5	6	7	9	10	11	12	14	15	16	17	19	20	21	22	24	25	26	27	28	30	31	32	33	34	36	37	38	39	40	41	43	44	45	46	47	49	50	51	52														
195		2	3	5	6	7	8	9	11	12	13	14	16	17	18	19	20	22	23	24	25	26	28	29	30	31	32	34	35	36	37	38	39	40	42	43	44	45	46	47	48	50	51	52													
200		2	3	4	6	7	8	9	10	11	13	14	15	16	17	19	20	21	22	23	25	26	27	28	29	30	32	33	34	35	36	37	38	39	41	42	43	44	45	46	47	48	49	51	52												
205		2	3	4	5	7	8	9	10	11	12	13	15	16	17	18	19	20	21	23	24	25	26	27	28	29	31	32	33	34	35	36	37	38	39	41	42	43	44	45	46	47	48	49	50	51										
210		2	3	4	5	6	7	9	10	11	12	13	14	15	16	18	19	20	21	22	23	24	25	27	28	29	30	31	32	33	34	35	36	38	39	40	41	42	43	44	45	46	47	48	49	50	51									
215		2	3	4	5	6	7	8	9	10	11	12	14	15	16	17	18	19	20	21	22	24	25	26	27	28	29	30	31	32	33	34	36	37	38	39	40	41	42	43	44	45	46	47	48	49	50	51								
220		2	3	4	5	6	7	8	9	10	11	12	13	14	15	16	18	19	20	21	22	23	24	25	26	27	28	29	30	32	33	34	35	36	37	38	39	40	41	42	43	44	45	46	47	48	49	50	51							
225		2	3	4	5	6	7	8	9	10	11	12	13	14	15	16	17	18	19	20	22	23	24	25	26	27	28	29	30	31	32	33	34	35	36	37	38	39	40	41	42	43	44	45	46	47	48	49	50	51						
230		2	3	4	5	6	7	7	8	9	10	11	12	13	14	15	16	17	18	19	20	21	23	24	25	26	27	28	29	30	31	32	33	34	35	36	37	38	39	40	41	42	43	44	45	46	47	48	49	50	51					
235		2	3	4	4	5	6	7	8	9	10	11	12	13	14	15	16	17	18	19	20	21	22	23	24	25	26	27	28	29	30	31	32	34	35	36	37	38	39	40	41	42	43	44	45	46	47	48	49	50	51					
240		2	3	3	4	5	6	7	8	9	10	11	12	13	14	15	16	17	18	19	20	21	22	23	24	25	26	27	28	29	30	31	32	33	34	35	36	37	38	39	40	41	42	43	44	45	46	47	48	49	50					
245		2	3	3	4	5	6	7	8	9	10	11	11	12	13	14	15	16	17	18	19	20	21	22	23	24	25	26	27	28	29	30	31	32	33	34	35	36	37	38	39	40	41	42	43	44	45	46	47	48	49	50				
250		2	3	3	4	5	6	7	8	9	10	10	11	12	13	14	15	16	17	18	19	20	21	22	23	24	25	26	27	28	29	30	31	32	33	34	35	36	37	38	39	40	41	42	43	44	45	46	47	48	49	50				
255			2	3	4	5	6	6	7	8	9	10	11	12	13	14	15	16	17	17	18	19	20	21	22	23	24	25	26	27	28	29	30	31	32	33	34	35	36	37	38	39	40	41	42	43	44	45	46	47	48	49				
260			2	3	4	5	5	6	7	8	9	10	11	12	13	14	14	15	16	17	18	19	20	21	22	23	24	25	26	27	28	28	29	30	31	32	33	34	35	36	37	38	39	40	41	42	43	44	45	46	47	48	49			
265			2	3	4	4	5	6	7	8	9	10	11	11	12	13	14	15	16	17	18	19	20	21	22	22	23	24	25	26	27	28	29	30	31	32	33	34	35	36	37	38	38	39	40	41	42	43	44	45	46	47	48			
270			2	3	3	4	5	6	7	8	8	9	10	11	12	13	14	15	16	16	17	18	19	20	21	22	23	24	25	26	27	28	28	29	30	31	32	33	34	35	36	37	38	39	40	41	42	43	44	45	46	47	48			
275			2	3	3	4	5	6	7	7	8	9	10	11	12	13	14	14	15	16	17	18	19	20	21	22	22	23	24	25	26	27	28	29	30	31	32	33	33	34	35	36	37	38	39	40	41	42	43	44	45	46	47			
280			2	3	3	4	5	6	6	7	8	9	10	11	12	12	13	14	15	16	17	18	18	19	20	21	22	23	24	25	26	27	27	28	29	30	31	32	33	34	35	36	37	38	38	39	40	41	42	43	44	45	46		
285			2	3	3	4	5	5	6	7	8	9	10	10	11	12	13	14	15	16	16	17	18	19	20	21	22	23	24	24	25	26	27	28	29	30	31	32	32	33	34	35	36	37	38	39	40	41	42	43	44	44	45		
290			2	2	3	4	4	5	6	7	8	8	9	10	11	12	13	13	14	15	16	17	18	19	19	20	21	22	23	24	25	26	26	27	28	29	30	31	32	33	33	34	35	36	37	38	39	40	41	41	42	43	44		
295			2	2	3	4	4	5	6	7	7	8	9	10	11	11	12	13	14	15	15	16	17	18	19	20	21	21	22	23	24	25	26	26	27	28	29	30	31	32	33	34	34	35	36	37	38	39	40	41	41	42	43		
300			2	2	3	3	4	5	6	6	7	8	9	9	10	11	12	12	13	14	15	16	16	17	18	19	20	21	21	22	23	24	25	25	26	27	28	29	30	31	32	33	34	35	36	36	37	38	39	40	41	42	43		

equations approach the accuracy of hydrostatic weighing, skinfolds, or girth measurements.

An advantage of bioelectrical impedance is that results are highly reproducible. Unlike other techniques, in which experienced technicians are necessary to obtain valid results, almost anyone can administer bioelectrical impedance. And, although the test results may not be completely accurate, this instrument is valuable in assessing body composition changes over time.

If this instrument or some other type of equipment for body composition assessment is available to you, you can use it to determine your percent body fat. You may want to compare the results with other techniques. Following all manufacturer's instructions will ensure the best possible result.

WAIST-TO-HIP RATIO

Scientific evidence suggests that the way people store fat affects the risk for disease. Some individuals tend to store fat in the abdominal area (called the "apple" shape). Others store it primarily around the hips and thighs (gluteal femoral fat or "pear" shape).

Obese individuals with a lot of abdominal fat clearly are at higher risk for coronary heart disease, congestive heart failure, hypertension, adult-onset diabetes (Type II), and strokes than are obese people with similar amounts of total body fat that is stored primarily in the hips and thighs. Relatively new evidence also indicates that, among individuals with high abdominal fat, those whose fat deposits are around internal organs (visceral fat) are at even greater risk for disease than those whose abdominal fat is primarily beneath the skin (subcutaneous fat).

Because of the higher risk for disease in individuals who tend to store a lot of fat in the abdominal area, as contrasted with the hips and thighs, a waist-to-hip ratio test was designed by a panel of scientists appointed by the National Academy of Sciences and the Dietary Guidelines Advisory Council for the U.S. Departments of Agriculture and Health and Human Services. The waist measurement is taken at the point of smallest circumference, and the hip measurement is taken at the point of greatest circumference.

The waist-to-hip ratio differentiates the "apples" from the "pears." Most men are apples, and most women are pears. The panel recommends that men need to lose weight if the waist-to-hip ratio is 1.0 or higher. Women need to lose weight if the ratio is .85 or higher (see Table 9.6). More conservative estimates indicate that the risk starts to increase when the ratio exceeds .95 and .80 for men and women, respectively. For example, the waist-to-hip ratio for a man with a 40-inch waist and a 38-inch hip would be 1.05 (40 ÷ 38). This ratio may indicate higher risk for disease.

TABLE 9.6 ▼ Disease Risk According to Waist-to-Hip Ratio

Waist-to-Hip Ratio		
Men	Women	Disease Risk
≤0.95	≤0.80	Very Low
0.96–0.99	0.81–0.84	Low
≥1.00	≥0.85	High

BODY MASS INDEX

Another technique scientists use to determine thinness and excessive fatness is the Body Mass Index (BMI). This index incorporates height and weight to estimate critical fat values at which the risk for disease increases.

BMI is calculated by multiplying your weight in pounds by 705, dividing this figure by your height in inches, and then dividing by the same height again (or weight in kilograms divided by the square of the height in meters). For example, the BMI for an individual who weighs 172 pounds and is 67 inches tall would be 27 (172 × 705 ÷ 67 ÷ 67).

According to BMI, the lowest risk for chronic disease is in the 22 to 25 range (see Table 9.7). Individuals are classified as overweight between 25 and 30. BMIs above 30 are defined as obesity and below 20 as underweight.

BMI is a useful tool to screen the general population, but, similar to height/weight charts, it fails to differentiate fat from lean body mass or where most of the fat is located (see waist-to-hip ratio). Using BMI, athletes with a large amount of muscle mass (body builders, football players) easily can fall in the moderate or even high-risk categories. Therefore, body composition and waist-to-hip ratios are better

TABLE 9.7 ▼ Disease Risk According to Body Mass Index (BMI)

BMI	Disease Risk
<20.00	Moderate to Very High
20.00 to 21.99	Low
22.00 to 24.99	Very Low
25.00 to 29.99	Low
30.00 to 34.99	Moderate
35.00 to 39.99	High
≥40.00	Very High

procedures to determine health risk and recommended body weight.

DETERMINING RECOMMENDED BODY WEIGHT

After finding out your percent body fat, you can determine your current body composition classification according to Table 9.8. In this table you will find the health fitness and the high physical fitness percent fat standards.

For example, the recommended health fitness fat percentage for a 20-year-old female is 28% or less. The health fitness standard is established at the point at which there seems to be no harm to health in terms of percent body fat. A high physical fitness range for this same woman would be between 18% and 23%.

The high physical fitness standard does not mean you cannot be somewhat below this number. Many highly trained male athletes are as low as 3%, and some female distance runners have been measured at 6% body fat (which may not be healthy).

Although people generally agree that the mortality rate is greater for obese people, some evidence indicates that the same is true for underweight people. "Underweight" and "thin" do not necessarily mean the same thing. A healthy thin person has total body fat around the high fitness percentage, whereas an underweight person has extremely low body fat, even to the point of compromising the essential fat.

The 3% essential fat for men and 12% for women seem to be the lower limits for people to maintain good health. Below these percentages normal physiologic functions can be seriously impaired. Some experts point out that a little storage fat (over the essential fat) is better than none at all.

As a result, the health and high fitness standards for percent fat in Table 9.8 are set higher than the minimum essential fat requirements, at a point beneficial to optimal health and well-being. Finally, because lean tissue decreases with age, one extra

TABLE 9.8 ▼ Body Composition Classification According to Percent Body Fat

			MEN		
Age	Excellent	Good	Moderate	Overweight	Obese
≤19	12.0	12.1-17.0	17.1-22.0	22.1-27.0	≥27.1
20-29	13.0	13.1-18.0	18.1-23.0	23.1-28.0	≥28.1
30-39	14.0	14.1-19.0	19.1-24.0	24.1-29.0	≥29.1
40-49	15.0	15.1-20.0	20.1-25.0	25.1-30.0	≥30.1
≥50	16.0	16.1-21.5	21.1-26.0	26.1-31.0	≥31.1
			WOMEN		
Age	Excellent	Good	Moderate	Overweight	Obese
≤19	17.0	17.1-22.0	22.1-27.0	27.1-32.0	≥32.1
20-29	18.0	18.1-23.0	23.1-28.0	28.1-33.0	≥33.1
30-39	19.0	19.1-24.0	24.1-29.0	29.1-34.0	≥34.1
40-49	20.0	20.1-25.0	25.1-30.0	30.1-35.0	≥35.1
≥50	21.0	21.1-26.5	26.1-31.0	31.1-36.0	≥36.1

High physical fitness standard
Health fitness standard

percentage point is allowed for every additional decade of life.

Your recommended body weight is computed based on the selected health or high fitness fat percentage for your age and gender. Your decision to select a "desired" fat percentage should be based on your current percent body fat and your personal health/fitness objectives. To compute your own recommended body weight:

1. Determine the pounds of body weight in fat (FW). Multiply body weight (BW) by the current percent fat (%F) expressed in decimal form (FW = BW × %F).
2. Determine lean body mass (LBM) by subtracting the weight in fat from the total body weight (LBM = BW − FW). (Anything that is not fat must be part of the lean component.)
3. Select a desired body fat percentage (DFP) based on the health or high fitness standards given in Table 9.8.
4. Compute recommended body weight (RBW) according to the formula: RBW = LBM ÷ (1.0 − DFP).

As an example of these computations, a 19-year-old female who weighs 160 pounds and is 30% fat would like to know what her recommended body weight would be at 22%:

Gender: female
Age: 19
BW: 160 lbs.
%F: 30% (.30 in decimal form)

1. FW = BW × %F
   FW = 160 × .30 = 48 lbs.
2. LBM = BW − FW
   LBM = 160 − 48 = 112 lbs.
3. DFP: 22% (.22 in decimal form)
4. RBW = LBM ÷ (1.0 − DFP)
   RBW = 112 ÷ (1.0 − .22)
   RBW = 112 ÷ (.78) = 143.6 lbs.

In Figures 9.4 and 9.5 you will have the opportunity to determine your own body composition, recommended body weight, and disease risk according to waist-to-hip ratio and BMI.

Other than hydrostatic weighing, skinfold thickness seems to be the most practical and valid technique to estimate body fat. If skinfold calipers are available, use this technique to assess percent body fat. If calipers are unavailable, you can estimate your percent fat according to the girth measurements technique or another technique available to you. (You may wish to use several techniques and compare the results.)

If you are on a diet/exercise program, you should repeat the computations about once a month to monitor changes in body composition. This is important because lean body mass is affected by weight reduction programs and amount of physical activity. As lean body mass changes, so will your recommended body weight. To make valid comparisons, the same technique should be used between pre- and post-assessments.

Changes in body composition resulting from a weight control/exercise program were illustrated in a co-ed aerobics course taught during a 6-week summer term. Students participated in aerobic dance routines four times a week, 60 minutes each time. On the first and last days of class, several physiological parameters, including body composition, were assessed. Students also were given information on diet and nutrition, and they basically followed their own weight control program.

At the end of the 6 weeks, the average weight loss for the entire class was 3 pounds (see Figure 9.6). But because body composition was assessed, class members were surprised to find that the average fat loss was actually 6 pounds, accompanied by a 3-pound increase in lean body mass.

When dieting, body composition should be reassessed periodically because of the effects of negative caloric balance on lean body mass. As is discussed in Chapter 10, dieting alone does decrease lean body mass. This lean body mass loss can be reduced or eliminated by combining a sensible diet with physical exercise.

I. **Percent Body Fat According to Skinfold Thickness**

Men

Chest (mm): _____

Abdomen (mm): _____

Thigh (mm): _____

Total (mm): _____

Percent Fat: _____

Women

Triceps (mm): _____

Suprailium (mm): _____

Thigh (mm): _____

Total (mm): _____

Percent Fat: _____

II. **Percent Fat According to Girth Measurements**

Men

Waist (inches): _____

Wrist (inches): _____

Difference: _____

Body Weight: _____

Percent Fat: _____

Women

Upper Arm (cm): _____   Constant A = _____

Age: _____   Constant B = _____

Hip (cm): _____   Constant C = _____

Wrist (cm): _____   Constant D = _____

BD* = A − B − C + D

BD = _____ − _____ − _____ + _____ =

Percent Fat = (495 ÷ BD) − 450 = (495 ÷ _____) − 450 =

*Body density

III. **Recommended Body Weight Determination**

A. Body Weight (BW): _____

B. Current Percent Fat (%F)**: _____

C. Fat Weight (FW) = BW × %F

FW = _____ × _____ =

D. Lean Body Mass (LBM) = BW − FW = _____ − _____ =

E. Age: _____

F. Desired Fat Percent (DFP − see Table 3.7): _____

G. Recommended Body Weight (RBW) = LBM ÷ (1.0 − DFP**)

RBW = _____ ÷ (1.0 − _____) =

**Express percentages in decimal form (e.g., 25% = .25)

FIGURE 9.4 ▼ Anthropometric measurements for body composition assessment and recommended body weight determination.

Waist-to-Hip Ratio

Waist (inches): _____

Hip (inches): _____

Ratio (waist ÷ hip): _____

Disease Risk (see Table 9.6): _____

Body Mass Index

Weight (pounds): _____

Height (inches): _____

BMI = Weight × 705 ÷ Height ÷ Height

BMI = _____ × 705 ÷ _____ ÷ _____

BMI =

Disease Risk (see Table 9.7): _____

FIGURE 9.5 ▼ Weight and health: Disease risk assessment.

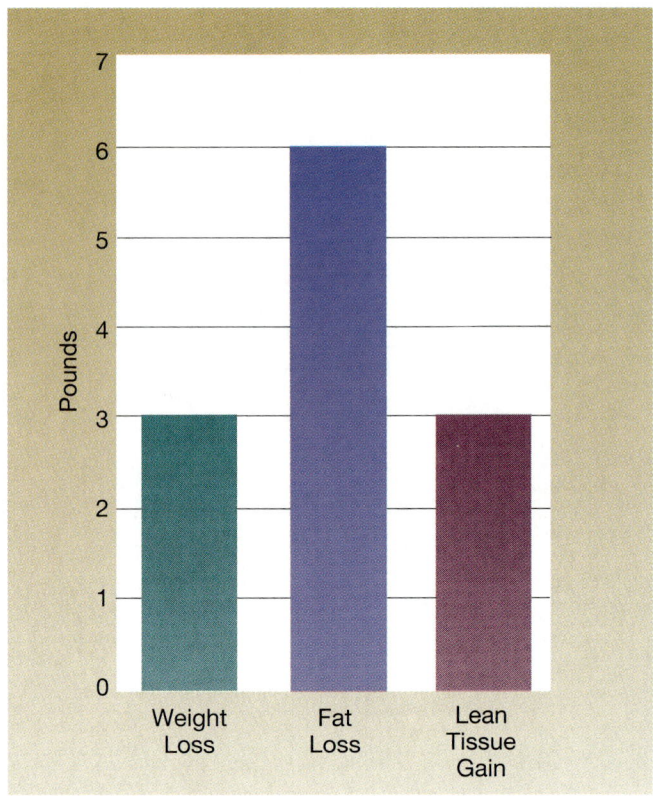

FIGURE 9.6 ▼ Effects of a six-week aerobics program on body composition.

10

Weight Management, Eating Disorders, and Wellness

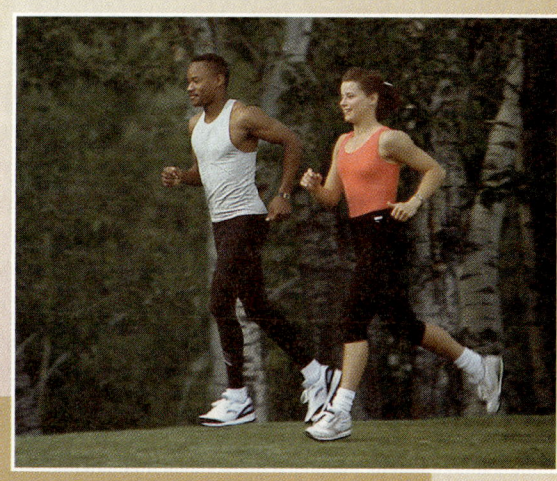

Objectives

▼ Learn the health consequences of obesity.

▼ Understand fad diets and other myths and fallacies regarding weight control.

▼ Become familiar with eating disorders, their associated medical problems and behavior patterns, and understand the need for professional help in treating these conditions.

▼ Understand the physiology of weight loss, including set-point theory and the effects of diet on basal metabolic rate.

▼ Recognize the role of a lifetime exercise program as the key to a successful weight loss and maintenance program.

▼ Learn how to implement a sound weight reduction and weight maintenance program.

▼ Learn behavior modification techniques that help in adhering to a lifetime weight maintenance program.

Achieving and maintaining recommended body weight is a major objective of a good fitness and wellness program. Next to poor cardiovascular fitness, too much body fat is the problem encountered most often in fitness and wellness assessments.

According to the 1992 Prevention Index, an annual survey of the effort Americans are making to promote good health, 63% of adults in the United States were over their recommended weight range. Evidence suggests that the prevalence is still increasing. In the last decade, the average weight of American adults increased by about 15 pounds.

In the meantime, the diet industry continues to thrive. About half of all women and a fourth of all men in the United States are on diets at any given moment. In 1990, Americans spent about $40 billion attempting to lose weight. More than $10 billion went to memberships in weight reduction centers and another $30 billion to diet food sales.

Obesity is a health hazard of epidemic proportions in most developed countries around the world. An estimated 35% of the adult population in industrialized nations is obese. Obesity by itself has been associated with several serious health conditions and accounts for 15% to 20% of the annual mortality rate in the United States.

Obesity is a major risk factor for diseases of the cardiovascular system, including coronary heart disease, hypertension, congestive heart failure, high levels of blood lipids, atherosclerosis, strokes, thromboembolic disease, osteoarthritis, varicose veins, and intermittent claudication. Other research points toward a possible link between obesity and cancer of the colon, rectum, prostate, gallbladder, breast, uterus, and ovaries.

In addition, obesity has been associated with diabetes, ruptured intervertebral discs, gallstones, gout, respiratory insufficiency, and complications during pregnancy and delivery. Further, it can lead to psychological maladjustment and a higher accidental death rate. Life insurance companies are quick to point out that overweight males have a 150% greater mortality rate than the average mortality rate.

Scientific evidence also points toward a higher mortality rate for excessively underweight people. Although the social pressure to be thin has decreased slightly in recent years, the pressure to attain model-like thinness is still with us and contributes to the gradual increase in the number of people who develop eating disorders (anorexia nervosa and bulimia are discussed later in this chapter).

Extreme weight loss also can lead to serious medical problems. Common conditions associated with eating disorders include heart damage, gastrointestinal problems, shrinkage of internal organs, immune system abnormalities, disorders of the reproductive system, loss of muscle tissue, damage to the nervous system, and even death.

Unfortunately, only about 10% of all people who begin a traditional weight loss program (without exercise) are able to lose the desired weight. Worse, only one in 200 is able to keep the weight off for a significant time.

Traditional diets have failed because few of them incorporate lifetime changes in food selection and exercise as the keys to successful weight loss. The $40 billion diet industry tries to capitalize on the idea that weight can be lost quickly without taking into consideration the consequences of fast weight loss or the importance of lifetime behavioral changes to ensure proper weight loss and maintenance.

▼ THE DIETING MYTH

Traditional dieting by itself seldom promotes permanent weight loss, for several reasons. First, too many fad diets mislead people with weight problems. Proponents of these diets continue to deceive people and claim they will lose weight by following all instructions.

Most diets are low in calories and deprive the body of certain nutrients, generating a metabolic imbalance that can even cause death. Under these conditions, a lot of the weight lost is in the form of

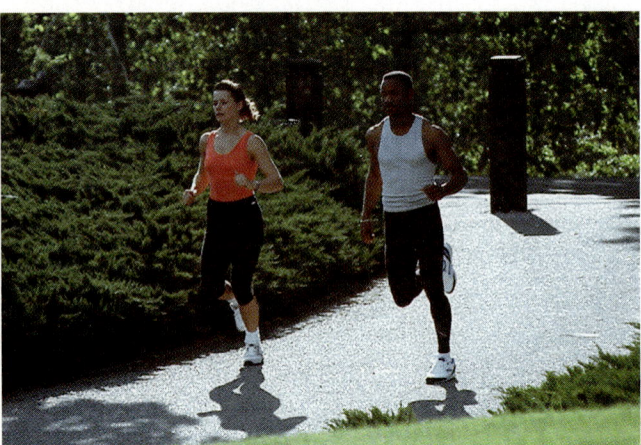

Maintaining recommended body weight is important to prevent disease and improve quality of life.

water and protein and not fat. On a crash diet, close to half the weight loss is in lean (protein) tissue.

When the body uses protein instead of a combination of fats and carbohydrates as a source of energy, weight is lost as much as 10 times faster.[1] A gram of protein produces half the amount of energy that fat does. In the case of muscle protein, one-fifth of protein is mixed with four-fifths water. Each pound of muscle yields only one-tenth the amount of energy of a pound of fat. As a result, most of the weight loss is in the form of water, which on the scale, of course, looks good. When a person resumes regular eating habits, though, most of the lost weight comes right back.

Some diets allow only certain specialized foods. If people would realize that no "magic" foods provide all the necessary nutrients, and that a person has to eat a variety of foods to be well-nourished, the diet industry would not be as successful. Most of these diets create a nutritional deficiency, which at times can be fatal.

The reason a few diets succeed is that people eventually get tired of eating the same thing day in and day out and, therefore, start eating less. If they happen to achieve the lower weight, once they go back to old eating habits without making permanent dietary changes, they quickly gain back the weight.

▼ EATING DISORDERS

Anorexia nervosa and bulimia are physical and emotional conditions in which a person becomes underweight and malnourished. These conditions usually arise from individual, family, or social pressures, in some combination. These medical disorders are increasing steadily in most industrialized nations in which society encourages low-calorie diets and thinness. People with eating disorders have an intense fear of becoming fat, which does not disappear even when they lose extreme amounts of weight.

ANOREXIA NERVOSA

Anorexia nervosa is a condition of self-imposed starvation to lose and then maintain low body weight. Approximately 19 of every 20 anorexics are young women. An estimated 1% of the female population in the United States is anorexic.

Anorexic individuals seem to fear weight gain more than death from starvation. They, too, have a distorted image of their body and think of themselves as being fat even when they are emaciated.

Although a genetic predisposition may exist, the anorexic person often comes from a mother-dominated home, with possible drug addictions in the family. The syndrome may begin following a stressful life event and the uncertainty of one's ability to cope efficiently.

Because the female role in society is changing more rapidly, women seem to be especially susceptible. Life experiences such as gaining weight, starting the menstrual period, beginning college, losing a boyfriend, having poor self-esteem, being socially rejected, starting a professional career, or becoming a wife or mother may trigger the syndrome.

These individuals typically begin a diet and at first feel in control and happy about the weight loss, even if they are not overweight. To speed up the weight loss, they frequently combine extreme dieting with exhaustive exercise and overuse of laxatives and diuretics.

Anorexics commonly develop obsessive and compulsive behaviors and emphatically deny the condition. They are preoccupied constantly with food, meal planning, grocery shopping, and unusual eating habits. As they lose weight and their health begins to deteriorate, anorexics feel weak and tired. They may realize they have a problem but will not stop the starvation and refuse to consider the behavior as abnormal.

Once they have lost a lot of weight and malnutrition sets in, physical changes become more visible. Some typical changes are amenorrhea (stopping menstruation), digestive problems, extreme sensitivity to cold, hair and skin problems, fluid and electrolyte abnormalities (which may lead to an irregular heartbeat and sudden stopping of the heart), injuries to nerves and tendons, abnormalities of immune function, anemia, growth of fine body hair, mental confusion, inability to concentrate, lethargy, depression, skin dryness, and lower skin and body temperature.

Many of the changes of anorexia nervosa can be reversed. Treatment almost always requires professional help, and the sooner it is started, the better are the chances to reverse and cure the disease. Therapy consists of a combination of medical and psychological techniques to restore proper nutrition, prevent medical complications, and modify the environment or events that triggered the syndrome.

Seldom are anorexics able to overcome the problem by themselves.

Unfortunately, anorexics strongly deny their condition. They are able to hide it and deceive friends and relatives quite effectively. Based on their behavior, many of them meet all of the characteristics of anorexia nervosa, but it goes undetected because both thinness and dieting are socially acceptable. Only a well-trained clinician is able to make a positive diagnosis.

BULIMIA

Bulimia, a pattern of binge eating and purging, is more prevalent than anorexia nervosa. For many years it was thought to be a variant of anorexia nervosa, but now it is identified as a separate condition. It afflicts mainly young people, and as many as one in every five women on college campuses may be bulimic, according to some estimates. Bulimia also is more prevalent than anorexia nervosa in males.

Bulimics usually are healthy-looking people, well-educated, near recommended body weight, who enjoy food and often socialize around it. In actuality, they are emotionally insecure, rely on others, and lack self-confidence and esteem. Recommended weight and food are both important to them.

As a result of stressful life events or the simple compulsion to eat, bulimics periodically engage in binge eating that may last an hour or longer, during which they may consume several thousand calories. A feeling of deep guilt and shame then sets in, along with intense fear of gaining weight. Purging seems to be an easy answer, as the binging cycle can continue without the fear of gaining weight.

The most common form of purging is self-induced vomiting, although strong laxatives and emetics are frequently ingested. Near-fasting diets and strenuous bouts of exercise also are commonly seen in bulimics. Medical problems associated with bulimia include cardiac arrhythmias, amenorrhea, kidney and bladder damage, ulcers, colitis, tearing of the esophagus, stomach, tooth erosion, gum damage, and general muscular weakness.

Unlike anorexics, bulimics realize their behavior is abnormal and feel great shame about it. Fearing social rejection, they pursue the binge-purge cycle in secrecy and during unusual hours of the day.

Bulimia can be treated successfully when the person realizes this destructive behavior is not the solution to life's problems. A change in attitude can prevent permanent damage or death.

Treatment for anorexia nervosa and bulimia can be sought on most school campuses through the school's counseling center or the health center. Local hospitals also offer treatment for these conditions. Support groups, frequently led by professional personnel and usually free of charge, are available in many communities.

PRINCIPLES OF WEIGHT CONTROL

Only a few years ago the principles governing a weight loss and maintenance program seemed to be fairly clear, but we now know the final answers are not yet in. Traditional concepts related to weight control have centered on three assumptions: (a) that balancing food intake against output allows a person to achieve recommended weight; (b) that fat people just eat too much; and (c) that the human body doesn't care how much (or little) fat is stored. Although these statements may have some truth, they are still open to much debate and research.

THE ENERGY-BALANCING EQUATION

The energy-balancing equation basically states that as long as caloric input equals caloric output, the person will not gain or lose weight. If caloric intake exceeds output, the individual gains weight. When output exceeds input, the person loses weight.

This principle is simple, and if daily energy requirements could be determined accurately, it seems reasonable that caloric intake could be balanced against output. This is not always the case, though, because genetic and lifestyle-related individual differences determine the number of calories required to maintain or lose body weight.

One pound of fat equals 3,500 calories. Assuming that a person's basic daily caloric expenditure is 2,500 calories, if this person were to decrease the daily intake by 500 calories per day, it should result in a loss of 1 pound of fat in 7 days ($500 \times 7 = 3,500$). As many dieters have experienced, however, even when caloric input is balanced carefully against estimated caloric output, weight loss does not always come as predicted. Furthermore, two people with similar measured caloric intake and output do not necessarily lose weight at the same rate.

The most common explanation regarding individual differences in weight loss and weight gain has been the variation in human metabolism from one person to another. We have all seen people who can eat "all day long" and not gain an ounce of weight, while others cannot even "dream" about food without gaining weight. Because many experts did not believe that human metabolism alone could account for such extreme differences, several theories have been developed that may better explain these individual variations.

SETPOINT THEORY

Results of several studies point toward a weight-regulating mechanism (WRM) in the hypothalamus of the brain, which regulates how much the body should weigh. This mechanism has a setpoint that controls both appetite and the amount of fat stored. It is hypothesized that the setpoint works like a thermostat for body fat, maintaining fairly constant body weight because it knows at all times the exact amount of adipose tissue stored in the fat cells.

Every person has his or her own certain body fat percentage (as established by the setpoint) that the body attempts to maintain. The genetic instinct to survive tells the body that fat storage is vital, and therefore it sets an acceptable fat level. This level remains somewhat constant or may climb gradually because of poor lifestyle habits. For instance, under strict calorie reduction, the body may make extreme metabolic adjustments in an effort to maintain its setpoint for fat. The basal metabolic rate may drop dramatically against a consistent negative caloric balance, and a person may be on a plateau for days or even weeks without losing much weight.

Dietary restriction alone will not lower the setpoint even though the person may lose weight and fat. When the dieter goes back to the normal or even below-normal caloric intake, at which the weight may have been stable for a long time, he or she quickly regains the fat loss as the body strives to regain a comfortable fat store.

Let's use a practical illustration. A person would like to lose some body fat and assumes that a stable body weight has been reached at an average daily caloric intake of 1,800 calories (no weight gain or loss occurs at this daily intake). In an attempt to lose weight rapidly, this person now goes on a strict low-calorie diet, or even worse, a near-fasting diet. Immediately the body activates its survival mechanism and readjusts its metabolism to a lower caloric balance.

After a few weeks of dieting at fewer than 400 to 600 calories per day, the body now can maintain its normal functions at 1,000 calories per day. Having lost the desired weight, the person terminates the diet but realizes the original intake of 1,800 calories per day will have to be lower to maintain the new lower weight.

To adjust to the new lower body weight, the intake is restricted to about 1,500 calories per day. The individual is surprised to find that, even at this lower daily intake (300 fewer calories), weight comes back at a rate of 1 pound every 1 to 2 weeks. Depending on the length and amount of the negative caloric balance, the metabolic rate may not kick back up to its normal level for several months after ending the diet.

From this explanation, individuals clearly should never go on very low-calorie diets. Not only will this lower the resting metabolic rate, but it also will deprive the body of basic daily nutrients required for normal function. Under no circumstances should a person go on a diet that calls for below 1,200 calories for women and 1,500 calories for men.

People need to realize that weight (fat) is gained over months and years, not overnight. Likewise, weight loss should be gradual, not abrupt. Individuals are more likely to keep excess weight off if they achieve the weight loss slowly and gradually.

Daily caloric intakes of 1,200 to 1,500 calories provide the necessary nutrients if properly distributed over the five basic food groups. The person always should try to meet the daily required servings from each group: bread, cereal, rice, pasta (6 to 11 servings); fruits (2 to 4 or more servings); vegetables (3 to 5 or more servings); milk, yogurt, and cheese (2 to 3 servings); and meat, poultry, fish, dry beans, eggs, and nuts (2 to 3 servings). Of course, the person will have to learn which foods meet the requirements for each group and yet are low in fat, sugar, and calories.

The most common question regarding the setpoint is how it can be lowered so the body will feel comfortable at a lesser fat percentage. Several factors seem to directly affect the setpoint. Aerobic exercise, a diet high in complex carbohydrates, nicotine, and amphetamines all have been shown to lower the fat thermostat. The last two, however, are more destructive than the overfatness, so they are not reasonable alternatives. As far as the extra strain on the heart is concerned, smoking one pack of cigarettes per day is estimated to be the equivalent of carrying 50 to 75 pounds of excess body fat.

On the other hand, a diet high in fats and refined carbohydrates, near-fasting diets, and perhaps even artificial sweeteners seem to raise the setpoint. Therefore, the only practical and sensible way to lower the setpoint and lose fat weight seems to be a combination of aerobic exercise and a diet high in complex carbohydrates and low in fat and sugar.

Because of the effects of proper food management on the body's setpoint, many nutritionists now believe the total number of calories should not be the main concern in a weight control program but, rather, the source of those calories. In this regard, most of the effort is spent in retraining eating habits, increasing the intake of complex carbohydrates and high-fiber foods, and decreasing the consumption of refined carbohydrates (sugars) and fats. In most cases, this change in eating habits brings about a decrease in total daily caloric intake.

A "diet" is no longer viewed as a temporary tool to aid in weight loss but, instead, as a permanent change in eating behaviors to ensure weight management and better health. The role of increased physical activity also must be considered, because successful weight loss, maintenance, and recommended body composition seldom are attainable without a moderate reduction in caloric intake combined with a regular exercise program.

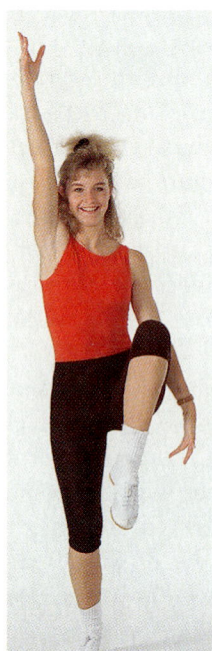
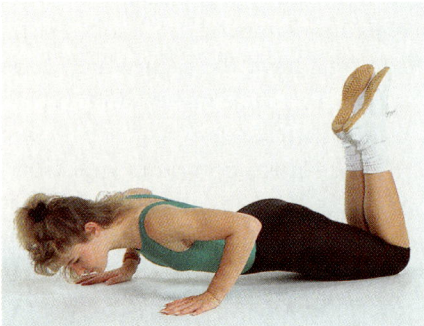

Regular participation in a combined lifetime aerobic and strength training-exercise program is the key to successful weight management.

RELATIONSHIP BETWEEN LEAN TISSUE AND METABOLISM

Fat can be lost by selecting proper foods, doing aerobic exercise, or restricting calories. When a person tries to lose weight by dietary restrictions alone, lean body mass (muscle protein, along with vital organ protein) always decreases.

The amount of lean body mass lost depends entirely on caloric limitation. In near-fasting diets, up to half of the weight loss might be lean body mass and the other half actual fat loss.[2] When diet is combined with exercise, close to 100% of the weight loss is in the form of fat, and lean tissue actually may increase (see Figure 10.1). Loss of lean body mass is never good because it weakens the organs and muscles and slows down the metabolism.

Contrary to some beliefs, aging is not the main reason for the lower metabolic rate. It is not so much that metabolism slows down as that people slow down. The aging process often is accompanied by reliance on amenities of life (remote controls, cellular telephones, intercoms, single-level homes, riding lawn mowers) that lull a person into sedentary living.

Basal metabolism is related directly to lean body weight. All other factors being equal, the more the lean tissue, the higher the metabolic rate. With sedentary living and less physical activity, the lean component decreases and fat tissue increases. At the same time, the organism continues to use the same

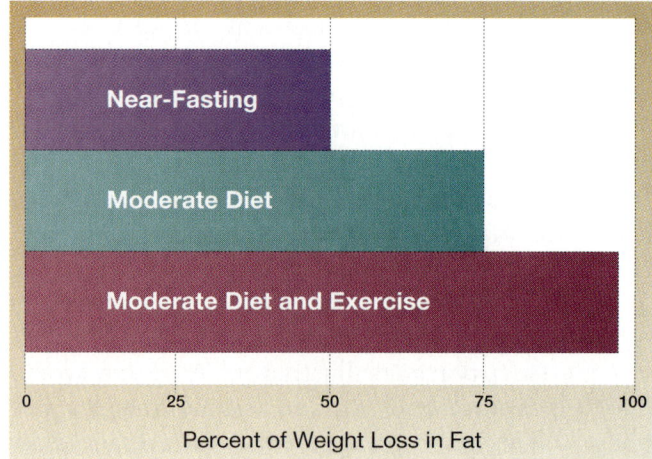

Adapted from Shephard, R. J. *Alive Man: The Physiology of Physical Activity*. Springfield, IL: Charles C. Thomas, 484–488. 1975.

FIGURE 10.1 ▼ Effects of different forms of weight loss on body composition.

amount of oxygen per pound of lean body mass. Because fat is considered metabolically inert from the point of view of caloric use, the lean tissue uses most of the oxygen, even at rest. As muscle and organ mass decreases, so do the energy requirements at rest.

Reductions in lean body mass are common in aging people (because of physical inactivity) and those on severely restricted diets. The loss of lean body mass also may account for the lower metabolic rate and the greater time it takes to kick back up.

A diet with caloric intake below 1,200 to 1,500 calories cannot guarantee that lean body mass will not be lost. Even at this intake level, some loss is inevitable unless the diet is combined with exercise. Many diets have claimed they do not alter the lean component, but the simple truth is that, regardless of what nutrients may be added to the diet, severe caloric restrictions always prompt a loss of lean tissue. Too many people constantly go on low-calorie diets. Every time they do, the metabolic rate keeps slowing down as more lean tissue is lost.

People in the 40s or older who weigh the same as they did when they were 20 commonly think they are at recommended body weight. During this span of 20 years or more, they may have "dieted" all too many times without participating in an exercise program. They regain the weight shortly after terminating each diet, but most of that gain is in fat.

Maybe at age 20 these individuals weighed 150 pounds and had only 15% to 16% fat. Now at age 40, even though they still weigh 150 pounds, they might be 30% fat. At recommended body weight, they wonder why they are eating very little and still having trouble staying at that weight.

▼ EXERCISE: THE KEY TO SUCCESSFUL WEIGHT LOSS AND MAINTENANCE

Based on the preceding discussion, exercise emerges as the key to weight loss and weight maintenance. Not only will exercise maintain lean tissue, but advocates of the setpoint theory say that exercise resets the fat thermostat to a new, lower level.

For a lot of people, the change in setpoint is rapid, but in some cases it may take time. A few overweight individuals have exercised faithfully almost daily, 60 minutes at a time, for a whole year, before weight change is significant. People with a "sticky" setpoint have to be patient and persistent.

If a person is trying to lose weight, a combination of aerobic and strength-training exercises works best. Aerobic exercise is the best to offset the setpoint, and the continuity and duration of these types of activities cause many calories to be burned in the process. Strength-training exercises, though, have the greatest impact on increasing lean body mass.

The role of aerobic exercise in successful lifetime weight management cannot be underestimated. This role was clearly shown in a 1989 research study by Dr. Konstantin Pavlou and colleagues, published in the *American Journal of Clinical Nutrition*.[3] As illustrated in Figure 10.2, the results indicated that individuals who combined a diet with a 12-week aerobic exercise program (three times per week, 35 to 60 minutes per session) achieved greater weight loss.

Even more significant in this investigation, only the individuals who participated in an 18-month post-diet aerobic exercise program were able to keep the weight off. Those who discontinued exercise gained weight. Furthermore, all of the individuals who initiated or resumed exercise during the 18-month follow-up were able to lose weight again. Individuals who only dieted and never exercised regained 60% and 92% of their weight loss at the 6- and 18-month follow-ups, respectively.

The effectiveness of a combined aerobic/strength-training program in aiding with weight loss was demonstrated in a 1991 study published in *Fitness Management* by Dr. Wayne Westcott.[4] Two exercise groups — a 30-minute aerobic group and a 15-minute aerobic plus 15-minute strength-training (30 minutes total) group — participated in an 8-week, 3 days per week study. Both groups followed a dietary plan consisting of approximately 60% carbohydrates, 20% fats, and 20% proteins.

The aerobic group lost an average of 3½ pounds, 3 of which were fat and the remaining 1/2 pound in the form of lean tissue. The combined aerobic strength-training group lost an average of 8 pounds. Body composition changes, however, indicated that the latter group actually lost 10 pounds of fat and gained 2 pounds of lean tissue (see Figure 10.3). The researcher concluded that a sensible strength-training program produces better weight loss, as well as muscle mass and metabolic rate maintenance.

As mentioned in Chapter 7, it is estimated that each additional pound of muscle tissue can raise the basal metabolic rate between 30 and 50 calories per day. Using the conservative estimate of 30 calories

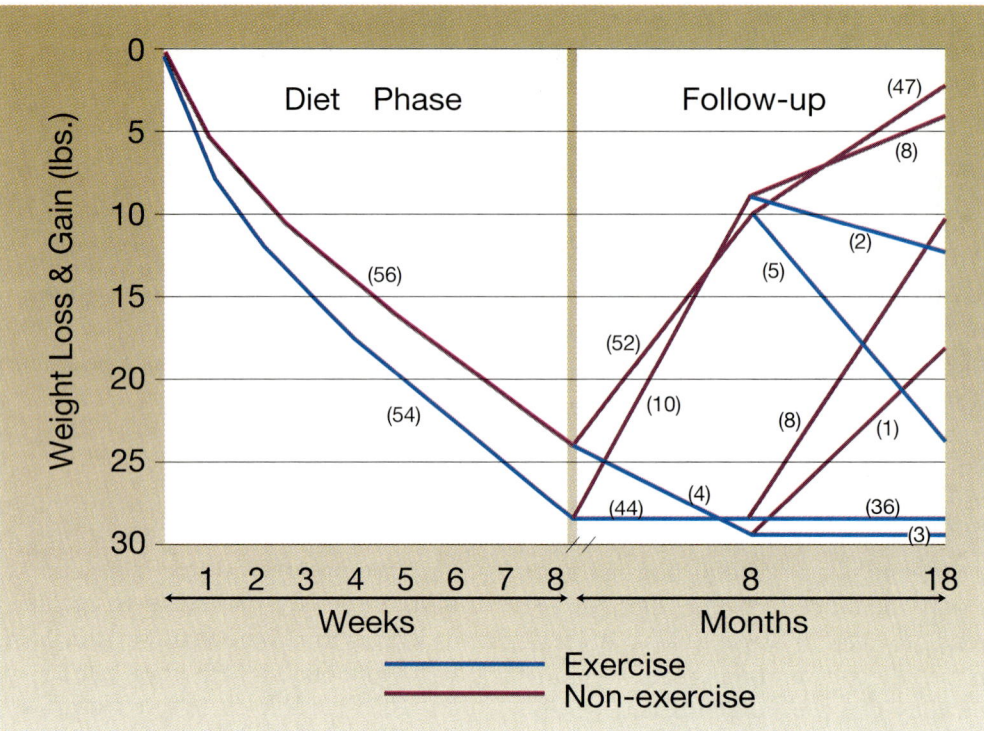

Adapted from K. N. Pavlou, S. Krey, and W. P. Steffee. "Exercise as an Adjunct to Weight Loss and Maintenance in Moderately Obese Subjects." *American Journal of Clinical Nutrition*, 49 (1989), 1115-1123.

FIGURE 10.2 ▼ Role of aerobic exercise during 12 weeks of weight loss and an 18-month follow-up on weight loss maintenance (numbers in parenthesis indicate number of participants).

per day, a person who adds 5 pounds of muscle tissue as a result of strength training increases the basal metabolic rate by 150 calories per day, which equals 54,750 calories per year, or the equivalent of 15.6 pounds of fat.

Strength training is recommended especially for people who think they are at their ideal body weight, yet their body fat percentage is higher than recommended. Keep in mind that the number of calories burned during a typical hour-long strength training session is much less than during an hour of aerobic exercise. Because of the high intensity of weight training, frequent rest intervals are required to recover from each set of exercise. The average person actually lifts weights only 10 to 12 minutes in each hour of exercise.

Weight can be lost through a regular strength-training program, but it is much slower than with aerobics. In the long run, however, the person enjoys the benefits of gains in lean tissue. Guidelines for developing aerobic and strength-training programs are given in Chapter 7.

Because exercise leads to an increase in lean body mass, body weight often remains the same or even increases after beginning an exercise program, while inches and percent body fat decrease. More lean tissue means more functional capacity of the human body. With exercise, most of the weight loss becomes apparent after a few weeks of training, when the lean component has stabilized.

Research has shown that there is no such thing as spot-reducing or losing "cellulite," as some people refer to the fat deposits that bulge out in certain areas of the body. These deposits are nothing but enlarged fat cells from accumulated body fat. Just doing several sets of daily sit-ups will not get rid of fat in the midsection of the body.

When fat comes off, it does so throughout the entire body, not just the area exercised. The greatest proportion of fat may come off the biggest fat deposits, but the caloric output of a few sets of sit-ups has practically no effect on reducing total body fat. A person has to exercise much longer to really see results.

Other touted means toward quick weight loss — rubberized sweatsuits, steam baths, mechanical vibrators — are misleading. When a person wears a sweatsuit or steps into a sauna, the weight lost is not

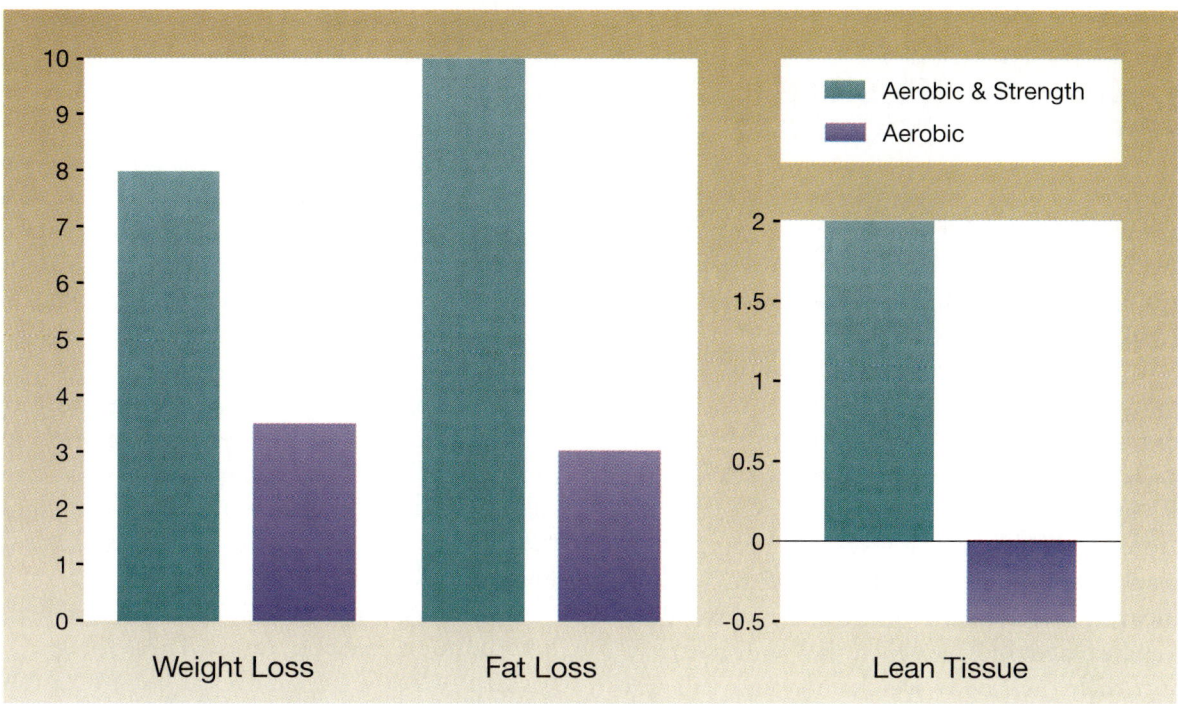

Both groups exercised 30 minutes per session, three times per week, for 12 weeks. The aerobic-plus-strength group performed 15 minutes of aerobic exercise and 15 minutes of strength training.

Source: Wescott, W. L. "You Can Sell Exercise for Weight Loss". *Fitness Management,* 7(12):33–34, 1991.

FIGURE 10.3 ▼ Effects of two forms of exercise on weight loss.

fat; it is merely a significant amount of water. Sure, it looks nice when you step on the scale immediately afterward, but this represents a false loss of weight. As soon as you replace body fluids, you quickly gain back the weight.

Wearing rubberized sweatsuits not only hastens the rate of body fluid loss, which is vital during prolonged exercise, but at the same time it raises core temperature. This combination puts a person in danger of dehydration, which impairs cellular function and in extreme cases even causes death.

Similarly, mechanical vibrators are worthless in a weight control program. Vibrating belts and turning rollers may feel good, but they require no effort whatsoever. Fat cannot be "shaken off"; it is burned off primarily in muscle tissue.

Although we now know that a negative caloric balance of 3,500 calories does not always result in a loss of exactly one pound of fat, the role of exercise in achieving a negative balance by burning additional calories is significant in weight reduction and maintenance programs. Sadly, some individuals claim the amount of calories burned during exercise is hardly worth the effort. Many people think that it is easier to cut their daily intake by some 200 calories than to participate in some sort of exercise that would burn the same amount of calories. The problem is that the willpower to cut those 200 calories lasts only a few weeks, and then it is right back to the old eating patterns.

If a person gets into the habit of exercising regularly, say three times a week, running 3 miles per exercise session (about 300 calories burned), it represents 900 calories in one week, 3,600 in one month, or 43,200 calories per year. This minimal amount of exercise could mean as many as 12 extra pounds of fat in a year, 24 in 2 years, and so on.

We tend to forget that our weight creeps up gradually over the years, not just overnight. Hardly worth the effort? And we have not even taken into consideration the increase in lean tissue, possible resetting of the setpoint, benefits to the cardiovascular system, and, most important, better quality of life! There is little argument that the fundamental reasons for overfatness and obesity are lack of physical activity and sedentary living.

IMPLEMENTING A SOUND AND SENSIBLE WEIGHT LOSS PROGRAM

Dieting never has been fun and never will be. People who are overweight and are serious about losing weight will have to make exercise a regular part of their daily life, along with proper food management and a sensible cut in caloric intake.

When increasing physical activity, some precautions are in order. Excessive body fat is a risk factor for cardiovascular disease. Depending on the extent of the weight problem, a medical examination and possibly a stress ECG (see Chapter 7) may be a good idea before undertaking the exercise program. A physician should be consulted in this regard.

Significantly overweight individuals also may have to choose activities in which they will not have to support their own body weight but that will still be effective in burning calories. Joint and muscle injuries are common in overweight individuals who participate in weight-bearing exercises such as walking, jogging, and aerobics.

Swimming may not be a good exercise either. More body fat makes the person more buoyant, and most people are not at the skill level to swim fast enough to get the best training effect. The tendency is to just "float" along, limiting the amount of calories burned as well as the benefits to the cardiovascular system.

Some better alternatives are riding a bicycle (either road or stationary), walking in a shallow pool, doing water aerobics, or running in place in deep water (treading water). These forms of water exercise are quickly gaining popularity and have proven to be effective in weight reduction without the "pain" and fear of injuries.

How long should each exercise session last? To develop and maintain cardiovascular fitness, 20 to 30 minutes of exercise at the ideal target rate, three to five times per week, is suggested (see Chapter 7). For weight-loss purposes, many experts recommend exercising at least 45 to 60 minutes at a time, five to six times a week.

A person should not try to do too much too fast. Unconditioned beginners should start with about 15 minutes three times per week, and then gradually increase the duration by approximately 5 minutes each week and the frequency by 1 day per week during the next 3 to 4 weeks.

One final benefit of exercise for weight control is that it allows fat to be burned more efficiently. Because both carbohydrates and fats are sources of energy, when the glucose levels begin to drop during prolonged exercise, more fat is used as energy substrate.

Equally important is that fat-burning enzymes increase with aerobic training. Fat is lost primarily by burning it in muscle. Therefore, as the concentration of the enzymes increases, so does the ability to burn fat.

In addition to exercise and adequate food management, sensible adjustments in caloric intake are recommended. Most research finds that a negative caloric balance is required to lose weight. Perhaps the only exception is with people who are eating too few calories.

People on long-term, low-calorie diets also have low basal metabolic rates. These people actually need to increase their daily caloric intake (combined with an exercise program) to get the metabolism to kick back up to a normal level.

The reasons for prescribing a lower caloric figure to lose weight are:

1. New behaviors take time to develop, and some people have trouble changing and adjusting to new eating habits.

2. Many individuals are in such poor physical condition that they take a long time to increase their activity level enough to offset the setpoint and burn enough calories to aid in loss of body fat.

3. Some dieters have difficulty succeeding unless they can count calories.

4. Many people simply will not alter their food selection. For those who will not change their food selection (which still increases the risk for chronic diseases), much more physical activity, a negative caloric balance, or a combination of the two is the only solution to lose weight successfully.

Using Tables 10.1 and 10.2, you can estimate your daily caloric requirement. As this is only an estimated value, individual adjustments related to many of the factors discussed in this chapter may be necessary to establish a more precise value. Nevertheless, the estimated value does offer a beginning guideline for weight control or reduction.

The average daily caloric requirement without exercise is based on typical lifestyle patterns, total body weight, and gender. Individuals who hold jobs that require heavy manual labor burn more calories during the day than those who have sedentary jobs (such as working behind a desk).

To find your activity level, refer to Table 10.1 and rate yourself accordingly. Because the number given in Table 10.1 is per pound of body weight, multiply your current weight by that number. For example, the typical caloric requirement to maintain body weight for a moderately active male who weighs 160 pounds is 2,400 calories (160 lbs × 15 cal/lb).

You can add to the previous caloric requirement the number of calories burned as a result of exercise. Table 10.2 provides the estimated caloric expenditure (per pound of body weight per minute of physical activity) based on the perceived exertion of the activity.

For instance, a person exercising at a somewhat hard intensity burns .070 calories per pound of body weight per minute of activity (cal/lb/min). With a body weight of 160 pounds, this man burns 11.2 calories each minute (160 × .070). In 30 minutes, he burns approximately 336 calories (30 × 11.2). These additional 336 calories can be added to the daily expenditure on exercise days.

Because of the many factors that play a role in weight control, the previous value is only an estimated daily requirement. Furthermore, to lose weight, we cannot predict that exactly 1 pound of fat will be lost in 1 week by reducing daily intake by 500 calories (500 × 7 = 3,500 calories, or the equivalent of 1 pound of fat).

The estimated daily caloric figure computed above provides only a target guideline for weight control. Periodic readjustments are necessary because individuals differ, and the estimated daily cost changes as you lose weight and modify your exercise habits.

The recommended number of calories to be subtracted from the daily intake to obtain a negative caloric balance depends on the typical daily requirement. At this point, the best recommendation is to moderately decrease the daily intake, never below 1,200 calories for women and 1,500 for men.

A good rule to follow is to restrict the intake by no more than 500 calories if the daily requirement is below 3,000 calories. For caloric requirements in excess of 3,000, as many as 1,000 calories per day may be subtracted from the total intake. The daily distribution should be approximately 60% carbohydrates (mostly complex carbohydrates), less than 30% fat, and about 12% protein.

The time of day when food is consumed also may play a part in weight reduction. A study conducted at the Aerobics Research Center in Dallas, Texas, indicated that when a person is on a diet, weight is lost most effectively if most of the calories are consumed before 1:00 p.m. and not during the evening meal. This center recommends that when a person is attempting to lose weight, intake should consist of a minimum of 25% of the total daily calories for breakfast, 50% for lunch, and 25% or less at dinner.

Other experts have reported that, if most of the daily calories are consumed during one meal, the

TABLE 10.2 ▼ Estimated Caloric Expenditure Based on Perceived Exertion of Physical Activity

Perceived Exertion		Caloric Expenditure (Cal/lb/min)
Very, very light	(7)*	0.030
Very light	(9)	0.040
Fairly light	(11)	0.050
Somewhat hard	(13)	0.070
Hard	(15)	0.090
Very hard	(17)	0.100
Very, very hard	(19)	0.110

*Numbers in parenthesis indicate the rate of perceived exertion (RPE), see Figure 7.2, Chapter 7.

Adapted from "Caloric Expenditure of Selected Physical Activities," contained in W. W. K. Hoeger and S. A. Hoeger, *Principles and Labs for Physical Fitness & Wellness* (Englewood: Morton Publishing, 1994), p. 78.

TABLE 10.1 ▼ Average Caloric Requirement Per Pound of Body Weight Based on Lifestyle Patterns and Gender

Lifestyle Rating*	Calories per Pound of Body Weight	
	Men	Women
Sedentary (limited physical activity)	13.0	12.0
Moderate Physical Activity	15.0	13.5
Hard Labor (strenuous physical effort)	17.0	15.0

*Pregnant and lactating women add 3 calories to these values.

body may perceive that something is wrong and will slow down the metabolism so it can store a greater amount of calories in the form of fat. Also, eating most of the calories in one meal causes a person to go hungry the rest of the day, making it harder to adhere to the diet.

To monitor daily progress, you should keep track of your daily food and caloric intake. For a more precise record, the information should be recorded immediately after each meal or snack. Meeting the basic requirements from each food group should get top priority. According to the person's progress, adjustments can be made in the typical daily requirement or the exercise program, or both.

TIPS FOR A LIFETIME WEIGHT MANAGEMENT PROGRAM

Achieving and maintaining recommended body composition is by no means impossible, but it does require desire and commitment. If adequate weight management is to become a priority in life, people must realize that some retraining of behavior is crucial for success. Modifying old habits and developing new positive behaviors take time.

Individuals have applied the following management techniques to successfully change detrimental behavior and adhere to a lifetime weight control program. In developing a retraining program, people are not expected to use all of the strategies listed but should select the ones that apply to them.

1. **Make a commitment to change.** People must recognize that they have a problem and decide by themselves whether they really want to change. The reasons for change must be more compelling than those for continuing present lifestyle patterns. If a sincere commitment is there, the chances for success already are enhanced.

2. **Set realistic goals.** Most people with a weight problem would like to lose weight in a relatively short time but do not realize that the weight problem developed over a span of several years. A sound weight reduction and maintenance program can be accomplished only by establishing new lifetime eating and exercise habits, both of which take time.

3. **Incorporate exercise into the program.** Choosing enjoyable activities, places, times, equipment, and people to work with helps a person adhere to an exercise program. Details on developing a complete exercise program are found in Chapter 7.

4. **Incorporate more physical activity in your daily schedule.** Every increase in the amount of daily activity helps with weight management. To increase daily activity, walk rather than drive to nearby places, use stairs instead of elevators and escalators, do not use remote controls, avoid using the telephone when within walking distance, do not use self-propelled lawnmowers, take additional short walks during the day, and the like.

5. **Develop healthy eating patterns.** Eat three regular meals a day consistent with the body's nutritional requirements. Try to eat over 75% of your daily caloric allowance before 1:00 p.m.

6. **Stay busy.** People tend to eat more when they sit around and do nothing. Occupying the mind and body with activities not associated with eating helps take away the desire to eat. Try walking, cycling, playing sports, gardening, sewing, or visiting a library, a museum, a park. Develop other skills and interests, or try something new and exciting to break the routine of life.

7. **Cook wisely.**
   - Use less fat and refined foods in food preparation.
   - Trim all visible fat off meats, and remove skin from poultry before cooking.
   - Skim the fat off gravies and soups.
   - Bake, broil, and boil instead of frying.
   - Sparingly use butter, cream, mayonnaise, and salad dressings.
   - Avoid shellfish, coconut oil, palm oil, and cocoa butter.
   - Prepare plenty of bulky foods.
   - Add whole-grain breads and cereals, vegetables, and legumes to most meals.
   - Try fruits for dessert.
   - Beware of soda, fruit juices, and fruit-flavored drinks.
   - Drink a lot of water, at least six glasses a day.

8. **Avoid social binges.** Social gatherings typically entice self-defeating behavior. Practice visual imagery before attending social gatherings: Visualize yourself in that gathering. Do not feel pressured to eat or drink, and don't rationalize in these situations. Choose low-calorie foods, and entertain yourself with other activities such as dancing and talking.

9. **Monitor changes and reward accomplishments.** Feedback on fat loss, lean tissue gain, and weight loss is a reward in itself. Awareness of changes in body composition also helps reinforce new behaviors. Being able to exercise without interruption for 15, 20, 30, 60 minutes, swimming a certain distance, running a mile — all these accomplishments deserve recognition. Meeting objectives calls for rewards, but not related to eating. Buy new clothing, a tennis racquet, a bicycle, exercise shoes, or something else that is special and you would not have acquired otherwise.

10. **Think positive.** Avoid negative thoughts on how difficult changing past behaviors might be. Instead, think of the benefits you will reap, such as feeling, looking, and functioning better, plus enjoying better health and improving the quality of your life. Attempt to stay away from negative environments and people who will not be supportive. Avoid those who do not have the same desires and who encourage self-defeating behaviors.

▼ IN CONCLUSION

Taking off excessive body fat and keeping it off for good cannot be done quickly and simply. Weight management is accomplished through a lifetime commitment to physical activity and proper food selection. When taking part in a weight (fat) reduction program, people also have to moderately decrease their caloric intake and implement strategies to modify unhealthy eating behaviors.

During the process of behavior modification, relapses into past negative behaviors are almost inevitable. The three most common reasons for relapse are: (a) stress-related factors (major life changes, depression, job changes, illness); (b) social reasons (entertaining, eating out, business travel); and (c) self-enticing behaviors (placing yourself in a situation to see how much you can get away with: "One small taste won't hurt"; leading to "I'll eat just one slice"; and finally, "I haven't done so well, so I might as well eat some more."

Making mistakes is human and does not necessarily mean failure. Failure comes to those who give up and do not use previous experiences to build upon and, in turn, develop skills that will prevent self-defeating behaviors in the future. "Where there's a will, there's a way," and those who persist will reap the rewards.

▼ NOTES

1. Remington, D., A. G. Fisher, and E. A. Parent. *How to Lower Your Fat Thermostat*. Provo, UT: Vitality House International, Inc., 1983.

2. Shephard, R. J. *Alive Man: The Physiology of Physical Activity*. Springfield, IL: Charles C. Thomas, 484-488, 1975.

3. Pavlou, K. N., S. Krey, and W. P. Steffe. "Exercise as an adjunct to weight loss and maintenance in moderately obese subjects." *American Journal of Clinical Nutrition* 49:1115-1123, 1989.

4. Wescott, W. L. "You can sell exercise for weight loss." *Fitness Management*, Vol 7(12):33-34, 1991.

Are You A Psychological Overeater?

Psychological overeaters generally fall into several distinct categories. Finding yourself in one of these categories is no cause for panic. Becoming aware of when, why, and where you overeat can help you avoid the triggers that lead to nonstop nibbling. To find out where you fit in, answer the questions below as follows:

0 = never   1 = once in a while   2 = fairly often   3 = regularly

The category with the highest score gives you your basic overeating style.

Nervous Night Eater

_____ I often skimp on meals until nightfall, then I stuff my face non-stop.
_____ I crave sweet, salty, or high-fat snacks.
_____ I often munch in front of the TV starting with the evening news on through the late show.
_____ I often conduct midnight raids on the refrigerator.
_____ I have trouble getting to sleep or staying asleep.
_____ I drink more than three cups of coffee a day.
_____ On a scale of 1 to 10, I'd say my stress level rates a 9 or 10.
_____ I've been called a worrywart.

Compulsive Eater

_____ I often skip sit-down meals and usually eat on the run.
_____ I'm rarely without some type of food in my mouth.
_____ I'd rather eat food — even when I'm not hungry — than waste it.
_____ I crave foods that are sweet, starchy, and soft (but I'll eat anything).
_____ I usually sneak food when no one is around to see me eat it.
_____ My favorite beverage is diet soda — lots of it.
_____ I'm cheery on the outside, but inside I feel lonely and blue.
_____ My love life is either stressful or nonexistent.

Closet Binge Eater

_____ About three times a month, I suddenly pig out uncontrollably.
_____ When I binge, I gobble food fast and steadily, easily polishing off an entire bag of cookies.
_____ I binge in private and usually at night.
_____ My binges usually are triggered when I'm upset or stressed out.
_____ Immediately after bingeing I feel calm, but later ashamed and furious at myself.
_____ After a binge, I often fast or crash diet.
_____ Often after bingeing, my stomach aches or I have trouble sleeping.
_____ I often feel angry and depressed but don't know why.

Hand-Me-Down Eater

_____ My family devours king-size portions of rich food at every meal.
_____ My parents and siblings are overweight.
_____ My family frequently snacks together in front of the TV.
_____ The most exercise my family gets is reaching for seconds on pie.
_____ Both my mother and I love to cook.
_____ Having a well-stocked pantry makes me feel secure and loved.

(Continued)

Are You A Psychological Overeater? (Continued)

_____ My mother always serves an extravagant dinner with rich desserts.
_____ My family celebrates even minor occasions with lavish feasts.

Thin/Fat
_____ I was overweight as a teenager and now am deathly afraid of gaining weight.
_____ It's a never-ending battle to stay thin.
_____ I eat nothing but low-calorie meals.
_____ I nag those close to me if they gain even a pound or two because I detest fat people.
_____ My life would be ruined if I were to gain weight.
_____ I can tell you the fat and calorie count of nearly every food.
_____ Fat people are weak and have no will power.
_____ Bingeing is the furthest thing from my mind.

Chronic Dieter
_____ I've tried all the latest diets and read all the diet books, but none of them are any good.
_____ Within a few months of losing weight, I'm back to my former fat self.
_____ I often crash-diet before a party or important social event.
_____ I know more than most people about diets, nutrition, and psychological causes for weight gain.
_____ I can tell you exactly how and why I lost and regained every pound.
_____ I've memorized the calorie count for foods from A to Z.
_____ Weight-loss groups and doctors have all failed me.
_____ I'm into quick and easy weight loss.

Environmental Eater
_____ I can't resist the aromas emanating from a bakery.
_____ Just reading about luscious dessert recipes makes me drool.
_____ TV food commercials send me to the refrigerator.
_____ Eating food goes along with the territory of my job — power lunches, social dinners, etc.
_____ I eat more than most people at meals.
_____ When dining out, I rarely pass up the pastry dessert cart.
_____ I've begun to develop love handles on my waist and batwings under my arms.
_____ I rarely turn down an extra helping or a meal, even if I'm not hungry — if it's there, I'll eat it.

Couch Potato
_____ I prefer curling up with a bag of chips to physical activity.
_____ The most exercise I get these days is lifting a fork to my mouth.
_____ It takes fewer and fewer calories to maintain the same weight.
_____ I wouldn't be caught dead in workout gear.
_____ Walking to stores at the mall is an effort.
_____ I'm stressed and anxious most of the time.
_____ I sit behind a desk all day.
_____ Once I could have danced all night, but since I've gained weight, I can barely shuffle to the TV.

Adapted from John Feltman and the editors of *Prevention* Magazine, "Improving Your Eating Style," *Food and Nutrition* (Emmaus, PA: Rodale Press, 1993). Used by permission.

Setting Your Dietary Priorities

More than 300 top nutrition experts in a poll conducted by Medical Consensus Surveys, a research arm of *Prevention* Magazine, were asked to rate 44 nutritional actions (all purported to benefit health) as follows: extremely important, very important, important, not important but may help, or probably worthless. The nutritionists' responses then were compiled and statistically weighted to create a list of dietary "top priorities" for preserving and boosting your health.

Priority/Ranking	Action
Very High Priority	
79	Control calorie intake to control your weight
76	Reduce all dietary fats
75	Control fat intake to control your weight
High Priority	
71	Increase physical activity to enable greater nutrient intake
71	Enjoy your food
70	Balance your diet among the five food groups
69	Ensure adequate intake of vitamins and minerals to meet the RDAs
65	Replace saturated fats with monosaturated and polysaturated fats
65	If not pregnant or trying to conceive, limit your alcohol intake to one or two drinks per day
63	Replace whole-milk products with low-fat and nonfat dairy products
63	Avoid raw eggs, raw meat, and raw seafood
62	Increase total fiber to at least 20 grams per day
62	Eat more complex carbohydrates, such as grains, rice, beans, potatoes, bread, and pasta
61	Eat more fish in place of meat
59	Ensure adequate intake of soluble fiber
57	Avoid very low calorie diets
56	Cut meat portions to 3 to 4 ounces
55	Reduce dietary cholesterol
54	Ensure adequate intake of insoluble fiber
54	Eat at least five fruits and vegetables per day
54	Eat breakfast
51	Reduce sodium intake
Moderate Priority	
49	Increase intake of cruciferous vegetables, such as broccoli, cauliflower, kale, and others
49	Avoid eating large meals and snacking excessively in the evening when activity levels tend to be low
48	Switch from butter to margarine
48	Restrict intake of tropical oils
47	Drink six to eight 8-ounce glasses of water (or decaffeinated, low-calorie, and low-fat fluids) every day
47	Avoid nitrates and nitrites (smoked and cured foods)
44	Reduce trans-fatty acids (e.g., stick margarine, hydrogenated vegetable shortening)
43	Reduce sugar intake
41	Eat three square meals a day with a minimum of snacking in between
41	Eat only when you're hungry (regardless of whether it's mealtime or not) and only to satiety
40	Limit your daily caffeine consumption to the amount in 4 cups of coffee
38	Peel or wash fruit before eating to avoid pesticides
37	Increase beta-carotene intake
37	Switch from stick margarine to soft (tub) and liquid margarine
37	Have a regular nutritional assessment
30	Eliminate alcohol from your diet
29	Restrict your intake of phosphorus
Low Priority	
24	Increase intake of vitamin E beyond the RDA without exceeding safe limits
23	Increase intake of vitamin C beyond the RDA without exceeding safe limits
16	Make breakfast the biggest meal of the day
14	Avoid irradiated foods
13	Avoid overgrilled (i.e., charred) or blackened foods

Note: The numbers in the left column represent the relative importance of each positive action, based on a scale of 0 (not important) to 100 (extremely important).

11

CARDIOVASCULAR WELLNESS

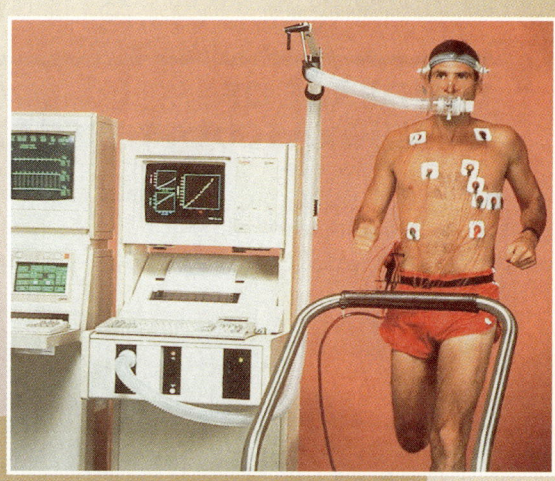

Objectives

- ▼ Define cardiovascular disease and coronary heart disease.
- ▼ Teach the importance of a healthy lifestyle in preventing cardiovascular disease.
- ▼ Discuss the major risk factors that lead to the development of coronary heart disease.
- ▼ Present guidelines for cardiovascular disease prevention.

At the beginning of the 20th century, the most common health problems in the United States were infectious diseases such as tuberculosis, diphtheria, influenza, kidney disease, polio, and other diseases of infancy. Progress in the field of medicine largely eliminated these diseases. Nevertheless, as the American people started to enjoy the "good life" (sedentary living, alcohol, fatty foods, excessive sweets, tobacco, drugs), a parallel increase was seen in chronic diseases such as cancer, diabetes, emphysema, cirrhosis of the liver, and, in particular, diseases of the cardiovascular system.

As the incidence of chronic diseases grew, it became clear that prevention was the best medicine. Consequently, a new fitness and wellness trend gradually developed over the last three decades. People began to realize that good health is largely self-controlled and that the leading causes of premature death and illness in the United States could be prevented by adhering to positive lifestyle habits.

▼ INCIDENCE OF CARDIOVASCULAR DISEASE

Cardiovascular disease is the leading cause of death in the United States, accounting for more than 42% of the total mortality rate in 1990. The disease encompasses all pathological conditions that affect the heart and the circulatory system (blood vessels). Some examples of cardiovascular diseases are coronary heart disease, peripheral vascular disease, congenital heart disease, rheumatic heart disease, atherosclerosis, strokes, hypertension (high blood pressure), and congestive heart failure.

Although heart and blood vessel disease is still the number-one health problem in the United States, the incidence has declined by 36% in the last two decades (see Figure 11.1). The main reasons for this dramatic decrease are health education and better treatment modalities. More people now are aware of the risk factors for cardiovascular disease and are changing their lifestyles to lower their own potential risk for this disease.

According to the 1990 estimates by the American Heart Association, over 70 million Americans were afflicted by diseases of the cardiovascular system, including nearly 64 million with hypertension and more than 6 million with coronary heart disease. Many of these individuals have more than one type of cardiovascular disease.

In addition, the 1991 estimated cost of heart and blood vessel disease exceeded $101 billion. Heart attacks alone cost American industry approximately 132 million workdays annually, including $15 billion in lost productivity because of physical and emotional disability.

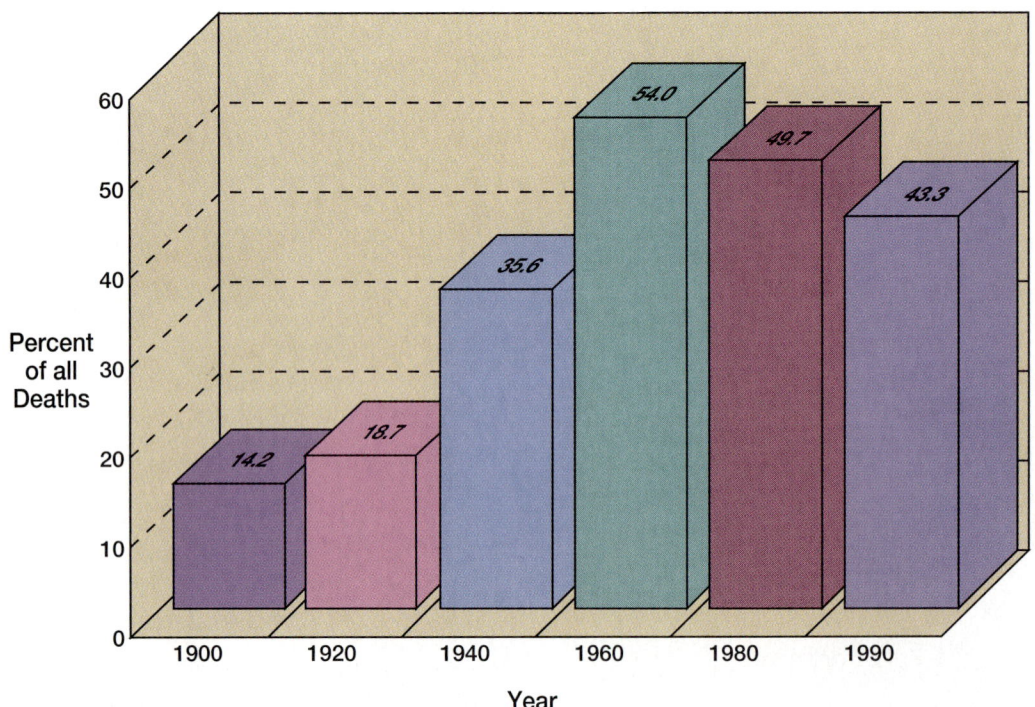

FIGURE 11.1 ▼ Incidence of cardiovascular disease in the United States for selected year: 1900–1990.

CORONARY HEART DISEASE

The major form of cardiovascular disease is coronary heart disease (CHD), a condition in which the arteries that supply the heart muscle with oxygen and nutrients are narrowed by fatty deposits such as cholesterol and triglycerides. Narrowing of the coronary arteries diminishes the blood supply to the heart muscle, which can precipitate a heart attack (see Figure 11.2).

CHD is the single leading cause of death in the United States, accounting for approximately a third of all deaths and more than half of all cardiovascular deaths. Oddly enough, almost all of the risk factors for CHD are preventable and reversible, and individuals can control them by modifying their lifestyle.

More than 1.5 million people have heart attacks each year, and more than half a million of them die as a result. About half the time, the first symptom of coronary heart disease is the heart attack itself, and 40% of the people who have a first heart attack die within the first 24 hours. In one of every five cardiovascular deaths, sudden death is the initial symptom.

About half of those who die are men in their most productive years, between ages 40 and 65. Furthermore, the American Heart Association estimates that in excess of $700 million a year is spent in replacing employees who had heart attacks.

The leading risk factors contributing to CHD are:

- Physical inactivity
- Low HDL-cholesterol
- Elevated LDL-cholesterol
- Smoking

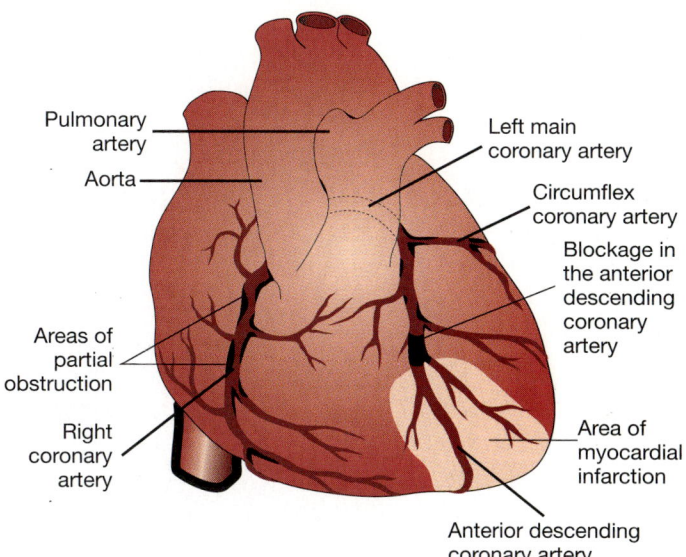

FIGURE 11.2 ▼ Myocardial infarction (heart attack) as a result of acute reduction in blood flow through the anterior descending coronary artery.

- High blood pressure
- Abnormal stress or resting electrocardiogram
- Family history of heart disease
- Personal history of heart disease
- Diabetes
- Excessive body fat
- Elevated triglycerides
- Tension and stress
- Age

Although genetic inheritance plays a role in CHD, the most important determinant is personal lifestyle. With the exception of age, family history of heart disease, and certain electrocardiogram (ECG) abnormalities, the risk factors are preventable and reversible.

Studies have documented further that multiple interrelations usually exist between risk factors. Physical inactivity, for instance, often contributes to an increase in (a) body weight (fat), (b) cholesterol, (c) triglycerides, (d) tension and stress, (e) blood pressure, and (f) risk for diabetes. The interrelationships among leading cardiovascular risk factors are depicted in Figure 11.3.

PHYSICAL INACTIVITY

Physical inactivity is responsible for low levels of cardiovascular endurance, previously defined as the ability of the lungs, heart, and blood vessels to

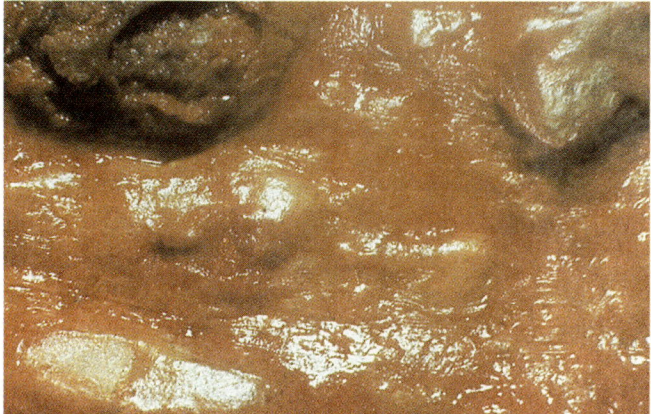

Buildup of fatty plaque on inner lining of an artery from atherosclerosis.

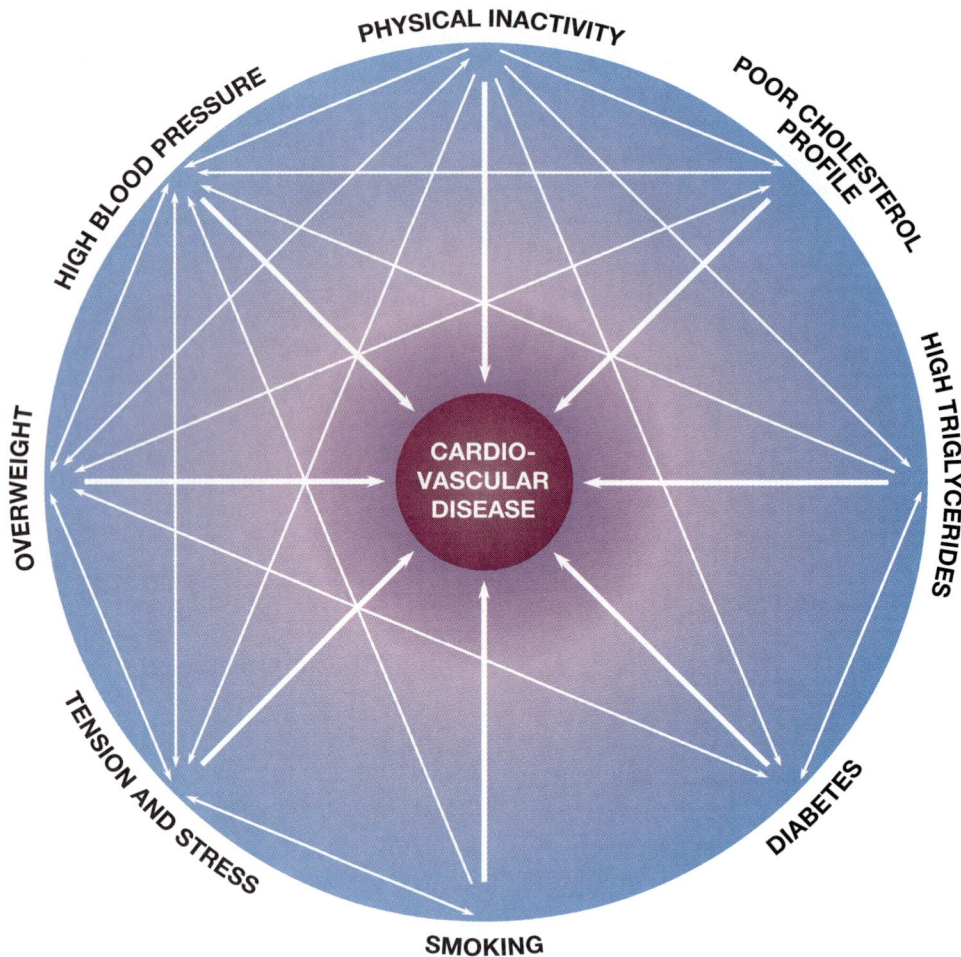

FIGURE 11.3 ▼ Interrelationships among leading cardiovascular risk factors.

deliver enough oxygen to the cells to meet the demands of prolonged physical activity. Improving cardiovascular endurance through aerobic exercise may have the greatest impact in reducing overall risk for heart disease. Although specific recommendations can be followed to improve each risk factor, a regular aerobic exercise program helps control most of the major risk factors that lead to heart disease. Dr. Kenneth Cooper, pioneer of the aerobic movement in the United States, says the evidence of the benefits of aerobic exercise in reducing heart disease is far too impressive to be ignored.

Aerobic exercise: (a) increases cardiovascular endurance, (b) decreases and controls blood pressure, (c) reduces body fat, (d) lowers blood lipids (cholesterol and triglycerides), (e) improves HDL-cholesterol, (f) helps control diabetes, (g) increases and maintains good heart function, sometimes improving certain ECG abnormalities, (h) motivates toward smoking cessation, (i) alleviates tension and stress, and (j) counteracts a personal history of heart disease.

Research at the Institute for Aerobics Research in Dallas, Texas, clearly shows the tie between cardiovascular fitness and mortality, regardless of age and other risk factors (see Figure 11.4).[1] A higher level of physical fitness benefits even those who have other risk factors such as high blood pressure and serum cholesterol, cigarette smoking, and a family history of heart disease.

Although the findings show that the higher the level of cardiovascular fitness, the longer the life, the largest drop in premature death is seen between the unfit (group 1) and the moderately fit (groups 2 and 3). Even small improvements in cardiovascular endurance, greatly decrease the risk for cardiovascular mortality. Most adults who take part in a moderate exercise program can attain these fitness levels easily.

The American Heart Association acknowledged the importance of physical activity in preventing

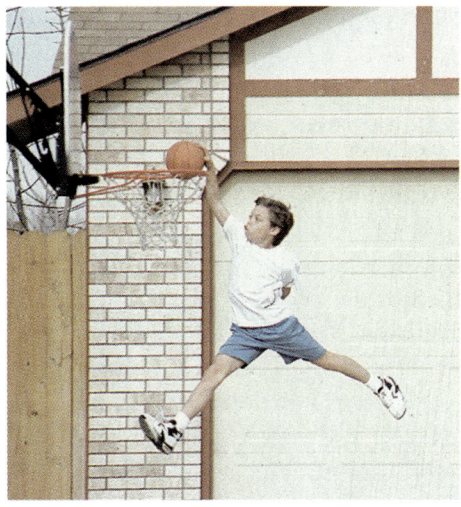
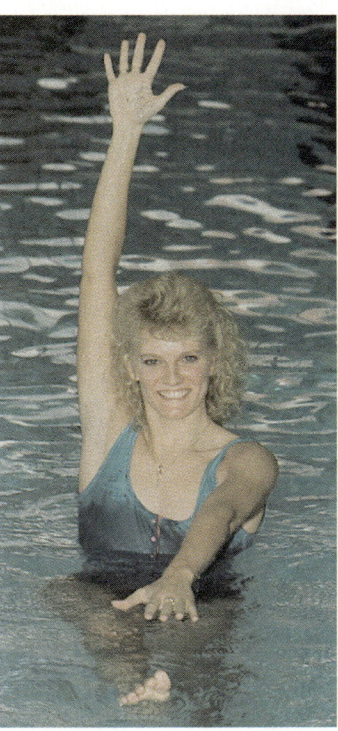
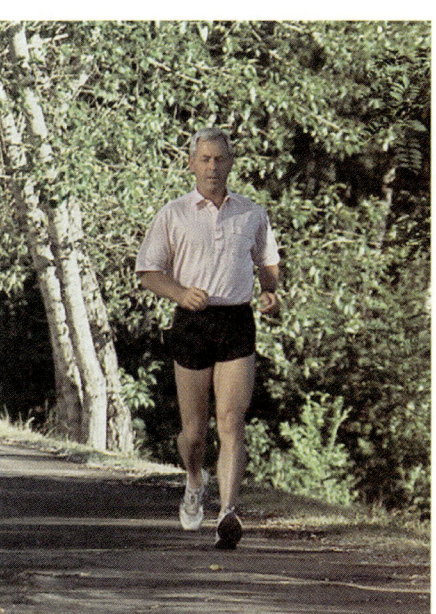

Lifetime participation in aerobic activities is one of the most important factors in preventing cardiovascular disease.

CHD when it added physical inactivity as one of the four major risk factors for this disease in 1992. The other three factors are smoking, high blood pressure, and abnormal cholesterol.

Subsequent research published in 1993 in the *New England Journal of Medicine* substantiated the importance of exercise in CHD prevention.[2] Dr. Ralph Paffenbarger and his colleagues indicated that

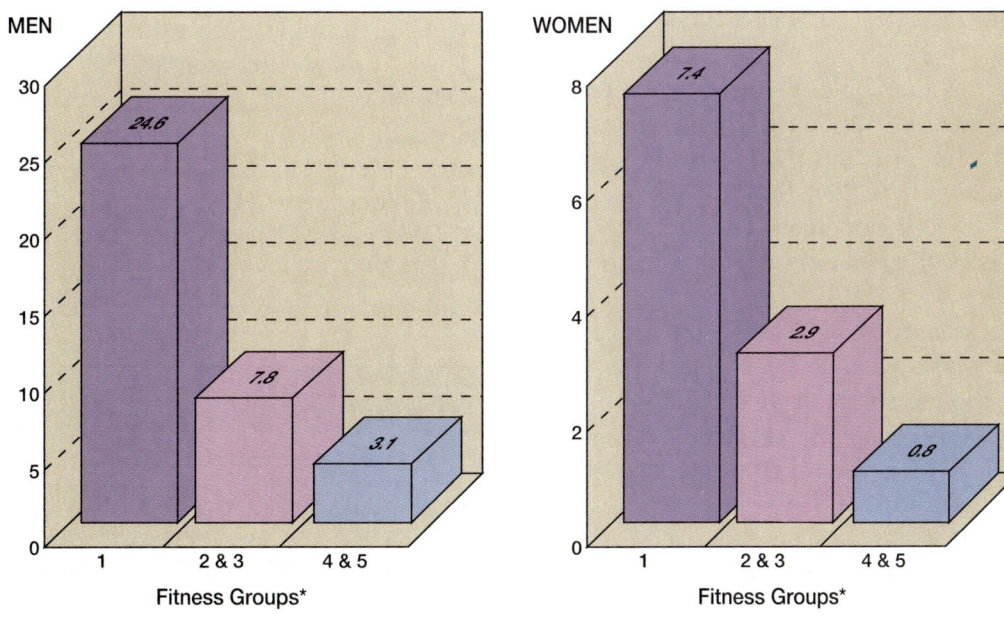

*Least fit group = 1, Most fit group = 5

From S. N. Blair, H. W. Kohl, III, R. S. Paffenbarger, Jr, D. G. Clark, K. H. Cooper, and L. W. Gibbons, "Physical Fitness and All-Cause Mortality: A Prospective Study of Healthy Men and Women." *Journal of the American Medical Association,* 262 (1989), 2395–2401.

FIGURE 11.4 ▼ Age-Adjusted Cardiovascular Death Rates per 10,000 Person-Years of Follow-up (1970–1985) by Physical Fitness Groups in the Aerobics Center Longitudinal Study, Dallas, Texas (one person-year indicates one person followed up 1 year later).

starting a moderate to vigorous physical activity program was as important as quitting smoking, managing blood pressure, or controlling cholesterol. The increase in physical activity resulted in the same decrease in relative risk for death from CHD as giving up cigarette smoking.

Even though aerobically fit individuals have a lower incidence of cardiovascular disease, a regular aerobic exercise program by itself does not guarantee a lifetime free of cardiovascular problems. Poor lifestyle habits, such as smoking, eating too many fatty/salty/sweet foods, being overweight, and having high stress levels, increase cardiovascular risk and will not be eliminated completely through aerobic exercise.

ABNORMAL CHOLESTEROL PROFILE

Cholesterol is a waxy substance, technically a steroid alcohol, found only in animal fats and oil. This fatty substance is essential for specific metabolic functions in the body, but an abnormal cholesterol profile contributes to atherosclerotic plaque, a buildup of fatty tissue in the walls of the arteries. As the plaque builds up, it blocks the blood vessels that supply the heart muscle (myocardium) with oxygen and nutrients, and these obstructions can trigger a myocardial infarction or heart attack (see Figure 11.2).

Cholesterol is carried in the bloodstream by molecules of protein known as high-density lipoproteins (HDLs), low-density lipoproteins (LDLs), and very low-density lipoproteins (VLDLs). Subcategories of these lipoproteins have been identified recently, but the discussion here focuses only on these major categories.

Cholesterol has received much attention lately because direct relationships have been established between high total cholesterol, high LDL-cholesterol and low HDL-cholesterol, and the rate of CHD in both men and women. Unfortunately, the heart disguises its problems quite well and typical symptoms of heart disease, such as angina pectoris or chest pain, do not start until the arteries are about 75% blocked. In many cases, the first symptom is sudden death.

The general recommendation by the National Cholesterol Education Program (NCEP) is to keep total cholesterol levels below 200 mg/dl. Other health professionals recommend that total cholesterol in individuals age 30 and younger should not be higher than 180 mg/dl, and for children the level should be below 170 mg/dl. Cholesterol levels between 200 and 239 mg/dl are borderline high, and levels of 240 mg/dl and above indicate high risk for disease (see Table 11.1).

Cholesterol is transported primarily in the form of LDL and HDL. The low-density molecules tend to release cholesterol, which then may penetrate the lining or inner membrane of the arteries and speed up the process of atherosclerosis. The National Cholesterol Education Program (NCEP) guidelines state that an LDL-cholesterol value below 130 mg/dl is desirable, between 130 and 159 mg/dl is borderline-high, and 160 mg/dl and above carries high risk for cardiovascular disease.

HDL-cholesterol, on the other hand, tends to attract cholesterol, which is carried to the liver to be metabolized and excreted. HDLs act as "scavengers," removing cholesterol from the body and preventing plaque from forming in the arteries. The more HDL-cholesterol, the better. HDL-cholesterol is the "good cholesterol" and offers some protection against heart disease.

New evidence suggests that low levels of HDL-cholesterol could be the best predictor of CHD and may be more significant than the total value. Substantial research supports the evidence that a low level of HDL-cholesterol has the strongest relationship to CHD at all levels of total cholesterol, including levels below 200 mg/dl. The recommended HDL-cholesterol value to minimize the risk for CHD is 45 mg/dl or higher. Guidelines for the various types of cholesterol are given in Table 11.1.

For the most part, HDL-cholesterol is determined genetically. Generally, women have higher values than men. This is one of the reasons heart disease is less common in women. Black children and adult

TABLE 11.1 ▼ Cholesterol Guidelines

	Amount	Rating
Total Cholesterol	<200 mg/dl	Desirable
	200–239 mg/dl	Borderline high
	≥240 mg/dl	High risk
LDL-Cholesterol	<130 mg/dl	Desirable
	130-159 mg/dl	Borderline high
	≥160 mg/dl	High risk
HDL-Cholesterol	≥45 mg/dl	Desirable
	36–44 mg/dl	Moderate risk
	≤35 mg/dl	High risk

black men have higher values than caucasians. HDL-cholesterol also decreases with age.

Increasing HDL-cholesterol improves the cholesterol profile and decreases the risk for CHD. Habitual aerobic exercise, weight loss, and quitting smoking all have been shown to raise HDL-cholesterol. Beta-carotene and drug therapy also promote higher HDL-cholesterol levels.

HDL-cholesterol and a regular aerobic exercise program are clearly related, but the exercise program has to be intense to decrease LDL and increase HDL. Twenty minutes of aerobic exercise three times per week may not be enough to alter a lipid profile very much. Individual responses to aerobic exercise differ but, generally, the more the exercise, the higher the HDL-cholesterol level. Aerobic exercise five to six times a week and up to 60 minutes a session in the proper heart rate target zone may be needed to see results.

The antioxidant effect of vitamins C and E and beta-carotene also can lower the risk for CHD. Antioxidants prevent oxygen from combining with other substances it may damage. During metabolism, oxygen is used to convert carbohydrates and fats into energy. In doing so, oxygen is transformed into stable forms of water and carbon dioxide. A small amount of oxygen, however, ends up in an unstable form, called free radicals. These free radicals attack and damage proteins and lipids, in particular the cell membrane and DNA.

Free radicals are thought to play a key role in the development of conditions such as heart disease, cancer, and emphysema. Researchers believe antioxidants offer protection by absorbing free radicals before they can cause damage and also by interrupting the sequence of reactions once damage has begun, thwarting certain chronic diseases.

New information suggests that a single unstable free radical can damage LDL particles. Vitamin C seems to inactivate free radicals, and vitamin E protects LDL from oxidation. Beta-carotene not only absorbs free radicals, keeping them from causing damage, but it also seems to increase HDL levels.

Certain cholesterol-lowering drugs also may help raise HDL levels. Clinical data have shown an improvement when HDL-cholesterol is increased with colestipol plus niacin and the diet is low in fat and saturated fat.

Although the average American consumes between 400 and 600 mg of cholesterol daily, the body actually manufactures more than that. Approximately 1000 mg of cholesterol per day is produced from saturated fats. Saturated fats are found mostly in meats and dairy products but seldom in foods of plant origin. Poultry and fish contain less saturated fat than beef does, but they should be eaten in moderation (about 3 to 6 ounces per day). Unsaturated fats are mainly of plant origin and cannot be converted to cholesterol.

Because of individual differences, a few people can have higher-than-normal intakes of saturated fats and still maintain normal cholesterol levels. Conversely, some people with a lower intake can have abnormally high cholesterol levels.

If LDL-cholesterol is higher than recommended, it can be lowered by losing body fat, manipulating the diet, and taking medication. A diet low in fat, saturated fat, and cholesterol, and high in complex carbohydrates and fiber is recommended to decrease LDL-cholesterol. The NCEP recommends replacing saturated fat with monounsaturated fat (for example, olive, canola, peanut, and sesame oils), because the latter does not cause a reduction in HDL-cholesterol.

Many experts believe that to have a significant effect in lowering LDL-cholesterol, total fat consumption must be significantly lower than the current 30% of total daily caloric intake guideline. Saturated fat consumption ideally should be less than 10% of the total daily caloric intake, and average cholesterol consumption should be much lower than 300 mg per day. Research studies on the effects of a 30%-fat diet have shown that it has little or no effect in lowering cholesterol, and CHD actually continues to progress in people who have the disease.

The good news comes from a 1991 study published by Dr. James Barnard in the *Archives of Internal Medicine*.[3] In this investigation the participants followed a 10% or less fat-calorie diet combined with a regular aerobic exercise program, primarily walking. In the diet, cholesterol intake was limited to less than 25 mg/day. The report indicated that the participants lowered their cholesterol by an average of 23% in only 3 weeks. The author of the study concluded that the exact percent fat guideline (10% or 15%) is unknown but that 30% total fat calories is definitely too much when attempting to lower cholesterol.

A daily 10%-total-fat diet requires that the person limit fat intake to an absolute minimum. Some health care professionals contend that a diet like this is difficult to follow indefinitely. People with high cholesterol levels may not need to follow that diet indefinitely but should adopt the 10%-fat diet while attempting to lower cholesterol. Thereafter, eating a 30%-fat diet may be adequate to maintain recommended cholesterol levels. Based on a 1991 national survey, current fat consumption in the United States averages 37% of total calories.

HIGH TRIGLYCERIDES

Triglycerides also are known as free fatty acids. In combination with cholesterol, they speed up formation of plaque. These fatty acids are carried in the bloodstream primarily by VLDLs and chylomicrons.

Although triglycerides are found in poultry skin, lunch meats, and shellfish, they are manufactured mainly in the liver, from refined sugars, starches, and alcohol. High intake of alcohol and sugars (honey included) raises triglyceride levels. They can be lowered by cutting down on these foods along with reducing weight (if overweight) and doing aerobic exercise. An optimal blood triglyceride level is less than 100 mg/dl (see Table 11.2).

Some people consistently have slightly elevated triglyceride levels (above 140 mg/dl) and HDL-cholesterol levels below 35 mg/dl. About 80% of these individuals have a genetic condition called LDL phenotype B (approximately 40% of the U.S. population falls in this category). Although the blood lipids may not be notably high, these people are at higher risk for atherosclerosis and CHD.

People who never have had a blood chemistry test should do so. An initial test always is useful to establish a baseline for future reference. The blood test should include the HDL-cholesterol component.

Although no definite guidelines have been set, after a person has an initial normal baseline test and keeps recommended dietary and exercise guidelines, a blood analysis every 3 years prior to age 35 should suffice. After age 35, individuals should have a blood lipid test every year, in conjunction with a regular preventive medicine physical examination.

TABLE 11.2 ▼ Triglycerides Guidelines

Amount	Rating
<125 mg/dl	Desirable
126–499 mg/dl	Borderline high
≥500 mg/dl	High risk

SMOKING

Cigarette smoking is the single largest preventable cause of illness and premature death in the United States. When considering all related deaths, tobacco is responsible for 450,000 unnecessary deaths per year. About 50,000 of those who die are nonsmokers who were exposed to second-hand smoke. Smoking has been linked to cardiovascular disease, cancer, bronchitis, emphysema, and peptic ulcers. In relation to coronary disease, not only does smoking speed up the process of atherosclerosis, but the risk of sudden death following a myocardial infarction also increases threefold.

Smoking prompts the release of nicotine and another 1,200 toxic compounds or so into the bloodstream. Similar to hypertension, many of these substances destroy the inner membrane that protects the walls of the arteries. Once damage to the lining occurs, cholesterol and triglycerides can be deposited readily in the arterial wall. As the plaque builds up, it obstructs blood flow through the arteries.

Furthermore, smoking encourages the formation of blood clots, which can completely block an artery already narrowed by atherosclerosis. In addition, carbon monoxide, a byproduct of cigarette smoke, decreases the blood's oxygen-carrying capacity. A combination of obstructed arteries, nicotine, and less oxygen in the heart muscle heightens the risk for a serious heart problem.

Smoking also increases heart rate, raises blood pressure, and irritates the heart, which can trigger fatal cardiac arrhythmias (irregular heart rhythms). Another harmful effect is a decrease in HDL-cholesterol, the "good" type that helps control blood lipids. Smoking actually presents a much greater risk of death from heart disease than from lung disease.

Pipe and cigar smoking and chewing tobacco also increase the risk for heart disease. Even if no smoke is inhaled, toxic substances are absorbed through the membranes of the mouth and end up in the bloodstream.

PERSONAL AND FAMILY HISTORY

Individuals who have had cardiovascular problems are at higher risk than those who never have had a problem. People with this history should control the other risk factors as much as they can. Because most risk factors are reversible, this will greatly decrease the risk for future problems. The more time that has passed since the cardiovascular problem occurred, the lower is the risk for recurrence.

Genetic predisposition toward heart disease has been clearly demonstrated and seems to be gaining in importance. All other factors being equal, a person with blood relatives who have or had heart disease before age 60, runs a greater risk than someone who has no such history. The younger the age at which the incident happened to the relative, the greater is the risk for the disease.

In many cases, we have no way of knowing whether a person's true genetic predisposition or simply poor lifestyle habits led to a heart problem. A person may have been physically inactive, overweight, smoked, and had bad dietary habits, leading to a heart attack. Because we cannot differentiate these factors reliably, a person with a family history of cardiovascular problems should watch all other factors closely and maintain as low a risk level as possible. In addition, an annual blood chemistry analysis is recommended strongly to make sure the body is handling blood lipids properly.

HIGH BLOOD PRESSURE (HYPERTENSION)

Blood pressure is a measure of the force exerted against the walls of the blood vessels by the blood flowing through them. Blood pressure is assessed using a sphygmomanometer and a stethoscope. The sphygmomanometer consists of an inflatable bladder contained within a cuff and a mercury gravity manometer or an aneroid manometer from which the pressure is read. The pressure is measured in milliliters of mercury and usually expressed in two numbers. Ideal blood pressure should be 120/80 or below (see Table 11.3). The higher number reflects the pressure exerted during the forceful contraction of the heart or systole (therefore, the name "systolic" pressure), and the lower pressure is taken during the heart's relaxation, or diastolic phase, when no blood is being ejected.

TABLE 11.3 ▼ Blood Pressure Guidelines

Rating	Systolic	Diastolic
Ideal	≤120	≤80 mmHg
Borderline high	121–139	81–89 mmHg
Hypertension	≥140	≥90 mmHg

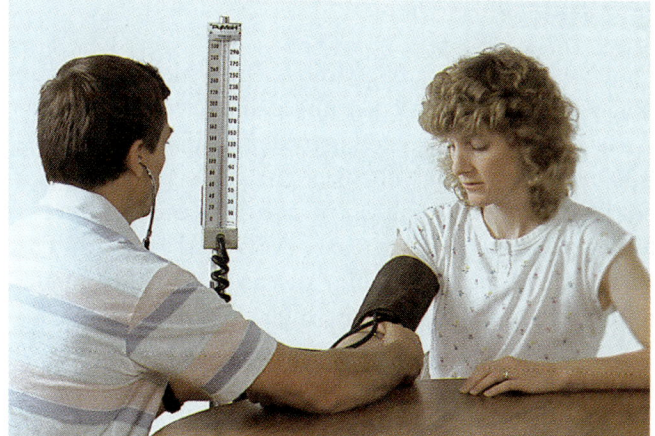

Blood pressure assessment using a mercury gravity manometer.

Based on current American Heart Association estimates, almost 64 million adults and close to 3 million children (6 to 17 years old) in the United States are hypertensive. Hypertension has been viewed as the point at which the pressure doubles the mortality risk, about 160/96. Statistical evidence clearly indicates, however, that blood pressure readings above 140/90 increase the risk of disease and premature death. Therefore, the American Heart Association considers all blood pressures above 140/90 as hypertension.

Even though the threshold for hypertension has been set at 140/90, many experts believe that the lower the blood pressure, the better. Even if the pressure is around 90/50, as long as individuals do not have any symptoms of low blood pressure or hypotension, they do not need to be concerned. Typical hypotension symptoms are dizziness, lightheadedness, and fainting.

Blood pressure may fluctuate during a regular day. Many factors affect blood pressure, and one single reading may not be a true indicator of your real pressure. For example, physical activity and stress increase blood pressure, whereas rest and relaxation decrease it. Consequently, several measurements should be taken before diagnosing elevated pressure.

As a disease, hypertension has been called the silent killer. It does not hurt, it does not make you feel sick, and unless you check it, years may go by before you even realize you have a problem. High blood pressure is a risk factor not only for CHD but also for congestive heart failure, strokes, and kidney failure.

DIABETES

Diabetes mellitus is a condition in which the blood glucose is unable to enter the cells because the pancreas either totally stops producing insulin or does not produce enough to meet the body's needs. As a result, glucose absorption by the cells and the liver is low, leading to high glucose levels in the blood. The incidence of cardiovascular disease and death in the diabetic population is quite high. People with chronically elevated blood glucose levels also may have problems in metabolizing fats, which can make them more susceptible to atherosclerosis, increase the risk for coronary disease, and lead to other conditions such as vision loss and kidney damage.

Fasting blood glucose levels above 120 mg/dl may be an early sign of diabetes and should be brought to the attention of a physician. Many health care practitioners consider blood glucose levels around 150 to 160 mg/dl as borderline diabetes (see Table 11.4).

The two major types of diabetes are: Type I, or insulin-dependent diabetes, and Type II, or non-insulin-dependent diabetes. Type I also is called juvenile diabetes because it is found mainly in young people. In insulin-dependent diabetes, the pancreas produces little or no insulin. In non-insulin-dependent (Type II) diabetes, often referred to as adult-onset diabetes, the insulin-producing cells function adequately but the body is unable to use insulin properly.

Although there is a genetic predisposition to diabetes, adult-onset diabetes is related closely to overeating, obesity, and lack of physical activity. In most cases, this condition can be corrected through a special diet, a weight-loss program, and a regular exercise program. A diet high in water-soluble fibers (found in fruits, vegetables, oats, and beans) is helpful in treating diabetes. An aerobic exercise program — walking, cycling, or swimming four to five times per week — often is prescribed because it increases the body's sensitivity to insulin. Individuals who have high blood glucose levels should consult a physician to decide on the best treatment.

According to research by Dr. Susan Helmrich and colleagues published in 1991 in the *New England Journal of Medicine*,[4] aerobic exercise helps prevent diabetes in middle-aged men. The protective effect is even greater in those with risk factors such as obesity, high blood pressure, and family propensity.

This preventive effect is attributed to lowered body fat and better sugar and fat metabolism through a regular exercise program. At 3,500 calories expended per week through exercise, the risk was cut in half when compared to sedentary men. The preventive effect, the study suggests, should hold for women, too.

EXCESSIVE BODY FAT

Body composition is the ratio of lean body weight to fat weight. If the body contains too much fat, the person is considered obese. Obesity long has been recognized as a primary risk factor for CHD.

Until a few years ago, experts believed that CHD actually was brought on by some of the other risk factors that usually accompany obesity (higher blood lipids, hypertension, diabetes, lower level of cardiovascular fitness). More recent evidence, however, suggests that too much body fat is a serious coronary risk factor in and of itself. Even when all of the other risk factors are within a good range, people with body fat percentages higher than the recommended standard have a higher incidence of coronary disease.

Attaining recommended body composition is important not only in decreasing cardiovascular risk but also in reaching a better state of health and wellness. The only positive thing that can be said about excess body fat is that it can be lost through a combination of diet and exercise. Dieting by itself seldom works.

People who have a weight problem and desire to achieve recommended weight can do so by (a) increasing their physical activity; (b) consuming a diet low in fat and refined sugars and high in complex carbohydrates and fiber; and (c) moderately reducing their total caloric intake while still providing all of the necessary nutrients to sustain normal body functions. Recommendations for weight management are discussed in Chapter 10.

TENSION AND STRESS

Tension and stress (the topic of Chapter 2) have become a normal part of life. Everyone has to deal

TABLE 11.4 ▼ Blood Glucose Guidelines

Amount	Rating
≤120	Desirable
121–159	Borderline high
≥160	High

daily with goals, deadlines, responsibilities, pressures. Almost everything in life (whether positive or negative) is a source of stress. The stressor itself is not what creates the health hazard but, rather, the individual's response to it.

The human body responds to stress by producing more catecholamines (hormones) to prepare the body for fight or flight. These hormones elevate heart rate, blood pressure, and blood glucose levels, enabling the person to take action.

If the person "fights or flees," the higher levels of catecholamines are metabolized and the body is able to return to a "normal" state. But, if a person is under constant stress and unable to take action (such as with the death of a close relative or friend, loss of a job, trouble at work, financial insecurity), the catecholamines remain elevated in the bloodstream.

People who are unable to relax put a constant low-level strain on the cardiovascular system that could manifest itself in heart disease. In addition, when a person is in a stressful situation, the coronary arteries that feed the heart muscle constrict, reducing the oxygen supply to the heart. If the blood vessels are significantly blocked by atherosclerosis, abnormal heart rhythms or even a heart attack may follow.

AGE

Age is a risk factor because of the greater incidence of heart disease in older people. This tendency may be induced partly by other factors stemming from changes in lifestyle as we get older (less physical activity, poor nutrition, obesity, and so on).

Young people should not think they will escape heart disease. The process begins early in life. This was clearly shown in American soldiers who died during the Korean and Vietnam conflicts. Autopsies conducted on soldiers killed at 22 years of age and younger revealed that approximately 70% had early stages of atherosclerosis. Other studies have found elevated blood cholesterol levels in children as young as 10 years old.

Even though the aging process cannot be stopped, it certainly can be slowed down. Physiological versus chronological age is an important concept in preventing disease. Some individuals in their 60s or older have the body of a 20-year-old. And 20-year-olds often are in such poor condition and health that they almost seem to have the body of a 60-year-old. Risk factor management and positive lifestyle habits are the best ways to slow down the natural aging process.

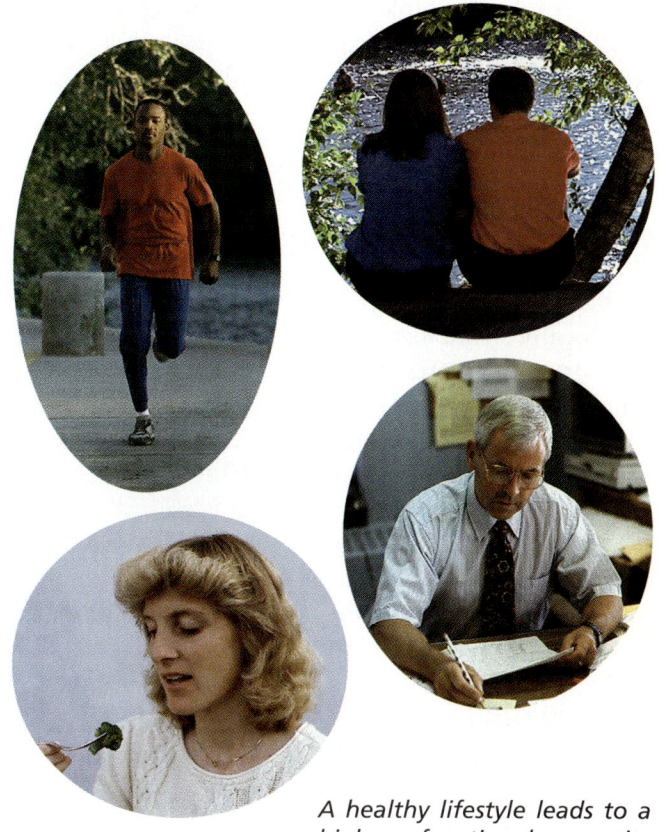

A healthy lifestyle leads to a higher functional capacity throughout life.

▼ GUIDELINES FOR PREVENTING CARDIOVASCULAR DISEASE

As discussed, most cardiovascular risk factors are preventable and reversible. Overall risk factor management is the best guideline to lower the risk. A regular aerobic exercise program in combination with proper nutrition, avoidance of tobacco, blood pressure control, stress management, and weight control are the key elements in preventing disorders of the cardiovascular system.

LIFETIME AEROBIC EXERCISE

Lifetime aerobic exercise is one of the most important activities in preventing and reducing cardiovascular problems. The basic principles for cardiovascular exercise were given in Chapter 7. In general, however, only moderate aerobic exercise is required to greatly reduce the risk of cardiovascular disease. Work at the Aerobics Research Institute in Dallas demonstrated that even small amounts of aerobic exercise can reduce cardiovascular risk considerably. A simple 40-minute walking (or equivalent) program, six to seven times per week, seems to have a strong inverse relationship with premature cardiovascular mortality.

NUTRITION RECOMMENDATIONS

Nutrition was the topic of Chapter 8. Here, we specifically relate it to cardiovascular disease prevention. In this regard, the diet should contain ample amounts of fruits, vegetables, and grains. Because of their antioxidant effect, foods high in vitamins C and E and beta-carotene should be a regular part of the diet. Foods high in sugar and salt should be avoided. Alcohol should only be consumed in moderation.

As a rule of thumb, the following guidelines are recommended to prevent LDL-cholesterol and total cholesterol elevation:

1. Consume fewer than three eggs per week.
2. Eat red meats (3 oz per serving) fewer than three times per week, and no organ meats (such as liver and kidneys).
3. Do not eat commercially baked foods.
4. Drink low-fat milk (1% or less fat, preferably) and low-fat dairy products.
5. Do not use coconut oil, palm oil, or cocoa butter.
6. Eat fish, especially those high in Omega-3 fatty acids (fresh or frozen mackerel, herring, tuna, salmon, lake trout) twice a week.
7. Bake, broil, grill, poach, or steam food instead of frying.
8. Refrigerate cooked meat prior to adding to other dishes. In this manner, fat hardened in the refrigerator can be removed before mixing the meat with other foods.
9. Avoid fatty salad dressings and sauces made with butter, cream, or cheese.
10. Maintain recommended body weight.

The combination of a healthful diet, a sound aerobic exercise program, and weight control is the best prescription for controlling blood lipids. If this approach does not work, the person should consult a physician and get a blood test to break down the lipoproteins into the various subcategories. A breakdown into the various subcategories may be difficult to obtain as most laboratories across the country do not perform these blood tests. Starting in 1991, however, the American Heart Association established six Lipid Disorder Training Centers that administer comprehensive blood tests. Your local American Heart Association can provide further information.

SMOKING CESSATION

Cigarette smoking, low levels of fitness, a poor cholesterol profile, and high blood pressure are the four major risk factors for CHD. Nonetheless, the risk for both cardiovascular disease and cancer starts to decrease the moment you quit smoking. The risk approaches that of a lifetime nonsmoker 10 and 15 years, respectively, after cessation.

Quitting cigarette smoking is no easy task. Only about 20% of smokers who try to quit for the first time succeed each year. The addictive properties of nicotine and smoke make quitting difficult. Smokers have physical and psychological withdrawal symptoms when they stop smoking. Even though giving up smoking can be extremely difficult, it is by no means impossible.

The most crucial factor in quitting cigarette smoking is the person's sincere desire to do so. More than 95% of the successful ex-smokers have been able to quit on their own, either by quitting cold turkey or by using self-help kits available from organizations such as the American Cancer Society, the American Heart Association, and the American Lung Association. Only 3% of ex-smokers have quit as a result of formal "stop smoking" programs. Chapter 13 contains a stop-smoking program.

BLOOD PRESSURE CONTROL

Of all hypertension, 90% has no definite cause. Referred to as *essential hypertension*, this type is

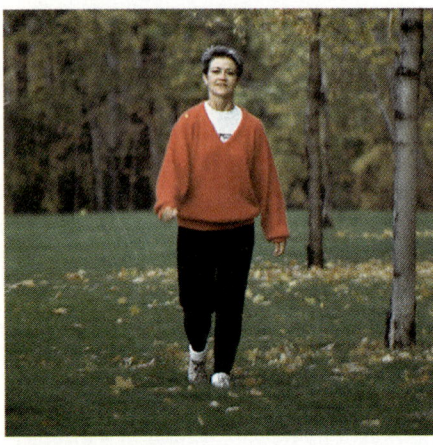

A moderate aerobic exercise program greatly reduces the risk for premature cardiovascular death.

treatable. Aerobic exercise, weight reduction, a low-sodium/high-potassium diet, stress reduction, no smoking, a diet designed to decrease blood lipids, lower caffeine and alcohol intake, and antihypertensive medication have been used effectively to treat essential hypertension. The other 10% of hypertension is caused by pathological conditions such as narrowing of the kidney arteries, glomerulonephritis (a kidney disease), tumors of the adrenal glands, and narrowing of the aortic artery. With this type of hypertension, the pathological cause has to be treated first to correct the blood pressure problem.

A major factor contributing to high blood pressure in about half of all hypertensive people is too much sodium in the diet (salt, or sodium chloride, contains approximately 40% sodium). With high sodium intake, the body retains more water, which increases the blood volume and, in turn, drives up blood pressure. Although sodium is essential for normal body functions, only 200 mg, or one-tenth of a teaspoon of salt, is required daily. Even under strenuous conditions of job and sports participation that produce heavy perspiration, the amount of sodium required is seldom more than 3,000 mg per day. Yet, sodium intake in the typical American diet ranges between 6,000 and 20,000 mg per day!

When treating high blood pressure (unless it is extremely high), many sports medicine physicians suggest trying a combination of aerobic exercise, weight loss, and reduced sodium before they recommend medication. In most instances, this treatment brings blood pressure under control.

Aerobic exercise often is prescribed in treating hypertensive patients. Several well-documented studies have indicated that nearly 90% of hypertensive patients who begin a moderate aerobic exercise program can expect a notable decrease in blood pressure after only a few weeks of training. The research data also show that exercise, not weight loss, is the major contributor to lower blood pressure. If aerobic exercise is discontinued, these changes are not maintained.

The best tip, though, is to take a preventive approach. Keeping blood pressure under control is easier than trying to bring it down once it is high. Blood pressure should be checked regularly, regardless of whether it is or is not elevated. Regular physical exercise, weight control, a low-salt diet, no smoking, and stress management are the basic guidelines for blood pressure control.

STRESS MANAGEMENT

Individuals who are under a lot of stress and do not cope well with it need to take measures to counteract the effects of stress in their lives. One of the best suggestions is to identify the sources of stress and learn how to cope with them. People need to take control of themselves, examine and act upon the things that are most important in their lives, and ignore less meaningful details. Relaxation techniques for stress management are presented in Chapter 2.

Physical exercise is one of the best ways to relieve stress. When a person takes part in physical activity, the body metabolizes excess catecholamines and is able to return to a normal state. Exercise also steps up muscular activity, which leads to muscular relaxation after completing the physical activity. Many executives prefer the evening hours for their physical activity programs, stopping after work at a health or fitness club. By doing this, they are able to "burn up" the excess tension accumulated during the day and enjoy the evening hours.

▼ RESTING AND STRESS ELECTROCARDIOGRAMS

The electrocardiogram (introduced in Chapter 7) provides a valuable measure of the heart's function. The ECG records the electrical impulses that stimulate the heart to contract. In reading an ECG, five general areas are interpreted: heart rate, heart rhythm, the heart's axis, enlargement or hypertrophy of the heart, and myocardial infarction or heart attack.

On a standard 12-lead ECG, 10 electrodes are placed on the person's chest. From these 10 electrodes, 12 "pictures" or leads of the electrical impulses are studied from 12 different positions as they travel through the heart muscle (myocardium).

By looking at ECG tracings, abnormalities in heart functioning can be identified. Based on the findings, the ECG may be interpreted as normal, equivocal, or abnormal. An ECG does not always identify problems, so a normal tracing is not an absolute guarantee. On the other hand, an abnormal tracing does not necessarily signal a serious condition.

ECGs are taken at rest, during stress of exercise and during recovery. An exercise ECG also is known as a graded exercise stress test or a maximal exercise tolerance test. Similar to a high-speed road test on a car, a stress ECG reveals the heart's tolerance to

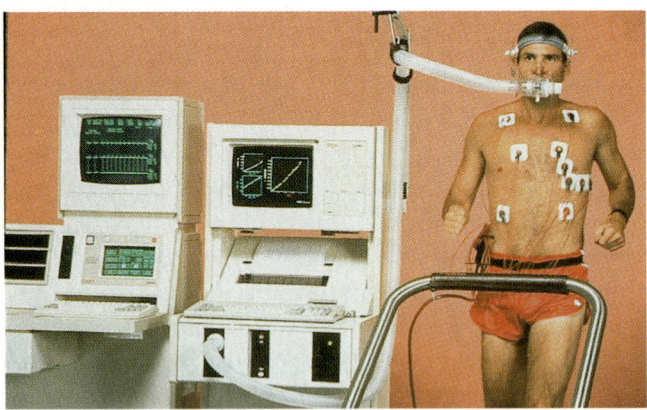

Graded treadmill exercise tolerance test with electrocardiographic monitoring (exercise stress test).

high-intensity exercise. It is a much better test to discover CHD than is a resting ECG.

Stress ECGs also are used to assess cardiovascular fitness levels, to screen individuals for preventive and cardiac rehabilitation programs, to detect abnormal blood pressure response during exercise, and to establish actual or functional maximal heart rate for exercise prescription.

Not every adult who wishes to start or continue in an exercise program needs a stress ECG. The following criteria can be applied to determine when this type of test should be administered:

1. Men over age 40 and women over age 50.
2. A total cholesterol level above 200 mg/dl, or an HDL-cholesterol below 35 mg/dl.
3. Hypertensive and diabetic patients.
4. Cigarette smokers.
5. Individuals with a family history of CHD, syncope, or sudden death before age 60.
6. People with an abnormal resting ECG.
7. All individuals with symptoms of chest discomfort, dysrhythmias, syncope, or chronotropic incompetence (a heart rate that increases slowly during exercise and never reaches maximum).

At times the stress ECG has been questioned as a reliable predictor of CHD. Even so, it remains the most practical, inexpensive, noninvasive procedure available to diagnose latent (undiagnosed/unknown) CHD. The test is accurate in diagnosing CHD about 65% of the time. Part of the problem is that many times those who administer stress ECGs do it without clearly understanding the test's indications and limitations.

The sensitivity of a stress test increases along with the severity of the disease. More accurate results also are found for people at high risk for cardiovascular disease, in particular men over 40 and women over 50 with a poor cholesterol profile, high blood pressure, or a family history of heart disease. Test protocols, number of leads, electrocardiographic criteria, and the skill of the technicians administering the test also affect its sensitivity. Despite its limitations, a stress ECG test still is a useful tool in identifying people at high risk for exercise-related sudden death.

▼ A FINAL WORD

Most of the risk factors for CHD are reversible and preventable. The fact that a person has a family history of heart disease and possibly some of the other risk factors because of neglect in lifestyle does not mean this person is doomed. A healthier lifestyle — free of cardiovascular problems — is something over which you have much control. You are encouraged to be persistent. Willpower and commitment are necessary to develop patterns that eventually will turn into healthy habits and contribute to your total well-being.

▼ NOTES

1. Blair, S. N., H. W. Kohl III, R. S. Paffenbarger, Jr, D. G. Clark, K. H. Cooper, and L. W. Gibbons. "Physical fitness and all-cause mortality: A prospective study of healthy men and women." *Journal of the American Medical Association* 262:2395-2401, 1989.

2. Paffenbarger, R. S., Jr., R. T. Hyde, A. L. Wing, I. Lee, D. L. Jung, and J. B. Kampert. "The association of changes in physical-activity level and other lifestyle characteristics with mortality among men." *The New England Journal of Medicine* 328:538-545, 1993.

3. Barnard, R. J. "Effects of life-style modification on serum lipids." *Archives of Internal Medicine* 151:1389-1394, 1991.

4. Helmrich, S. P., D. R. Ragland, R. W. Leung, and R. S. Paffenbarger. "Physical activity and reduced occurrences of non-insulin-dependent diabetes mellitus." *The New England Journal of Medicine* 325:147-152, 1991.

Chapter 12

Cancer Prevention and Wellness

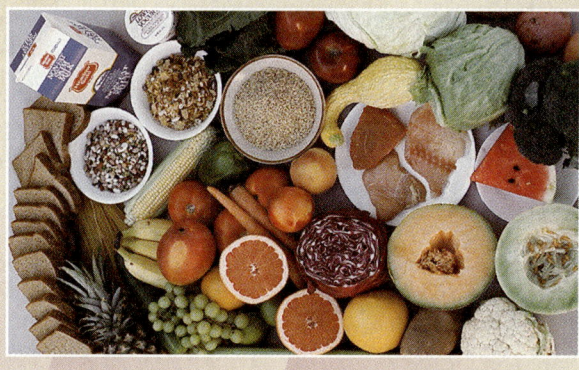
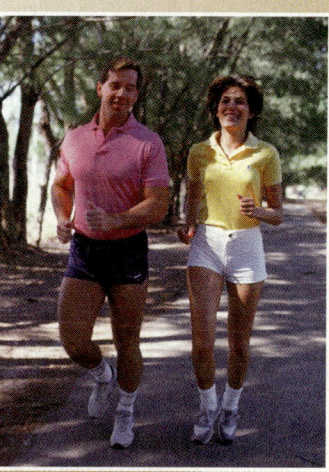

Objectives

▼ Understand that cancer is of many different types, each with its own characteristics and causes.

▼ Differentiate the major types of cancer.

▼ Recognize precancerous conditions and warning signs of cancer.

▼ Differentiate the three basic kinds of skin cancers.

▼ Learn about the gender-specific cancers, their incidence, and risk factors.

▼ List guidelines for preventing cancer, including dietary suggestions.

▼ Understand the role of self-examinations (and how to conduct these) and examination by physicians.

More than half a million Americans die from cancer each year, making it second only to heart disease as the leading killer in this country. The American Cancer Society estimates that almost a third of all Americans alive today eventually will be diagnosed with cancer — a rate that almost certainly could be reduced dramatically through behavioral and lifestyle changes.

A group of more than a hundred diseases, cancer is characterized by cells that grow at an uncontrolled rate, mature in an abnormal way, and spread to invade nearby tissues. A process called *metastasis* occurs when cancer cells from one growth break off, enter the bloodstream or lymph system, and are carried to another (often distant) part of the body, where the cells "set up housekeeping" and a second cancerous growth begins. The cancer has metastasized, or spread, in more than half of all cancer victims by the time they are diagnosed with cancer, a factor that makes treatment more complicated.

Cancer starts when an *initiator* alters DNA, the cell's basic genetic material, in a way that allows the cell to dictate its own rate of growth. The alteration can occur in minutes or days. Initiators include radiation, chemicals, and viruses. Having a cell with altered DNA, however, does not guarantee cancer. Fortunately, special enzymes travel up and down the DNA to repair breaks and changes in it.

Anything that speeds up the rate of cell division lessens the chance that repair enzymes will find the altered part of the DNA in time. Once a cell multiplies and incorporates its newly altered DNA into its genetic instructions, the cell no longer realizes its DNA has been changed.

Compounds that increase cell division are called promoters. They are thought to promote cancer either by reducing the time available for repair enzymes to act or by encouraging cells with altered DNA to develop and grow. Development and growth of these altered cells may take up to 20 years. Common promoters are thought to be estrogen, alcohol, and dietary fat in excess.

Even after an altered cell has multiplied, cancer does not necessarily result. First, a cell mass must grow large enough to affect body metabolism. During this initial stage of growth, the immune system may find the altered cells and destroy them. Or the cancer cells themselves may be so defective that their own DNA limits their ability to grow, and they die anyway.

Actually, most of us probably have cancerous or precancerous (potentially cancerous) cells in our bodies at some time. Many of them die because of mutation. Many more are destroyed by a healthy immune system. Occasionally, though, the immune system is unable to dominate, and cancer develops.

Survival depends on how early the cancer is diagnosed, the tissues involved, strength of the immune system, and potential treatment options. Cures have been discovered for some kinds of cancer. The American Cancer Society estimates that four of every five cancer victims can beat the odds and survive. An estimated 5 million Americans who have had cancer are still alive today. Approximately 3 million of them are considered cured (having survived 5 years or longer without any further signs of the cancer).

Just as the term *cancer* encompasses many different forms, the probable causes of cancer are many. We know that cancer is caused by certain substances in the environment. We also know that cigarette smoking and dietary factors play a role. So do heredity (the inherited tendency for certain kinds of cancer) and race. Researchers are beginning to learn that some cancers can be caused by viruses. (Viruses that increase the risk for cancer include Epstein-Barr, human papilloma, Hepatitis B, and T-cell leukemia/lymphoma). And, although some controversy still surrounds the notion, increasing evidence suggests that attitudes and emotions might increase susceptibility to cancer and could cause physiological changes in the body that can lead to the development of cancer.

▼ CANCER INCIDENCE AND RISK FACTORS

According to statistics from the American Cancer Society, someone in the United States dies of cancer every minute. It strikes people of all ages and is the leading killer of children between ages 3 and 14. More than half a million people in the United States die from cancer each year, and more than a million are diagnosed each year. The American Cancer Society pointed out recently that one of every five deaths from any cause in the United States is from cancer.

The incidence of cancer varies slightly between men and women. The most common cancers in men are prostate, colon/rectal, bladder, and lymphomas, in that order. The most common cancers in women are breast, colon/rectal, lung, uterine, and ovarian.

Deaths from cancer, by site and gender, are shown in Figure 12.1.

The important thing to remember about cancer statistics is that they can be changed. The American Cancer Society estimates that two of every five people who die from cancer could have been saved if they had been diagnosed sooner. And we can go a long way toward preventing cancer. As one example, the National Academy of Sciences says that 60% of cancer in women and 40% of cancer in men is caused by diet. That's a sobering fact, and one you can do something about.

You can't control some causes of cancer — heredity and race, for instance. But you can actively reduce many identified risk factors, and that's a decision that can help you beat the odds of developing cancer. Proven risk factors are discussed in the following pages.

TOBACCO

Cigarette smoking has been called the number-one preventable cause of death in the United States. According to estimates by the American Cancer Society, cigarette smoking directly causes approximately 30% of all cancers in this country and approximately 75% of all lung cancers among Americans. It also is a leading cause of bladder cancer.

Smoking — which also contributes to other serious diseases such as emphysema, heart disease, and stroke — introduces carbon monoxide and lethal *carcinogens* (cancer-causing substances) into the body. Your chance of getting cancer as a result of cigarette smoking is related to how long you have smoked, how many packs a day you smoke, and how deeply you inhale the smoke.

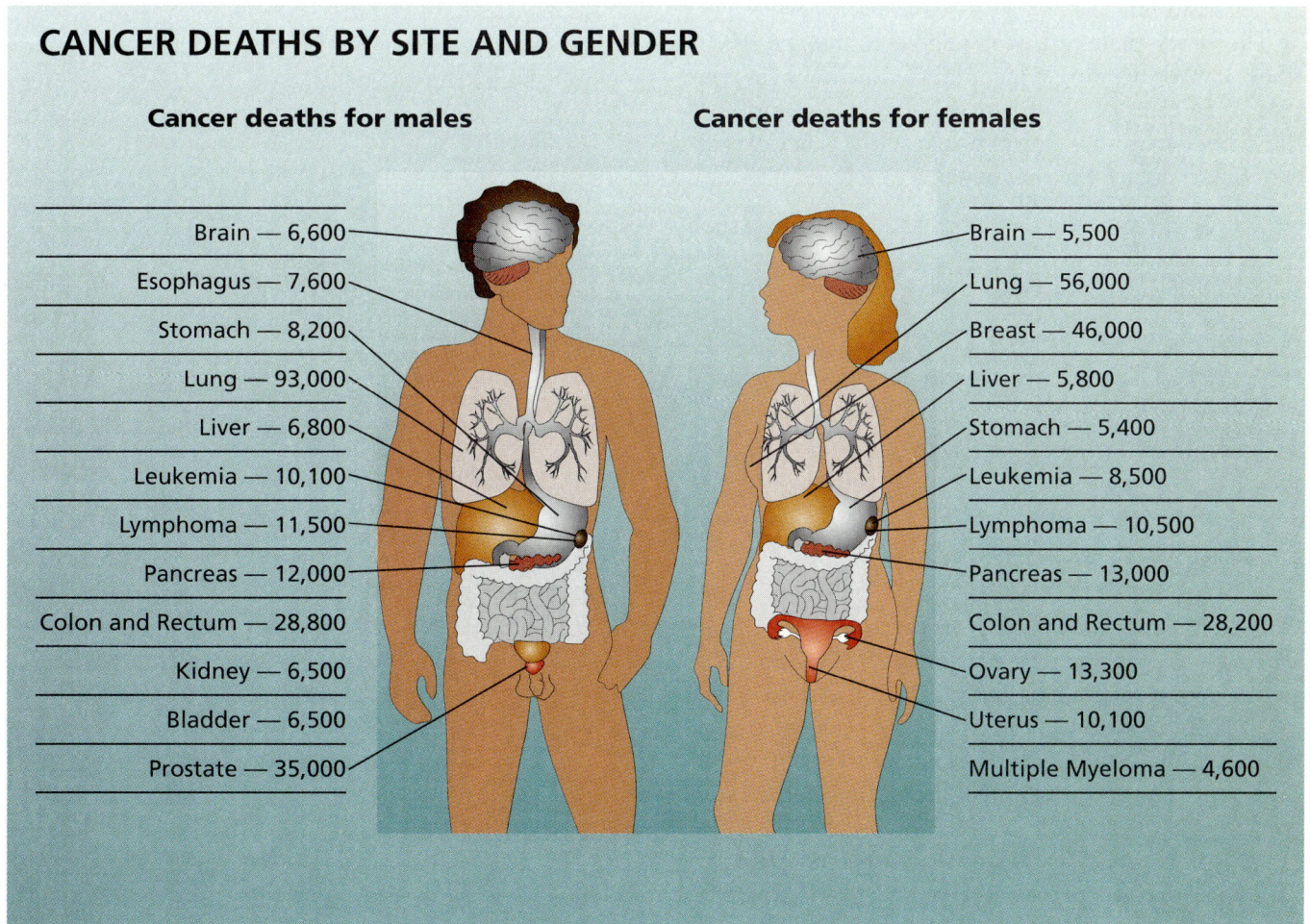

FIGURE 12.1 ▼ Cancer deaths by site and gender.

Smokeless tobacco also poses significant risk for cancer, despite the persistent myth that it's okay to "chew" if you don't smoke. Smokeless or chewing tobacco is a leading cause of cancer of the mouth, throat, esophagus, and larynx.

DIET

As mentioned, diet is estimated to be a major factor in 60% of cancers in women and 40% of cancers in men. Although more research is needed, some scientists believe diet actually may play as important a role as cigarette smoking in boosting the risk of developing cancer.

Although researchers aren't sure why, a diet high in saturated fats (the same kind of diet that leads to heart disease) increases the risk for cancer as well. Specific culprits are tropical oils (such as coconut oil and palm oil) and animal fats (fatty meats, whole milk, cheese, and other "animal source" foods). Scientists generally agree that cancer risk increases substantially if more than 30% of one's daily calories comes from fat.

The other dietary factor related to cancer risk is fiber. If the diet doesn't contain enough fiber, your risk of certain kinds of cancers, especially cancer of the colon, increases dramatically. Other dietary factors that increase the risk of cancer include:

▶ Foods cured or pickled with salt or nitrites (such as luncheon meats).
▶ Smoked foods.
▶ Charcoal-broiled foods.
▶ Foods containing cyclamates (a type of artificial sweetener).
▶ Vitamin and mineral deficiency.
▶ Excessive alcohol.

CARCINOGENS

Cancer-causing substances, or carcinogens, include materials ranging from electromagnetic radiation or radon gas to chemicals such as vinyl chloride and arsenic. In most cases, the risk of cancer is related to the dose: One-time massive exposure to a carcinogen may cause cancer, as can prolonged, long-term exposure to small amounts.

As carcinogens are identified, experts generally take measures to protect the public from exposure. Strict building codes ban the use of asbestos. The drug diethylstilbestrol (DES) — used to prevent miscarriages until the early 1960s — no longer can be prescribed. Accidental exposure, however, still occurs. Engineers and contractors who demolish or remodel old buildings, including schools, have to take extreme measures to prevent exposure to the asbestos used to "fireproof" the structures.

Possible Carcinogens (Cancer-Causing Substances)

▼ Aflatoxins (in rotting peanuts)
▼ Alcohol
▼ Alkylating agents
▼ Anabolic steroids
▼ Arsenic
▼ Asbestos
▼ Benzene
▼ Benzo(a)pyrene (in tobacco smoke)
▼ Beryllium
▼ Betel nuts
▼ Cadmium
▼ Chlornaphazine
▼ Chrome ores
▼ Chrysene (in tobacco smoke)
▼ Coke (a type of coal)
▼ Creosote oil
▼ Cyclamates
▼ Diethylstilbestrol (DES)
▼ Estrogen (synthetic)
▼ Ionizing radiation
▼ Immunosuppressive drugs
▼ Isopropyl oil
▼ Mesothorium
▼ Nickel carbonyl
▼ Nickel ores
▼ Nitrates
▼ Nitrites
▼ Nitrosamines
▼ Oral contraceptives
▼ Paraffin oil (crude)
▼ Penacetin
▼ Radiation
▼ Radium
▼ Radioactive dust/gas
▼ Radon
▼ Soots
▼ Tars
▼ Tar fumes
▼ Tobacco
▼ Ultraviolet light
▼ Vinyl chloride
▼ Wood dust
▼ X-rays

ENVIRONMENTAL POLLUTANTS

Certain environmental pollutants have been shown to cause cancer. Others, at high enough levels, are suspected strongly of causing cancer. The chemicals in the water we drink, the hydrocarbons emitted in automobile exhaust, and the agents in some insecticides and pesticides have been shown to cause cancer at certain levels. Even though few people are exposed to a high dosage of these pollutants, researchers are concerned about the effects of chronic, low-level exposure.

VIRUSES

The first virus known to cause cancer was identified in 1911 by a scientist who injected it into chickens, causing cancerous tumors. Since that time, exhaustive research has been conducted in the attempt to identify viruses that may cause cancers in humans.

One group of viruses — three variants of the human papilloma virus (HPV), which causes genital warts — is suspected of causing cervical cancer and other genital malignancies. According to research findings published in the *American Journal of Epidemiology*, these cancer-causing viruses can be sexually transmitted.

Researchers aren't sure of the precise role viruses may play in causing cancer but believe that approximately 2% of all cancers in the United States may be related to viruses. In some cases, researchers believe, the virus may be responsible for *causing* or initiating the cancer; once the disease takes hold, the virus no longer is in the picture. In other situations, the viruses may not actually *cause* the cancer but may increase the risk of developing cancer.

Scientists also have identified a particular kind of virus called *retroviruses*. These viruses invade a cell's chromosome, or genetic structure, and are passed on to each succeeding generation of cells as the cells divide. The human immunodeficiency virus (HIV), which causes AIDS, is a retrovirus.

Controversy still surrounds the notion of cancer-causing viruses. Most scientists conclude that certain viruses may cause cancer only under certain circumstances. For example, Epstein-Barr virus (EBV), which causes mononucleosis in the United States, generally causes a cancer called *Burkitt's lymphoma* among children in Africa. Scientists now are researching the possibility that EBV, or similar viruses responsible for herpes, may sharply increase the risk of Hodgkin's disease, cervical cancer, and some forms of leukemia.

HEREDITY

Genetic factors definitely can increase the risk of developing certain kinds of cancers, and heredity is a factor in an estimated 10% of all cancers in the United States. Figures reported in the *Washington Post* estimate that approximately 14 million Americans are at risk because they inherited the tendency for certain malignancies. Cancers caused by hereditary factors often begin in childhood and can increase the likelihood of developing the cancer by as much as 30 times normal odds.

In a few cases, the cancer itself is inherited. One example is retinoblastoma, a cancer of the eye that occurs in infants and young children. More often, what is inherited is not the actual cancer but, rather, the predisposition for that cancer, the tendency to develop that cancer. Exciting new research has identified, for example, a gene that predisposes its carriers to cancer of the colon. Once the gene is identified, a person carrying the gene can take certain precautions and undergo aggressive early screening to improve the odds of preventing or successfully treating the disease.

The risk for certain leukemias can be genetically passed from parent to child. The tendency for lung, colon, breast, uterine, prostate, bone, brain, stomach, and adrenal gland cancers also can be inherited.

Signs of Inherited Cancers

How can you tell if a cancer developed because of genetic tendencies? Four patterns generally identify hereditary cancers:

▶ Many family members develop the same kind of cancer.

▶ The cancer strikes victims at an earlier age than usual; for example, breast cancer typically occurs in the 60s but may strike a woman in her 40s who inherited the tendency.

▶ The cancer strikes more than once — in both breasts, for example, or in two different places in the liver.

▶ The person has an unusual gender pattern; for example, a cancer unusual in women will affect the women in a family.

STRESS

An individual's response to stress has been linked to the risk for developing cancer, as well as certain other diseases (such as heart disease). Chronic stress and the hormones it unleashes on the body interfere with the immune system's ability to recognize cancerous cells and destroy them.

Joseph G. Courtney of the University of California, Los Angeles, School of Public Health and his co-workers joined forces with researchers in Sweden and their large database on Stockholm-area patients with colorectal cancer. In September, 1993, issue of *Epidemiology*, Courtney's team confirmed that on-the-job aggravation seems to put people at higher risk for developing colon and rectal cancers. Those who reported a history of workplace problems over the past 10 years faced 5.5 times the colorectal-cancer risk of adults who reported no such problems.

Although controversy still surrounds the idea, researchers have identified a "cancer-prone" personality, a collection of traits that seem to occur in people who later develop cancer. Called the *Type C personality*, it is characterized by unusual compliance and the tendency to internalize conflict. It also is marked by the individual's inability to deal with stress in a healthy way.

CHRONIC IRRITATION

Evidence indicates that chronic irritation of cells or tissues can lead to cancer. The following all have been linked to certain kinds of cancers and seem to increase the risk for cancer.

- Chronic low-grade infections.
- Repeated bladder infections.
- Repeated ulceration of tissues.
- Chronic infection of scar tissue.
- Constant irritation of a mole or other benign growth.
- Certain kinds of injuries.
- Long-term irritation of gallstones against the gallbladder.

ESTROGEN-REPLACEMENT THERAPY

When the level of estrogen, normally produced by the ovaries, tapers off as a woman reaches menopause, physicians may prescribe estrogen replacement therapy to ease or delay the troublesome symptoms of menopause. Evidence shows that estrogen-replacement therapy also can help prevent osteoporosis, a loss of bone tissue that affects mostly older women. Research has indicated, however, that estrogen-replacement therapy increases the risk of endometrial cancer (a cancer of the lining of the uterus) and may increase the risk of breast cancer.

The risk factors just discussed are general risk factors for cancer. Knowing the specific risk factors for certain kinds of cancers can help you reduce your odds of developing one of the more common cancers.

TYPES OF CANCER

Cancers have been classified according to six general types. These are carcinomas, carcomas, lymphomas, melanomas, leukemias, and neuroblastomas.

1. **Carcinomas.** Spread through the bloodstream and lymph system, carcinomas — the most common kind of cancers — affect the tissues that line most body cavities and that cover body surfaces.

The Seven Warning Signs of Cancer

1. A change in bowel or bladder habits.
2. A sore that does not heal.
3. Unusual bleeding or discharge.
4. Thickening or a lump in the breast or elsewhere.
5. Indigestion or difficulty in swallowing.
6. An obvious change in a wart or mole.
7. A nagging cough or hoarseness.

Examples are lung cancer, breast cancer, skin cancer, colon cancer, and uterine cancer. (If the cancer occurs in a gland, it is called an *adenocarcinoma*.)

2. **Sarcomas.** Spread through the bloodstream, sarcomas affect the connective tissues of the body, such as the muscles, bones, and cartilage. Sarcomas are less common than carcinomas, but they grow and spread more quickly and form more solid tumors.
3. **Lymphomas.** Spread through the lymph system, lymphomas are cancers of the lymphatic, or infection-fighting, cells. Lymph nodes in the groin, armpits, and neck can be affected. An example of lymphoma is Hodgkin's disease.
4. **Melanomas.** Spread through the bloodstream, melanomas affect the skin. They generally begin as a mole that later becomes cancerous. They grow and spread rapidly.
5. **Leukemias.** Spread through the bloodstream, leukemias affect the tissues that manufacture blood, especially the spleen and the bone marrow.
6. **Neuroblastomas.** Spread through the bloodstream, neuroblastomas affect the nervous system or the adrenal glands. Relatively uncommon, they occur most often in children under age 10.

SITES OF CANCER

Cancers also can be classified according to site. Some common sites are discussed on the following pages, and Table 12.1 summarizes pertinent data on these cancers.

SKIN CANCER

More than half a million Americans are diagnosed with some form of skin cancer every year, and it causes approximately 8,000 deaths annually. According to available figures, skin cancer accounts for approximately 40% of all cancers. The three basic kinds of skin cancers are:

1. **Basal cell carcinoma.** This is the most common, and least serious, of the skin cancers. It usually does not spread, and it grows slowly. Most basal cell carcinomas occur on the face, neck, and hands — areas of chronic sun exposure.

> ### Precancerous Skin Conditions
> Precancerous conditions are those in which a benign, or noncancerous, condition becomes cancerous for one reason or another. Generally, physicians recommend that the following precancerous skin conditions be surgically removed or repaired to prevent their becoming cancerous, regardless of how low the risk may be:
>
> ▼ Benign tumors
>
> ▼ Chronic scaly patches on the skin
>
> ▼ Brown or black warts
>
> ▼ Moles subject to chronic irritation (such as those on the waist that are constantly rubbed by a waistband or belt)
>
> ▼ A lump on the lip, tongue, or inside the cheek
>
> ▼ A scaly patch on the inside of the cheek

2. **Squamous cell carcinoma.** This type of cancer grows faster than the basal cell type and involves deeper layers of skin, but it rarely spreads to other parts of the body.
3. **Malignant melanoma.** This rapidly growing cancer is the most dangerous skin cancer and almost always spreads to other organs. Of the 8,000 people who die from skin cancer each year, approximately 6,000 succumb to malignant melanoma.

Basal and squamous cell carcinomas are detected and treated quite easily. Malignant melanoma can be treated successfully if it is diagnosed and treated early. If not treated early, metastasis makes treatment extremely difficult.

The risk factors for skin cancer include:

▶ Sun exposure (most dangerous are ultraviolet B rays, at their strongest between 10 a.m. and 2 p.m.).

▶ Fair skin that burns easily and rarely tans.

▶ Fair skin that sometimes tans.

▶ Blonde or red hair.

▶ Artificial sources of ultraviolet rays, such as tanning booths and sunlamps.

▶ History of one or more severe sunburns.

▶ A dark brown or black wart.

TABLE 12.1 ▼ Common Cancers

	Risk Factors	Warning Signals	Early Detection	Treatment	5-Year Survival with Treatment
Lung cancer (est. 170,000 new cases a year; 149,000 deaths)	Cigarette smoking for 20 or more years; exposure to certain industrial substances, particularly asbestos; second-hand smoke; radiation; radon.	Persistent cough, sputum streaked with blood, chest pain, recurring bronchitis or pneumonia.	Difficult to detect early. Diagnosis based on chest x-ray, sputum testing, fiberoptic bronchoscopy (direct examination of the lungs by means of a specially lighted tube).	Surgery, radiation therapy, chemotherapy.	The leading cause of cancer death among both men and women.
Breast cancer (est. 183,000 new cases a year; 46,300 deaths)	Over age 50, personal or family history of breast cancer, no children, first child after age 30, dense breast tissue, obesity, high fat intake, alcohol, estrogen replacement therapy after menopause.	Breast changes: lumps, thickening, swelling, puckering, dimpling, skin irritation, nipple distortion, scaliness, discharge, pain, tenderness.	Monthly breast self-examination. Professional breast exam every 3 years for women ages 20-40 and every year over age 40. Yearly mammography for all women over 50, every 1 or 2 years for women 40-49; baseline mammogram for those 35-39. Tissue biopsy confirms diagnosis.	Surgery, from lumpectomy (local removal of tumor) to a modified radical mastectomy (removal of breast and lymph glands, leaving underlying muscle intact); radiation; chemotherapy; or all three. For metastatic breast cancer, autologous bone marrow transplantation.	Until recently, the leading cause of cancer death in women; now surpassed by lung cancer.
Uterine and cervical cancer (46,000 new cases a year; 10,100 deaths)	For cervical cancer: early age of first intercourse, multiple sex partners, genital herpes, human papilloma virus infection, significant exposure to second-hand smoke. For uterine cancer: infertility, failure to ovulate, prolonged estrogen therapy, obesity.	Unusual vaginal bleeding or discharge.	Pap smear every 3 years after two initial negative tests 1 year apart.	Surgery, radiation, or a combination of the two. In precancerous stages, cervical cells may be destroyed by extreme cold or intense heat. Precancerous endometrial changes are treated with the hormone progesterone.	Cervical cancer mortality has declined 70% during the last 40 years with wider application of the Pap smear. Postmenopausal women with abnormal bleeding should be checked.
Ovarian cancer (est. 20,700 new cases a year)	Family history of ovarian cancer; personal history of breast cancer; obesity; infertility (because the abnormality that interferes with conception may also play a role in cancer development); low levels of transferase, an enzyme involved in metabolism of dairy foods.	Often no obvious symptoms until advanced stages. Painless swelling of abdomen; irregular bleeding; lower abdominal pain; digestive and urinary abnormalities; fatigue; backache; bloating; weight gain.	Women with family history: annual pelvic and abdominal exams; blood test for a tumor marker called CA125 every 6 months; annual pelvic ultrasound. (In cases of very high risk, some oncologists recommend prophylactic removal of ovaries no later than age 35.)	Surgery, sometimes in combination with chemotherapy or radiation.	85% if detected and treated early; 23% in advanced cases.

Colon and rectum cancer (est. 152,000 new cases a year; 57,000 deaths)	Personal or family history of colon and rectal cancer or polyps (growths) in the colon or rectum; inflammatory bowel disease; high-fat, low-fiber diet.	Unusual bleeding from rectum, blood in stool, a change in bowel habits.	Digital rectal exam (once a year after age 40); stool-blood slide test that detects blood in feces (every year after age 50); proctosigmoidoscopy, a rectal exam using a hollow, lighted tube (every 3-5 years after age 50, following 2 consecutive normal annual exams). Diagnosis may require a colonoscopy (viewing the entire colon) or a barium enema.	Surgery, sometimes in combination with chemotherapy or radiation.	Considered a highly curable disease when digital and proctoscopic examinations are included in routine checkups.
Skin cancer (Melanoma) (est. 32,000 new cases a year; 6,800 deaths)	Excessive exposure to sun, fair complexion, occupational exposure to carcinogens. (Inherited skin disorders, such as xeroderma pigmentosum and familial atypical multiple mole melanoma, account for 10% of cases.)	Unusual skin condition, especially a change in size or color of a mole; appearance of darkly pigmented growth or spot; oozing, scaliness, bleeding; appearance of a bump; change in sensation, itchiness, tenderness, or pain.	Examine moles on your skin once a month.	Surgery, radiation, electrodesication (tissue destruction by heat), cryosurgery (tissue destruction by cold), or a combination of therapies.	Melanoma is readily detected by observation and diagnosed by simple biopsy.
Oral cancer (including pharynx) (est. 29,800 new cases a year; 7,700 deaths)	Heavy smoking of cigarettes, cigars, pipes; excessive drinking; use of chewing tobacco.	A sore that bleeds easily and doesn't heal; a lump or thickening; a reddish or whitish patch; difficulty chewing, swallowing, or moving the tongue or jaws.	Regular exams by your dentist or primary-care physician.	Surgery and radiation.	Many more lives should be saved because the mouth is easily accessible to visual examination by physicians and dentists.
Leukemia (est. 29,300 new cases a year; 18,600 deaths)	Down syndrome and other inherited abnormalities; excessive exposure to radiation and to certain chemicals, such as benzene.		Difficult to detect early because its symptoms are often similar to those of less serious conditions, such as flu. Diagnosis is based on blood tests and bone-marrow biopsy.	Chemotherapy, drugs, blood transfusions, and antibiotics; bone-marrow transplants.	Leukemias are cancers of blood-forming tissues and are characterized by the abnormal production of immature white blood cells. Acute leukemia strikes mainly children and is treated by drugs that have extended life from a few months to as much as 10 years. Chronic leukemia strikes usually after age 25 and progresses less rapidly.
Testicular cancer (6,100 new cases a year)	Young men under age 35.		Testicular self-examinations.	Surgical removal of the diseased testis, radiation therapy, chemotherapy, removal of nearby lymph nodes.	96% if the cancer is localized; 89% overall.
Prostate cancer (est. 165,000 new cases a year; 35,000 deaths)	Risk increases with age, black men more susceptible than whites. Suspected risk factors: family history, high-fat diet, exposure to heavy metal cadmium, high number of sexual partners, history of frequent STDs.	Frequent urination, difficulty urinating, blood in the urine, lower back pain.	Rectal exam; new blood test available.	Surgical removal of prostate, conventional radiation, or implanting "seeds" of radioactive iodine in the prostate; hormone therapy.	Occurs mainly in men over 60; can be detected by digital rectal exam at annual checkup.

Adapted from the American Cancer Society, *Cancer Facts and Figures*, 1993.

- Birthmarks or congenital moles (although these do not always become cancerous, they should be watched closely and removed if they begin to grow or change in appearance).
- Moles that are irritated chronically (moles at the waistline, bra line, or other areas where clothing constantly rubs them).
- Occupational exposure to creosote, coal tar, pitch, arsenic, or radium.

Currently, young women have the highest rate of skin cancer, about twice that of men. Researchers believe tanning habits are at fault. Scientists also are concerned about the gradual deterioration of the earth's ozone layer. The ozone layer is what screens out a percentage of the harmful ultraviolet rays, and, as it thins, the skin is more exposed to those rays, boosting the risk of skin cancer for everyone.

The sharp increase in incidence of skin cancer has researchers alarmed. Over the past decade, it has increased 93%. If current rates continue, researchers estimate that one in 90 Americans will have skin cancer by the year 2000. Danger signs of skin cancer are given in Figure 12.2.

LUNG CANCER

The leading cancer killer, lung cancer afflicts approximately 157,000 Americans each year; approximately 142,000 of them die annually. Lung cancer occurs almost exclusively among cigarette smokers. According to the U.S. Department of Health and Human Services, the cellular changes and tissue damage that lead to lung cancer have been observed in 93% of active smokers and 6% of former smokers but only 1% of those who have never smoked. Researchers estimate that more than three-fourths of all lung cancer could be eliminated if people did not smoke.

Once a disease predominantly affecting men, lung cancer in women has risen along with increased smoking rates among women. Today, lung cancer is

---

Danger Signs of Skin Cancer

The American Academy of Dermatology advises: Know your spots and do a spot check. Also, have your skin checked by a doctor for any changes once a year. If you notice one of the following changes in your skin, you should see your family doctor or dermatologist immediately:

▼ **Basal-cell or squamous-cell carcinomas:** any lesion that is new, starts growing, starts changing, bleeds, is scabby, or doesn't heal.

▼ **Melanoma:**

A. *Asymmetry:* One half of a mole or lesion doesn't look like the other half.

B. *Border:* A mole has an irregular, scalloped, or not clearly defined border.

C. *Color:* The color varies or is not uniform from one area of a mole or lesion to another, whether the color is tan, brown, black, white, red, or blue.

D. *Diameter:* The lesion is larger than 6 millimeters or larger than a pencil eraser.

▼ **Actinic kerotosis:** a precancerous skin lesion that is dry, scaly, reddish, and slightly raised.

Melanoma Warnings

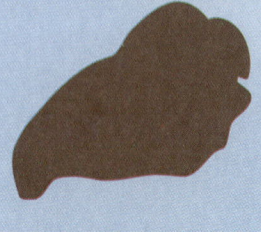
Asymmetrical

Border irregular

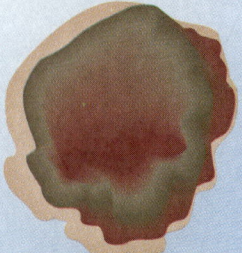
Color varied

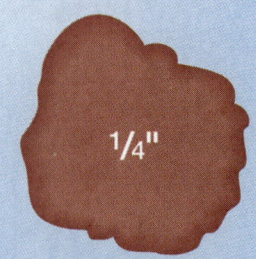
Diameter larger than 1/4"

Adapted from *FDA Consumer*, May 1991.

FIGURE 12.2 ▼ Danger signs of skin cancer.

steadily decreasing in men and steadily increasing in women.

Unfortunately, lung cancer spreads rapidly, and it is rarely detected early, as it usually does not cause symptoms or show up on an x-ray until it is quite advanced. By that time, damage is usually too extensive to treat successfully. When symptoms do occur, they might be manifested by persistent hoarseness, a nagging cough, repeated bouts of pneumonia or bronchitis, or spitting up blood.

The number-one risk factor for lung cancer is cigarette smoking. Most at risk are those who have smoked more than 20 years. Recent research has shown that secondary smoke — cigarette smoke inhaled by nonsmokers who live or work with smokers — also significantly increases the risk of lung cancer. The Centers for Disease Control estimate that 3,000 nonsmokers die each year from lung cancer caused by second-hand tobacco smoke. Other risk factors for lung cancer include:

- Exposure to asbestos.
- Severe air pollution.
- Exposure to carcinogenic chemicals.
- Exposure to certain metals (cadmium, cobalt, chromium, silver, nickel, and steel).
- Exposure to arsenic or radioactive ores.
- Exposure to radon gas.

All other risk factors for lung cancer are much more marked if the individual also smokes.

COLON AND RECTAL CANCER

Cancer of the colon and rectum — also called *colorectal cancer* — is the second leading cancer killer in the United States. About 155,000 new cases are diagnosed each year, and almost 60,000 Americans die of colorectal cancer annually. If detected early, colorectal cancer usually can be treated successfully because it grows and spreads quite slowly. Bleeding from the rectum, bright red blood in the stools, or a change in bowel habits can indicate colorectal cancer. Risk factors include:

- A personal or family history of polyps (benign growths) in the colon or rectum.
- A family history of colorectal cancer.
- A diet high in fats and low in fiber.
- Inflammatory bowel problems (such as colitis).

Age is also considered a risk factor. The risk for colorectal cancer increases sharply after age 40. Researchers believe that at least half, and possibly *all*, cases of colorectal cancer can be attributed to a genetic tendency for polyps in the colon or rectum combined with a high-fat, low-fiber diet.

BREAST CANCER

The second leading killer of women, breast cancer kills almost 50,000 American women each year. Estimates are that one in nine American women eventually will develop breast cancer at some time in her life.

Early detection is the key to successful treatment. Heightened awareness of the disease, together with breast self-examination and regular mammograms, has improved survival rates because cancers are being diagnosed earlier. General symptoms of breast cancer include a thickening or lump in the breast, distortion or dimpling of a breast, swollen lymph nodes under the arm, or retraction, pain, discharge, or scaliness of the nipple. General risk factors for breast cancer include:

- A grandmother, mother, or sister with breast cancer.
- Early onset of menstruation (before age 12).
- Delayed onset of menopause (after age 55).
- First pregnancy after age 30.
- Obesity.
- A woman who has never been pregnant.
- A woman who has never breast-fed.
- Age (dramatic increase after age 50).

A report from the Utah Population Database suggests that 17%–19% of breast cancer cases may be attributable to a family history of the disease. Also, women with a first-degree relative with colon cancer had a 30% increase in risk for breast cancer. A family history of breast cancer, however, does not necessarily affect the prognosis or outcome adversely.

Hormone replacement therapy (HRT, usually for post-menopausal women) may be associated with a higher risk, although the available data are difficult to interpret. Some researchers believe the progestin component of HRT may have a greater impact on risk than the estrogen component. The studies of oral contraceptives to date show no significant increase in risk. Because of the remaining uncertainty, though, some gynecologists advise against long-term use of oral contraceptives in young women who have not borne children.

What about diet? Despite earlier findings that a high-fat diet raises the risk, recent studies have found little support for a role of dietary fat in the onset of breast cancer. Evidence is mounting that daily alcohol consumption increases the risk, however. Daily consumption of vitamin A — as little as one carrot or less — may reduce risk.

Other studies reveal interesting findings, but these have not been confirmed yet. According to one of these, the longer a woman breast-feeds and the more babies she nurses, the less is her risk for breast cancer. Diethylstibestrol (DES) taken during pregnancy increases a woman's risk for breast cancer later in life, but this risk probably is small and does not increase with time. Environmental factors — specifically pesticide residues in food — also have been implicated, but this is the most difficult area to study systematically.

Many factors probably contribute to a woman's risk of developing breast cancer, but the known risk factors account for only a small percentage of breast cancer cases. The majority of patients (60%–70%) have no known risk factors for the disease except older age. Age is the most influential known risk factor.

CERVICAL CANCER

The death rate from cancer of the cervix has decreased more than 70% during the past four decades because of early detection — mainly in the form of Pap smears and regular gynecological examinations. Today, approximately 60,000 women are diagnosed with invasive cervical cancer each year in the United States. With early diagnosis, treatment usually is successful. Unusual vaginal bleeding or discharge is often an early symptom. Risk factors for cervical cancer can be:

▶ Early age at first intercourse.
▶ Multiple sex partners.
▶ A history of viral genital infections.
▶ Cigarette smoking.

Recent research has shown that the human papilloma virus, a sexually transmitted virus responsible for genital warts, can cause cervical cancer.

UTERINE CANCER

Uterine cancer, which involves the endometrium, or lining, of the uterus, affects approximately 48,000 women in the United States each year. Because of detection, the death rate from uterine cancer has fallen dramatically. Only about 4,000 deaths a year in this country are attributed to uterine cancer. With early detection, treatment generally is successful. Symptoms of uterine cancer might be unusual vaginal discharge, unusual vaginal bleeding, or bleeding between menstrual periods. Risk factors for uterine cancer include:

▶ Late onset of menopause.
▶ History of infertility/failure to ovulate.
▶ Prolonged estrogen replacement therapy.
▶ Obesity.
▶ Diabetes.

OVARIAN CANCER

Although ovarian cancer claims a relatively few 13,000 American women each year, it is a particularly difficult cancer because it typically reveals no symptoms until in its latest stages and it can be difficult to diagnose. The survival rate 5 years after diagnosis averages 40%. Late symptoms include abdominal swelling or bloating, persistent abdominal gas, and unexplained stomachaches or indigestion.

Age is a factor. The risk increases with age and is highest for women in their 60s. For unknown reasons, the rates are higher among Jewish women. This form of cancer also strikes Americans, Scandinavians, and Scots at three times the rate it hits Japanese women.

Other risk factors include:

▶ A grandmother, mother, or sister with ovarian cancer.
▶ Never had children (doubles the risk).
▶ Use of oral contraceptives.
▶ Occurrence of colorectal, breast, or uterine cancer (doubles the risk).
▶ Early onset of ovulation.

TESTICULAR CANCER

Although testicular cancer is not one of the most common types of cancer in the United States, it is the most common cancer in young men between ages 15 and 34. Of all cancer deaths in that age group, 12% are from testicular cancer. For reasons that aren't clear to researchers, the incidence of testicular cancer in this age group has been increasing steadily. If this cancer is found in its early stages, however, the chances for cure are nearly 100%.

Early detection is the key to successful treatment. Many men discover the cancer themselves through self-examination. The major warning sign is an often painless thickening or hard lump in the testicle. Other signs include pain or a sensation of heaviness in the affected testicle, an accumulation of fluid or blood in the scrotum, and a dull ache in the groin that may involve the lower abdomen. Risk factors for testicular cancer include:

▶ An undescended testicle (risk can be 40 times as high).

▶ A testicle that did not descend until after age 6 (risk can be 40 times as high).

▶ A grandfather, father, or brother with testicular cancer.

PROSTATE CANCER

The leading cancer in American men and the third leading cause of cancer death in men (after lung and colon cancer), prostate cancer strikes more than 160,000 men in the United States every year. More than 30,000 die from it.

Prostate cancer often is detected early because it generally provokes an array of symptoms fairly early in its development. The symptoms, however, can be mistaken for signs of other, more common ailments, such as a prostate or bladder infection. If detected early, prostate cancer can be treated successfully about 84% of the time. A new blood test that measures the amount of prostate-specific antigen (PSA) in the blood can be used to help diagnose prostate cancer.

Signs and symptoms of prostate cancer include pain in the pelvis, lower back, or upper thighs; blood in the urine or semen; pain or burning during urination; frequent urination; and weak or interrupted urine, difficulty starting or stopping the flow of urine, or inability to urinate.

The risk of prostate cancer increases with age. At highest risk are men over age 65, in whom more than 80% of all prostate cancers are diagnosed. Another substantial risk factor is race: African-American men have the highest rate of prostate cancer in the world. Oddly enough, the cancer is relatively rare in Africa and is much more common in North America and northwest Europe than it is in Central and South America or the Near East.

Other risk factors can include:

▶ A family history of prostate cancer.

▶ Occupational exposure to cadmium.

▶ A high-fat diet.

BLADDER CANCER

Approximately 50,000 new cases of bladder cancer are diagnosed each year in the United States, and close to 10,000 Americans die from it each year. If the cancer is detected while it is still confined to the bladder — before it has metastasized to involve other organs — almost nine in 10 can be cured.

The most common signs of bladder cancer are more frequent urination and blood in the urine. The cancer is four times more common in men than in women. Other risk factors include:

▶ Cigarette smoking (smoking is believed to cause almost half the bladder cancers in men and approximately 40% of the bladder cancers in women).

▶ Occupational exposure to leather and rubber.

▶ Occupational exposure to dyes.

▶ Living in an urban area.

PANCREATIC CANCER

Although pancreatic cancer is not one of the most common cancers, its incidence has more than doubled in the past two decades, making it the fifth most common cancer killer in Americans. More than 25,000 Americans die each year of pancreatic cancer, and more than 70,000 new cases are diagnosed each year. The survival rate from pancreatic cancer is low. The disease spreads rapidly, and few survive more than 3 years. In addition, pancreatic cancer is a "silent" disease, usually progressing without symptoms until extremely advanced stages.

The risk for pancreatic cancer increases with age. The highest risk is between ages 65 and 79. Men are at higher risk, as are African-Americans. Other risk factors include:

▶ Smoking cigarettes.

▶ Consuming alcohol.

▶ Eating a high-fat diet.

▶ Being exposed to gasoline and some chemical cleaners on the job.

ORAL CANCER

Oral cancer has increased substantially over the past two decades, which correlates with the popularity of smokeless tobacco (chewing tobacco). Twice as many men as women get oral cancer; more than 30,000 Americans are diagnosed with it each year, and approximately 8,500 die. These figures are rising.

Signs of oral cancer generally include a sore that fails to heal or that bleeds easily; a reddish or whitish patch that does not go away; a lump or thickening in the cheek, tongue, or lips; and difficulty chewing or swallowing. Risk factors include:

▶ Use of smokeless tobacco (chewing tobacco).

▶ Smoking cigarettes, cigars, or a pipe.

▶ Excessive alcohol consumption.

▼ GUIDELINES FOR PREVENTING CANCER

Now for the good news: Researchers estimate that as much as 85% of all cancer is related to lifestyle and environmental factors over which we have control. By changing your lifestyle and taking control over your environment, you have a pretty good chance of beating the odds of getting cancer. Your general risk for cancer can be cut dramatically by:

▶ Avoiding substances known to cause cancer (such as tobacco) and overuse of alcohol.

▶ Avoiding overexposure to sunlight.

▶ Avoiding overeating and eating an anti-cancer diet.

▶ Doing appropriate self-examinations and getting regular checkups to boost your chances of early detection.

Table 12.2 summarizes major preventive measures.

SMOKING CESSATION

According to former U.S. Surgeon General C. Everett Koop, the single best thing you can do to lower your risk for cancer is to stop smoking. Smoking causes 85% of all lung cancers and three of 10 cancers overall. If you're smoking now, stop. (That goes for any tobacco in any form, not just cigarette smoking.) If you don't smoke, don't start.

If you smoke now, will quitting do any good? Yes, say the experts. Your lungs will start to heal as soon as you stop smoking. Your risk will be slightly higher than if you never smoked, but eventually your risk can be the same as nonsmokers. Although the American Cancer Society warns that there are no "safe" cigarettes, you can cut the amount of carcinogens you get by switching to a filtered, low-tar, low-nicotine cigarette while you quit. A smoking cessation program is presented in Chapter 13.

LIMITED SUN EXPOSURE

The major cause of skin cancer is too much sun, so if you want to lower your risk for skin cancer, you have to limit your exposure to the sun. Sunscreens protect against the ultraviolet rays of the sun. The sun protection factor (SPF) tells you the protection you're getting. An SPF of 10, for example, lets you stay in the sun 10 times as long as you normally would without burning. If your skin normally starts to redden after 20 minutes, a sunscreen with an SPF of 10 lets you stay in the sun 200 minutes before you start to burn. After that time, you'll begin to burn. You can't simply apply more and expect longer protection.

Always use a sunscreen if you're going outside for longer than 15 minutes, even if you think you won't be getting that much sun exposure. Choose a sunscreen that provides adequate protection for your skin type (see the accompanying chart). Apply it at least 30-45 minutes before exposure to the sun. Apply the sunscreen frequently if you're in and out of the water (look for a waterproof or

TABLE 12.2 ▼ Preventing Cancer

Smoking	Cigarette smoking is responsible for 85% of lung cancer cases among men and 75% among women — about 83% overall. Smoking accounts for about 30% of all cancer deaths. Those who smoke two or more packs of cigarettes a day have lung cancer mortality rates 15 to 25 times greater than nonsmokers.
Sunlight	Almost all of the more than 600,000 cases of nonmelanoma skin cancer diagnosed each year in the United States are considered to be sun-related. Sun exposure is a major factor in the development of melanoma, and the incidence increases for those living near the equator and at high altitudes.
Alcohol	Oral cancer and cancers of the larynx, throat, esophagus, and liver occur more frequently among heavy drinkers of alcohol.
Smokeless tobacco	Use of chewing tobacco or snuff increases risk of cancer of the mouth, larynx, throat, and esophagus and is highly habit-forming.
Estrogen	For mature women, estrogen treatment to control menopausal symptoms increases risk of endometrial cancer. Estrogen use by menopausal women calls for careful discussion between the woman and her physician.
Radiation	Excessive exposure to ionizing radiation can increase cancer risk. Most medical and dental x-rays are adjusted to deliver the lowest dose possible without sacrificing image quality. Excessive radon exposure in homes may increase risk of lung cancer, especially in cigarette smokers. If levels are found to be too high, remedial actions should be taken.
Occupational hazards	Exposure to several different industrial agents (nickel, chromate, asbestos, vinyl chloride, etc.) increases risk of various cancers. Risk from asbestos is greatly increased when combined with cigarette smoking.
Nutrition	Risk for colon, breast, and uterine cancers increases in obese people. High-fat diets may contribute to the development of cancers of the colon, and prostate. High-fiber foods may help reduce risk of colon cancer. A varied diet containing plenty of vegetables and fruits rich in vitamins A and C may reduce risk for a wide range of cancers. Salt-cured, smoked, and nitrite-cured foods have been linked to esophageal and stomach cancer. Heavy use of alcohol, especially when accompanied by cigarette smoking or chewing tobacco, increases risk of cancers of the mouth, larynx, throat, esophagus, and liver.

Adapted from the American Cancer Society.

water-resistant screen). Apply the screen heavily to areas where your skin is thin, such as your nose, face, neck, and hands. Use sunscreen even on cloudy days (clouds don't block the ultraviolet rays) and during the winter when you're outside. Sunscreen is especially important the closer you are to the equator and if you're at a high altitude, which affords less protection from UV rays.

To further cut your risk for overexposure to the sun:

▶ Even when using a sunscreen, avoid being in the sun between 10 a.m. and 3 p.m. UV rays are at their most intense then. You can burn even if you're sitting in the shade. Plan outdoor activities during the earlier morning or early evening hours, when sun is less intense and temperatures are cooler.

▶ If you have to stay outside for long periods, wear protective clothing — long pants, a long-sleeved shirt, a hat with a brim or visor. Wear tightly woven cottons, and avoid white or thin fabrics. Don't sit in the sun in wet clothing.

▶ Don't assume that because your skin isn't red, it isn't getting burned. A sunburn becomes most evident 6 to 24 hours after being in the sun.

▶ Avoid surfaces that reflect the sun's rays more intensely: concrete, snow, expanses of metal, expanses of sand. More than half the sun's rays

Skin Types

A fair-skinned person (Type 1) in the sun at noon and at an elevation of about 5000 feet stands a good chance of beginning to burn within 10 minutes. The times are determined by multiplying the sun-protection factor (SPF) number by 10 minutes. For example, SPF 15 x 10 min. = 150 min. = 2 hrs. 30 min. To determine how long a given SPF will protect your skin, this 6-point standard scale used by dermatologists gives guidelines for your exposure limits.

Type 1: fair skin with blue or green eyes and light blond or red hair; typical time for skin to burn: 10-20 minutes.

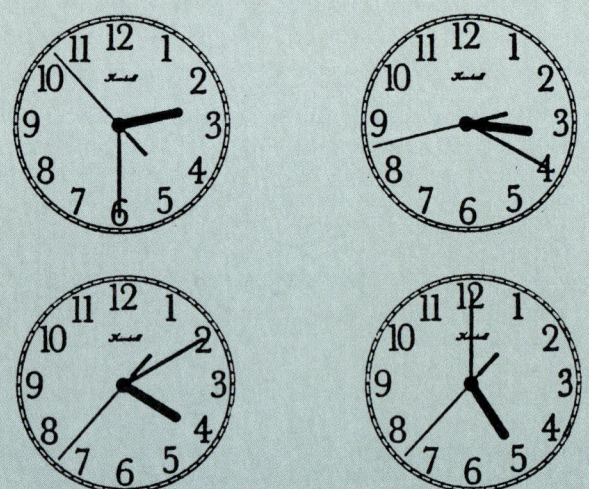

Type 2: fair skin with deep blue, hazel or brown eyes and ash blond, deep red, or light brown hair; typical burn time: 15-30 minutes.

Type 3: medium skin with brown eyes and brown hair; typical burn time: 20-40 minutes.

Type 4: light to medium brown skin with dark brown eyes and hair; typical burn time: 25-50 minutes.

Type 5: light to golden brown skin with dark brown eyes and black hair; typical burn time: 30-60 minutes.

Type 6: brown to deepest brown skin with dark brown eyes and black hair; typical burn time: 40-75 minutes.

---

can be concentrated onto your skin, resulting in severe burns and skin damage.

▶ Stay out of the sun or take extra precautions if you are taking antibiotics (especially penicillin or tetracycline), birth control pills, insulin (especially oral insulin), diuretics, and some medications used to lower blood pressure. They increase the damage from ultraviolet rays.

▶ Don't drink alcohol if you will be exposed to sunlight. Alcohol, too, increases the damage from ultraviolet rays.

▶ Don't patronize tanning salons or booths, and don't use a sunlamp. Tanned skin is damaged skin. There is no such thing as a "safe" tan.

Most important, do whatever you can to avoid a sunburn. The risk of skin cancer from exposure to sunlight is cumulative. Each time you are unprotected and exposed to sunlight, some amount of damage accrues. With increasing damage, you also increase your risk of developing skin cancer. Sunburns are especially dangerous. Experts say that even one bad sunburn during childhood can double your risk for getting skin cancer later on.

AN ANTI-CANCER DIET

The American Cancer Society and the National Academy of Science have jointly released the following dietary guidelines for reducing cancer risk. They bear repeating here.

▶ Maintain a normal weight. A 12-year study involving almost a million Americans showed that those who were overweight — especially those who were 40% or more overweight — ran substantially higher risks for cancer. According to the study, those who are obese run a one-and-a-half times greater risk for cancer of the breast and colon, two times higher risk for cancer of the prostate, three times greater risk for cancer of the gallbladder, and five times greater risk for uterine cancer. The American Cancer Society recommends limiting calories and increasing exercise to maintain an ideal weight.

▶ Reduce the amount of fat you eat. The American Cancer Society recommends reducing the percentage of calories that come from fat to 30%, and even lower if you need to lose weight. Cut down on foods high in fats, such as red meats, whole milk and whole milk products, cheeses, butter, pastries, candies, and oils. Trim all visible fat from your meat before cooking it, remove skin and fat from chicken before cooking, avoid frying foods, and use low-fat methods of cooking (broiling, poaching, baking). Skim all visible fats from soups, stews, and gravies; if you can, refrigerate them overnight, then remove the hardened fat that rises to the surface.

▶ Eat more high-fiber foods, such as whole-grain cereals, whole-grain breads, bran cereals, legumes (including kidney beans), lima beans, pinto beans, rice, popcorn, and brown rice. Leave well-scrubbed skins on fruits and vegetables. Eat foods with visible hulls, seeds, and textured skins, such as strawberries, raspberries, and peaches.

▶ Eat food rich in vitamins A and C every day. Good sources of vitamin A are fresh foods that are dark green or deep yellow in color: spinach, broccoli, carrots, sweet potatoes, squash, apricots, and peaches. Good sources of vitamin C are citrus fruits (such as oranges, grapefruit, and tangerines), strawberries, cantaloupes, tomatoes, and green peppers.

▶ Eat cruciferous vegetables such as cabbage, broccoli, cauliflower, Brussels sprouts, and kohlrabi, as they seem to provide protection against a number of cancers.

▶ Cut down on salt-cured, smoked, and nitrite-cured foods. Limit the amount of bacon, ham, hot dogs, beef jerky, smoked fish, smoked meats, and salt-cured fish you eat. Don't smoke your own foods. When you barbecue, keep temperatures low enough so food doesn't get charred.

▶ If you drink, use alcohol in strict moderation. Alcohol significantly increases your risk for a number of cancers, especially if you also smoke cigarettes. A study reported in the *New England Journal of Medicine* linked alcohol consumption with breast cancer. Women who had as few as three alcoholic drinks a week had a 30% higher chance of developing breast cancer than women who seldom or never drank. Researchers at the National Cancer Institute went even farther, putting the risk at 50% higher for women who drink any alcohol at all and as much as 100% higher for women who have three drinks or more a week.

In addition to these guidelines, the following dietary suggestions can further reduce your risk of cancer:

▶ Get plenty of calcium. It seems to help neutralize carcinogenic substances in the digestive tract. Low-fat milk is a good source.

▶ Avoid foods that have been treated heavily with chemicals or pesticides or processed with a lot of additives. Wash fruits and vegetables well before you eat them.

▶ Refrigerate foods that need it, especially fruits and vegetables. Evidence shows that fruits and vegetables naturally produce nitrites, a process that refrigeration slows down.

▶ Cut down on cholesterol — something you do anyway if you're eating a diet low in fat. Two studies reported in the *New England Journal of Medicine* maintain that high cholesterol levels in the blood contribute to colorectal cancer.

Table 12.3 summarizes the dietary measures that may lower your risk for cancer. The key seems to be variety and moderation.

APPROPRIATE SELF-EXAMS

One of the keys to successful cancer treatment is early detection. You should examine yourself regularly for skin, breast, or testicular cancer.

Skin Self-Exams

One of the easiest and quickest self-exams is a brief survey to detect possible skin cancers.

▶ Make a drawing of yourself. Include a full front view, a full back view, and close-up views of your head (both sides), the soles of your feet, the tops of your feet, and the backs of your hands.

▶ After you get out of the bath or shower, examine yourself closely in a full-length mirror. On your sketch make note of any moles, warts, or other skin marks you find anywhere on your body. Pay particular attention to areas that are exposed to the sun constantly, such as your face, the tops of your ears, and your hands.

▶ Briefly describe each mark on your sketch: its size, what color, texture, and so on.

▶ Repeat the exam about once a month. If you notice changes in any of the marks, contact your physician.

TABLE 12.3 ▼ Anti-Cancer Dietary Measures

Substance	Associated Cancers	Comments	Steps to Take
Fiber	May *decrease* risk of colorectal cancer.	Different types of fiber may affect cancer risk differently. Benefits also may be due to lower fat intakes usually associated with high-fiber diets.	Eat 4 to 5 servings a day of a variety of vegetables, fruits, whole-grain cereals, and legumes. Maximize fiber in vegetables and fruits by eating them unpeeled.
Fruits and vegetables	May *decrease* risk of colorectal and breast cancers.	Good sources of fiber (see above). Cruciferous vegetables, such as broccoli, cabbage, and Brussels sprouts, also contain indoles — nitrogen compounds which, in some studies, have knocked out carcinogens that can lead to breast cancer.	To maximize indole intake, eat vegetables raw, steamed, or microwaved; boiling leaches up to half the indoles.
Fat	May *increase* risk of breast, colon, and prostate cancers.	Lowering fat intake will almost automatically lower caloric intake and boost fiber intake — steps that also will lower cancer risk.	Decrease calories from fat to 25% to 30% of total daily calories. (Current average intake is 40% of total calories.)
Alcohol	Heavy use *increases* risk of cancers of the oral cavity, larynx, and esophagus; moderate use may *increase* breast cancer risk.	Cigarette smoking in conjunction with alcohol drinking greatly increases cancer risk. Alcohol use also can cause liver cirrhosis, which may lead to liver cancer.	Drink only occasionally and sparingly.
Salt-cured, smoked, barbecued and nitrite-preserved foods	May *increase* risk of stomach, esophageal, and lung cancers.	Smoking and charcoal-grilling foods produces tars that are similar to those in cigarette smoke, and are absorbed by the food. Manufacturers have substantially decreased nitrites used in meat preservation.	Opt for other cooking methods; limit intake of salt-cured and nitrite-preserved foods.
Beta-carotene and antioxidant vitamins (A, C, and E)	Inconclusive	Vitamin E and beta-carotene have been associated with lower rates of cancer in humans; a lesser effect has been noted with the other antioxidant nutrients. More research is needed.	Eat a balanced and varied diet to ensure that you get the RDA for all vitamins; do not take megadose vitamin supplements.
Selenium	Inconclusive	Limited evidence shows this trace element may protect against breast and colon cancers; however, it is highly toxic in high doses.	Taking selenium supplements can be dangerous; you get all the selenium you need from a varied diet.
Artificial sweeteners	Inconclusive	High levels of saccharin cause bladder cancer in rats, but no evidence of this in humans. Long-term effects of aspartame are unknown.	Moderate use poses no risk.
Coffee and caffeine	None	Both coffee and caffeine have received a clean bill of health.	Moderate use of coffee and caffeine does not appear to be a risk.
Food additives	None	Chemical additives found to be carcinogenic in animals have been banned; insufficient evidence that additives currently in use have any cancer risk or benefit.	None

Reprinted with permission of the *Johns Hopkins Medical Letter Health After 50*, © MedLetter Associates, 1992.

Self Exam

1 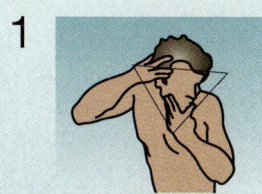 Examine your face, especially the nose, lips, mouth, and ears – front and back. Use one or both mirrors to get a clear view.

2 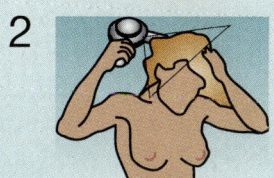 Thoroughly inspect your scalp, using a blow dryer and mirror to expose each section to view. Get a friend or family member to help, if you can.

3 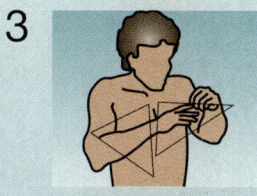 Check your hands carefully: palms and backs, between the fingers, and under the fingernails. Continue up the wrists to examine both front and back of your forearms.

4 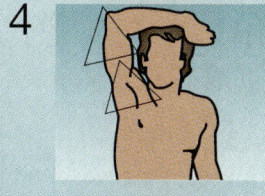 Standing in front of a full-length mirror, begin at the elbows and scan all sides of your upper arms. Don't forget the underarms.

5 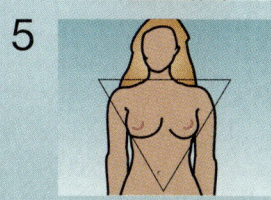 Next focus on the neck, chest, and torso. Women should lift breasts to view the underside.

6 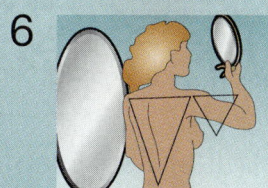 With your back to the full-length mirror, use the hand mirror to inspect the back of your neck, shoulders, upper back, and any part of the back of your upper arms you could not view in step 4.

7 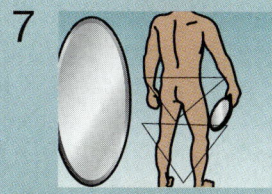 Still using both mirrors, scan your lower back, buttocks, and backs of both legs.

8 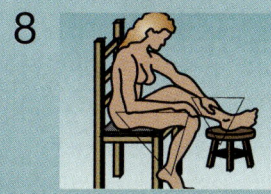 Sit down; prop each leg in turn on another stool or chair. Use the hand mirror to examine the genitals. Check front and sides of both legs, thigh to shin; ankles, tops of feet, between toes, and under toenails. Examine soles of feet and heels

Reprinted with permission from *Family Practice Recertification*, Vol. 14, No. 3, March, 1992.

Breast Self-Exams

Early detection of breast cancer is vital to successful treatment, and a woman who does regular monthly self-exams has a much better chance of detecting changes that could indicate problems. When you're doing self-exams regularly, you can detect a growth when it's about the size of a pea; a physician doing a breast exam probably won't detect it until it's two to three times that size.

Perform the exam regularly, once a month. A week after your menstrual period is the best time, as your breasts won't be subject to the swelling that sometimes precedes menstruation, and it will be a regular reminder. If you don't have periods, pick a day you can remember easily (such as the first day of the month).

The American Cancer Society recommends a three-stage self-exam:

1. **While you're in the bathtub or shower:** Using the flat part of your fingers, use your right hand to examine your left breast, your left hand to examine your right breast. Move gently over each breast, checking for hard knots, lumps, or thickening of tissue.

2. **While you're standing in front of a mirror:** Stand in front of a mirror with your arms at your sides. Look at your breasts. They should be fairly symmetrical and even. Few women have breasts that are precisely the same, but you should make note of any substantial differences.

    Next, lift your arms above your head, and check your breasts again. Note any changes in the contour, any swelling, any dimpling, or any nipple changes.

    Finally, put your hands on your hips and press so your chest muscles flex. Check again. Note any differences in contour, dimpling, or swelling.

    This kind of exam, repeated every month, will give you a good idea of what's normal for you and will help you quickly spot any changes.

3. **While you're lying down:** You'll need to examine both breasts, one at a time. To examine your right breast:

    ▶ Place a pillow or folded towel under your right shoulder to elevate and flatten your breast, distributing breast tissue more evenly against your chest wall. Rest your head on your right arm.

    ▶ With the flat pads of the fingers of your left hand, press gently in small circular motions, starting at the outside edge of your breast and continuing in to your nipple. Imagine that your breast is a clock face: Start at 12 o'clock on the outside edge, and work all the way around your breast to 12 o'clock again. Then move in toward your nipple about an inch, and repeat. Keep going around the "clock face" until you reach your nipple. A firm ridge of tissue beneath each breast is normal. You are checking for knots, hard lumps, indentations, thickening, swellings, or masses. Take the time to check every part of your breast. It will require at least three circles around the "clock face."

    ▶ Using the flat pads of the fingers of your left hand, check your armpit area thoroughly for lumps, swellings, thickening, or painful lymph nodes.

    ▶ Finally, squeeze your nipple gently between your thumb and index finger of the left hand. Note any pain, scaliness, or discharge.

Repeat the exam on your left breast, using the pillow or padded towel under your left side and conducting the exam with your right hand.

The key to breast self-examination is to do the exam regularly. Cancer is detected soonest when you notice a change from one month to the next. Immediately report to your doctor any changes or anything unusual. And don't forego your yearly medical exam.

Testicular Self-Exam

Testicular cancer detected early can be treated successfully a good deal of the time. The key to early detection is a simple, 3-minute self-exam done once a month. Choose a day each month (the first day usually is easy to remember), and do the exam as soon as you get out of a warm bath or shower, as your testicles and scrotal skin are most relaxed then. You need to examine both testicles, one at a time.

▶ Using both hands, roll the testicle gently between your thumbs and fingers. You'll feel a rope like structure toward the back of the testicle. That's the epididymis, and it's normal. Most cancers occur toward the front of the testicle, and they will feel like a pea-sized lump or hard knot.

Breast Exam

1 Raising one arm at a time over your head, use the fingertips of the opposite hand to check for any changes, lumps, or thickening.

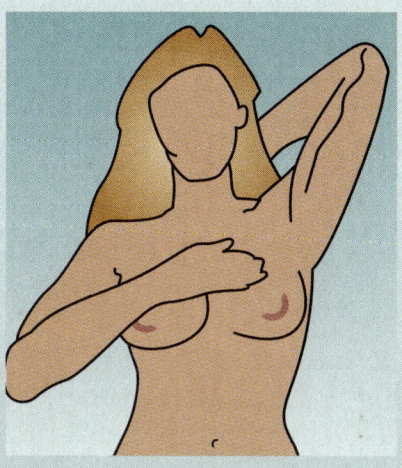

2 Start near the nipple and work outward in widening circles.

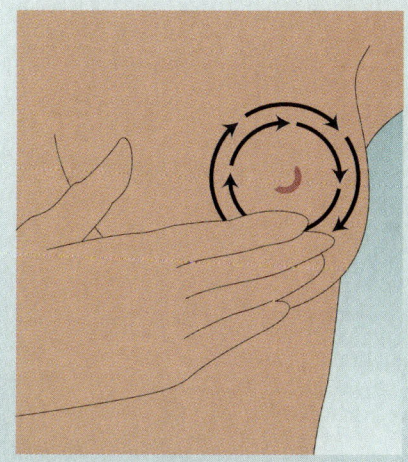

3 Visually examine your breasts in a mirror with your arms at your sides.

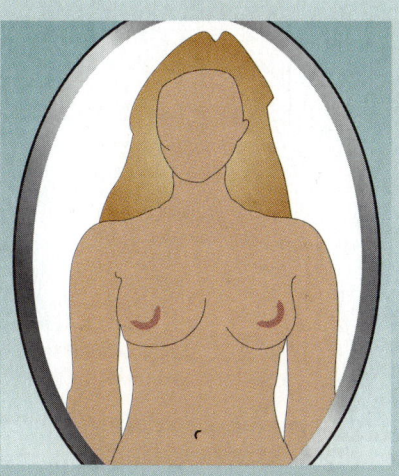

4 Visually examine your breasts in a mirror with your arms raised above your head.

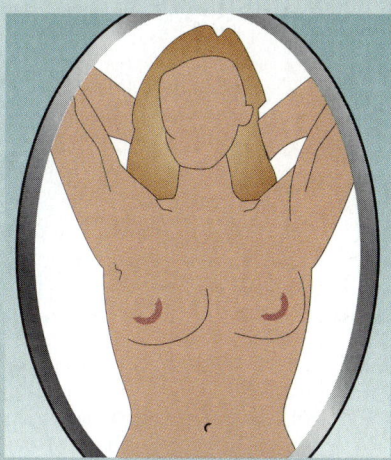

5 Check your nipples by squeezing them gently. Unless you have recently had a baby, any discharge is abnormal.

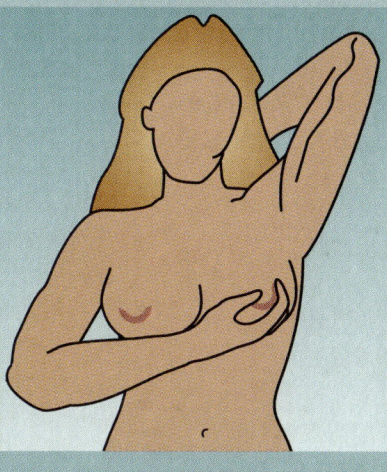

6 Place a pillow under your shoulder and your arm under your head. With your other hand, feel your breast and armpit for lumps, thickening, or other changes.

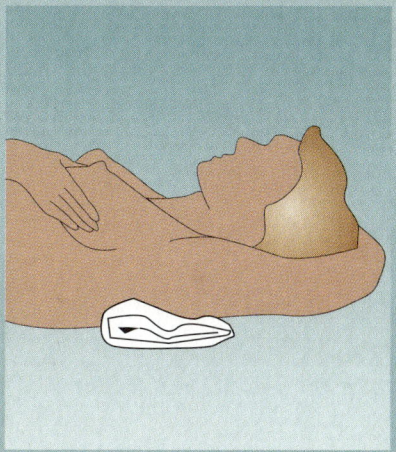

Adapted from *Family Practice Recertification* 14(3), March 1992. Used by permission.

Testicular Self-Exam

How do I do this examination?

Here's how to go about it: Roll each testicle between your thumb and first three fingers until you have felt the entire surface (see Figure below). The testicles should feel round and smooth, like hard-boiled eggs.

These are the things you have to be on the lookout for:

▼ Lumps
▼ Irregularities
▼ A change in the size of the testicle
▼ Pain in the testicle
▼ A dragging or heavy sensation.

How often do I have to do this exam?

Do it at least once a month. It helps to pick a regular day of the month — the day of your birthday, the first of the month, the first Sunday, or some other day that's easy for you to remember. You can do the exam more often if you like.

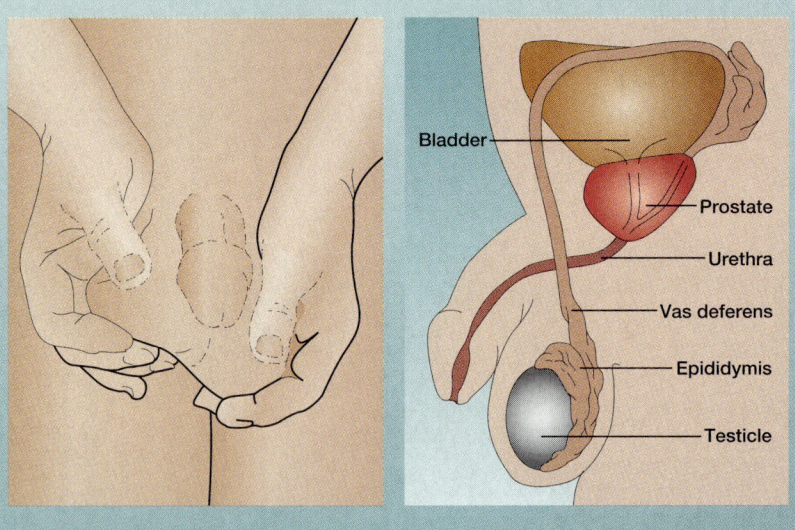

Reprinted with permission from *Patient Care*, © Medical Economics Publishing, Inc., Montvale, New Jersey, 07645. All rights reserved.

▶ Repeat the exam on the other testicle.
▶ Immediately report to your doctor any nodules or lumps.

AGE-APPROPRIATE CHECKUPS

In addition to self-exams you do at home, your physician can do examinations and tests to enable early detection of cancer. The exams in Table 12.4 are the final weapon in your arsenal against cancer.

If you are at high risk for a certain cancer, you should have screening tests more often. Check with your physician. Sexually active women should have annual Pap smears and pelvic exams as soon as sexual activity begins.

TABLE 12.4 ▼ Medical Checkups

Examination	Age and Frequency
▼ Cancer-related checkup (skin, thyroid gland, mouth, lymph glands, ovaries, prostate gland, testicles)	▼ Age 20 to 40: every 3 to 4 years. ▼ Beginning at age 40: once a year
▼ Breast	▼ Ages 20 to 40: physician exam every 3–4 years ▼ Ages 35–39: one baseline mammogram ▼ Ages 40–50: exam and mammogram every 2 years ▼ Age 50 and older: exam and mammogram annually
▼ Colon and rectum	▼ Ages 40 and up: digital rectal exam annually ▼ Ages 50 and up: stool blood test annually ▼ Ages 50 and up: proctology exam every 2 years after two negative annual exams
▼ Uterus	▼ Ages 20 to 40: pelvic exam every 3 years ▼ Ages 40 and up: pelvic exam annually
▼ Cervix	▼ Ages 20 to 40: pelvic exam and Pap smear once every 2 years after two consecutive negative tests ▼ Age 40 and up: annual exams regardless of age; if sexually active with more than one partner
▼ Prostate	▼ Ages 40 and up: digital exam annually and PSA protein test

What Is Your Risk of Developing Certain Cancers?

For each question, select the response that best describes you; record the point value in the space provided. Total your points for each section separately.

Lung Cancer

1. Sex _____
   - 2 Male
   - 1 Female
2. Age _____
   - 1 39 or younger
   - 2 40-49
   - 5 50-59
   - 7 60 and over
3. _____
   - 8 Smoker
   - 1 Nonsmoker
4. Type of smoking _____
   - 10 Current smoker of cigarettes or little cigars
   - 3 Pipe and/or cigar, but not cigarettes
   - 2 Ex-cigarette smoker
   - 1 Nonsmoker
5. Amount of cigarettes smoked per day _____
   - 1 0
   - 5 Less than 1/2 pack
   - 9 1/2-1 pack
   - 15 1-2 packs
   - 20 2 or more packs
6. Type of cigarette* _____
   - 10 High tar/nicotine
   - 9 Medium tar/nicotine
   - 7 Low tar/nicotine
   - 1 Nonsmoker
7. Duration of smoking _____
   - 1 Never smoked
   - 3 Ex-smoker
   - 5 Up to 15 years
   - 10 15-25 years
   - 20 25 or more years
8. Type of industrial work _____
   - 3 Mining
   - 7 Asbestos
   - 5 Uranium and radioactive products

Lung total _____

*Tar/nicotine levels:
High: 20 + mg. tar/1.3 + mg. nicotine
Medium: 16-19 mg. tar/1.1-1.2 mg. nicotine
Low: 15 mg. or less tar/1.0 mg. or less nicotine

Colon and Rectal Cancer

1. Age _____
   - 10 39 or younger
   - 20 40-59
   - 50 60 and over
2. Has anyone in your immediate family ever had: _____
   - 20 Colon cancer
   - 10 One or more colon polyps
   - 1 Neither
3. Have you ever had: _____
   - 100 Colon cancer
   - 40 One or more colon polyps
   - 20 Ulcerative colitis
   - 10 Cancer of the breast or uterus
   - 1 None
4. Bleeding from the rectum (other than obvious hemorrhoids or piles) _____
   - 75 Yes
   - 1 No

Colon and rectal total _____

Skin Cancer

1. Frequently work or play in the sun _____
   - 10 Yes
   - 1 No
2. Work in mines, around coal tars, or around radioactivity _____
   - 10 Yes
   - 1 No
3. Complexion — fair skin or light skin _____
   - 10 Yes
   - 1 No

Skin total _____

Breast Cancer (Women Only)

1. Age group _____
   - 10 20-34
   - 40 35-49
   - 90 50 and over
2. Racial group _____
   - 5 Asian
   - 20 African-American
   - 25 Non-Hispanic White
   - 10 Hispanic
3. Family history _____
   - 30 Mother, sister, aunt, or grandmother with breast cancer
   - 10 None
4. Your history _____
   - 25 Previous lumps or cysts
   - 10 No breast disease
   - 100 Previous breast cancer
5. Maternity _____
   - 10 First pregnancy before age 25

(Continued)

What Is Your Risk of Developing Certain Cancers? (continued)

15 First pregnancy after age 25
20 No pregnancies

Breast total _____

Cervical Cancer (Women Only)

1. Age group _____
   10 Younger than 25
   20 25-39
   30 40-54
   30 55 and over
2. Racial group _____
   10 Asian
   20 African American
   10 Non-Hispanic White
   20 Hispanic
3. Number of pregnancies _____
   10 0
   20 1 to 3
   30 4 and over
4. Viral infections _____
   10 Herpes and other viral infections or ulcer formations on the vagina
    1 Never
5. Age at first intercourse _____
   40 Younger than 15
   30 15-19
   20 20-24
   10 25 and over
    5 Never
6. Bleeding between periods or after intercourse _____
   40 Yes
    1 No

Cervical total _____

Analysis

If your *lung* total is:

24 or less You have a low risk for lung cancer.
24-49 You may be a light smoker and would benefit from quitting.
50-74 As a moderate smoker, your risks for lung and upper respiratory tract cancer are increased. If you stop smoking now, these risks will decrease.
75 or over As a heavy cigarette smoker, your risks for lung and upper respiratory tract cancer are greatly increased. You should stop smoking now. See your physician if you have possible signs of lung cancer (nagging cough, hoarseness, persistent sore in the mouth or throat).

If your *colon and rectal* total is:'

29 or less You are at low risk for colon and rectal cancer.
30-69 You are at moderate risk. Testing by your physician may be indicated.
70 or over You are at high risk. You should see your physician for the following tests: digital rectal exam, stool occult blood test, and (where applicable) proctoscopic exam.

Numerical risks for *skin* cancer are difficult to state. For instance, a person with a dark complexion can work longer in the sun and be less likely to develop cancer than a light-complected person. Furthermore, a person wearing a long-sleeved shirt and wide-brimmed hat may work in the sun and be less at risk than a person who wears a bathing suit for only a short period. The risk goes up greatly with age. If you answered "yes" to any question, you need to protect your skin from the sun or any other toxic material. Changes in moles, warts, or skin sores are important and should be seen by your physician.

If your *breast* total is:

100 or less You are at low risk. You should do monthly breast self-examination (BSE) and have your breasts examined by a physician as part of a cancer-related checkup.
100-199 You are at moderate risk. You should practice monthly BSE and have your breasts examined by a physician as part of a cancer-related checkup. Periodic mammograms should be included, as directed by your physician.
200 or over You are at high risk. You should practice monthly BSE and have professional examinations more often. See your physician for the examinations recommended for you.

If your *cervical* total is:

40-69 You are at low risk. Your physician will advise you about how often you should have a Pap test.
70-99 You are at moderate risk. More frequent Pap tests may be required.
100 or more You are at high risk. You should have a Pap test and pelvic exam as advised by your physician.

From American Cancer Society, Texas Division.

WELLNESS ▼ *Guidelines for a Healthy Lifestyle*

13

Addictive Behavior and Wellness

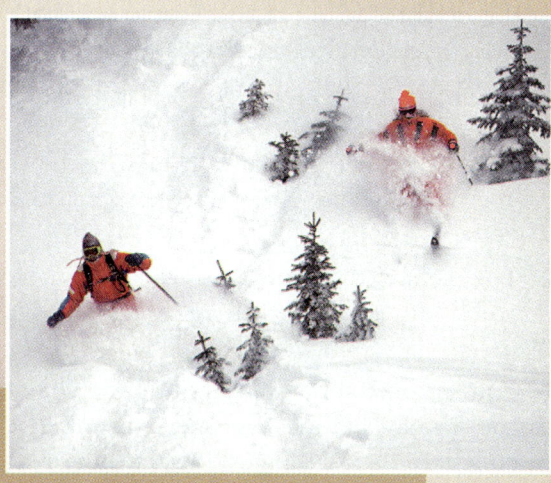

Objectives

▼ Define "addiction" and differentiate it from "habit."
▼ Learn the warning signs of addiction.
▼ Cite the threats to the six dimensions of wellness.
▼ Understand the nonaddictive personality.
▼ Delineate addictive personality traits.
▼ List factors leading to addiction.
▼ Learn the major risk factors of addiction to: caffeine, tobacco, alcohol, marijuana, cocaine.
▼ List guidelines for managing and changing addictive behavior.

Everyone knows what a habit is. We all have them. You might have the habit of flopping down in front of the television as soon as you get home every day, or of biting your nails when you're bored. Most habits are harmless, but when a habit escalates into an addiction, it threatens wellness.

Broadly defined, an addiction is *an abnormal or disordered relationship with an object* (such as tobacco or alcohol) or an event or behavior (such as shoplifting or gambling). Addiction goes far beyond dependence on drugs, which is what is normally associated with it. Some estimates are that well over 30% of all Americans are addicts of some kind.

How can you tell that something is no longer a habit, that it has become a full-blown addiction? A number of signs point to addictive behavior:

▶ You can't seem to get satisfaction from the behavior. No matter how much you get, it's just never enough. You're constantly frustrated by the need to do more or get more. (That frustration, incidentally, is much different from the motivation that stems from challenge and determination.)

▶ You don't get pleasure from the behavior. It doesn't contribute to an overall sense of well-being.

▶ The behavior becomes predictable. You know you'll do a certain thing a certain way. The pattern never changes.

▶ You become inflexible about the behavior. You run 2 miles before class every morning, and you balk at a friend's suggestion that you play tennis instead. If your friend won't run with you, you run anyway — either before you play tennis or instead of playing tennis.

▶ You feel a lower sense of self-worth or self-esteem because of what you're doing, but you can't seem to stop.

▶ You don't necessarily enjoy the behavior, but you feel driven to do it anyway. You might be disgusted by your obsession to look at pornographic magazines, and might think it's a dirty habit, but you can't seem to stop, regardless of your feelings. Your behavior even might make you sick, but you can't seem to change.

▶ You stay locked in the behavior as a way of escaping demands or stresses, not because you see the behavior as an exhilarating challenge.

▶ The behavior dulls your senses, provides an escape, or otherwise helps you get away from stress, unhappiness, boredom, or frustration. Whenever you get a chance for challenge or reward, you resort to the addictive behavior instead of taking a chance on some other behavior.

Addiction threatens all six dimensions of wellness: physical, emotional, social, intellectual, occupational, and spiritual.

1. *Physical wellness.* People who are addicted to an object or an event generally fail to take good care of themselves because they are preoccupied with the addictive behavior. They might not get enough sleep, may skip meals, could even put themselves in dangerous situations. Certain addictive behaviors damage the body itself. As examples, bulimia damages the throat and alcoholism damages the liver. The stress accompanying some addictions can injure virtually every organ and system in the body.

2. *Emotional wellness.* Addictive behavior lowers self-esteem. The addict usually feels guilty, anxious, angry, depressed, and ashamed. Many addicts suffer unexplained mood swings or episodes of rage and violence. Many also find themselves confronted with unresolved issues they thought were no longer an issue.

3. *Social wellness.* Other than the interaction the addiction requires, an addict usually is a loner who gradually cuts off relationships with family members, friends, colleagues, or classmates. Addiction brings with it a powerful preoccupation that takes priority over people, places, and events outside the addictive behavior.

4. *Intellectual wellness.* Addiction impairs reasoning, judgment, and logic. Things that used to provide intellectual challenge or stimulation — coursework in a graduate class, exploration of nearby geological sites, debates over a proposed nuclear waste dump — no longer matter.

5. *Occupational wellness.* All of the addict's focus is on the addictive behavior, which leaves little time for school or a job. Absenteeism increases; quality takes a dive; relationships with professors, other students, colleagues, and supervisors suffer.

6. *Spiritual wellness.* Because of the time and energy demands of an addiction, addicts have difficulty maintaining the same priorities and values they once had. Addicts gradually lose a sense of self and a feeling of being "connected" to the people and the world around them. They can't focus on something greater than self, nor can they appreciate themselves in a meaningful way.

THE ADDICTIVE PERSONALITY

The notion of an addictive personality has been somewhat controversial. One school of thought flatly believes there is no such thing as an addictive

Could You Be An Addict?

Directions: The following test, designed by Dr. Lawrence Hatterer, a clinical associate professor of psychiatry at Cornell University Medical School, will help you understand addictive behavior better so you can recognize it in yourself or perhaps in people you know. If you answer "yes" to half or more of the questions, you may have a problem and should seek immediate professional help.

		YES	NO
1.	I'm a person of excesses. I can't regulate what I do for pleasure and often use a substance or indulge in an activity heavily, in order to get high.	☐	☐
2.	I'm an extremely self-involved person. People tell me I'm into myself too much.	☐	☐
3.	I'm compulsive. I must have what I want when I want it, regardless of the consequences.	☐	☐
4.	I'm either excessively dependent on or independent of others.	☐	☐
5.	I'm preoccupied. I spend a lot of time thinking or fantasizing about an activity or a substance. Also, I will work my day around doing it or go to pains to make sure it's available.	☐	☐
6.	I deny that I do this and lie about it to others who ask me.	☐	☐
7.	I have been involved in this behavior for at least a year.	☐	☐
8.	I've told myself I could easily stop, even though I've shown no signs of slowing down.	☐	☐
9.	Once I start indulging in this behavior or substance, I find I have trouble stopping.	☐	☐
10.	One or more members of my family also are involved in some kind of excessive behavior or substance abuse.	☐	☐
11.	I find I gravitate mostly toward people who have the same behavior or take the same substance as I do.	☐	☐
12.	I seem to be developing a tolerance to the behavior or substance. I have had a need to steadily increase the amounts I take or the time I spend doing it.	☐	☐
13.	I have found that my excessive use of highs has only made my problems worse.	☐	☐
14.	If someone tries to keep me from obtaining the substance or practicing the activity, I get angry and reject or abuse them.	☐	☐
15.	I experience withdrawal symptoms if I cannot indulge in the substance or activity.	☐	☐
16.	This has gotten in the way of my functioning. I've missed something important — days at school or work, time with friends, family, children — because of it.	☐	☐
17.	The substance/activity is destroying my home life. I know I'm hurting those closest to me.	☐	☐
18.	I've failed in many goals in life, lost money, given up many social and occupational contacts, all because of my excessive behavior.	☐	☐
19.	I've tried to stop or cut down on my excesses but have been unsuccessful.	☐	☐
20.	I've physically endangered myself or others in accidents that were a direct result of my excessive behavior.	☐	☐

Margot Gilman, reprinted with permission from *McCall's Magazine*. © 1986 by The McCall Publishing Company.

personality. Other researchers believe no set of personality traits leads to addiction but have identified a "constellation of traits" that disposes someone to addiction. The more of these characteristics a person has, and the stronger each trait or condition is, the more vulnerable that person is to addiction.

THE NONADDICTIVE PERSONALITY

Some traits of people who are *not* likely to have addictive behavior are:

▶ They have the ability to face problems head-on with optimism and realism, and they work to overcome their problems. They recognize their own limitations and pace themselves accordingly to maximize their ability to cope.

▶ They are able and eager to look at their circumstances realistically. They set realistic goals, and they work toward achieving their goals in a structured, reasonable way. They escape the frustration and disappointment that come with unreached goals.

▶ They aren't too hard on themselves. They recognize their limitations and weaknesses but also appreciate their strengths and good qualities. They structure their lives so they can maximize their strengths without having to "escape" their weaknesses.

▶ They have a keen interest in other people, allow others the freedom to pursue their own interests, and have at least a few deep relationships with other people. They have the ability to love and be loved and consider others' feelings, desires, and needs as they fashion their own behavior. They are not controlled by others but are sensitive to others.

▶ They are happy, spontaneous, creative, and like to try new things.

▶ They see a lot of positive things in life and are eager to discover more. They appreciate things in their lives and have a fresh sense of humor that allows them to retain some perspective about what happens to them.

TRAITS THAT MAKE PEOPLE PRONE TO ADDICTION

The book *A Wellness Way of Life* points out that the objects, events, or behaviors involved in addiction aren't necessarily bad, but an addict has an unhealthy or abnormal relationship with those objects, events, or behaviors. For example, food provides us with nutrition and energy, but food addicts eat compulsively and endanger their health. Sex provides intimacy, but a sex addict becomes preoccupied with pornography or an ever-expanding gamut of sexual partners. Drugs can cure disease, but drug addicts harm themselves by abusing the substance.

In his book *The Addictive Personality: Roots, Rituals, and Recovery,* author Craig Nakken defined the addictive personality as belonging to people who have been taught not to trust people, who do not have healthy relationships, and who never have learned to connect to other people, their own emotions, and the world around them.

Despite controversy surrounding the notion of an "addictive personality," most professionals agree that the following traits make individuals vulnerable to addictive behavior:

▶ A genetic factor may predispose a person to addictive behavior. This factor seems especially prevalent with the tendency for alcohol and drug abuse.

▶ They feel powerless and victimized by their surroundings. An addictive behavior can engender a feeling of strength or aggression they can't cultivate on their own.

▶ They display antisocial behavior and have a strong sense of alienation from other people. They lack confidence, which makes them unable to communicate well and, in turn, makes them particularly susceptible to peer pressure (shown to be a strong determinant in drug and alcohol abuse). They are unable to seek comfort from others.

▶ An opposite set of traits also has been shown to make people more prone to addictive behavior. These people are less mature than others and are not able to deal with situations as maturely as their counterparts. They tend to become dependent, conforming, and compliant, even when they think their own needs are being compromised. They do anything possible to avoid conflict, are extremely fearful of being criticized, and try desperately to please others.

▶ They *seem* outgoing and sociable but have a great deal of trouble developing any kind of interpersonal relationship. They fear other people and stay detached. They seem to fear deep involvement, usually because they feel incapable of handling relationships.

▶ They recognize problems, but instead of tackling them head-on, they feel overwhelmed and incapable. They lack problem-solving skills. They do anything they can to deny the problem, hide from the problem, or run away from the problem — something that usually develops into an addictive behavior.

▶ When threatened by a problem, they try to escape — sometimes through fantasy or daydreaming but always through something that helps them forget about the problem.

▶ They don't have the ability to set realistic, reasonable goals and go about achieving them systematically. Instead, they set unrealistic, or even impossible, goals, then drive toward those goals erratically. When they don't achieve their goals, they sink into depression.

▶ They worry about their own capabilities and have low self-esteem. They fear the future and what it might hold, feel unsure about their ability to measure up, and dread what lies ahead.

▶ They do not deal well with stress. They allow stress to build up without knowing how to cope with it, and when things get really tough, the addictive behavior may be the only way out.

▶ They don't deal well with frustration and feel threatened particularly by even low levels of frustration. Much of that stems from deep feelings of inferiority. They have felt inferior since early childhood and have been unable to aggressively meet problems head-on. With a constant fear of being overwhelmed, embarrassed, or compromised, they turn to addictive behavior to escape or to get a false sense of power over their environment.

▶ They lack normal levels of spontaneity, creativity, and eagerness for life. As a result, they get bored, and they turn to an addiction to relieve the boredom.

▶ They often come from high-risk backgrounds. Higher rates of addictive behavior, especially drug and alcohol abuse, are found in populations of the economically disadvantaged, latchkey children, abuse victims, people with physical or mental handicaps, school dropouts, pregnant teenagers, runaways, the homeless, and children of alcoholics.

▶ They often are risk-takers who are impulsive and have unusually high levels of energy. They look for excitement and stimulation and turn to an addictive behavior to get it.

▼ THE RISK FACTORS OF ADDICTION

As mentioned, addictive behavior covers a wide spectrum: eating disorders, compulsive gambling, shoplifting, compulsive spending, alcoholism, sexual addiction, to name a few. Factors leading to addiction include the following:

▶ The behavior is reinforced.
▶ The addiction is an attempt to meet basic human needs, such as physical needs, the need to feel safe, the need to belong, the need to feel important, or the need to reach one's potential.
▶ The addiction relieves stress.
▶ The addiction results from peer pressure.
▶ The addiction can be present within the person's value system (a person whose values wouldn't let him or her shoot heroine may be able to rationalize compulsive eating or obsessive television watching, for example).
▶ A serious physical illness is present, and the addiction may provide escape from pain or the fear of disfigurement.
▶ There is pressure to perform or succeed.
▶ The person hates himself or herself.
▶ A genetic link is present. Heredity may dictate your susceptibility to some addictions.
▶ Brain activity may vary. Some addictions may be attributable to intense brainwave speed.
▶ Society allows addiction. Advertising even *encourages* it (you can sleep better with a pill; beer helps you enjoy sports more fully, parties are more fun with alcohol, and so on).

The same general traits and behaviors are involved in all kinds of addictions, whether they involve food, sex, gambling, shopping, or drugs. Most common, however, are addictions to caffeine, tobacco, marijuana, and cocaine.

CAFFEINE

Caffeine is probably the most widely used drug in the United States. An estimated 82%-92% of Americans regularly consume caffeine. It is found in coffee, tea, cocoa, chocolate, colas, a variety of soft drinks, and a number of prescription and over-the-counter drugs. Caffeine is a common ingredient in nonprescription drugs for cold and allergy relief, pain relief, weight control, alleviation of fluid retention, and alertness. Caffeine occurs naturally in coffee, tea, and chocolate, and it is added to other products during manufacturing.

In one survey, only approximately 1% of the men, women, and children questioned had not used caffeine in some form over the 3-day period before the survey. The most common source of caffeine is coffee. Kids who use products containing caffeine, however, can build up an unhealthy level relatively fast. The capsule you take for a headache can give you more than you'd imagine: One Excedrin or two Anacin contain as much caffeine as two cups of instant coffee.

Regular coffee drinkers are at greater risk for heart disease, coronary artery disease, and heart attack. One study showed that drinking five cups of coffee a day may increase the risk of heart attack. Another study found that women who drink one-half to four cups of tea a day are twice as likely to have premenstrual syndrome (PMS). Much more moderate amounts of caffeine — sometimes no more than the amount in one cup of coffee — may pose a risk in some individuals, too, and can cause the following effects:

▶ Increase in heart rate, blood pressure, and blood cholesterol levels.
▶ Increase in metabolism and the amount of oxygen the body's cells require.
▶ Increase in urinary output.
▶ Impairment of fine-motor control.
▶ Dizziness.
▶ Headaches.
▶ Insomnia.
▶ Irritability, anxiety, and agitation.
▶ Indigestion.

Chronic use of caffeine can lead to a toxic condition known as *caffeinism*. Symptoms of caffeinism include rapid breathing and heart rate, trembling, agitation, nausea, loss of appetite, and in some cases may lead to convulsions and hallucinations.

TOBACCO

Tobacco products — cigarettes, cigars, pipes, smokeless tobacco — all contain the drug *nicotine*, a poisonous addictive substance inhaled when smoking tobacco and absorbed through the lining for the mouth when chewing it. People who smoke only pipes and cigars seem to have fewer health risks from smoking than those who smoke cigarettes, but they still run a much higher risk than people who don't smoke at all.

Facts About Second-Hand Tobacco Smoke

Every year in America, an estimated 3,000 nonsmokers die from lung cancer caused by second-hand tobacco smoke. If you breathe it regularly, you're probably at risk.

▼ Exposure to second-hand smoke causes 30 times as many lung cancer deaths as all regulated air pollutants combined.

▼ Second-hand smoke leads to coughing, phlegm, chest discomfort, reduced lung function, and reddening, itching and watering of your eyes.

▼ More than 4,000 chemical compounds have been identified in tobacco smoke; at least 43 are known to cause cancer in humans or animals.

▼ Exposure to second-hand smoke contributes up to 300,000 infections annually in children younger than 18 months. Infections include potentially serious conditions such as pneumonia and bronchitis. Between 7,500 and 15,000 children are hospitalized as a result of these infections.

▼ Second-hand smoke triggers 8,000 to 26,000 new cases of asthma in children and worsens symptoms in 400,000 to 1 million asthmatic children.

▼ Infants are three times more likely to die from Sudden Infant Death Syndrome (SIDS) if their mothers smoke during and after pregnancy.

▼ There is no safe level of exposure to second-hand cigarette smoke.

From Centers for Disease Control and Prevention, Atlanta, GA, and Environmental Protection Agency.

Why Do You Smoke?

	Always	Frequently	Occasionally	Seldom	Never
A. I smoke cigarettes in order to keep myself from slowing down.	5	4	3	2	1
B. Handling a cigarette is part of the enjoyment of smoking it.	5	4	3	2	1
C. Smoking cigarettes is pleasant and relaxing.	5	4	3	2	1
D. I light up a cigarette when I feel angry about something.	5	4	3	2	1
E. When I have run out of cigarettes I find it almost unbearable until I can get them.	5	4	3	2	1
F. I smoke cigarettes automatically without even being aware of it.	5	4	3	2	1
G. I smoke cigarettes to stimulate me, to perk myself up.	5	4	3	2	1
H. Part of the enjoyment of smoking a cigarette comes from the steps I take to light up.	5	4	3	2	1
I. I find cigarettes pleasurable.	5	4	3	2	1
J. When I feel uncomfortable or upset about something, I light up a cigarette.	5	4	3	2	1
K. I am very much aware of the fact when I am not smoking a cigarette.	5	4	3	2	1
L. I light up a cigarette without realizing I still have one burning in the ashtray.	5	4	3	2	1
M. I smoke cigarettes to give me a "lift."	5	4	3	2	1
N. When I smoke a cigarette, part of the enjoyment is watching the smoke as I exhale it.	5	4	3	2	1
O. I want a cigarette most when I am comfortable and relaxed.	5	4	3	2	1
P. When I feel "blue" or want to take my mind off cares and worries, I smoke cigarettes.	5	4	3	2	1
Q. I get a real gnawing hunger for a cigarette when I haven't smoked for a while.	5	4	3	2	1
R. I've found a cigarette in my mouth and didn't remember putting it there.	5	4	3	2	1

Scoring Your Test:

Enter the numbers you have circled on the test questions in the spaces provided below, putting the number you have circled to question A on line A, to question B on line B, etc. Add the three scores on each line to get a total for each factor. For example, the sum of your scores over lines A, G, and M gives you your score on "Stimulation," lines B, H, and N give the score on "Handling," etc. Scores can vary from 3 to 15. Any score 11 and above is high; any score 7 and below is low.

```
A _____ + G _____ + M _____ = _____   Stimulation
B _____ + H _____ + N _____ = _____   Handling
C _____ + I _____ + O _____ = _____   Pleasure Relaxation
D _____ + J _____ + P _____ = _____   Crutch: Tension Reduction
E _____ + K _____ + Q _____ = _____   Craving: Psychological Addiction
F _____ + L _____ + R _____ = _____   Habit
```

A score of 11 or above on any factor indicates that smoking is an important source of satisfaction for you. The higher you score (15 is the highest), the more important a given factor is in your smoking. See page 296 for strategies for dealing with why you smoke.

From *A Self-Test for Smokers*. U.S. Department of Health and Human Services, 1983.

Nicotine Dependence Are You Hooked?

Answer each question in the list below, giving yourself the appropriate points.	0 points	1 point	2 points
____ 1. How soon after you wake up do you smoke your first cigarette?	After 30 minutes	Within 30 minutes	—
____ 2. Do you find it difficult to refrain from smoking in places where it is forbidden, such as the library, theater, doctor's office?	No	Yes	—
____ 3. Which of all the cigarettes you smoke in a day is the most satisfying?	Any other than the first one in the morning	The first one in the morning	—
____ 4. How many cigarettes a day do you smoke?	1-15	16-25	26+
____ 5. Do you smoke more during the morning than during the rest of the day?	No	Yes	—
____ 6. Do you smoke when you are so ill that you are in bed most of the day?	No	Yes	—
____ 7. Does the brand you smoke have a low, medium, or high nicotine content?	Low	Medium	High
____ 8. How often do you inhale the smoke?	Never	Sometimes	Always
____ Total			

Scoring
More than 6 points — very dependent
Less than 6 points — low to moderate dependence.

From American Lung Association: Fagerstrom Test.

Experts estimate that approximately one-third of the population in the United States uses tobacco every day and more than 50 million Americans smoke more than 500 billion cigarettes every year. Although the percentage of the U.S. population that smokes has definitely declined over the last two and a half decades, the percentage of heavy smokers (those who smoke more than 25 cigarettes a day) actually has *increased*, most dramatically among women.

In 1990, about 28% of men and 23% of women smoked cigarettes. Rates of smoking varied, based on gender, age, racial or ethnic group, and education level. Adults with less than a 12th-grade education are more than twice as likely to smoke as are those with college degrees.

Drug addicts are another major group of tobacco users. Some studies have found that over 90% of heroin addicts and 80% of alcoholics are heavy cigarette smokers. Other recent studies suggest that smokers are more likely than nonsmokers to have suffered from depression. These findings lead some researchers to suggest that underlying psychological or physiological traits may predispose people to drug use, including tobacco.

Former U.S. Surgeon General C. Everett Koop, in his annual report to the nation, declared cigarette smoking to be the chief, single, avoidable cause of death in our society, and the most important health issue of our time. According to the *Public Citizen Health Letter*, cigarettes cause more premature deaths than AIDS, alcohol, cocaine, heroin, fires, automobile accidents, and suicide combined. An estimated 6 minutes of life is lost for every cigarette smoked. A 25-year-old who smokes two packs a day will shave almost 9 years from life expectancy, experts predict. Figure 13.1 depicts smoking-attributed deaths in the United States by year and gender.

Besides the risk of earlier death, the proven health risks of smoking include:

▶ Lung cancer (approximately 83% of all lung cancer is caused directly by cigarette smoking, and of the 17% that occurs in nonsmokers, one in five results from inhaling secondary cigarette smoke).

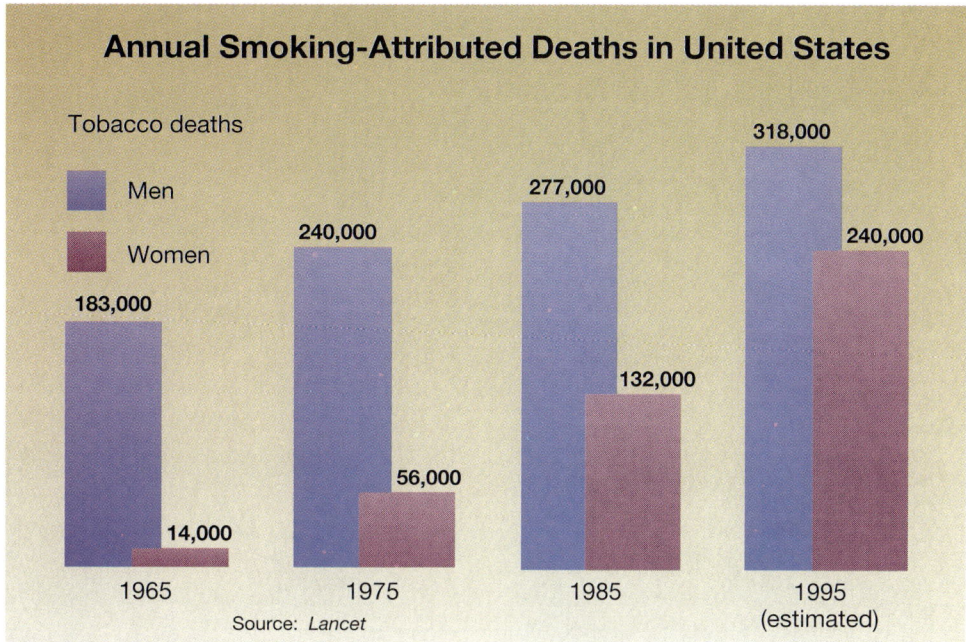
FIGURE 13.1

- Oral cancer (cancer of the mouth, palate, larynx, pharynx, and esophagus in cigarette smokers; and cancer of the lip, tongue, and jaw in pipe smokers).

- Cancer of the pancreas (two to five times higher in smokers).

- Cancer of the bladder (smoking is the greatest risk factor in bladder cancer; more than half of all men who get cancer of the bladder are cigarette smokers).

- Chronic obstructive pulmonary disease (emphysema, asthma, and chronic bronchitis; an estimated 90% of all cases are smokers, and smokers run 25 times higher risks).

- Heart attacks, strokes, and coronary artery disease, including damage to the inner surface of coronary arteries (more than a quarter of a million deaths from heart disease each year are attributed directly to cigarette smoking).

- Peptic ulcer (death rates from peptic ulcer are much higher in smokers, because the condition is much harder to treat among smokers).

- Risk of miscarriage, stillbirths, death during infancy, and low birthweight babies (children born to women who smoke are still physically and socially underdeveloped at the age of 7).

- Increase in risk for sudden infant death (SID) syndrome in babies born to mothers who smoke; children of smoking parents have higher rates of asthma and middle-ear infections.

Because many consider smokeless (chewing) tobacco to be a safer alternative, its use has increased dramatically over the past two decades. Today, more than 12 million Americans use smokeless tobacco, half of them regularly. Smokeless tobacco *isn't* safe. It causes oral cancer as well as a variety of mouth and gum diseases, including loss of taste, gingivitis, pyorrhea, tooth loss, unusual wear on tooth surfaces, and leukoplakia (precancerous thick, rough, white patches on the tongue, gums, or inner cheek). Smokeless tobacco also has been shown to increase blood pressure.

A person can reverse the damage of cigarette smoking by quitting. The benefits of quitting start almost immediately, and 15 years after quitting smoking, the risk of death and disease will be no higher than if the person had never smoked at all (assuming the person is not already ill when quitting). Some think that nothing else a person can do for health can have such immediate, far-reaching dividends as quitting smoking. Figure 13.2 shows the specific health effects of smoking.

286 WELLNESS ▼ *Guidelines for a Healthy Lifestyle*

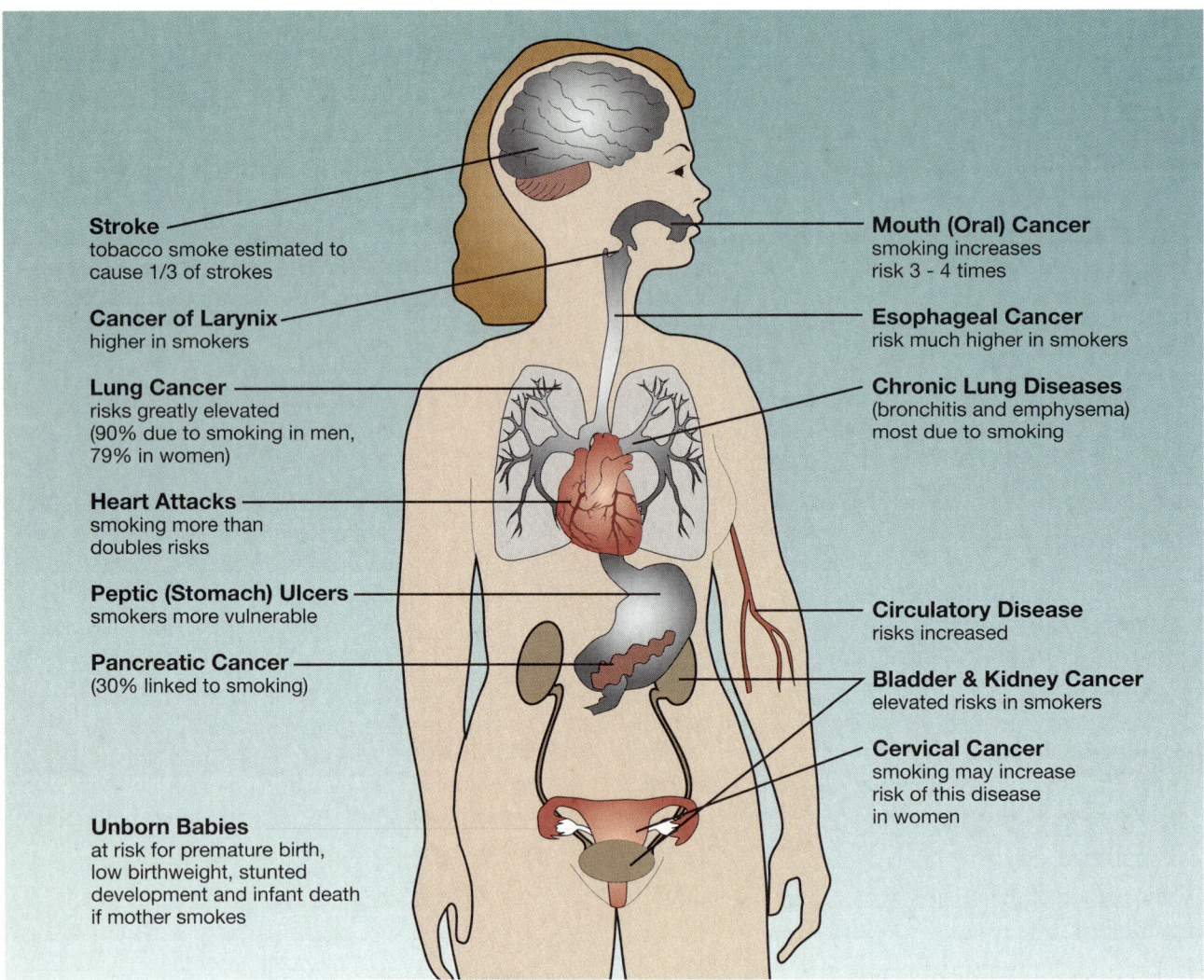

FIGURE 13.2 ▼ The health effects of smoking.

▼ Healthy People 2000 Objectives For Tobacco Use

The U. S. Department of Health and Human Services has listed these goals for tobacco use in the United States by the year 2000:

▼ Reduce cigarette smoking to less than 15 percent of all adults (special target groups are blue-collar workers, adults who have not graduated from high school, military personnel, pregnant women and women of reproductive age, Blacks, Hispanics, Native Americans, Alaska natives, and southeast Asian men)

▼ Reduce cigarette smoking among children so less than 15 percent go on to smoke as adults

▼ Have at least half the adult smokers stop for at least one day a year

▼ Have at least 60 percent of women who smoke cigarettes stop while they are pregnant

▼ Expose no more than 20 percent of children aged six and under to cigarette smoke at home

▼ Have no more than 6 percent of males aged twelve to twenty-four use smokeless tobacco

▼ Establish all elementary, middle, and secondary schools as tobacco-free environments and include tobacco prevention in all curricula

▼ Establish smoke-free environments in 75 percent of the nation's workplaces

▼ Enact comprehensive clean indoor air acts that prohibit smoking in all fifty states

ALCOHOL

The most widely used drug in the United States, alcohol is thought to be the cause of more than half of all fatal automobile accidents in the United States. Someone is injured every minute, and someone dies every 23 minutes from an alcohol-related accident. One in every two of us will be involved in an alcohol-related accident at some time in our lives.

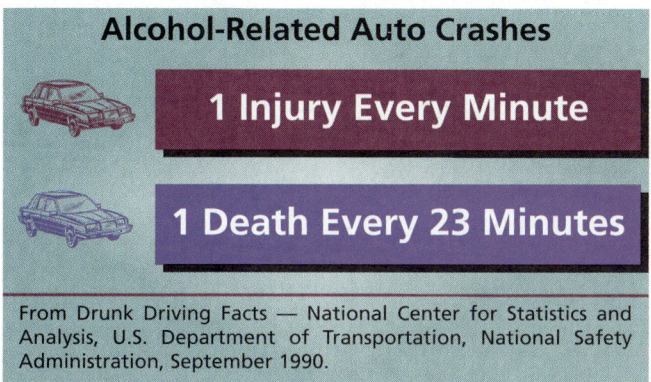

And that's not all. Our entire society suffers the consequences of alcohol abuse, in terms of crimes, medical expenses, and emotional health. Figure 13.3 graphically shows the role of alcohol in many societal problems.

Alcohol poses a tough dilemma. It's socially acceptable among many people who use alcohol to celebrate a victory, ease tension in a difficult situation, bring on relaxation after a hard day, or even inspire a little romance. Almost half of all sixth-graders have tried wine coolers, yet only a fifth of those surveyed knew that wine coolers contained alcohol. And even though the legal drinking age is 21 in all 50 states, more than 90% of all high school seniors drink at least some alcohol; more than a third reported having five or more drinks in one sitting during the previous 2 weeks, and 4% drink every day.

Although society generally tolerates the moderate use of alcohol, many Americans don't stop there. An estimated 12 million Americans — a fourth of them under age 17 — have what's classified as a "drinking problem." Projections for alcohol abuse and alcohol dependence for the year 2000 are given in Figure 13.4.

People drink for many reasons, but what has fascinated researchers are the reasons people are able to avoid having problems with alcohol. According to the National Institute on Alcohol Abuse and Alcoholism, a lot depends on how you were exposed to alcohol as you grew up. Officials at the Institute say you're least likely to have a problem with alcohol if

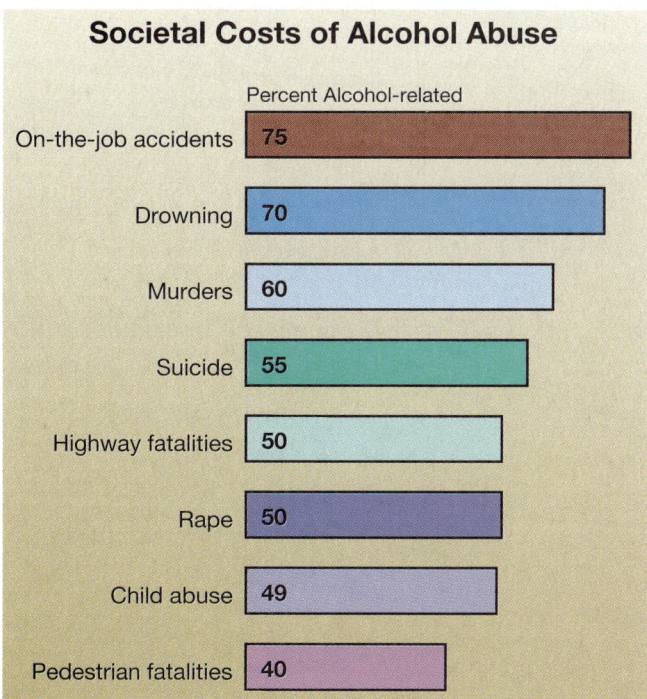

FIGURE 13.3 ▼ Percent of common problems that are related to alcohol.

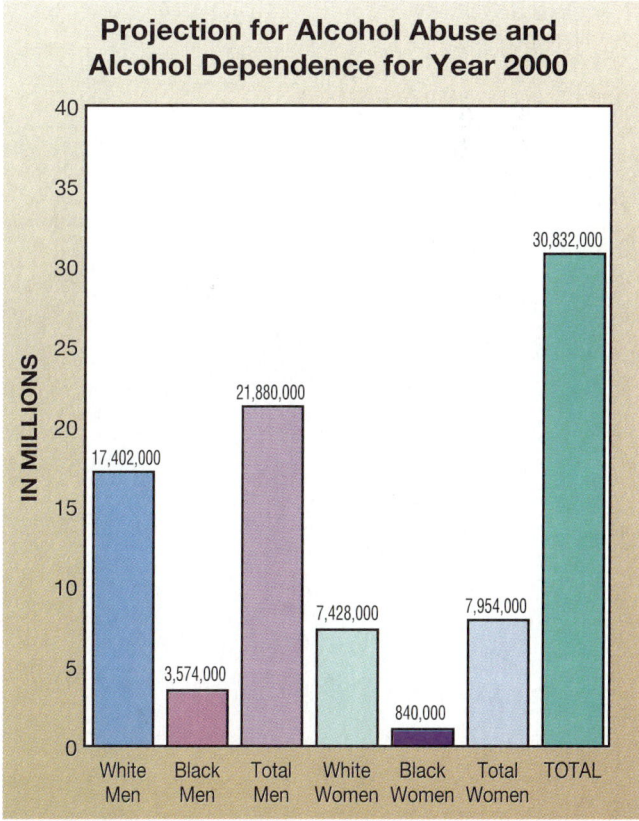

FIGURE 13.4 ▼ Projected alcohol abuse in the United States by the year 2000.

your parents had responsible drinking habits and these attitudes:

▶ Alcohol is a food and should be used in small quantities at mealtimes.

▶ Alcohol is a beverage. It's not the focus of a group activity.

▶ Drinking doesn't prove you're more grown up or "more of a man."

▶ Getting drunk is not acceptable.

▶ No one has to drink. Abstinence is a legitimate choice.

An obvious problem associated with drinking is intoxication. The "morning after" usually is marred by fatigue, weakness, nausea, vomiting, dehydration, extreme sensitivity to light and sound, severe headache, bloodshot eyes, and the inability to remember part or all of what went on while you were drunk.

Long-term risks associated with alcohol include:

▶ Permanent damage to brain cells and small brain size. Alcohol abuse can cause Korsakoff's syndrome (loss of memory, psychosis, learning loss, and degeneration of brain matter) and Wernicke's syndrome (visual impairment and confusion).

▶ Nerve damage and interference with neurotransmitters, causing loss of sensation.

▶ Damage to muscle fibers.

▶ Alcoholic cardiomyopathy (degeneration of the heart muscle).

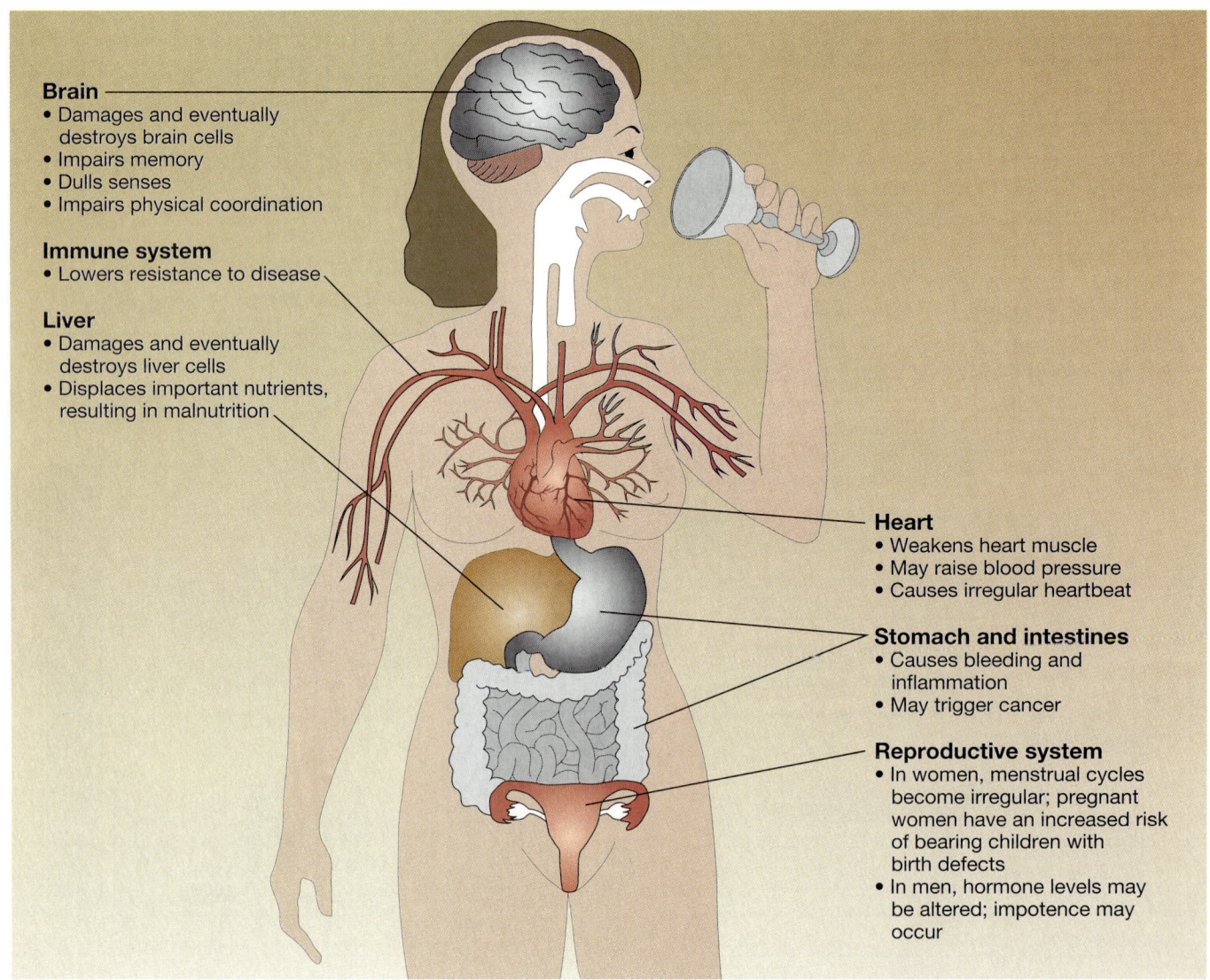

FIGURE 13.5 ▼ Long-term risks associated with chronic alcohol use.

- High blood pressure, heart attack, damage to coronary arteries, irregular heartbeat, disruption of blood flow to the heart, and angina (chest pain, usually on exertion).
- Anemia.
- Greater risk for pneumonia, emphysema, tuberculosis, and other lung diseases.
- Cirrhosis of the liver, cancer of the liver, or chronic enlargement of the liver.
- Breast cancer (women who drink at all run a 50% higher risk; women who have three drinks a day run a 100% higher risk).
- Cancer of the mouth, tongue, pharynx, esophagus, stomach, and intestines.
- Esophageal varices (varicose veins in the esophagus; death can come rapidly if the varices rupture).
- More risk for peptic ulcers or bleeding of the stomach lining because of irritation.
- Inflammation of the pancreas or interference with its ability to produce insulin.
- Malnutrition (because the small intestine may be unable to absorb nutrients).
- Less immunity and ability to fight infection.

Experts now think even a few drinks during the entire term of a pregnancy can be harmful to the fetus. Tests show the blood alcohol content is much higher in the fetus than in the mother who drank the alcohol. Most people believe the greatest harm is done during the first 3 months of pregnancy, when the fetus is most susceptible, but that alcohol any time during fetal development can cause damage. Even one episode of heavy drinking can injure the baby.

Women who drink while they are pregnant run the risk of giving birth to a baby with fetal alcohol syndrome (FAS), estimated to be the third leading cause of birth defects and mental retardation in newborns. FAS, which usually results from regular or moderate to heavy drinking during pregnancy, is characterized by low birthweight, small head size, mental retardation, poor motor development, long-term developmental disabilities, and a distinctive set of facial malformations (short eye openings, low nasal bridge, thin upper lip, and absence of a groove above the upper lip).

> **Healthy People 2000 Objectives For Alcohol Use**
>
> The U.S. Department of Health and Human Services has the following goals for the year 2000:
> - Reduce deaths from alcohol-related motor vehicle accidents to 8.5 per 100,000 people.
> - Reduce deaths from cirrhosis to no more than six per 100,000 people.
> - Have less than 28% of high school seniors and less than 32% of college students engage in episodes of heavy drinking.
> - Reduce average annual alcohol consumption to less than 2 gallons of alcohol per adult (it's 2.5 gallons now).
> - Establish alcohol and drug treatment programs for traditionally underserved people in all 50 states.
> - Establish drug and alcohol policies in at least 60% of the workplaces with 50 or more employees.
> - Establish effective driver's license suspension or revocation laws in all 50 states for people caught driving under the influence of alcohol or drugs.
> - Establish laws that more effectively limit access to alcohol by minors in all 50 states.
> - Restrict promotion of alcoholic beverages to young audiences in at least 20 states.
> - Establish laws in all 50 states that reduce legal blood alcohol concentration to .04% in adults and .00% in those younger than 21.
> - Establish routine drug/alcohol screening and referrals for treatment among at least 75% of the nation's primary health care providers.

MARIJUANA

Made from the dried, crushed leaves and flowers of the *cannabis sativa* plant, marijuana — which looks a lot like tobacco — most often is rolled into papers and smoked like cigarettes. Although marijuana is a chemically complex plant, with more than 400 identified substances, the one that has made marijuana popular is its chief psychoactive agent, THC (delta-9-tetrahydrocannabinol).

Interestingly, the marijuana today's college students smoke is much more potent than what their parents smoked 20 or 30 years ago. Experts estimate that the plants cultivated today have three times the

Natural Versus Unnatural Highs

In contrast to natural and healthy highs, unnatural highs result from self-imposed attempts to escape; upon returning to normal functioning, an increasing disappointment with normal day-to-day living occurs. The heaviest impact in being involved in unnatural highs, however, is on relationships.

The most basic relationship that any of us have as adults is with ourselves. Father John Powell has discussed a three-step process toward maturity that begins with our relationship with ourselves. The three steps in this process generally occur in the following order to ensure integrated growth toward maturity:

▼ Accept yourself.
▼ Be yourself.
▼ Forget yourself.

These steps can be viewed as part of an upward-pointing spiral with gradually widening cycles representing growth as we continue to more fully accept ourselves, learn to truly be ourselves, and forget ourselves in the service of others. This, in turn, allows us to accept ourselves more deeply and continue with the cycle. Natural highs can occur at any point in the cycle and provide support and encouragement to continue the growth.

Let's briefly examine the destructive nature of chemical dependency as it relates to this process of growth. Carl Jung once described alcoholism to Alcoholics Anonymous founder, Bill Wilson, as "a spiritual disease which has at its base a drive for wholeness. . . ." Chemical dependency might be understood as an attempt to be happy with who we are, to feel whole and complete, and to accept ourselves.

The first use of chemicals for most people occurs as part of an attempt to be accepted. Once individuals accept themselves as okay just the way they are, they are more capable of truly being themselves in their own uniqueness.

Harry Guntrip has described mental health as the capacity to live life to the fullest in ways that enable us to realize our own natural potentialities and that unite us with, rather than divide us from, all the human beings who make up our world. He has said, "Nothing is more sad than to see a human being facing his basic withdrawnness, and complaining with a terrible sense of frustration that he cannot express himself, cannot get in touch with other people, and cannot love." Father Joseph Martin, well known for his films and lectures on chemical dependency, states, "An alcoholic is a creature who is cut off from the very purpose for which he was created to love and to be loved" (from his video presentation, "Alcoholism and the Family").

Chemical highs give people a superficial sense of acceptance in such a way as to not allow true self-acceptance to take place. In consequence, there is no foundation for truly being oneself and developing one's own talents. In fact, the process is hindered through decreased mental and physical capacity and an increased narrowing of interests. As chemical dependency progresses unchecked, it eventually will cause huge losses in all areas of life — and eventually the loss of life itself.

An AA poem clearly illustrates the destructive nature of the misguided, however well-intentioned, use of alcohol and other drugs.

We drank for happiness
and became unhappy.
We drank for joy
and became miserable.
We drank for sociability
and became argumentative.
We drank for friendship
and made enemies.
We drank for sleep
and awakened without rest.
We drank for strength
and felt weak.
We drank "medicinally"
and acquired health problems.
We drank for relaxation
and got the shakes.
We drank for bravery
and became afraid.
We drank to make conversation easier
and slurred our speech.
We drank to feel heavenly
and ended up feeling like hell.
We drank to forget
and were forever haunted.
We drank for freedom
and became slaves.
We drank to erase problems
and saw them multiply.
We drank to cope with life
and invited death.

Viktor Frankl has described happiness as an experience that cannot be sought directly but can come only as a byproduct of serving others.

Chemical dependency treatment assists individuals to begin to experience growth and satisfaction by replacing unhealthy dependence on chemicals with healthy and more mature understanding and appreciation of the interdependence among themselves, others, and a higher power. Through abstinence, and involving themselves in the process of accepting themselves, being themselves, and forgetting themselves, natural highs begin to occur. Thoreau stated it beautifully: "Sometimes we are clarified and calmed healthily, as we never were before in our lives, not by an opiate, but by some unconscious obedience to the all-just laws, so that we become like a still lake of purest crystal, and without an effort our depths are revealed to ourselves. All the world goes by and is reflected in our deeps."

From *Professional Counselor*, December 1993

amount of THC as those cultivated just 10 years ago.

Marijuana use has declined steadily over the last decade. More than a third of the nation's college students 10 to 15 years ago smoked marijuana regularly, and a third of those smoked it daily. Today, marijuana use seems to be at its lowest level since statistics were first recorded in 1975. Unfortunately, though, it's still a "major player" in the drug scene on today's college campuses; more than a third of the students smoke it occasionally. Almost half of all high school seniors also report smoking marijuana occasionally; one in five smokes marijuana an average of once a month.

Marijuana is fat-soluble, stored in the fatty tissues of the brain, body, and reproductive organs. As a result, the immediate effects of marijuana intoxication usually last several hours. Marijuana actually can stay in the system as long as a month. The body has difficulty completely eliminating the marijuana, and the effects are cumulative, building up over time. What this means is that if you smoke a joint every weekend, which may not seem all that bad, your body is constantly permeated with the drug.

Marijuana has been on a roller coaster as far as the media are concerned. Publicity has ranged from virtual "scare tactics" about the monstrous effects of the drug to a casual attitude that marijuana is "not that bad." The truth lies somewhere in between. As far as researchers can tell, marijuana use has the following risks and long-term effects:

▶ Lowers brain and motor functions.
▶ Changes cell membranes, especially those in the brain and reproductive tracts, interfering with the cell's ability to absorb energy.
▶ Interferes with immunity and compromises the immune system's ability to fight infection.
▶ Speeds the heart rate and increases blood pressure, leading to long-term cardiac damage (this is a problem particularly for people who already have arteriosclerosis, angina, or some other heart disease).
▶ Causes lung damage more intense than that caused by cigarette smoking. Studies show that marijuana smoke causes four times the lung damage as the same amount of tobacco smoke. Marijuana is higher in tars and contains more carcinogens.
▶ Impairs oxygen and carbon dioxide exchange in the lungs.
▶ Depresses the sex drive and causes impotence.
▶ Lessens male fertility by decreasing the sperm count, reducing sperm motility (movement), and damaging sperm (causing irregularly shaped sperm).
▶ Reduces female fertility by inhibiting ovulation.
▶ Puts pregnant women at higher risk for miscarriage or stillbirth.
▶ Can cause birth defects in babies born to mothers who smoke it during pregnancy (especially low birthweight, prematurity, and congenital deformities similar to those of fetal alcohol syndrome).

Perhaps one of the most serious risks from marijuana use is its status as a "gateway" drug. Those who use marijuana regularly are much more likely to try other, more dangerous drugs, such as cocaine.

COCAINE

Also known as "coke" or "snow," cocaine is a crystalline powder extracted from the leaves of the coca plant grown in Central and South America. It probably is the most powerfully addictive of any of the illicit drugs and can be injected, smoked (freebasing), or inhaled through the nose. It acts as both a powerful local anesthetic and a central nervous system stimulant. In fact, mixtures of novocaine and caffeine have been sold on the street as cocaine.

According to estimates, more than 20 million Americans have used cocaine at least once, and more than a million are dependent on it. Cocaine use has increased dramatically since it became widely available in the United States during the 1970s. In one study, approximately a fourth of all college students reported using it at least once; approximately one in five had used it at least once during the year preceding the survey; and almost one in 10 used it at least once a month.

The effects of cocaine can be immediate and devastating. According to the National Institute on Drug Abuse, more than 200,000 drugs were involved in cases admitted to hospital emergency rooms during a recent year. Of those cases, 26% involved cocaine.

A particularly dangerous and addictive form of cocaine is crack, which derives its name from a popping or crackling sound when it is smoked. Crack is manufactured by mixing the drug with ammonia,

How Different Drugs Affect the Body

	Alcohol	Amphetamines ("Speed," "Bennies," "Black Beauties," "Uppers")	Cocaine ("Crack")	LSD (and other hallucinogens)
Type of Drug (Chemical)	▶ *ethyl alcohol* (ethanol), a clear liquid (in beer, wine, spirits); ▶ made from grain, fruit, vegetables or synthetically ▶ favored for its relaxing, intoxicating properties since antiquity ▶ beers contain about 5% alcohol, wines to 12% and spirits about 40% (about 13.6 g per drink) ▶ a sedative-hypnotic and central nervous system (CNS) depressant	▶ synthetically produced: *amphetamine* (Speed), *dextroamphetamine* (Dexedrine), *methylamphetamine* or "Ice," *methylphenidate* (Ritalin), etc. ▶ used as pills, inhaled or injected (Speed) ▶ CNS stimulants that resemble action of adrenaline (natural body hormone)	▶ derived from South American coca bush (still chewed in Andes to offset fatigue) ▶ crack is mixture of cocaine and baking soda ▶ *cocaine hydrochloride* is white powder ("coke," "C," "flake," "snow") ▶ formerly used in many medicines (until 1920) ▶ stimulant action — like amphetamine, but now legally classed as a narcotic	▶ derived from mushrooms *(psilocybin)* or cactus *(mescaline)* or synthetically — e.g., *lysergic acid* (LSD) or "acid" and *phencyclidine* (PCP) — "hog," "angel dust" ▶ structures resemble *catecholamines* — normal brain neurotransmitters ▶ hallucinogens can distort reality and produce severe delusions
Short Term Effects (after a single dose)	▶ effects vary with size, sex, and amount of food in stomach; ▶ initial relaxation and loss of inhibitions ▶ increased sociability ▶ impaired coordination ▶ slowing down of reflexes and mental processes ▶ attitude changes, increased risk-taking and bad judgment/danger in driving car, operating machinery ▶ sleepiness	▶ nervous system briefly stimulated ▶ reduces appetite ▶ increases energy, offsets fatigue ▶ talkative restlessness, greater alertness ▶ faster breathing ▶ rise in heart rate and blood pressure (with risk of burst blood vessels and heart failure) ▶ temperature raised, mouth dry, skin sweaty ▶ pupils dilated ▶ alleviates nose-stuffiness (original medicinal use)	▶ short-acting, powerful CNS stimulant, also a local anesthetic ▶ effects vary depending whether drug is "snorted" (inhaled), injected, put in mouth, rectum or vagina, or smoked (as crack) ▶ transient euphoria and increased energy ▶ appetite-loss ▶ rise in heart-rate and breathing ▶ dilated pupils ▶ agitated, restless talkativeness ▶ brief rise in sex drive	▶ unpredictable effects — at first like amphetamine ▶ excitation, arousal ▶ temperature raised ▶ altered sense of smell, shape, size, color, distance ▶ exhilaration, "mind-expansion" or anxiety — depending on user ▶ rapid pulse, dilated pupils, blank stare ▶ exaggerated power sense with possibly violent behavior ▶ later — dramatic perceptual distortions ▶ occasionally convulsions
With Larger Doses and Longer Use	▶ blackouts (memory loss) ▶ facial flushing; slurred speech ▶ staggering gait, stupor ▶ rise in blood pressure ▶ pancreatitis, hepatitis, stomach ulcers, injuries (broken bones) ▶ effects magnified by other depressants (e.g., opiates, barbiturates, tranquilizers, antihistamines, sleep aids, cold remedies) ▶ alone or combined with other drugs can increase accident rates ▶ overdose may be fatal, from respiratory distress	▶ bizarre behavior, talkativeness, restlessness, tremors, excitability ▶ sense of power, superiority, aggression ▶ illusions and hallucinations ▶ some users become paranoid, suspicious, panicky, violent ▶ raised blood pressure ▶ insomnia	▶ permanently stuffy nose (if snorted) and risk of perforated nasal septum ▶ brief euphoric effect followed by "crash" — depression ▶ anesthetic effect can depress brain function ▶ bizarre, erratic, perhaps violent actions ▶ paranoid "psychosis" (disappears if drug is discontinued) ▶ sensation of "crawling under the skin" ▶ convulsions, disturbed heart action, even death	▶ anxiety, panic attacks, paranoid delusions, occasionally psychosis (like schizophrenia) ▶ injury or accidents due to drug-induced delusions or distance misjudgment ▶ increased risk of fetal abnormalities ▶ tolerance develops rapidly but also disappears fast with renewed drug sensitivity ▶ with PCP, high fever, muscle spasm, erratic behavior, psychosis lasting weeks or more
Long-Term Effects (prolonged repeated use)	▶ harms many body organs: pancreas, GI tract, blood circulation, heart, liver, kidney, brain ▶ may produce liver cirrhosis, ulcers, memory loss, impotence ▶ increased risk of cancers (mouth, larynx, throat, maybe breast) ▶ vitamin depletion ▶ damages offspring ▶ dependence frequent	▶ malnutrition, emaciation (owing to appetite loss) ▶ anxiety states ▶ "amphetamine-psychosis" (with schizophrenia-like hallucinations) ▶ kidney damage ▶ susceptibility to infection ▶ sleep disorders ▶ *psychological* dependence	▶ weight loss, malnutrition ▶ destroyed nose tissues (if sniffed) ▶ restlessness, mood swings, insomnia, *extreme* excitability, suspiciousness/paranoia, delusions ("psychosis") ▶ depression ▶ impotence ▶ risk of heart attacks ▶ strong *psychological* dependence	▶ long-term medical effects not known ▶ may include muscle tenseness, "flashbacks" — brief, spontaneous recurrence of prior LSD (hallucinogenic) experiences ▶ prolonged, profound depression ▶ panic attacks ▶ no *physical* dependence
Withdrawal Symptoms	▶ insomnia, headache ▶ nausea ▶ shakiness, tremors ▶ sweating, seizures	▶ long sleep, chills ▶ ravenous hunger ▶ depression	▶ little or no withdrawal sickness; sleepiness ▶ extreme exhaustion ▶ possibly "cocaine blues" (depression)	▶ few withdrawal effects, possible "flashbacks," anxiety

Reprinted with permission from Health News. Health News is a bimonthly publication of the University of Toronto Faculty of Medicine. Subscriptions and back issues can be obtained by writing to *Health News*, 109 Vanderhoof Ave., Suite 205, Toronto, Ontario M4G 2H7 or by calling (416) 696-8818.

THIRTEEN ▼ Addictive Behavior and Wellness

Nicotine	Caffeine	Cannabis (marijuana, "pot," "grass," hashish)	Narcotic (Opioid) analgesics (painkillers)	Solvents (Inhalants)
▶ derived from tobacco ▶ used medicinally in South America ▶ tobacco smoke contains 4,000 chemicals but nicotine is the most addictive ▶ a typical Canadian cigarette contains one mg nicotine but amount absorbed varies with smoker ▶ stimulates central nervous system	▶ derived from tea, coffee beans, kola nuts, chocolate ▶ used in many medicines (e.g., with painkillers, cold/cough, pain remedies, antihistamines) ▶ average cup of coffee contains 60-75 mg caffeine, colas about 35 mg (per 250 ml) ▶ CNS stimulant	▶ derived from *cannabis sativa* or hemp plant; preparations vary in potency; "hash" most potent, marijuana least ▶ smoked in "joints" or chewed (sometimes with food) ▶ medicinally used for epilepsy, glaucoma, against nausea ▶ classed as hallucinogen	▶ poppy derivatives (opium, codeine, morphine, heroin) and synthetics (Demerol, Methadone, Dilaudid, Percodan) ▶ smoked, eaten, or injected ▶ ancient painkillers used medicinally ▶ deaden pain, produce euphoria and drowsiness	▶ volatile organic hydrocarbons from petroleum and natural gas (e.g., gasoline, toluene, hexane, chloroform, carbon tetrachloride, nail polish remover or acetone, lighter fluid, paint thinners, cleaning fluid, airplane cement, plastic glue) ▶ hallucinogenic effects
▶ speeds pulse ▶ stimulates, then reduces brain and nervous system activity ▶ blood pressure rises ▶ sense of relaxation ▶ reduced urine output ▶ impairs cleansing action of lung's cilia (hairs) ▶ greater alertness and concentration abilities (claimed)	▶ stimulates brain, speeds nerve-cell transmission ▶ elevates mood and alertness ▶ stimulates mental activity ▶ speeds up breathing, metabolism ▶ enhances mental performance ▶ postpones fatigue ▶ shortens sleep ▶ more urine output ▶ rise in blood fats ▶ increases stomach acidity ▶ decreases appetite	▶ produces dreamlike euphoria, laughter, relaxation ▶ alters sense of space, time ▶ increases heart rate ▶ reddens eyes ▶ dreamy, "stoned" look ▶ at later stages, users are quiet, reflective, sleepy ▶ combined with alcohol, increased effects, distorted behavior ▶ impairs short-term memory, thinking, and ability to drive car or perform complex tasks	▶ briefly stimulate, then depress higher brain centers ▶ give quick pleasure surge (for few minutes) then stupor (which mutes hunger, pain, sex-drive) ▶ taken by mouth, effects slower, no initial pleasure surge ▶ pupils tiny, body warm, limbs heavy ▶ mouth dry, skin itchy ▶ users may "nod" off, alternately awake or asleep, oblivious to surroundings	▶ exhilaration, light-headedness, excitability, disorientation ▶ confusion, slurred speech, dizziness ▶ distorted perception ▶ visual and auditory hallucinations ▶ muscular control impaired ▶ possible nausea, increased saliva, sneezing ▶ reflexes dampened ▶ recklessness, feelings of power, invincibility
▶ lung damage ▶ damaged blood circulation ▶ slowed wound-healing ▶ vitamin C depletion ▶ shortness of breath ▶ more upper respiratory infections ▶ cancer-formation risks	▶ nervousness, hand tremors ▶ delayed sleep onset, reduces "depth" of sleep, insomnia ▶ abnormally rapid heartbeat ▶ jitteriness ▶ mild delirium possible ▶ convulsions (rare) ▶ suspected cancer-causing agent	▶ slowed digestive (gastrointestinal) activity ▶ time misjudgment ▶ sharpened or distorted sense of color, sound ▶ thinking slow and confused ▶ apathy, loss of motivation/drive ▶ large doses can produce severe confusion, panic attacks ▶ hallucinations (even psychosis)	▶ extremities heavy ▶ permanent drowsiness ▶ pupils become pin-points ▶ skin cold, moist, bluish ▶ progressively slower breathing ▶ depressed breathing ▶ *supervised pain-killing doses* let people remain quite clear-headed and safe ▶ dangers increase with alcohol intake	▶ drowsiness and possible unconsciousness ▶ severe disorientation ▶ risks increase with fume concentration ▶ irregular heartbeat, heart action disturbed ▶ large doses may cause heart failure — e.g., "sudden sniffing death" (especially with spot removers or airplane cement)
▶ narrowed blood vessels, risk of heart attack, stroke ▶ bronchitis, emphysema ▶ raised risk of cancers of mouth, lung, larynx, throat, bladder, pancreas, possibly cervix ▶ stomach ulcers ▶ impairs fetal growth ▶ strong dependence	▶ raised blood cholesterol level ▶ risk of stomach ulcers ▶ suspected cancer-inducing agent ▶ *possible* damage to unborn baby ▶ regular coffee use (more than 5 cups daily) can lead to dependence (getting "hooked" on drug)	▶ loss of drive, reduced energy ▶ regular heavy use increases risk of — bronchitis, lung cancer — reduced sex hormones — impaired learning — memory loss — possible decrease in immunity ▶ *psychological* dependence	▶ constipation ▶ moodiness ▶ risk of endocarditis (heart infection) and other infections (AIDS) from needle-sharing ▶ hormone upsets (menstrual irregularities) ▶ liver damage ▶ damaged offspring ▶ strong dependence	▶ pallor, thirst, nose, eye, mouth sores ▶ irritability, hostility, forgetfulness ▶ may damage liver, kidney and brain ▶ nosebleeds, impaired blood cell formation ▶ depression, weight-loss ▶ other drugs compound damage ▶ dependence possible
▶ anxiety, jitteriness ▶ inability to concentrate ▶ increased appetite	▶ severe headache ▶ irritability ▶ tiredness	▶ withdrawal symptoms mild — possible nausea, insomnia, anxiety, irritability	▶ striking withdrawal effects (4-5 hours after last dose), sweating, anxiety, diarrhea, "gooseflesh," shivering, tremors	▶ restlessness, anxiety, irritability, headaches ▶ stomach upsets ▶ delirium (rare)

baking soda, and water, then heating it until the hydrochloride evaporates. Crack cocaine reaches the brain within 4 to 6 seconds, creating intense euphoria. Addiction to crack is so powerful that it has been defined as one of the most serious drug problems in the country. Cocaine has been known to cause sudden death. In a well-known case, Boston Celtics star Len Bias collapsed and died from cocaine shortly after being signed to the team.

Cocaine use has the following risks and long-term effects:

- Rapidly increases heart rate and blood pressure (can cause strokes or bleeding in the brain, even in young, healthy people).
- Increases breathing rate.
- Can cause heart and respiratory failure, including fluid buildup in the lungs.
- Raises body temperature.
- Lowers immune system response.
- Damages upper respiratory system if inhaled (damage to mucous membranes of nose, chronic runny nose, sores, chronic sore throat, and chronic hoarseness, eventually destroying the septum).
- Curbs appetite (can lead to malnutrition).
- Damages the liver.
- Causes impotence.
- Induces "cocaine psychosis," characterized by paranoia, delusions, and violence.

Babies born to cocaine users have significant developmental problems before birth. Fluctuations in the mother's blood pressure cause the blood vessels in the baby's brain to deteriorate, eventually resulting in strokes. Babies who are born cocaine-addicted can suffer developmental retardation, visual problems, and respiratory and liver disease.

OTHER ADDICTIVE DRUGS AND CAUTIONS

Other drugs, legal and illegal, carry risk factors as well. The relative use of the most commonly used drugs in the United States is depicted in Figure 13.6.

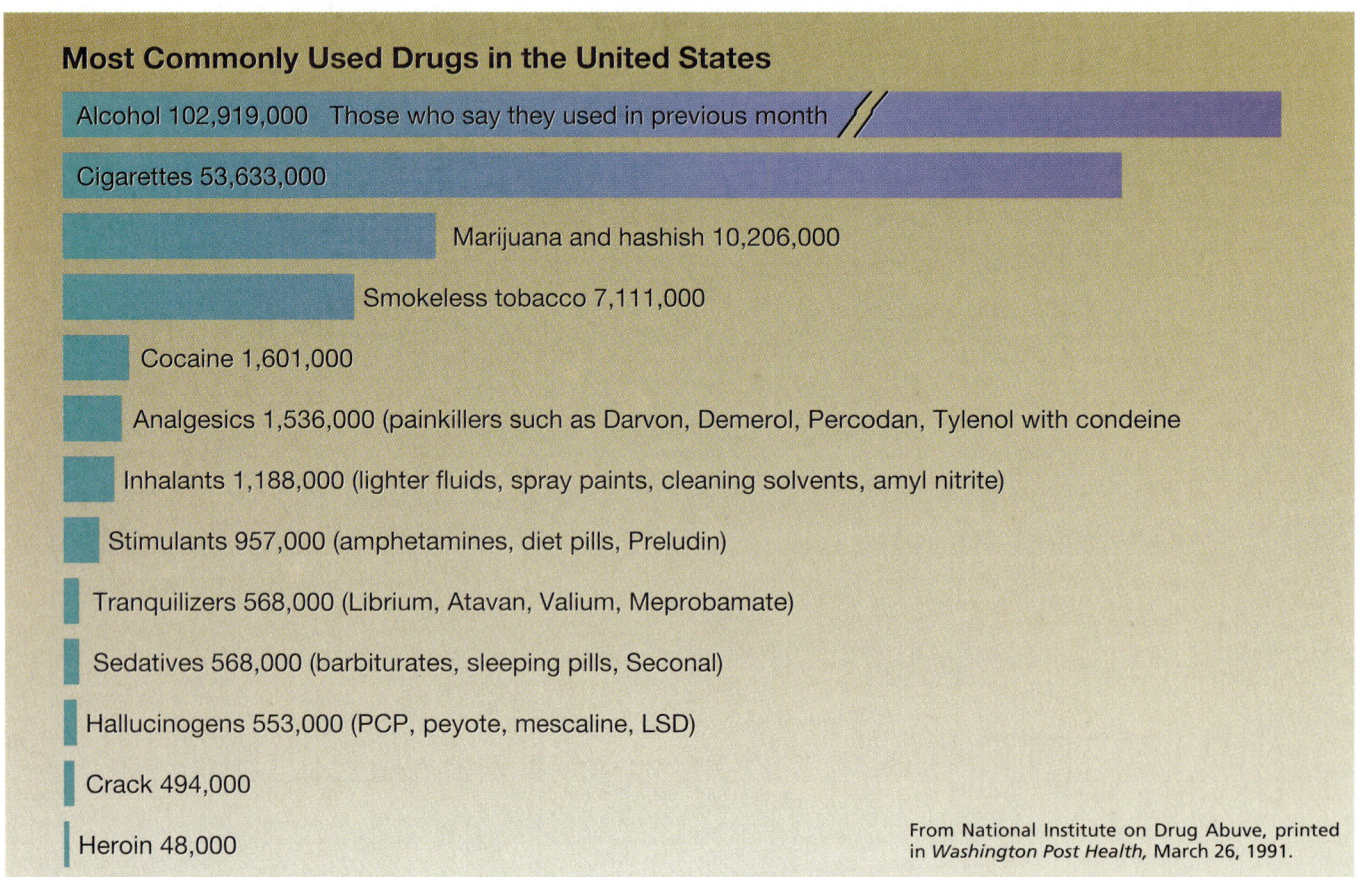

FIGURE 13.6 ▼ Drugs most commonly used in the United States.

If you're taking any kind of medication — even over-the-counter drugs such as a cold medicine — you could get into serious trouble if you drink. Alcohol blocks the actions of some drugs, and vastly increases the effects of many others, resulting in something similar to a severe overdose. We cannot list all the drugs here, but be especially cautious if you're taking:

- Pain pills, both narcotic (e.g., Darvon) and non-narcotic (e.g., aspirin).
- Over-the-counter cold medication.
- Antihistamines for colds or allergies.
- Antibiotics.
- Sleeping pills.
- Diet pills.
- Tranquilizers.
- Medication for depression.

Alcohol also can have serious, even fatal, consequences if you drink while you're taking the medications commonly prescribed for high blood pressure, water retention, epilepsy, diabetes, hemophilia, or heart disease.

To be safe, abstain from alcohol completely. If you don't, talk to your doctor or pharmacist about possible drug-alcohol interactions *before* you have a drink.

▼ WELLNESS GUIDELINES FOR MANAGING ADDICTIVE BEHAVIOR

Regardless of what kind of addictive behavior you're struggling with, five general steps can help you change your behavior:

1. *Watch yourself.* Changing an addiction requires you to first know what you're up against. Define your addiction and where it fits into your life, a process that requires some self-watching. If you're trying to stop smoking, for example, first figure out how many cigarettes you smoke every day. Figure out when you smoke and if anything in particular makes you want to reach for a cigarette. Keep a "behavioral diary" a few weeks, recording the times you engage in the behavior, the circumstances surrounding it, and your emotions at the time.

2. *Manage yourself.* Study the diaries you kept, and look for patterns. Does a specific time of day cause problems for you? Do your emotions play a critical role? Do certain activities cause you to indulge your addiction? Analyze what you've learned, and devise a plan. If you have a hard time passing up a cigarette when you pass the vending machine in your building, plan an alternative route. If you always smoke a cigarette at 10 a.m., plan to be in someone else's office or busy yourself with something you can't leave.

    Another technique of self-management is to change the consequences of your behavior. If you think smoking a cigarette helps you relax, that's a *positive* reinforcement. Instead, decide you're going to have to give up something you enjoy — watching a favorite television show, going out to eat with friends Friday night — for every cigarette you smoke.

    Still another technique of self-management is *visualization.* Visualize what you're going to be like (or look like) if your addiction continues. Use your imagination, and get into some really vivid scenes. Now visualize how you'll look, feel, or be if you can conquer your addictive behavior.

3. *Face reality.* You can't play games your whole life (such as avoiding the cigarette vending machine). Eventually you'll have to face reality, expose yourself to temptation, and overcome it.

    Start by going cold turkey. Completely avoid the addictive substance. After about a month, when you feel ready, start facing small temptations. As you face smaller ones successfully, you'll be ready for the larger ones. This kind of practice takes time. Go at it slowly, one step at a time. Keep reading your diaries and watching yourself, identifying the things that act as cues or signals, then figuring out which are the most dangerous for you. Begin with the least dangerous, and expose yourself to it. Keep practicing until you've mastered that step, then move on. *A note of caution:* If your addiction involves drugs, alcohol, or any health- or life-threatening behavior, work on abstaining; don't try to "condition" yourself.

4. *Develop alternative pleasures.* You probably get some pleasure from your addiction — a feeling of euphoria, an escape from stress, or entertainment. Figure out what it is. Now figure out a new,

positive way of getting the same thing. Make a list of positive things you can do that will bring you pleasure — reading a good book, roller blading with friends, taking a weekend trip. Then indulge; you will have an easier time breaking away from your addictive behavior if you have something pleasant to replace it with.

5. *Prevent relapse.* The most important thing to do is to realize you could fall back into your addictive behavior. Stay on guard. Plan ahead. If you know you'll be in a situation that will be difficult, develop some strategies. If you can, avoid the people, places, and things that spell trouble for you. If you do slip up, don't give up. See it as a temporary mistake, and stick to your plans for success.

Specific techniques and suggestions can help you overcome an addiction to tobacco and can help you establish responsible behavior when it comes to alcohol.

OVERCOMING TOBACCO ADDICTION

No one method of quitting works for everyone. Your reasons for smoking and your habits are unique to you. So is your life circumstance. Some people suggest that if you are severely depressed, going through a major life crisis, or having *severe* emotional problems, you should aim at reducing the number of cigarettes you smoke instead of completely quitting until your situation is back on track.

If you smoke two or more packs of cigarettes a day, you might do better if you try first to cut down the number of cigarettes you smoke, then gradually stop the habit completely.

You might try some of the following techniques or suggestions as you work to stop smoking:

▶ The U.S. Surgeon General report stresses that there are no safe cigarettes and no safe way to

▼ Strategies For Dealing With Why You Smoke

Why You Smoke	Substitutes
Stimulation You smoke to keep from slowing down, for a lift, to pep you up.	Find something else to pep you up — a hobby, brisk walks, simple exercises.
Handling You like the ritual of smoking, to have something in your hands and mouth.	Pick something else to handle: coins, pen or pencil, "worry beads"; try doodling, or chew on paper straws or minted toothpicks.
Relaxation You enjoy smoking; it's a reward, a time you feel good about yourself.	Consider the harm cigarettes cause you and the reward of quitting. Substitute social or physical activity; prove self-control and feel good about yourself.
Crutch You smoke to deal with problems and negative feelings.	Prove to yourself smoking doesn't solve problems. Reduce tension other ways: Take deep breaths, call a friend, talk over feelings. Work on keeping your "cool."
Craving You feel "hooked" and begin to think of the next cigarette before you put out present one. You're aware of the need to smoke.	Recognize that quitting will be difficult and prepare to "see it through." Plan to try to stop "cold turkey," abstaining completely. The day before quitting, smoke to the point of distaste.
Habit You smoke automatically, often without realizing what you're doing.	Become aware of every cigarette you smoke and ask yourself why you're smoking and if you really want it. Wrap up your cigarettes or put them in a place difficult to get.

smoke. While you are quitting, though, try to choose a brand that is lower in tar and nicotine than the brand you use now, smoke fewer cigarettes each day, inhale less deeply, and put out the cigarette after you've smoked only half of it.

▶ Set a goal. Determine a date when you want to have quit smoking. Start now to quit, and tell those around you about it.

▶ Check with your doctor. Some prescription drugs can help take away the craving for nicotine. One popular drug is available in chewing gum form; it contains small doses of nicotine and helps many people overcome their addiction. Your doctor probably will suggest chewing a piece of the gum each time you have the urge to smoke. (The gum isn't a cure-all. It can cause sores in your mouth, provoke nausea, and should not be used by pregnant or nursing women.)

▼
Six-Step Smoking Cessation Approach

The following six-step plan has been developed as a guide to help you quit smoking. The total program should be completed in 4 weeks or less. Steps 1 through 4 should take no longer than 2 weeks. A maximum of 2 additional weeks are allowed for the rest of the program.

Step One. Decide positively that you want to quit. Prepare a list of the reasons you smoke and why you want to quit.

Step Two. Initiate a personal diet and exercise program. Exercise and lower body weight create more awareness of healthy living and increase motivation for giving up cigarettes.

Step Three. Decide on the approach you will use to stop smoking. You may quit cold turkey or gradually decrease the number of cigarettes you smoke daily. Many people have found that quitting cold turkey is the easiest way to do it. Although it may not work the first time, after several attempts all of a sudden smokers are able to overcome the habit without too much difficulty. Tapering off cigarettes can be done in several ways. You may start by eliminating cigarettes you do not necessarily need or switch to a brand lower in nicotine or tar every couple of days, or smoke less of each cigarette, or simply cut down the total number of cigarettes you smoke each day.

Step Four. Set the target date for quitting. In choosing the target date, a special date may add a little extra incentive. An upcoming birthday, anniversary, vacation, graduation, family reunion — all are examples of good dates to free yourself from smoking.

Step Five. Stock up on low-calorie foods — carrots, broccoli, cauliflower, celery, popcorn (butter-and salt-free), fruits, sunflower seeds (in the shell), sugarless gum, and plenty of water. Keep such food handy on the day you stop and the first few days following cessation. Replace this food for cigarettes when you want one.

Step Six. This is the day you will quit smoking. On this day and the first few days thereafter, do not keep cigarettes handy. Stay away from friends and events that trigger your desire to smoke. Drink large amounts of water and fruit juices, and eat low-calorie foods. Replace smoking time with new, positive substitutes that will make smoking difficult or impossible. When you desire a cigarette, take a few deep breaths and then occupy yourself by talking to someone else, washing your hands, brushing your teeth, eating a healthy snack, chewing on a straw, doing dishes, playing sports, going for a walk or bike ride, going swimming, and so on.

If you have been successful and stopped smoking, a lot of events can still trigger your urge to smoke. When confronted with such events, people rationalize and think, "One won't hurt." It will not work! Before you know it, you will be back to the regular nasty habit. Therefore, be prepared to take action in those situations. Find adequate substitutes for smoking. Remind yourself of how difficult it has been and how long it has taken you to get to this point. Keep in mind that it will only get easier rather than worse as time goes on.

From *Fitness & Wellness*, 2nd ed. Werner W. K. Hoeger and Sharon A. Hoeger. Englewood, CO: Morton Publishing Co., 1993. Used by permission.

- Learn relaxation techniques, and use them to help you overcome the urge to smoke.

- Progressively switch to brands of cigarettes that have less and less nicotine. As your body's demand for nicotine diminishes, it will be easier to stop smoking without suffering difficult withdrawal symptoms.

- Change your brand of cigarettes. Buy a brand that doesn't taste good.

- Each time you resist smoking, put aside the money you would have spent on that pack of cigarettes. Keep it in a separate account. When you've succeeded in quitting, take a trip, buy a new stereo, or use the money for something you've always wanted.

- As you quit, you'll struggle with common withdrawal symptoms, such as irritability, headaches, dry mouth, hunger, constipation, and trouble going to sleep. Anticipate these symptoms and plan ahead to compensate. Soak in a hot bath or use relaxation techniques when you're feeling irritable or get a headache. Chew gum or sip fruit juice to moisten a dry mouth. Keep plenty of low-fat, low-calorie snacks (such as raw fruits and vegetables or air-popped popcorn) on hand to ease hunger. Include plenty of fiber (such as whole-grain breads and cereals) in your diet to overcome irregularity. Use relaxation techniques to help you fall asleep.

- Have substitutes on hand for times you want a cigarette. Chew sugarless gum, eat raw carrot sticks, suck on hard candy, chew on pieces of fresh ginger, or nibble on sunflower seeds.

- Avoid situations, people, and routines that make it easy for you to smoke. If you always smoke after you eat a meal, for example, finish with a piece of fresh fruit instead, then swish your mouth out with a great-tasting mouthwash.

- Start a program of brisk exercise once a day.

- Many communities have smoking cessation programs and support groups. Consider joining a local group to get the support you need. Look in the yellow pages under "Smoker's Treatment," ask your physician to recommend a group, or call the local chapter of the American Cancer Society.

Conclusions of the Report of the U.S. Surgeon General on Short-Term Benefits of Smoking Cessation

▼ Among former smokers, the decline in risk of death compared with continuing smokers begins shortly after quitting and continues for at least 10 to 15 years.

▼ Smoking cessation halves the risks for cancers of the oral cavity and the esophagus, compared with continued smoking, as soon as 5 years after cessation, with further reduction over a longer period of abstinence.

▼ The risk of cervical cancer is substantially lower among former smokers in comparison with continuing smokers, even in the first few years after cessation.

▼ The excess risk of coronary heart disease (CHD) caused by smoking is reduced by about half after 1 year of smoking abstinence and then declines gradually.

▼ After smoking cessation, the risk of stroke returns to the level of never smokers; in some studies this has occurred within 5 years, but in others as long as 15 years of abstinence were required.

▼ For those without overt chronic obstructive pulmonary disease (COPD), smoking cessation improves pulmonary function about 5% within a few months after cessation.

▼ Pregnant smokers who stop smoking at any time up to the 30th week of gestation have infants with higher birth weight than do women who smoke throughout pregnancy. Quitting in the first 3 to 4 months of pregnancy and abstaining throughout the remainder of pregnancy protects the fetus from the adverse effects of smoking on birth weight.

▼ Smokers with gastric or duodenal ulcers who stop smoking improve their clinical course relative to smokers who continue to smoke.

OVERCOMING ALCOHOL ADDICTION

Alcoholism is a complex problem that requires careful treatment by professionals. Support groups, such as Alcoholics Anonymous, also can be extremely

Do You Have a Problem with Alcohol?

To determine if you have a problem with alcohol, answer yes (Y) or no (N) to the following questions about your drinking behavior. Refer to the scale at the end of the quiz for evaluation of your answers.

____ 1. Do you occasionally drink heavily after a disappointment or a quarrel or when your parents or boss gives you a hard time?

____ 2. When you have trouble or feel pressured at school or at work, do you always drink more heavily than usual?

____ 3. Have you noticed that you are able to handle more liquor than you did when you were first drinking?

____ 4. Did you ever wake up the "morning after" and discover that you could not remember part of the evening before, even though your friends tell you that you did not pass out?

____ 5. When drinking with other people, do you try to have a few extra drinks that others don't notice?

____ 6. Are there certain occasions when you feel uncomfortable if alcohol is not available?

____ 7. Have you recently noticed that when you begin drinking, you are in more of a hurry to get the first drink than you used to be?

____ 8. Do you sometimes feel a little guilty about your drinking?

____ 9. Are you secretly irritated when your family or friends discuss your drinking?

____ 10. Have you recently noticed an increase in the frequency of your memory blackouts?

____ 11. Do you often find that you wish to continue drinking after your friends say they have had enough?

____ 12. Do you usually have a reason for the occasions when you drink heavily?

____ 13. When you are sober, do you often regret things you did or said while drinking?

____ 14. Have you tried switching brands or following different plans for controlling your drinking?

____ 15. Have you often failed to keep the promises you've made to yourself about controlling or cutting down on your drinking?

____ 16. Have you ever tried to control your drinking by changing jobs or moving to a new location?

____ 17. Do you try to avoid family or close friends while you are drinking?

____ 18. Are you having an increasing number of financial and academic problems?

____ 19. Do more people seem to be treating you unfairly without good reason?

____ 20. Do you eat very little or irregularly when you are drinking?

____ 21. Do you sometimes have the shakes in the morning and find that it helps to have a drink?

____ 22. Have you recently noticed that you cannot drink as much as you once did?

____ 23. Do you sometimes stay drunk for several days at a time?

____ 24. Do you sometimes feel very depressed and wonder whether life is worth living?

____ 25. Sometimes after a period of drinking, do you see or hear things that aren't there?

____ 26. Do you get terribly frightened after you have been drinking heavily?

If you answer *yes* to two or three of these questions, you may wish to evaluate your drinking in these areas. *Yes* answers to *several* of these questions may indicate one of the following stages of alcoholism:

▼ Questions 1–8 (early stage): Drinking is a regular part of your life.

▼ Questions 9–21 (middle stage): You are having trouble controlling when, where, and how much you drink.

▼ Questions 22–26 (beginning of the final stage): You no longer can control your desire to drink.

National Council on Alcoholism.

helpful to people who are trying to combat alcoholism. Alcoholism is a lifelong condition. You can be treated and become a "recovering" alcoholic who no longer uses alcohol, but the underlying condition is always there. If you think you may be alcoholic or have a serious drinking problem, see your physician.

If you do not have a drinking problem but want to make sure you use alcohol responsibly:

▶ Learn how much alcohol you can drink safely — how much you can enjoy without becoming impaired or intoxicated — then stick to that level. Set an actual number of drinks, and don't go over that number.

▶ Drink slowly. Enjoy what's going on instead of focusing on your drink. You might try alternating a drink with some plain mixer, soda, sparkling water, or fruit juice.

▶ Eat something whenever you drink. Alcohol is absorbed from the stomach more slowly if you've eaten something.

▶ If you're at a party, ask for a nonalcoholic beverage. Most people will be happy to provide sodas, juices, or sparkling water for those who don't want to drink.

▶ If you are hosting an activity, consider alcohol as a secondary aspect of the activity, not its focal point. Provide nonalcoholic alternatives for people to drink; don't push people who resist alcohol; and establish firm rules about intoxication (you won't tolerate it).

▶ If you drink any alcohol at all, *don't drive*. Ask a friend to drive you home, call a taxi, or arrange to spend the night where you are. Likewise, don't let someone else drive if that person has been drinking.

▶ Do not drink alcohol if you are taking any kind of prescription or over-the-counter medication.

▶ Do not drink alcohol if you are pregnant or nursing.

If you think you *may* have a drinking problem, here are some danger signs:

▶ You're preoccupied with alcohol. You think about it or plan it even when you're not drinking.

▶ You drink to escape your problems or relieve stress.

▶ You need a drink to help you go to sleep.

▶ You need a drink to help you get going in the morning.

▶ You get drunk often or stay drunk several days at a time.

▶ You sneak drinks or drink alone.

▶ You make excuses for why you drink.

▶ You hide the amount you drink from your mate, children, friends.

▶ You gulp your drinks.

▶ You have had blackouts, periods during which you can't remember what happened.

▶ You've had accidents frequently because of drinking.

▶ You've been ill a lot because of drinking.

▶ You've missed work or school because of drinking.

▶ You've had financial or legal problems because of drinking.

▶ Your personality or behavior changes after you drink.

▶ Once you sober up, you regret the things you did while you were drinking.

▶ Other people tell you that you drink too much.

▶ You think you drink too much.

▶ You feel guilty about your drinking.

▶ You've tried to stop drinking but can't.

▶ You don't want to talk about the negative effects of drinking.

OVERCOMING DRUG ADDICTION

As with alcohol abuse, professional help usually is needed in overcoming addiction to drugs. If you think you may have a drug problem and want to quit, the following tips may be helpful.

1. Pre-understanding (thinking of stopping)
   ▶ Note feelings and circumstances that trigger a "trip" or binge (e.g., stress, hostility, anxiety, anger).
   ▶ List noticeable problems associated with drug taking at school, work, home, or in public (e.g., less concentration, memory lapses, reduced performance, accidents, family rows).

2. Understanding (recognizing one's drug problem)
   ▶ Admit possible health and other adverse effects (possibly already evident to others).

Are You An Addict?

The following questions were written by recovering addicts in Narcotics Anonymous.

	Yes	No
1. Do you ever use alone?	☐	☐
2. Have you ever substituted one drug for another, thinking that one particular drug was the problem?	☐	☐
3. Have you ever manipulated or lied to a doctor to obtain prescription drugs?	☐	☐
4. Have you ever stolen drugs or stolen to obtain drugs?	☐	☐
5. Do you regularly use a drug when you wake up or when you go to bed?	☐	☐
6. Have you ever taken one drug to overcome the effects of another?	☐	☐
7. Do you avoid people or places that do not approve of you using drugs?	☐	☐
8. Have you ever used a drug without knowing what it was or what it would do to you?	☐	☐
9. Has your job or school performance ever suffered from the effects of your drug use?	☐	☐
10. Have you ever been arrested as a result of using drugs?	☐	☐
11. Have you ever lied about what or how much you use?	☐	☐
12. Do you put the purchase of drugs ahead of your financial responsibilities?	☐	☐
13. Have you ever tried to stop or control your using?	☐	☐
14. Have you ever been in a jail, hospital, or drug rehabilitation center because of your using?	☐	☐
15. Does using interfere with your sleeping or eating?	☐	☐
16. Does the thought of running out of drugs terrify you?	☐	☐
17. Do you feel it is impossible for you to live without drugs?	☐	☐
18. Do you ever question your own sanity?	☐	☐
19. Is your drug use making life at home unhappy?	☐	☐
20. Have you ever thought you couldn't fit in or have a good time without using drugs?	☐	☐
21. Have you ever felt defensive, guilty, or ashamed about your using?	☐	☐
22. Do you think a lot about drugs?	☐	☐
23. Have you had irrational or indefinable fears?	☐	☐
24. Has using affected your sexual relationships?	☐	☐
25. Have you ever taken drugs you didn't prefer?	☐	☐
26. Have you ever used drugs because of emotional pain or stress?	☐	☐
27. Have you ever overdosed on any drugs?	☐	☐
28. Do you continue to use despite negative consequences?	☐	☐
29. Do you think you might have a drug problem?	☐	☐

Are you an addict? This is a question only you can answer. Members of Narcotics Anonymous found that they all answered different numbers of these questions "yes." The actual number of *yes* responses isn't as important as how you feel inside and how addiction has affected your life. If you are an addict, you must first admit that you have a problem with drugs before any progress can be made toward recovery.

Reprinted from *Am I an Addict?*, revised copyright © 1986, World Service Office, Inc. Reprinted by permission of World Service Office, Inc. All rights reserved.

- Make a drug diary — when, with whom, how, and in what circumstances drugs are taken. When added up, the amount consumed may come as a surprise!
- Devise a balance sheet of pros and cons of drug-taking (e.g., pleasures/rewards versus negative effects).
- Determine whether drug consumption is already damaging your health (often sufficient to motivate a serious quitting attempt).
- Decide that no one else is to blame. The drug-taking is one's own decision. It can be beaten by one's own efforts.
- Ask your family doctor or other expert for advice. Medical caregivers often can explain the risks of a specific drug, motivate, and support quitting efforts.
- Realize that certain symptoms (e.g., anxiety, sleeplessness, paranoia, phobias, hostility) may have been viewed wrongly as the *cause* rather than the *consequence* of drug use.
- Check out places to get help — experts, clinics, detox centers — and how to learn new coping skills.

3. Action (making an effort to stop or cut back)
    - Set realistic goals for change (e.g., short-term quit strategies — "a week without drugs," "not this weekend") Cut back or abstain for a day, week, month at a time.
    - Try self-help tactics using manuals, quit guides, and advice from drug addiction agencies.
    - Plan to counter temptation. List drug-taking "cues" and how to avoid or sidestep them.
    - Adopt an open, frank approach when seeking advice. This is most likely to enlist maximum understanding and a frank, supportive response.
    - Anticipate relapses. Become wary of feelings, events, places that might trigger a relapse.
    - Do not regard a relapse as a failure or loss of "all that's been gained" but, rather, as a learning experience — one step on the way to doing better next time.
    - Be prepared for several tries before breaking a drug habit.
    - Enlist cooperative support from family and friends. The families of quitters also may need counseling.

Consider these alternatives instead of drugs:
- If you need physical relaxation, try athletics, exercise, or outdoor hobbies.
- Stimulate your senses. Train yourself to be more aware of nature and beauty.
- If you're anxious, depressed, or uptight, turn to people — friends, professional counselors, support groups.
- Volunteer in programs where you can help others and not focus on yourself.
- If you want to escape boredom, stimulate your mind through reading, classes, creative games, discussion groups, memory training, or travel.
- Pursue training in music, art, singing, or writing. Attend more concerts, ballets, or museum shows.
- Volunteer in political campaigns, or join lobbying and political-action groups.
- Explore various philosophical theories through classes, seminars, and discussion groups.
- If you're looking for adventure, sign up for a wilderness survival outing; take up boardsailing or rock climbing.

14

Sexually Transmitted Disease: Prevention and Wellness

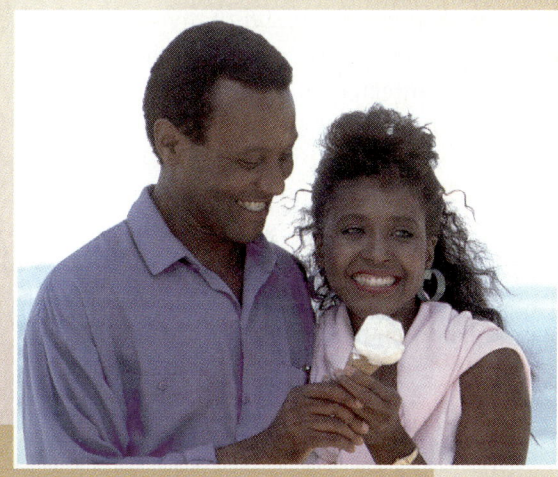

Objectives

▼ Understand how sexually transmitted diseases are passed from one person to another.

▼ Be aware of the incidence of STDs in their various forms.

▼ Learn the reasons for the prevalence of STDs.

▼ Learn the symptoms, risks, and treatment for various STDs: chlamydia, gonorrhea, genital warts, herpes, viral hepatitis (not technically an (STD), pelvic inflammatory disease, pubic lice and scabies, syphilis, and AIDS.

▼ Know general guidelines for reducing the risks of contracting STDs.

Sexually transmitted diseases, including AIDS, are exactly what their name implies: They are *transmitted*, or passed from one person to another, through sexual contact. Several sexually transmitted diseases also can be passed in infected blood. Generally, the organisms that cause sexually transmitted diseases are fragile and can't exist outside the protective environment of the human reproductive tract. Therefore, you can't be infected by toilet seats, soap dishes, towels, or doorknobs. Some sexually transmitted diseases can be treated and cured. Others have no cure. All of them can be prevented by appropriate sexual behavior.

Sexually transmitted diseases (STDs) have been around a long time. They are mentioned in the Old Testament, and epidemics were recorded as early as the time of Columbus. Today, the more than 25 STDs identified by researchers are among the most prevalent infectious diseases in the United States. More than a million new cases are reported to the Centers for Disease Control (CDC) every year. Because many people who are infected show no symptoms, the CDC estimates that the number of Americans infected in any one year may be as high as 10 million. Most people with STDs are those in the most sexually active group: between ages of 15 and 30. The diseases are no respecter of race, creed, gender, education, or socioeconomic status. Table 14.1 lists estimated new cases of STDs in 1993.

Many STDs have reached epidemic proportions, even though many of them can be cured with proper medication. STDs are rampant for a number of reasons:

TABLE 14.1 ▼ Estimated New Cases of Sexually-Transmitted Diseases in 1993

Disease	Number of Cases
HIV	50,000
Genital herpes	500,000
Syphilis	120,000
Hepatitis B	300,000
Gonorrhea	1,500,000
Trichomonosis	3,000,000
Chlamydia	4,000,000
Human papilloma virus (HPV)	1,200,000

▶ Some STDs cause no symptoms, so victims are unaware that they are infected. Others cause only mild symptoms that can be easily confused with other ailments.

▶ When birth control pills became widely available, many people stopped using condoms as a form of birth control, and, though condoms prevent STDs, birth control pills do not.

▶ As a trend, people are becoming sexually active at an earlier age and are having more than one sexual partner.

▶ Some people infected with STDs who have no symptoms continue to have sex and spread the disease.

▶ The statistical trend toward marrying later has resulted in more sexual activity for longer periods.

▶ Some STDs cannot be treated; others have developed strains that resist antibiotics.

▶ Fear of social stigma, disapproval, and condemnation stops some people from seeking treatment even when they suspect they might be infected. Others become complacent because of the past successes of penicillin and other antibiotics.

▶ Many victims deny the possibility of infection, believing "It can never happen to me," or they believe STDs affect only "high-risk" groups.

▼ Myths About STDs

Remember the old myth about catching "something" from a toilet seat? It's just that — a myth! So are these:

▼ You can get an STD in a swimming pool or hot tub.
▼ You can get an STD from using someone else's towel or washcloth.
▼ If your partner doesn't have symptoms, you're safe.
▼ If your symptoms go away on their own, you're cured.
▼ You won't catch an STD if your partner is being treated.
▼ You can always tell if you have an STD.

STDs are caused by bacteria, viruses, parasites, and fungi. Infection can recur with every new exposure. The body generally does not build up a resistance to the organisms that cause the diseases. Most affect the genitals. Left untreated, many have serious complications that affect the entire body. AIDS which disables the immune system and leaves the body open to various opportunistic infections, eventually causes death.

Strictly speaking, anyone who engages in sexual activity is at risk for STDs. The more sexual partners, the greater is the risk. The risk also increases substantially if a person does not use condoms. Sexual behavior that tears or damages the vagina, anus, or penis increases the risk; anal intercourse is especially dangerous. Gay and bisexual men, their sexual partners, intravenous drug users, and their partners are at highest risk. An infected mother can pass the disease to her fetus or infant during gestation and birth.

General signs and symptoms of STDs include:

- Sores on or near the genitals
- Pain in the genitals
- A burning sensation in the genitals
- Discharge from the vagina or penis
- Itching around the genitals, in the vagina, in the rectum, around the anus, or in and around the mouth
- Abdominal pain
- Growths or warts in the genital area; may be skin-colored or dark, flat, or raised

Sores, warts, itching, rashes, and burning in areas of the body other than the genitals, vagina, rectum, and mouth generally don't indicate STDs. If you develop these symptoms and think you may have been exposed to an STD, however, you should see a physician. Understanding the incidence, signs and symptoms, and risks for specific STDs can help you reduce your risks of becoming infected.

CHLAMYDIA

The most common STD in the United States, chlamydia afflicts more than 4 million men and women each year. As many as half a million cases in women progress to pelvic inflammatory disease, which can cause sterility. An estimated 4% of all pregnant women are infected. If left untreated, chlamydia is chronic. The Centers for Disease Control estimate that chlamydia now is 10 times more prevalent than gonorrhea, which until recently was the most common STD in the United States.

Caused by a bacteria, chlamydia often occurs simultaneously with other sexually transmitted diseases, most commonly gonorrhea and herpes. Unidentified for many years, it used to be called simply "non-gonococcal urethritis" until the bacteria was identified and laboratory tests were developed to diagnose it.

Almost all men who are infected have symptoms; almost all women who are infected *do not* have symptoms unless the infection progresses into something more serious, such as pelvic inflammatory disease. Even when women do have symptoms, they often are mild and can disappear on their own even though the woman is still infected. When symptoms occur, they usually appear 1 to 3 weeks after infection.

Chlamydia infects the mucous membranes that line the genitals, rectum, anus, mouth, and eyes. It is transmitted by contact with infected mucous membranes and occurs most commonly between heterosexuals. The most common complications for newborns are pneumonia and conjunctivitis (an infection of the membranes in the eyes); more than 30,000 newborn babies are infected each year in the United States.

When to Get Checked For a Possible STD

- If you are sexually active
- If you know or suspect your sex partner is infected
- If you change sex partners often. (Wait about 4 weeks, then get tested.)
- If there are signs of:
  - a vaginal or penile discharge ("the drip")
  - rash, warty growths, pimple, itchiness or sore on genitals
  - persistent lower abdominal pain
  - pain when urinating
  - changes in menstrual flow, unusual bleeding (in women).

Women should get regular Pap smear tests to detect early signs of cervical cancer.

The most common symptoms in men include:

- Whitish or puslike discharge from the penis.
- Pain during urination; urination may be followed by a watery, clear discharge.
- Frequent urination.
- Urethral itching.
- Abdominal discomfort.

Women who experience symptoms may have:

- Whitish vaginal discharge.
- Itching or burning of the genitals.
- Mild pain during urination.
- Abdominal discomfort.
- Bleeding between periods.
- Symptoms of pelvic inflammatory disease (fever, painful intercourse, pelvic pain, vaginal discharge).

Complications of chlamydia in men include sterility and diseases of the urinary tract. In women, chlamydia is the leading cause of pelvic inflammatory disease, which also can cause sterility. Chlamydia that is untreated can damage the arteries, heart valves, and heart muscle in men and women alike. At particular risk for chlamydia are women with more than one sexual partner, women who do not use some kind of barrier (such as condoms) during intercourse, women under age 25 who have multiple sexual partners, and women under age 20 who are pregnant.

Treatment consists of a full course of antibiotics, usually tetracycline or erythromycin. Infected and diagnosed individuals should:

- Take all the antibiotics the doctor prescribes.
- Have a follow-up culture 2 weeks after you finish taking the antibiotics to make sure the bacteria have been completely destroyed.
- Avoid all sexual activity until the infection is gone, at least until the follow-up culture is clean.
- Tell all sexual partners to get tested for chlamydia; if one of the sexual partners is infected, a person can be reinfected.

GONORRHEA

Known most commonly as "the clap," gonorrhea infects almost 2 million Americans a year, according to reports given to the CDC. This makes gonorrhea the second most prevalent STD in the United States. Some estimate that the actual number of infected people in this country is four times that high.

Gonorrhea is caused by a bacteria that infects the cervix, rectum, urethra, or mouth. It is transmitted by intercourse, anal-genital sex, and oral-genital sex. Because the environment of the vagina is so conducive to growth of the bacteria that causes gonorrhea, women have an 80% chance of developing gonorrhea if they are exposed to the bacteria through intercourse. Men have only about a 20% chance. Left untreated, gonorrhea is chronic and progressive.

The symptoms of gonorrhea generally develop within 2 days to 2 weeks after infection, but, as with chlamydia, it may have no symptoms at all or only mild symptoms. Men tend to have more noticeable signs and symptoms, which include:

- A profuse, yellowish or milky, foul-smelling discharge from the penis.
- Burning, frequent urination.
- Fever.
- Abdominal pain.
- Swelling of the testicles.

If women develop symptoms, they usually are mild and include:

- Slight burning or pain in the genital area.
- Slight vaginal discharge.
- Abnormally heavy menstrual bleeding or bleeding between periods.

If the gonorrhea is transmitted during oral sex, a sore throat may develop. If it was transmitted during anal intercourse, pain, burning, and discharge from the anus may result.

Babies born to infected mothers may become blind. Because gonorrhea is so prevalent, the eyes of newborns are treated routinely with silver nitrate. Other complications include pneumonia and infections of the anus or rectum.

If left untreated, gonorrhea can cause permanent sterility in women and men alike. Other complications include heart damage, brain damage, liver damage, arthritis, skin lesions, and meningitis. The bacteria responsible for gonorrhea can survive in the reproductive tract for years, enabling a man or a woman without symptoms to infect multiple partners unknowingly.

Gonorrhea is most often treated with penicillin. If a chlamydia infection is also present, tetracycline is added. Unfortunately, some new strains of gonorrhea are resistant to penicillin and must be treated with newer drugs. Anyone who is infected and diagnosed with this STD should:

▶ Take the full course of antibiotics prescribed by a doctor, even though the symptoms probably will ease up within 12 hours and disappear within 3 days.

▶ Return for a follow-up culture a week after finishing the antibiotics.

▶ Avoid sexual intercourse or other sexual contact that could spread the infection until the doctor verifies that the infection is completely gone.

▶ Report the names of all sexual contacts who could have been infected; if they are not treated, reinfection could occur.

Gonorrhea is so common that some health officials recommend regular screening (usually once every 6 months) for all sexually active people.

▼ GENITAL WARTS

The third most prevalent STD in the United States, genital warts are caused by the human papilloma virus (HPV). An estimated 1.2 million Americans, most of them between ages 15 and 24, develop the infection each year. The most common symptom — warts on the penis (foreskin, glands, or shaft), scrotum, anus, cervix, or around the urethra — may develop as soon as 1 to 3 months after infection but may not appear until 8 months after infection. Outbreaks of warts are more common during pregnancy and in people with a weak immune system. Genital warts can be transmitted by skin-to-skin contact during intercourse or by oral-genital contact during oral sex.

Some people never develop symptoms of genital warts. In others, the warts are inside the vagina or rectum or on the cervix, so they may not be noticed unless a physician conducts an examination. In those who *do* develop symptoms, these usually start with localized irritation and itching, followed by the growth of warts. The warts may be soft or hard, flat, small, yellowish, and dry. In moist areas of the body, they usually are larger and shaped irregularly and may be white, pink, or gray. Genital warts often look like cauliflower. In women, they often clump together. If the infection was passed via oral sex, the warts may grow in and around the mouth.

The complications of genital warts are potentially deadly. Of the 65 different strains of HPV, 12 have been linked to cervical cancer. In fact, the HPV is associated with approximately 90% of all cervical cancer, and it may play a strong role in other genital cancers as well, including cancer of the penis.

Newborns infected by their mothers can develop warts in the mouth and bronchial passages. This can interfere with breathing.

Treatment can remove the warts, but it cannot kill the virus that causes the warts. Recurrence is extremely common. The typical treatment for genital warts is the drug podophyllin, which causes the wart to slough off. It normally is applied by a physician once a week for 5 or 6 weeks until the wart has disappeared completely. Podophyllin can't be used by pregnant women or to treat warts in the cervical area.

Warts that resist treatment with podophyllin sometimes can be removed by surgery, electrocautery (burning), or cryotherapy (freezing). All these options result in scarring.

A person diagnosed and treated for genital warts should:

▶ Follow the physician's instructions carefully; repeated treatment usually is necessary to remove the warts.

▶ Use any antibiotic ointments prescribed by the physician.

▶ Avoid sexual contact during an outbreak of warts.

▶ For women: Have a Pap smear every year to monitor the risk of cervical cancer.

▶ Never use over-the-counter wart removers. They are useless against genital warts and can cause tissue damage if applied to the genital area.

Again, treatment does not kill the virus that causes genital warts. Once infected, the person always carries the virus, even though it may be dormant for months or years at a time.

HERPES

Of the different strains of herpes simplex virus, the most common is herpes simplex-1, the culprit behind the common cold sore or fever blister. Other viruses in the herpes family cause chicken pox, shingles, and infectious mononucleosis. The herpes simplex-2 virus is what causes the STD, sometimes called *herpes genitalis*.

Once a person gets genital herpes, it remains forever. There's no cure, and there's no treatment. The virus always will reside in the body. That doesn't mean the blistering sores characteristic of a herpes outbreak are always present in the body. Some people have only one or two outbreaks a year; others may have them much more often. The virus can be spread, however, even when no lesions are visible. Herpes is transmitted by contact with an active sore or with the virus-containing secretions from the vagina or penis.

Approximately half a million new cases of herpes are reported to the CDC each year. Officials there estimate that more than 20 million Americans have the virus.

Usually within 10 days of infection, flulike symptoms arise that may include:

▶ Fever.

▶ Swollen glands, especially in the groin. Muscle aches and pains.

▶ Fatigue.

▶ Occasionally, shooting or stabbing pains in the abdomen and legs.

During this initial period, pain may be felt during intercourse or urination. The characteristic blisters that appear on the genitals or mouth follow the flu-like symptoms and progress through four stages:

▶ At the site where the virus entered the body, the skin starts to itch or tingle, turns red, and becomes extremely sensitive. This sensation, which generally precedes all outbreaks, is called the *prodrome*.

▶ One or more small, painful blisters or sores erupt on the glands and shaft of the penis, around the anus, at the opening of the vagina, on the clitoris, on the cervix, and on the labia. If oral-genital contact occurred, the sores may be in or around the mouth. The blisters rupture and the resulting painful, itching, open sores may weep a yellowish secretion or pus.

▶ Without treatment, the sores diminish; scabs form and fall off within one to 2 weeks. Pain, fever, and other symptoms subside.

▶ The virus lies dormant in the nerve endings for an unpredictable time. Recurrences of the blisters — which usually are less severe, of shorter duration, and without warning — occur in approximately two-thirds of the cases and can be caused by unrelated illness, fever, emotional stress, lack of sleep, exposure to cold or heat, sunburn, poor nutrition, and menstruation.

The most typical complication of herpes is *autoinoculation* — spreading the virus to other parts of one's own body, such as the mouth or eyes. Men don't seem to suffer any serious long-term complications. Women, on the other hand, run much higher risk for cervical cancer if they are infected with herpes.

Possibly the most serious complications involve babies born to mothers with herpes. If a woman with an active herpes lesion delivers a baby vaginally, the baby has a one-in-four chance of becoming infected and can be blind, have mental retardation, have damage to internal organs, and die. During active herpes, a woman should have a Caesarean section delivery to lower the risk of infecting the baby.

Herpes is caused by a virus, and it has no known cure. An antiviral drug, acyclovir, has helped relieve symptoms in some people during the initial outbreak only. Early indications are that continual use of acyclovir may help prevent recurrences. A person diagnosed with herpes should:

▶ Wash the hands thoroughly after touching infected areas, to avoid spreading the disease to other areas of the body.

▶ Keep the infected lesions clean and dry.

▶ Wear loose clothing to avoid irritating the infected areas; avoid scratching, rubbing, touching, or picking at sores.

▶ Avoid sexual contact of any kind during times when lesions are active.

▶ Use a latex condom to prevent spread of the infection when blisters are not present.

- Practice good health habits to avoid getting fatigued or stressed, which can lead to recurrences.
- For women; Have a Paps smear every 6 to 12 months to monitor the risk for cervical cancer. If pregnant, discuss the history of the infection with the doctor.

▼ VIRAL HEPATITIS

Hepatitis, an infection that causes inflammation of the liver, is caused by one or more viruses. Of the four identified types of hepatitis, the most common is hepatitis A, more often called "infectious hepatitis." Even though hepatitis A can be transmitted sexually, it is not considered to be an STD. It most often is spread through unsanitary conditions, poor hygiene, direct exposure to the virus, or infected food and water. An estimated half of all adults in the United States have developed antibodies to hepatitis A, and it can be prevented with gamma globulin injections within 10 days of exposure.

Hepatitis B, an STD that affects close to half a million Americans each year, is spread through exposure to the contaminated blood or body fluids of an infected person. Besides being spread through semen, it can be transmitted through breast milk, saliva, and perspiration.

People at high risk for contracting hepatitis B include intravenous drug users and their partners, as well as people with multiple sexual partners. Homosexual men are at particular risk for hepatitis B.

Signs and symptoms of hepatitis B develop within 6 months of infection and include:

- Milk fever.
- Loss of appetite.
- Nausea and vomiting.
- Diarrhea.
- Severe fatigue.
- Pain in the muscles and joints.
- Headache.
- Tenderness in the upper right section of the abdomen.

Within 2 weeks after symptoms first appear, signs of liver damage may become apparent, including:

- Jaundice (yellowish discoloration of the skin and whites of the eyes).
- Light gray or whitish stools.
- Dark urine.
- Tender, enlarged liver.

Because the symptoms of hepatitis B are so much like those of the flu or infectious mononucleosis, a blood test is needed for proper diagnosis. Long-term complications from hepatitis B, which can be devastating, include liver cancer, chronic progressive hepatitis, liver failure, cirrhosis of the liver, and death.

Hepatitis B has no cure, but an effective vaccine is available to make the person immune and prevent infection. Anyone in the high-risk group should ask for the vaccine. High-risk individuals include:

- Sexually active heterosexuals and homosexuals and their partners.
- Sexual partners of an infected person *or* a person living in the house with an infected person, even if not sexually involved.
- Intravenous drug users and their partners.
- People in the health-care professions.
- Natives of or travelers to Africa, Asia, Alaska, and the Pacific Islands.

People diagnosed with hepatitis B should:

- Get plenty of rest. Follow the physician's guidelines for limiting activity during the acute stage of infection.
- Do not use drugs, including alcohol, that are metabolized by the liver, as these substances can overly burden an already-stressed liver.
- Avoid sexual contact.
- If pregnant, discuss the disease with a physician. Do not breast-feed the baby.
- Have regular follow-up checkups to determine the risk of liver disease.

▼ PELVIC INFLAMMATORY DISEASE

As mentioned earlier, pelvic inflammatory disease (PID) can be caused by other sexually transmitted diseases, most commonly chlamydia and gonorrhea. The most dangerous of all STDs, it is a severe infection of the lining of the abdominal cavity that can be caused by other factors, including an intrauterine device (IUD) for birth control.

One of the factors that makes PID so dangerous is that it's so difficult to diagnose, and, unless it's treated immediately, it can cause scar tissue to form in the Fallopian tubes. A common result is sterility, because partially or completely blocked tubes prevent the egg from entering the uterus.

Signs and symptoms of PID include:

▶ Menstrual irregularities, including irregular cycles, profuse bleeding during menstruation, and vaginal bleeding between cycles.
▶ Severe menstrual cramps.
▶ Vaginal discharge.
▶ Pain or tenderness in the abdomen or lower back.
▶ Fever and chills.
▶ Nausea and vomiting.
▶ Loss of appetite.
▶ A burning sensation during urination.

As mentioned, some women who develop PID become sterile. Among those who do get pregnant, the risk of ectopic pregnancy (a fetus that attaches to the Fallopian tube instead of the uterus), miscarriage, and stillbirth is increased dramatically.

PID can be treated with antibiotics. Early treatment is essential. A person who is diagnosed and treated, should:

▶ Follow the complete course of antibiotics prescribed by a doctor, even if the symptoms disappear.
▶ Stop using an IUD.
▶ Avoid sexual activity until the infection has cleared.
▶ Ask that any sexual partners be treated; if they are not, reinfection can occur.
▶ Do not douche, as it can spread the infection.

▼ PUBIC LICE AND SCABIES

Commonly called "crabs," pubic lice are tiny parasites that move from partner to partner during sexual activity. Pubic lice actually are one of three different kinds of lice that attach to various parts of the body. Whereas pubic lice grip the pubic hair and feed on the small blood vessels of the underlying skin, other lice attach to skin or the hair of the head.

With a life cycle of approximately 2 months, pubic lice attach to the pubic hair, where females can lay as many as 10 eggs (nits) a day. The nits adhere to the pubic hair with a thick, sticky substance. Body warmth incubates the eggs until they hatch, and the new lice start feeding on the blood vessels as the old lice drop off. As they drop off, the lice are visible to the naked eye in bedding and clothing. The tiny mite that causes scabies has a similar life cycle, but the female mite burrows under the skin at night.

Common signs and symptoms of pubic lice include:

▶ Intense itching in the pubic area.
▶ Visible lice or whitish nits in the pubic hair.
▶ Swollen glands in the groin.

Common signs and symptoms of scabies include:

▶ Characteristic patterns of burrowing, most commonly on the buttocks, under the breasts, between the fingers and on the wrists.
▶ A discharge of pus from the burrowed areas.
▶ Intense itching.

Treatment options for pubic lice include Kwell, available only by prescription, and an over-the-counter preparation called A-200 Pyrinate. Both are applied to the pubic hair in a single dose; a fine-tooth comb is used to remove nits. Kwell also is used to treat scabies. Most advise against using Kwell during pregnancy, so pregnant women should check with a doctor.

Individuals diagnosed with scabies should follow the doctor's directions, as scabies also can be transmitted by close nonsexual contact. If diagnosed with pubic lice, the infected person should:

▶ Follow treatment directions carefully.
▶ Dip the comb in vinegar, then water, to dissolve the sticky substance holding nits to the pubic hair.
▶ Wash all clothing, bedding, and linens contacted prior to treatment. This is one STD in which an innocent victim *can* be infected by towels or sheets.
▶ Clean all upholstery and furniture contacted prior to treatment.

▶ Avoid sexual contact, and inform all sexual partners; if they are not treated, reinfection can occur.

▼ SYPHILIS

Fortunately, syphilis has been on the decline in the United States. Current estimates indicate fewer than 120,000 cases. Caused by a *spirochete* (corkscrew-shaped type of bacteria), syphilis is transmitted through intercourse, anal-genital contact, and oral-genital contact. It also can be transmitted by kissing a person who has a sore on the mouth, although this is not common. Syphilis has four specific stages:

1. *Primary stage.* Occurring 2 to 3 weeks after the bacteria enters the body, a painless, red-rimmed sore, called a *chancre*, develops at the site where the bacteria entered. The chancre may be as large as a dime but commonly is as small as a pinhead and may go unnoticed, especially if it is in the vagina, rectum, anus, or mouth. Within 3 to 6 weeks, the chancre clears up without treatment, so many infected people assume it was something else.

2. *Secondary stage.* Any time from 6 weeks to a year after the chancre heals, the symptoms of secondary syphilis appear. These symptoms, which may be mild to severe and can last anywhere from a few days to a few months, include:

   ▶ Low-grade fever.
   ▶ Nausea and loss of appetite.
   ▶ Whitish patches on the mouth and throat.
   ▶ Sore throat.
   ▶ Rash on the soles of the feet and palms of the hands.
   ▶ Headache.
   ▶ Swollen glands.
   ▶ Hair loss.
   ▶ Joint pain.
   ▶ Large sores on the genitals or around the mouth.

   Even if untreated, these symptoms usually run their course, then disappear. Disappearance of symptoms does not mean the infection is over. The disease remains dormant, and symptoms can reappear at any time. The person remains infectious during this stage even though symptoms have cleared up.

3. *Latent stage.* No outward symptoms are present during the latent stage, which may last as long as 30 years, and the person is no longer contagious. Even though nothing seems to be happening on the outside, the spirochetes attack the body's organs vigorously, causing substantial damage to the brain, heart, and central nervous system. Maladies characteristic of the latent stage include heart disease, senility, blindness, central nervous system deterioration, and death.

4. *Late (tertiary) stage.* During the final stage of untreated syphilis, the disease results in blindness, deafness, central nervous system destruction, paralysis, psychosis, and, finally, death.

Penicillin is the drug of choice in treating syphilis. With treatment, syphilis can be cured at any stage. A person diagnosed and treated for syphilis should:

▶ Follow the complete course of antibiotics as prescribed by a doctor, even if no symptoms are apparent.

▶ Discuss with the doctor the possibility of simultaneous STD infections, such as gonorrhea or chlamydia. If additional infections are present, higher doses of various antibiotics are necessary.

▶ Avoid sexual activity until cured.

▶ Have follow-up blood tests for a year after finishing antibiotic treatment.

▼ HIV AND AIDS

According to a January, 1994, article in the *Harvard Mental Health Letter*, "AIDS and Mental health,":

> The pandemic that has been sweeping the world for the last 10 years is a medical crisis. According to the best estimates, there will be more than 10 million cases of AIDS in the world and more than 500,000 in the United States by the end of 1994. More than 2 million Americans will have been infected with the virus and more than 400,000 will have died of the consistently fatal disorder. Neither a cure nor a vaccine is likely to be discovered soon.

HIV is a progressive disease. At first, people who become infected with HIV may not know they are infected. An incubation period of weeks, months, or years may go by during which no symptoms appear. The virus may live in the body 10 years or longer before symptoms develop.

As the infection progresses to the point at which certain diseases develop, the person is said to have AIDS. HIV itself doesn't kill. Nor do people die of AIDS. AIDS is the term used to define the final stage of HIV infection. Death is caused by a weakened immune system that is unable to fight off the opportunistic diseases that develop.

Earliest symptoms of the disease include unexplained weight loss, constant fatigue, mild fever, swollen lymph glands, diarrhea, and sore throats. Advanced symptoms include loss of appetite, skin diseases, night sweats, and deterioration of the mucous membranes.

Most of the illnesses AIDS patients develop are harmless and rare in the general population but are fatal to AIDS victims. The two most common fatal conditions in AIDS patients are *pneumocystis carinii pneumonia* (a parasitic infection of the lungs) and *kaposis sarcoma* (a type of skin cancer). The AIDS virus also may attack the nervous system, causing brain and spinal cord damage.

On the average, the individual develops the symptoms that fit the case definition of AIDS about 7 to 8 years following infection. From that point on, the person may live another 2 to 3 years. In essence, from the point of infection, the individual may endure a chronic disease 8 to 10 years.

The only means to determine whether someone has HIV is through an *HIV antibody test*. Being HIV positive does not necessarily mean the person has AIDS. Several years may go by before the person develops the diseases that fit the case definition of AIDS.

Upon HIV infection, the immune system's line of defense against the virus is to form antibodies that bind to the virus. On the average, the body takes 3 months to manufacture enough antibodies to show up positive in an HIV antibody test. Sometimes this may take 6 months or longer.

If HIV infection is suspected, a prudent waiting period of 3 to 6 months is suggested prior to testing. During this time, and from there on, individuals should refrain from further endangering themselves and others through risky behaviors. Some people choose to be tested to be reassured that their risky behaviors are acceptable. Even if the test turns up negative for HIV, this does not represent a "license" to continue risky behaviors. Once infected with the virus, a person never will become uninfected. There is no second chance. Everyone must protect himself or herself against this chronic disease. No one should be so ignorant as to believe that it can never happen to him or her!

Although professionals disagree as to how many carriers actually will develop AIDS, sooner or later most HIV-infected individuals will be diagnosed with AIDS. Even if a person has not developed AIDS, the virus can be passed on to others who could easily develop AIDS.

HIV TRANSMISSION

HIV is transmitted by the exchange of cellular body fluids including blood, semen, vaginal secretions, and maternal milk. These fluids may be exchanged during sexual intercourse, by using hypodermic needles previously used by infected individuals, between a pregnant woman and her developing fetus, by infection of babies from the mother during childbirth, less frequently during breast feeding, and rarely from a blood transfusion or organ transplant.

The risk of being infected with HIV from a blood transfusion today is slight. Prior to 1985, several cases of HIV infection came from blood transfusions because the blood was donated by HIV-infected individuals. Today, all individuals who donate blood are tested for HIV.

A myth regarding HIV is that it can be transmitted by donating blood. People cannot get HIV from giving blood. Health professionals use a brand-new needle every time they withdraw blood from a person. These needles are used only once and are thrown away immediately after each person has donated blood.

People do not get HIV because of who they are but because of what they do. HIV and AIDS can threaten anyone, anywhere: men, women, children, teenagers, young people, older adults, whites, blacks, hispanics, orientals, homosexuals, heterosexuals. bisexuals, druggies, Americans, Africans, Europeans. Nobody is immune to HIV. Figure 14.1 gives a comparison of HIV and AIDS cases by various groups.

HIV can be transmitted between males, between females, from male to female, or from female to male. HIV and AIDS are basically preventable. Almost all of the people who get HIV do so because they choose to engage in risky behaviors.

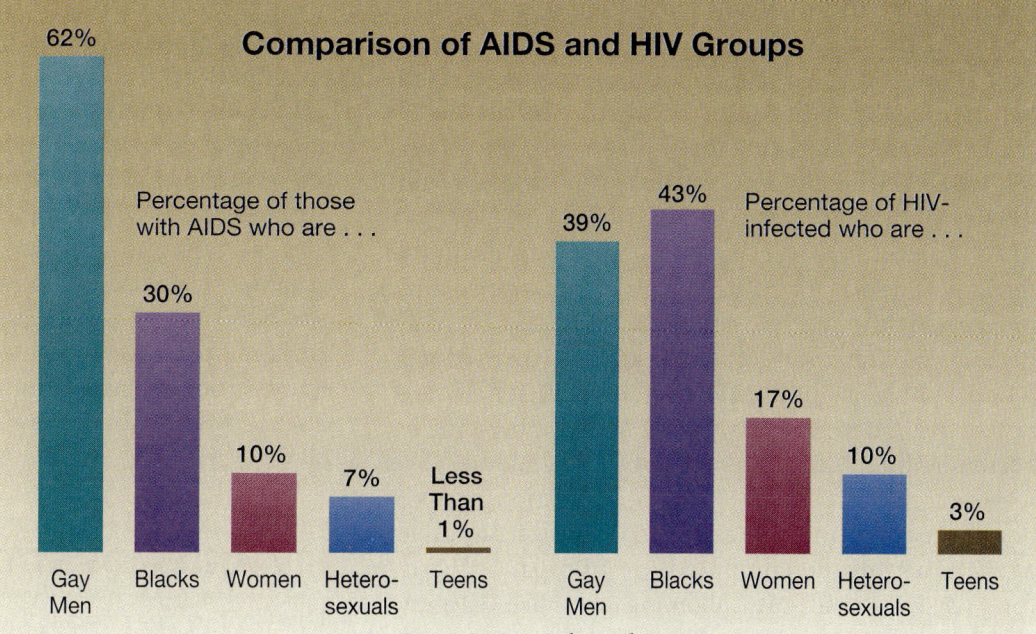

FIGURE 14.1 ▼ Comparison of people with HIV to those with full-blown AIDS; 22-state study shows the percentage of infections declining among gay men but rising sharply among black, teens and women.

From Centers for Disease Control and Prevention

RISKY BEHAVIORS

You cannot tell if people are infected with HIV or have AIDS by simply looking at them or taking their word. Not you, not a nurse, not even a doctor can tell without an HIV antibody test. Therefore, every time you engage in risky behavior, you run the risk of contracting HIV. The two most basic risky behaviors are:

1. *Having unprotected vaginal, anal, or oral sex with an HIV-infected person.* Unprotected sex means having sex without the proper use of a condom. A person should select only latex (rubber or prophylactic) condoms that say "disease prevention" on the package. Although you might have unprotected sex with an infected person and not get the virus, you can also get it by having unprotected sex only once with that infected person.

   Rubbing during sexual intercourse often damages mucous membranes and causes unseen bleeding (even in the mouth). During vaginal, anal, or oral sexual contact, infected blood, semen, or vaginal fluids can penetrate the mucous membranes that line the vagina, the penis, the rectum, the mouth, or the throat. From the membrane, HIV then can travel into the previously uninfected person's blood.

   Health experts believe unprotected anal sex is the riskiest type of sex. Even though bleeding is not visible in most cases, anal sex almost always causes tiny tears and bleeding in the rectum. This happens because the rectum does not stretch easily, the mucous membrane is quite thin, and small blood vessels lie directly beneath the membrane. Condoms also are more likely to break during anal intercourse because of the greater friction produced in a smaller cavity. All of these factors greatly enhance the risk of HIV transmission.

   Although latex condoms provide for "safer" sex if they are used correctly, they are not 100% foolproof. Abstaining from sex is the only 100% sure way to protect yourself from HIV infection and other STDs.

2. *Sharing hypodermic needles or other drug paraphernalia with someone who is infected.* Following an injection, a small amount of blood remains in the needle and sometimes in the syringe itself. If the person who used the syringe is infected with HIV and someone else uses that same syringe, regardless of the drug used (legal or illegal), that small amount of blood is sufficient to spread the virus. All used syringes should be destroyed and disposed of immediately after they are used.

   In addition, a person must be cautious when getting acupuncture, getting a tattoo, or having the ears pierced. If the needle used was used previously on someone who is HIV-inflected and it was not disinfected properly, the person risks getting HIV as well.

Infrequent use of drugs, including alcohol, also heightens the risk of spreading HIV. Otherwise prudent people often act irrationally and engage in risky behaviors when they are under the influence of drugs. Getting high can make you willing to have sex when you really didn't plan to, and thereby run the risk of HIV infection.

As pointed out earlier, HIV can be transmitted through a blood transfusion, an organ transplant, pregnancy (mother to fetus), and maternal milk (usually mother to child). Even though the nation's blood supply is quite safe (because all donors are tested for HIV), a very small risk is present in becoming infected from previously tested blood.

Because of the 3- to 6-month incubation period, donors recently infected with HIV can test negative at the time they donate blood (or an organ). Therefore, people who are planning to have surgery should store their own blood in advance so safe blood will be available if they need it.

Small concentrations of the virus have been found in saliva and teardrops, but there is no record of anyone getting HIV through French-kissing or from someone else's tears, coughs, or sneezes. In principle, if both people have open cuts in the lips, mouth, or gums, HIV could be transmitted through open-mouthed kissing, but such a case has never been documented.

The virus cannot be transmitted through perspiration (sweat) either. Sporting activities with no physical contact pose no risk to uninfected individuals, unless they have open wounds through which blood from an infected person can come in direct contact with the open wound of the uninfected person. The skin is an excellent line of defense against HIV. Blood from an infected person cannot penetrate the skin except through an opening in the skin. As an extra precaution, a person should use vinyl or latex gloves when performing work that requires direct contact with someone else's blood or open wound.

Some people fear getting HIV from health care professionals. The chances of getting infected during physical or medical procedures are practically nil. Health care workers take extra care to protect themselves and their patients from HIV.

HIV is not transmitted through casual contact. HIV cannot be caught by spending time, shaking hands, or hugging an infected person; from a toilet seat, dishes, or silverware used by an HIV patient; or by sharing a drink, food, a towel, or clothes with a person who has HIV.

What about dating? Dating and getting to know other people is a normal part of life. Dating, however, does not mean the same thing as having sex. Sexual intercourse as a part of dating can be risky, and one of the risks is AIDS. You can't tell if someone you are dating or would like to date has been exposed to HIV. The good news, though, is that as long as you avoid sexual activity and don't share drug needles, it doesn't matter whom you date.

Another myth regarding HIV transmission is that you can get it from insects or animals. The H in HIV stands for human. You cannot catch HIV from insects or animals. Animals do not get infected with HIV.

HIV AND AIDS STATISTICS

The Centers for Disease Control estimate that 1 million Americans are infected with HIV. Around the world an estimated 12 million people are infected. Because of the lengthy incubation period (7 to 8 years to develop AIDS) about 20% of the AIDS patients today are believed to have been infected as teenagers.

AIDS cases among adolescents in the United States increased 77% in the two years since 1991, and AIDS is now the sixth leading cause of death among all 15-24 year olds. According to World Health Organization, half of all persons with AIDS — 6 million of 12 million people worldwide — were infected with HIV when they were 15-24.

By the end of 1992, 253,448 AIDS cases had been diagnosed in the United States, and 171,980 had died from the diseases caused by HIV. The number of deaths is projected to double in 3 years. Most of the people who die are in the 20- to 45-year-old age group. By the year 2,000, deaths from HIV infection are expected to become the third leading cause of death, behind cardiovascular disease and cancer.

Approximately 66% of all AIDS cases in the United States have occurred in gay or bisexual men. AIDS among heterosexuals, nonetheless, is on the rise (see Figure 14.2). In fact, HIV is now spreading at a faster rate among heterosexuals. Many heterosexuals practice unprotected sex because they don't believe it can happen to their segment of the population. HIV is an epidemic that does not discriminate by sexual orientation. Worldwide, about 75% of the AIDS cases have been reported in heterosexuals.

A fighting spirit can apparently make a difference even in disease situations as serious as AIDS. The

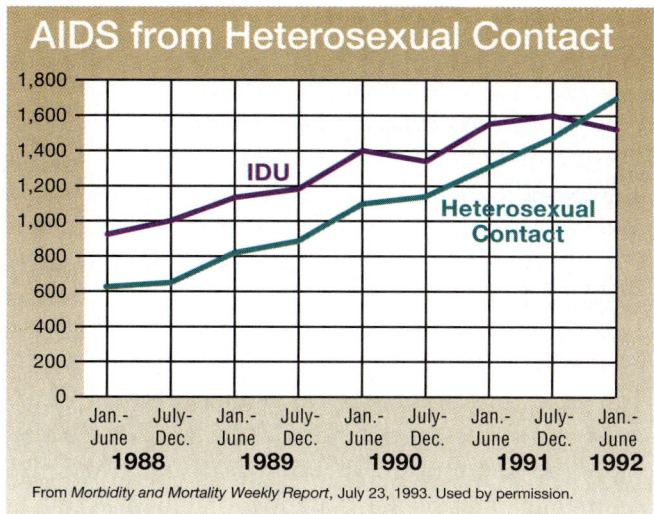

FIGURE 14.2 ▼ AIDS cases among U.S. women attributed to injecting drug use (IDU) and heterosexual contact, by half-year of diagnosis, 1988–1992.

message that AIDS patients usually get is one of giving up: as one researcher put it, "All that is emphasized to AIDS patients is that it is 100% fatal. Death, death, death." When someone with a powerful fighting spirit gets infected, the prognosis may be better.

HIV TESTING

A person can be tested for HIV in several ways. You may look up your local Public Health Department or AIDS Information Service (or related names) in the phone book. Testing is usually free of charge, and the results are kept confidential. Many states also conduct anonymous testing. Your name is never recorded. You can call several toll-free hotlines for more information on anonymous testing, treatment programs, support services, HIV and AIDS information, and STDs in general. All information discussed during a phone call to these hotlines is kept strictly confidential. The numbers to call are:

National AIDS Hotline: 1-800-342-AIDS or La Linea Nacional de SIDA: 1-800-344-SIDA, for Spanish speaking people.

STD Hotline: 1-800-227-8922.

National Institute on Drug Abuse (NIDA) Information and Treatment Referral: 1-800-622-HELP or 1-800-66-AYUDA for Spanish speaking only. NIDA also provides information on drug abuse and addictive behavior.

As with any other serious illness, AIDS patients deserve respect, understanding, and support. Refection and discrimination are traits of immature, hateful, and ignorant people. Education, knowledge, and responsible behaviors are the best ways to minimize fear and discrimination.

HIV TREATMENT

Even though several drugs are being tested to treat and slow down the disease process, AIDS has no known cure. Approximately 30 different approaches to an AIDS vaccine are being explored, and two have been approved for testing in humans. The best advice at this point is to take a preventive approach.

Although HIV has no cure, medications are available that allow HIV-infected patients to live longer. The sooner treatment is initiated following infection, the better are the chances for delaying the onset of AIDS.

Developing a vaccine to prevent HIV infection or AIDS seems highly unlikely in the next few years. People should not expect a medical breakthrough. Treatment modalities, however, should continue to improve and allow HIV-infected persons and AIDS patients to live longer and more productive lives.

Presently, several AIDS clinical trials are available in the United States. These projects are co-sponsored by the Centers for Disease Control, the Food and Drug Administration, the National Institute of Allergy and Infectious Diseases, and the National Library of Medicine. The purpose of AIDS clinical trials is to evaluate experimental drugs and various therapies for people at all stages of HIV infection. Interested individuals can call 1-800-TRIALS-A. As with all HIV testing, calls are completely confidential. Eligibility to participate in an AIDS clinical trial varies, and all applicants are evaluated individually. By calling the telephone number given, an interested person will receive information on the purpose and location of the trials (studies) that are open, eligibility requirements and exclusion criteria, and names and telephone numbers of contact persons.

HIV infections with HIV are rising nearly four times as fast in women as in men. While AIDS among men rose 2.5% between 1991 and 1992, the increase among women during the same period was 9.8%. Among adults, men with AIDS outnumber women about 8 to 1; in adolescents, the ratio is less than 3 men to 1 woman.

"Although in the United States, women currently represent a relatively small percentage of persons with HIV, they are the most rapidly growing segment of the HIV-infected population in this country," says Janet Arrowsmith-Lowe of the Center for Drug Evaluation and Research.

An estimated 18,500 healthy American youngsters were left motherless by AIDS by the end of 1991. Although black and hispanic women comprise 21% of the country's female population, they account for 74% of women diagnosed with AIDS.

Most women who now have AIDS became infected with HIV by injecting illegal drugs, but the rate of infection through sexual transmission has been rising dramatically. According to the CDC, cases diagnosed in 1992 marked the first time since the start of the epidemic that more women were infected through sex (50%) than through drug use (44%).

CDC reports, "Many women in the United States are unaware they are at risk for HIV infection, and HIV-infected women often remain undiagnosed until the onset of AIDS or until a perinatally infected child [infected before or during birth] becomes ill."

Myths About AIDS

You've probably heard one or more of these statements, but they're all untrue:
- You can get AIDS by donating blood.
- You can get AIDS through casual contact, such as shaking hands with or hugging an infected person.
- You can catch AIDS if an infected person coughs or sneezes on you.
- You can get AIDS from a mosquito.
- AIDS could spread rapidly through the general population.
- If you're not gay and don't shoot drugs, you're safe.
- Infected women can't transmit AIDS.
- If you don't have symptoms, you're not contagious.
- If you're HIV-positive, you'll know it from the symptoms.
- If you test positive for HIV, you have AIDS.
- Abstinence is the only way to protect yourself against AIDS.

ECONOMIC IMPACT OF HIV AND AIDS

Federal government spending for AIDS-related projects gradually increased to more than $900 million between 1982 and 1988. Costs continued to escalate to $1.3 billion in 1989, to $4.3 billion in 1992, and are expected to be in excess of $10.4 billion in 1994.

As of 1993, the annual U.S. health care cost to care for an HIV-positive individual who had not reached the AIDS stage was approximately $5,150. The yearly cost to treat an individual who had developed AIDS was about $32,000. The average cost from the onset of AIDS until death was $85,333. Assuming an incubation period of 7 years and an additional 3 years of AIDS, the direct treatment costs per person would average $121,383. This represents more than $30.5 billion to treat the 253,448 AIDS cases reported as of December 1992.

If the estimated 1 million people infected with HIV in the United State develop AIDS, direct health care costs for the disease will equal $121.383 billion. To place this figure in perspective, a person would have to spend $1 million per day for the next 332.5 years to spend the $121.382 billion.

Every American will help pay for these costs through taxes and a more expensive health care system. In the words of Dr. Russell Centanni, Professor of Biology at Boise State University: "Rather sobering for a preventable disease."

GUIDELINES FOR PREVENTING SEXUALLY TRANSMITTED DISEASES

Figure 14.3 graphically shows the risks identified with various STDs, by gender. With all the grim news about STDs, there is also some good news: You can do things to prevent their spread, and take precautions to keep yourself from becoming a victim.

The facts are in: The best prevention technique is a mutually monogamous sexual relationship, one in which two people have sexual relationships only with each other. That one behavior, says Dr. James Mason, director of the Centers for Disease Control in Atlanta, will remove you almost completely from any risk for developing an STD.

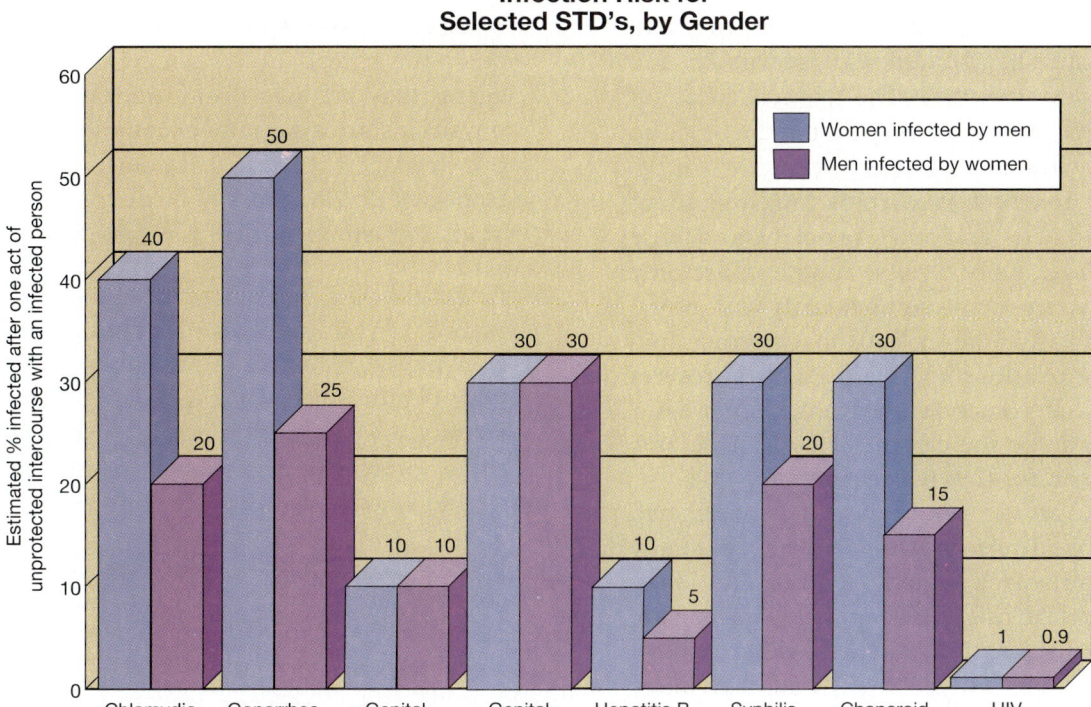

FIGURE 14.3 ▼ Infection risk for selected STDs, by gender.
From *Health & Sexuality* 2(2):3, 1991. Used by permission.

Unfortunately, in today's society it is becoming much more difficult to know at what point you can truly trust a person. You may be led to believe you are in a monogamous relationship when your partner actually: (a) may be cheating on you and gets infected, (b) ends up having a one night stand with someone who is infected, (c) got the virus several years ago before the present relationship and still doesn't know of the infection, (d) may not be honest with you and chooses not to tell you about the infection, or (e) is shooting up drugs and becomes infected. In any of these cases, HIV can be passed on to you.

Because your future and your life are at stake, and because you may never know if your partner is infected, you should give serious and careful consideration to postponing sex until you believe you have found a lifetime monogamous relationship. In doing so, you will not have to live with the fear of catching HIV or other STDs or deal with an unplanned pregnancy.

As strange as this may seem to some, many people postpone sexual activity until they are married. This is the best guarantee against HIV. Young people should understand that married life will provide plenty of time for fulfilling and rewarding sex.

If you choose to delay sex, do not let peers pressure you into having sex. Some people would have you believe you are not a real man or woman if you don't have sex. Manhood and womanhood are not proven during sexual intercourse but, instead, through mature, responsible, and healthy choices.

Other people lead you to believe that love doesn't exist without sex. Sex in the early stages of a relationship is not the product of love but is simply the fulfillment of a physical, and often selfish, drive. A loving relationship develops over a long time with mutual respect for each other.

Teenagers are especially susceptible to peer pressure leading to premature sexual intercourse. The result: more than a million teen pregnancies per year and a 43% pregnancy rate for all girls at least once as a teenager. Too many young people wish they had postponed sex and silently admire those who do. Sex lasts only a few minutes. The consequences of irresponsible sex, however, may last a lifetime. In some cases, they are fatal.

Then there are those who enjoy bragging about their sexual conquests and mock people who choose to wait. In essence, many of these conquests are only fantasies in an attempt to gain popularity with peers.

Sexual promiscuity never leads to a trusting, loving, and lasting relationship. Mature people respect others' choices. If someone does not respect your choice to wait, he or she certainly does not deserve your friendship or, for that matter, anything else.

There is no greater sex than that between two loving and responsible individuals who mutually trust and admire each other. Contrary to many beliefs, these relationships are possible. They are built upon unselfish attitudes and behaviors.

As you look around, you will find that many believe the same way you do. Seek them out and build your friendships and future around people who respect you for what you are and what you believe. You don't have to compromise your choices or values. In the end you will reap the greater rewards of a choice and lasting relationship, free of AIDS and other STDs.

What about those who do not have — or do not desire — a monogamous relationship? Some other things can be done to lower, but never completely eliminate, the risk for developing STDs in general:

1. Know your partner. The days are gone when anonymous bathhouse or singles-bars sex is safe. Limit your sexual relationships, and always practice safer sex.

2. Limit the number of sexual partners you have. Having one partner lowers your chance of infection. The more partners you have, the greater is your chance for infection.

3. If you are sexually promiscuous, consider having periodic physical checkups. Getting exposed to an STD by a person who does not have any symptoms and who is unaware of the infection is easy. Sexually promiscuous men and women between ages 15 and 35 are considered to be in a particularly high-risk group for developing STDs.

4. Use "barrier" methods of contraception to help prevent the disease from spreading. Condoms, diaphragms, the contraceptive sponge, and spermicidal suppositories, foams, and jellies can all deter the spread of certain STDs. Spermicidal agents may act as a disinfectant as well. Many physicians are especially encouraging promiscuous teenagers to use condoms. Traditionally, teenagers do not use any birth-control methods at all and remain at high risk for STDs.

5. Be responsible enough to abstain from sexual activity if you know you have an infection. Go to a physician or clinic for treatment, and ask your doctor when you can safely resume sexual activity. Abstain until it is safe. Just as you want to be protected in a sexual relationship, you should want to protect your partner as well.

6. Urinate immediately following sexual intercourse. This is not a reliable method, but it may help (especially men) flush bacteria and viruses from the urinary tract.

7. Wash thoroughly immediately after sexual activity. Washing with hot, soapy water will not guarantee safety against STDs, but it can prevent you from spreading certain germs on your fingers and may wash away bacteria and viruses that have not yet entered the body.

8. If you suspect your partner is infected with a STD, ask. He or she may not even be aware of the infection, so look for signs of infection, such as sores, redness, inflammations, a rash, growths, warts, or discharge. If you are unsure, abstain.

9. Consider abstaining from sexual relations if you have any kind of an illness or disease, even a common cold. Any kind of illness makes you more susceptible to other illnesses, and lower immunity can make you extra vulnerable to STDs. The same holds true for times when you are under extreme stress, when you are fatigued, and when you are overworked. Drugs and alcohol also can lower your resistance to disease.

10. Wear loose-fitting clothes made from natural fibers. Tight-fitting clothing made from synthetic fibers (especially underwear and nylon pantyhose) can create conditions that encourage the growth of bacteria and actually can aggravate STDs.

HIV RISK REDUCTION

Based upon recommendations from health experts, observing the following precautions can reduce your risk for getting HIV, and subsequently AIDS:

1. Postpone sex until you and your uninfected partner are prepared to enter into a lifetime monogamous relationship. In his book, *What You Can Do to Avoid AIDS*, Earvin "Magic" Johnson stated:[8]

    But if I had known what I do now when I was younger, I would have postponed sex as long as I could, and I would have tried to have it the first time with somebody that I knew I wanted to spend the rest of my life with. I certainly want my children to postpone sex. Now the rest of my life may be a lot shorter than I thought it was going to be, and I may not be around to see my son, Andre, grow up and to see what happens to the baby Cookie and I are having in the summer of '92, and, of course, I may not have the long life I want with Cookie.

2. Unless you are in a monogamous relationship and you know your partner is not infected (which you may never know for sure), practice safer sex every single time you have sex. This means you should use a latex condom from start to finish for each sexual act. If you think your partner should use a condom but refuses to do so, say no to sex with that person.

    Many experts believe greater protection can be obtained by placing a small amount of the spermicide nonoxynol–9 inside the condom at its tip and then lubricating the outside with additional spermicide. Nonoxynol–9 is used to kill the man's sperm for birth control purposes. In test tubes, it has been shown to kill STD germs and HIV. This spermicide, however, should not be used in place of a condom because it will not offer the same protection as the condom does by itself.

3. Avoid having multiple and anonymous sexual partners. Keep in mind that anyone you have sex with could be infected with HIV.

4. Don't have sexual contact with anyone who does not practice safer sex.

5. Avoid sexual contact with anyone who has had sex with people at risk for getting HIV, even if they are now practicing safer sex.

6. Don't have sex with prostitutes.

7. If you do have sex with someone who might be infected with HIV or whose history is unknown to you, avoid exchange of body fluids.

8. Don't share toothbrushes, razors, or other implements that could become contaminated with blood with anyone who is, or who might be, infected with HIV.

9. Be cautious regarding procedures such as acupuncture, tattooing, and ear piercing, in which needles or other nonsterile instruments may be used again and again to pierce the skin or mucous membranes. These procedures are safe if proper sterilization methods or disposable needles are followed. Before undergoing the procedure, ask what precautions are being taken.

10. If you are planning to undergo artificial insemination, insist on frozen sperm obtained from a laboratory that tests all donors for infection with HIV. Donors should be tested twice before accepting the sperm — once at the time of donation and again a few months later.

11. If you know you will be having surgery in the near future, and if you are able, consider donating blood for your own use. This will eliminate completely the already small risk of contracting HIV through a blood transfusion. It also will eliminate the more substantial risk for contracting other blood-borne diseases, such as hepatitis, from a transfusion.

Avoiding risky behaviors that destroy quality of life and life itself are critical components of a healthy lifestyle. Learning the facts so you can make responsible choices can protect you and those around you from startling and unexpected conditions. Using alcohol in moderation (or not at all), avoiding substance abuse, and preventing sexually transmitted diseases are key elements in averting both physical and psychological damage.

Comparing Selected Sexually Transmitted Diseases

Disease	Symptoms and Outlook	Complications	Diagnosis and Treatment
Syphilis Spirochete infection. Curable in early stages. Affects mainly those in their 20s. Transmitted by oral, genital, anal contact. After a decline, case numbers rising again in North America, mainly related to drug use or exchange of sex for drugs.	Painless sore (chancre) appears 3-6 weeks after infection on genitals, mouth or rectal area, most obvious in men, hardly noticed if vaginal. Heals without scarring. About 4-10 weeks later, 2nd stage: fever, rash, which disappears but may reappear.	If untreated, chronic, occasionally fatal. Third stage appears up to 30 years later with brain and spinal cord damage, blindness, insanity. Untreated, can cause miscarriage and birth defects; infants of infected mother may be born with syphilis (congenital syphilis).	Even if no symptoms, can diagnose by simple blood test; test results usually positive by time chancre (ulcer) appears. Antibiotics, taken as prescribed, a dependable cure in early stages.
Gonorrhea ("clap") Bacterial infection, transmitted by oral, vaginal, or anal sex. Prevalent in young women, teens. Untreated, can result in pelvic inflammatory disease (PID) and infertility. Up to half of women and men have no symptoms.	Symptoms (if any) within 7 days of contact: painful urination, thick vaginal or penile discharge, bleeding between periods, sore throat (if contracted via oral sex), rectal pain or discharge (if through anal sex).	May lead to tubal scarring, PID, ectopic pregnancy (outside womb, dangerous for mother). Can cause permanent sterility in both sexes. Eye infection and possible blindness in infected newborns.	Diagnosed by smear and lab culture. Antibiotics a reliable cure, but some strains now resistant to standard antibiotics (e.g., penicillin) so require *cefixime, ceftriaxone* or other new drugs.
Herpes Viral infection due to Herpes virus types I or II. Spreads via oral, vaginal, or anal sex, kissing. Can spread silently, via asymptomatic people. Most easily transmitted by direct contact with active sores or genital secretions.	Symptoms within 10 days: slight fever, tingling, shooting pains, swollen lymph glands, then painful blisters, anywhere on genitals — mainly penis, vulva, or anal areas. Subsides without treatment, but can recur. First outbreak usually worst, but sometimes unnoticed.	Virus remains permanently in nerves, stays dormant for months or years. Newborns may get herpes during birth, resulting in central nervous system damage or death. Caesarean delivery may be advised for babies of infected mothers.	Diagnosis from blisters (scraping or culture). *Acyclovir* tablets, not a cure, ease symptoms and reduce length of attack and its severity. Herpes support groups helpful in combatting psychological problems.
Chlamydia Bacterial infection, very common, in teens, 60%-80% without symptoms. Spreads via anal, vaginal, or oral sex with infected partners. Often occurs together with gonorrhea.	Like gonorrhea: painful urination, vaginal or penile discharge, abdominal pain, genital itching. But often mild, unnoticed in carriers, can disappear without treatment.	In women, leading cause of PID, ectopic pregnancy, infertility. In men, can produce urinary tract diseases and *prostatitis*. Babies of infected mothers prone to eye infections, pneumonia.	Diagnosed by culture or other tests. Antibiotic treatment a reliable cure (if caught early).
Genital Warts Caused by human papilloma-virus (HPV). Highly contagious, spread by intimate bodily contact, especially sexual activity, often accompanies other STDs.	Warts — tiny flat growths on and around genitals — usually itchy, pinkish, flat, irregularly surfaced, may increase in size. Often undetectable in women in vagina or on cervix, except by physician.	Certain HPV strains linked to cervical cancer in women (and possibly penile cancer in men). Infants born to mothers with HPV may develop warts.	Removal advised — chemically, by freezing, or with lasers. Women should have regular Pap smears to detect HPV infection and early cervical cancer changes.
Hepatitis B Virus passed on via blood, semen, vaginal secretions, saliva, needles, razors, toothbrushes. Can go from mother to infant at birth. Groups most at risk: those practicing anal sex, those with many partners, injection drug users, babies of infected mothers.	Usually subclinical with few or no symptoms. Possibly flulike malaise, fever, fatigue typically lasting 6 weeks, perhaps jaundice/skin and eye-white yellowing. May linger in body unnoticed.	60%-90% of infected children and 10% infected as adults become lifelong carriers, at risk of cirrhosis and liver cancer. Unsuspecting carriers can infect others. Fulminant, rapidly fatal form in one per 100 cases.	Detected by blood tests for viral markers. No cure. *Effective* safe vaccine recommended for all at risk — especially healthcare workers and those living with or close to known hepatitis B carriers.

Reprinted with permission from Health News. Health News is a bimonthly publication of the University of Toronto Faculty of Medicine. Subscriptions and back issues can be obtained by writing to *Health News*, 109 Vanderhoof Ave., Suite 205, Toronto, Ontario M4G 2H7 or by calling (416) 696-8818.

APPENDIX A

Nutritive Value of Selected Foods

Reprinted from *Principles & Labs For Physical Fitness and Wellness,* 3rd ed. Werne
W. K. Hoeger and Sharon A. Hoeger, Morton Publishing Company, 1994.

Code	Food	Amount	Weight gm	Calories	Protein gm	Fat gm	Sat. Fat gm	Cholesterol mg	Carbohydrate gm	Calcium mg	Iron mg	Sodium mg	Vit A I.U.	Thiamin (Vit B$_1$) mg	Riboflavin (Vit B$_2$) mg	Niacin mg	Vit C mg
1.	Almond Joy, candy bar	1.5 oz.	42	227	2.5	12	10.2	0	28	3	1.2	0	0	0.00	0.00	0.0	0
2.	Almonds, shelled	1/4 c	36	213	6.6	19	1.4	0	9	83	1.7	2	0	0.09	0.33	1.3	0
3.	Apple, raw, unpared	1 med	150	80	0.3	1	0.0	0	20	10	0.4	1	120	0.04	0.03	0.1	6
4.	Apple juice, canned or bottled	1/2 c	124	59	0.1	0	0.0	0	15	8	0.7	1	0	0.01	0.03	0.1	1
5.	Apple Pie, McDonald's	1	307	260	2	15	10.0	6	30	0	0.48	240	0	0.06	0	0	12
6.	Applesauce, canned, sweetened	1/2 c	128	116	0.3	0	0.0	0	31	5	0.7	3	50	0.02	0.01	0.0	2
7.	Apricots, canned, heavy syrup liq.	3 halves; 1¾ tbsp	85	73	0.5	0	0.0	0	19	9	0.3	1	1,480	0.02	0.02	0.3	3
8.	Apricots, dried, sulfured, uncooked	10 med halves	35	91	1.8	0	0.0	0	23	23	1.9	9	3,820	0.00	0.06	1.2	4
9.	Apricots, raw	3 (12 per lb)	114	55	1.1	0	0.0	0	14	18	0.5	1	2,890	0.06	0.04	0.6	11
10.	Arby Q, Arby's	1	190	389	18	15	5.5	29	48	84	6.1	1,268	0	0.27	0.41	9.2	0
11.	Arby Sauce, Arby's	.5 oz.	14	15	0	0	0.0	0	3	0	0.2	113	0	0.00	0.00	0.0	0
12.	Asparagus, cooked green spears	4 med	60	12	1.3	0	0.0	0	2	13	0.4	1	540	0.10	0.11	0.8	16
13.	Avocado, raw	1/2 med	120	185	2.4	19	3.2	0	7	11	0.6	4	310	0.12	0.22	1.7	15
14.	Bacon, cooked, drained	2 slices	15	86	3.8	8	2.7	30	1	2	0.5	153	0	0.08	0.05	0.8	0
15.	Bacon, lettuce, tomato sandwich	1	130	327	11.6	19	4.7	21	31	84	2.5	661	426	0.42	0.28	4.1	12
16.	Bagel	1 3½ in.	68	180	7.0	1	0.2	0	35	20	2.1	124	0	0.26	0.20	2.4	0
17.	Banana, raw	1 sm (7¾")	140	81	1.0	0	0.0	0	21	8	0.7	1	180	0.05	0.06	0.7	10
18.	Banana, nut bread	1 slice	50	169	3.0	8	1.5	33	22	18	0.9	172	49	0.09	0.09	0.8	1
19.	BBQ Sauce, McDonald's	1.12 oz.	32	50	0	0.6	0.2	0	12	0	0.0	350	200	0.00	0.00	0	2.4
20.	Beans, green snap, cooked	1/2 c	65	16	1.0	0	0.0	0	3	32	0.4	4	340	0.05	0.06	0.3	8
21.	Beans, lentils	1/4 c	50	53	3.9	0	0.0	0	10	12	1.0	0	10	0.03	0.04	0.4	0
22.	Beans, lima (Fordhook), froz., cooked	1/2 c	85	84	6.0	0	0.0	0	17	40	2.1	1	240	0.15	0.08	1.1	15
23.	Beans, red kidney, cooked	1 c	185	218	14.4	1	0.0	0	40	70	4.4	6	10	0.20	0.11	1.3	0
24.	Beans, refried	1/2 c	145	148	9.0	1	0.2	0	25	71	2.6	614	0	0.07	0.08	0.7	9
25.	Bean sprouts, mung, raw	1/2 c	52	18	2.0	0	0.0	0	4	10	0.7	3	10	0.07	0.07	0.4	10
26.	Beef, chuck, cooked,	3 oz.	85	212	25.0	12	7.8	80	0	11	3.1	43	20	0.05	0.19	3.8	0
27.	Beef, corned, canned	3 oz.	85	163	21.0	10	8.0	70	0	22	5.0	802	0	0.02	0.27	3.9	0
28.	Beef, ground, lean	3 oz.	85	186	23.3	10	5.0	81	0	10	3.0	57	20	0.08	0.20	5.1	0
29.	Beef, Lite Roast Deluxe, Arby's	1	182	294	18	10	3.5	42	33	156	3.0	826	200	0.27	0.52	8.4	8
30.	Beef, meatloaf	1 piece	111	246	20.0	15	6.1	125	6	37	2.4	434	181	0.08	0.23	4.1	1
31.	Beef N' Cheddar, Arby's	1	194	508	25	27	7.7	52	43	180	4.1	1,166	0	0.42	0.67	9.8	1
32.	Beef, round steak, cooked, trimmed	3 oz.	85	222	24.3	13	6.0	77	0	10	3.0	60	20	0.07	0.20	4.8	0
33.	Beef, rump roast	3 oz.	85	177	24.7	9	4.0	80	0	10	3.1	61	10	0.06	0.19	4.4	0
34.	Beef, sirloin, cooked	3 oz.	85	329	19.6	27	13.0	77	0	9	2.5	48	50	0.05	0.15	4.0	0
35.	Beef, T-bone steak	3 oz.	85	403	16.7	37	15.6	66	0	7	2.2	40	23	0.07	0.14	3.5	0
36.	Beef, thin, sliced	3 oz.	85	105	18.5	3	1.4	36	0	11	1.8	1,409	0	0.07	0.16	4.5	0
37.	Beer	12 fl. oz.	360	151	1.1	0	0.0	0	14	18	0.0	25	0	0.01	0.11	2.2	0
38.	Beer, light	12 fl. oz.	354	96	0.7	0	0.0	0	4	17	0.1	10	0	0.03	0.10	1.3	0
39.	Beets, red, canned, drained	1/2 c	80	32	0.8	0	0.0	0	8	15	0.6	164	15	0.01	0.02	0.1	2
40.	Beet greens, cooked	1/2 c	73	13	1.3	0	0.0	0	2	72	1.4	55	3,700	0.05	0.11	0.2	11
41.	Biscuits, baking powder	1 med	35	114	2.5	6	1.1	0	18	60	0.8	272	0	0.06	0.06	0.7	0
42.	Blueberries, fresh cultivated	1/2 c	73	45	0.5	0	0.0	0	11	10	0.8	1	75	0.02	0.05	0.4	10

APPENDIX A ▼ Nutritive Value of Selected Foods

#	Food	Serving	g	Cal													
43.	Bologna	1 slice (1 oz.)	28	86	3.4	8	3.0	15	0	2	0.5	369	0	0.05	0.06	0.7	0
44.	Bologna, turkey	2 slices	57	113	7.8	9	3.0	56	1	47	0.9	498	0	0.03	0.09	2.1	0
45.	Bouillon, broth	1 cube	4	5	0.8	0	0.0	0	0	0	0.0	960	0	0.00	0.00	0.0	0
46.	Brandy	1 oz.	28	69	0.0	6	0.1	0	11	0	0.0	1	0	0.00	0.00	0.0	1
47.	Bread, Corn	1 slice	78	161	5.8	6	0.1	0	23	94	0.9	490	120	0.10	0.15	0.5	0
48.	Bread, Cracked wheat	1 slice	25	65	2.3	1	0.2	0	12	16	0.7	106	0	0.10	0.10	0.8	0
49.	Bread, French enriched	1 slice	35	102	3.2	1	0.2	0	19	15	0.8	203	0	0.10	0.08	0.9	0
50.	Bread, Oatmeal	1 slice	25	65	2.1	1	0.2	0	12	15	0.7	124	0	0.12	0.07	0.9	0
51.	Bread, Pita pocket	1 piece	60	165	6.2	1	0.1	0	33	49	1.5	339	0	0.27	0.13	2.3	0
52.	Bread, Pumpernickel	1 slice	32	80	2.9	1	0.2	0	15	23	0.9	277	0	0.11	0.17	1.1	0
53.	Bread, Rye (American)	1 slice	25	61	2.3	0	0.1	0	13	19	0.4	139	0	0.05	0.02	0.4	0
54.	Bread, white enriched	1 slice	25	68	2.2	1	0.2	0	13	21	0.6	127	0	0.06	0.05	0.6	0
55.	Bread, whole wheat	1 slice	25	61	2.6	1	0.6	0	12	25	0.8	132	0	0.06	0.03	0.7	0
56.	Broccoli, cooked drained	1 sm stalk	140	36	4.3	0	0.0	0	6	123	1.1	14	3,500	0.13	0.28	1.1	126
57.	Broccoli, raw	1 sm stalk	114	38	4.1	0	0.0	0	7	117	1.3	17	2,835	0.10	0.23	0.9	125
58.	Brownies, with nuts	1	20	95	1.3	6	2.3	18	11	9	0.4	51	20	0.05	0.05	0.3	0
59.	Brussels sprouts, froz., cooked, drained	1/2 c	78	28	3.2	0	0.0	0	5	25	0.8	8	405	0.06	0.11	0.5	63
60.	Bulgur, wheat	1 c	135	227	8.4	1	0.0	0	47	27	1.8	809	0	0.07	0.04	3.2	0
61.	Burrito, bean	1	166	307	12.5	9.5	3.6	14	45	173	2.4	983	283	0.15	0.22	2.3	5
62.	Burrito, combination, Taco Bell	1	175	404	21.0	16	0.0	0	43	91	3.7	300	1,666	0.34	0.31	4.6	15
63.	Butter	1 tsp	5	36	0.0	4	0.4	12	0	1	0.0	46	160	0.00	0.00	0.0	0
64.	Buttermilk, cultured	1 c	245	88	8.8	0	1.3	5	12	296	0.1	319	10	0.10	0.44	0.2	2
65.	Cabbage, boiled, drained wedge	1/2 c	85	16	0.9	0	0.0	0	3	36	0.3	10	100	0.02	0.02	0.1	21
66.	Cabbage, raw chopped	1/2 c	45	11	0.6	0	0.0	0	3	22	0.2	9	60	0.03	0.03	0.2	21
67.	Cake, Angel food, plain	1 piece	60	161	4.3	0	0.0	0	36	5	0.1	170	0	0.01	0.08	0.1	0
68.	Cake, Carrot	1 piece	96	385	4.2	21	4.1	74	48	44	1.3	279	75	0.11	0.12	0.9	1
69.	Cake, Cheesecake	1 piece (3½")	85	257	4.6	16	9.0	150	24	48	0.4	189	216	0.03	0.11	0.4	4
70.	Cake, Chocolate, w/icing	1 piece	69	235	3.0	8	3.6	37	40	41	1.4	181	100	0.07	0.10	0.6	0
71.	Cake, Coffee	1 piece	72	230	4.5	7	2.5	47	38	44	1.2	310	120	0.14	0.15	1.3	0
72.	Cake, Devil's food, iced	1 piece	99	365	4.5	16	5.0	68	55	69	1.0	233	160	0.02	0.10	0.2	0
73.	Cake, Pound	1 piece	30	120	2.0	5	1.0	32	15	20	0.5	98	200	0.05	0.06	0.5	0
74.	Cake, White, choc. icing	1 piece	71	268	3.5	11	3.7	2	48	35	0.3	162	40	0.19	0.14	1.6	0
75.	Candy, hard	1 oz.	28	109	0.0	0	0.0	0	28	6	0.5	9	0	0.00	0.00	0.0	0
76.	Cantaloupe	1/4 melon 5" diam.	239	35	2.0	0	0.0	0	10	20	0.8	17	4,620	0.06	0.04	0.6	45
77.	Caramel (candy, plain or choc.)	1 oz.	28	113	1.1	3	1.6	0	22	42	0.4	64	0	0.01	0.05	0.1	0
78.	Carrots, cooked, drained	1/2 c	73	23	0.7	0	0.0	0	5	24	0.5	10	7,615	0.04	0.04	0.4	5
79.	Carrots, raw	1 carrot 7½" long	81	30	0.8	0	0.0	0	7	27	0.5	34	7,930	0.04	0.04	0.4	6
80.	Cashew, roasted, unsalted	2 oz.	57	326	9.2	27	5.4	0	16	23	2.3	10	0	0.24	0.10	1.0	0
81.	Cauliflower, cooked, drained	1/2 c	63	14	1.5	0	0.0	0	3	13	0.5	6	40	0.06	0.05	0.4	35
82.	Celery, green, raw, long	1 outer stalk 8"	40	7	0.4	0	0.0	0	2	16	0.1	50	110	0.01	0.01	0.1	4
83.	Cereal, All-Bran	1/4 c	21	53	3.0	0	0.1	0	16	17	3.4	242	947	0.28	0.33	3.8	11
84.	Cereal, Alpha Bits	1 c	28	111	2.2	1	0.0	0	25	8	1.8	219	1,875	0.40	0.40	5.0	0
85.	Cereal, Bran	1/2 c	30	72	3.8	1	0.0	0	22	25	3.0	247	2,000	1.00	0.80	3.0	20
86.	Cereal, Cheerios	1 c	23	89	3.4	1	1.2	0	16	38	3.6	246	949	0.32	0.32	4.0	12
87.	Cereal, Corn Chex	1 c	28	111	2.0	0	0.1	0	25	3	1.8	271	75	0.40	0.07	5.0	15
88.	Cereal, Corn Flakes	1 c	25	97	2.0	0	0.0	0	21	3	0.6	251	180	0.29	0.55	2.9	9
89.	Cereal, Cream of Wheat	1 c	244	140	3.6	1	0.1	0	29	54	10.9	5	0	0.24	0.07	1.5	0
90.	Cereal, Frosted Mini-Wheats	4 biscuits	31	111	3.2	0	0.0	0	26	10	2.0	9	2,050	0.40	0.50	5.5	16

Code	Food	Amount	Weight gm	Calories	Protein gm	Fat gm	Sat. Fat gm	Cholesterol mg	Carbohydrate gm	Calcium mg	Iron mg	Sodium mg	Vit A I.U.	Thiamin (Vit B₁) mg	Riboflavin (Vit B₂) mg	Niacin mg	Vit C mg
91.	Cereal, Fruit & Fibre w/dates	1 c	56	180	6.0	2	0.3	0	42	20	9.0	340	3,780	0.75	0.85	10.0	0
92.	Cereal, Granola, Nature Valley	1/2 c	57	252	5.8	10	7.0	0	38	36	1.9	116	41	0.20	0.10	0.4	0
93.	Cereal, Grape Nuts	1/2 c	57	202	6.6	0	0.0	0	47	22	2.5	394	3,815	0.80	0.80	10.0	0
94.	Cereal, Life	1 c	44	162	8.1	1	0.1	0	32	154	11.6	229	0	0.95	1.00	11.6	0
95.	Cereal, Nutri-Grain Wheat	1 c	44	158	3.8	1	0.1	0	37	12	1.2	299	2,915	0.60	0.70	7.7	23
96.	Cereal, Oatmeal, quick, cooked	1/2 c	120	66	2.4	1	0.2	0	12	11	0.7	262	0	0.10	0.03	0.1	0
97.	Cereal, Raisin Bran	1 c	49	160	4.0	1	0.2	0	40	25	24.0	293	2,500	0.51	0.57	6.7	0
98.	Cereal, Rice Krispies	3/4 c	22	85	1.4	0	0.0	0	19	3	1.4	255	971	0.30	0.30	3.8	11
99.	Cereal, Shredded Wheat	1 c	19	65	2.1	0	0.0	0	11	8	0.6	1	0	0.06	0.05	0.9	0
100.	Cereal, Special K	1 c	21	83	4.2	0	0.0	0	16	6	3.4	199	1,430	0.30	0.30	3.8	11
101.	Cereal, Sugar Corn Pops	1 c	28	108	1.4	0	0.0	0	26	1	1.8	103	1,875	0.40	0.40	5.0	15
102.	Cereal, Sugar Frosted Flakes	1 c	35	133	1.8	0	0.0	0	32	1	2.2	284	2,315	0.50	0.50	6.2	19
103.	Cereal, Sugar Smacks	1 c	37	141	2.7	1	0.1	0	32	4	2.4	100	2,500	0.49	0.57	6.7	20
104.	Cereal, Total	1 c	33	116	3.3	1	0.1	0	26	56	21.0	409	8,845	1.70	2.00	23.3	70
105.	Cereal, Wheat Chex	1 c	46	169	4.5	1	0.2	0	38	18	7.3	308	0	0.60	0.17	8.1	24
106.	Cereal, whole wheat, cooked	1/2 c	123	55	2.2	0	0.0	0	12	9	0.06	260	0	0.08	0.03	0.8	0
107.	Cereal, whole wheat flakes, ready-to-eat	1 c	30	106	3.1	1	0.0	0	24	12	2.0	310	1,410	0.35	0.42	3.5	11
108.	Cereal, 40% Bran Flakes	1 c	39	125	4.9	1	0.1	0	31	19	11.2	363	2,610	0.51	0.59	6.9	0
109.	Cereal, 100% Bran	1/2 c	33	89	4.2	2	0.3	0	24	23	4.1	229	0	0.80	0.90	10.4	31
110.	Champagne	4 oz.	113	87	0.2	0	0.1	0	2	6	0.4	7	0	0.00	0.01	0.1	0
111.	Cheese, American	1 oz. slice	28	100	6.0	8	5.6	27	0	188	0.1	307	343	0.01	0.10	0.0	0
112.	Cheese, Bleu	1 oz.	28	100	6.0	8	5.3	25	1	89	0.1	510	204	0.01	0.11	0.3	0
113.	Cheese, Cheddar	1 oz.	28	114	7.0	9	6.0	30	0	204	0.2	171	300	0.01	0.11	0.0	0
114.	Cheese, Cottage, 2%	1/2 c	113	103	15.5	2	1.4	10	4	78	0.2	459	79	0.03	0.21	0.2	0
115.	Cheese, Cottage, creamed	1/2 c	105	112	14.0	5	6.4	15	3	99	0.3	241	180	0.03	0.26	0.1	0
116.	Cheese, Creamed	1 oz.	28	99	6.0	8	3.0	31	1	167	0.3	71	320	0.02	0.14	0.0	0
117.	Cheese, Feta	1 oz.	28	75	4.5	6	4.2	25	1	140	0.2	316	180	0.04	0.23	0.3	0
118.	Cheese, Monterey jack	1 oz.	28	106	6.9	9	5.4	26	0	212	0.2	152	405	0.00	0.11	0.0	0
119.	Cheese, Mozzarella, skim	1 oz.	28	80	7.6	5	3.1	15	1	207	0.1	150	216	0.01	0.10	0.0	0
120.	Cheese, Parmesan	1 tbsp	5	23	2.1	2	1.0	4	0	69	0.1	93	45	0.00	0.02	0.0	0
121.	Cheese, Ricotta, part skim	1 oz.	28	39	3.2	2	1.4	9	1	77	0.1	35	160	0.01	0.05	0.0	0
122.	Cheese, Souffle	1 portion	110	240	10.9	19	9.5	189	7	221	1.1	400	880	0.06	0.26	0.2	0
123.	Cheese, Swiss	1 oz.	28	107	8.0	8	5.0	26	1	272	0.1	74	360	0.01	0.10	0.0	0
124.	Cheese puffs, Cheetos	1 oz.	28	158	2.2	10	4.8	5	14	17	0.4	344	130	0.01	0.03	0.2	0
125.	Cheeseburger, McDonald's	1 oz.	115	321	15.2	16	6.7	40	29	170	2.9	736	353	0.30	0.24	4.4	2
126.	Cherries	10	75	47	0.9	0	0.0	0	12	15	0.3	8	450	0.20	0.24	1.6	41
127.	Chicken, BK Broiler sandwich, Burger King	1 sandwich	168	379	24.0	18	3.0	53	31	48	2.3	764	350	0.42	0.22	9.2	5
128.	Chicken Breast Filet, Arby's	1	204	445	22	23.0	3.0	45	52	72	1.9	958	0	0.23	0.58	9.0	5
129.	Chicken breast, roast w/skin	1	98	193	29.2	8	2.1	83	0	14	1.0	69	91	0.07	0.12	12.5	0
130.	Chicken chow mein	1 c	250	255	31.0	11	3.6	75	10	58	2.5	718	250	0.08	0.23	4.3	10
131.	Chicken club sandwich, Wendy's	1	220	520	30	25	6.0	75	44	120	9.6	980	100	0.60	0.45	16.0	9
132.	Chicken Cordon Bleu, Arby's	1	225	518	30	27	5.3	92	52	204	2.1	1,463	0	0.42	0.68	10.2	5
133.	Chicken, drumstick Kentucky Fried	1	54	136	14.0	8	2.2	73	2	20	0.9	320	30	0.04	0.12	2.7	0
134.	Chicken, drumstick, roasted	1	52	112	14.1	6	1.6	48	0	6	0.7	47	52	0.04	0.11	3.1	0

APPENDIX A ▾ Nutritive Value of Selected Foods

#	Food	Serving	Wt (g)	Cal	Prot	Fat	Sat Fat	Chol	Carb	Ca	Fe	Na	Vit A	Thia	Ribo	Niac	Vit C
135.	Chicken McNuggets	6	111	329	19.5	21	5.2	64	15	11	1.3	521	92	0.16	0.14	7.7	2
136.	Chicken Nuggets, Wendy's	6 pc.	94	280	14	20	5.0	50	12	48	0.48	600	0	0.09	0.11	6.0	0
137.	Chicken, patty sandwich	1	157	436	24.8	23	6.1	68	34	44	1.9	2,732	47	0.13	0.26	9.2	4
138.	Chicken, wing, Kentucky Fried	1	45	151	11.0	10	2.9	70	4	0	0.6	300	0	0.03	0.07	0.0	0
139.	Chicken, roast, light meat without skin	3 oz.	85	141	27.0	3	0.4	45	0	10	1.2	54	51	0.03	0.09	9.9	0
140.	Chicken, roast, dark meat without skin	3 oz.	85	149	24.0	5	0.8	50	0	11	1.5	54	127	0.06	0.19	4.7	0
141.	Chicken, Roast Deluxe, Arby's	1	195	276	24	7	1.7	33	33	156	1.9	777	200	0.44	0.80	9.4	7
142.	Chicken Sandwich, breaded Wendy's	1	208	450	26	20	4.0	60	44	120	9.6	740	100	0.45	0.36	14.0	6
143.	Chicken Sandwich, Grilled, Wendy's	1	177	290	24	7	1.0	60	35	120	2.4	670	100	0.38	0.27	10.0	6
144.	Chicken Sandwich, McChicken	1	187	415	19	19	9.0	50	39	180	1.8	830	100	0.90	0.18	9.0	2
145.	Chili con carne	1 c	255	339	19.1	16	5.8	28	31	82	4.3	1,354	150	0.08	0.18	3.3	8
146.	Chocolate fudge	1 oz.	28	115	0.6	3	2.1	1	21	22	0.3	54	0	0.01	0.03	0.1	0
147.	Chocolate, milk	1 oz.	28	147	2.0	9	3.6	5	16	65	0.3	27	80	0.02	0.10	0.1	0
148.	Chocolate, milk w/almonds	1 oz.	28	150	2.9	10	4.4	5	15	61	0.6	23	30	0.03	0.13	0.3	0
149.	Clam, canned, drained	3 oz.	85	83	13.0	2	0.2	50	2	46	3.5	750	93	0.01	0.09	0.9	9
150.	Cocoa, hot, with whole milk	1 c	250	218	9.1	9	6.1	33	26	298	0.8	123	318	0.10	0.44	0.4	2
151.	Cocoa, plain, dry	1 tbsp	5	14	0.9	1	0.0	0	3	7	0.6	0	0	0.01	0.02	0.1	0
152.	Coconut, shredded, packed	1/2 c	65	225	2.3	23	20.0	0	6	8	1.1	165	0	0.03	0.01	0.3	2
153.	Cod, batter fried	3.5 oz.	100	199	19.6	10	3.9	55	8	80	0.5	100	2	0.02	0.02	1.8	0
154.	Cod, cooked	3 oz.	85	144	24.3	4	1.5	60	0	27	0.9	63	150	0.06	0.09	2.7	0
155.	Cod, poached	3.5 oz.	100	94	20.9	1	0.3	60	0	29	0.5	110	2	0.08	0.08	3.0	0
156.	Coffee	3/4 cup	180	1	0.0	0	0.0	0	0	1	0.2	2	0	0.00	0.00	0.1	0
157.	Coleslaw	1 c	120	173	1.6	17	1.0	5	16	53	0.5	144	190	0.06	0.06	0.4	35
158.	Collards, leaves without stems, cooked, drained	1/2 c	95	32	3.4	1	2.0	0	5	178	0.8	28	7,410	0.01	0.19	1.2	72
159.	Cookies, Chocolate chip homemade	2 2¼" diam.	20	103	1.0	6	1.7	14	12	7	0.4	70	20	0.02	0.02	0.2	0
160.	Cookies, Fig bars	4 bars	56	210	2.0	4	1.0	27	42	40	1.4	180	31	0.08	0.07	0.7	0
161.	Cookies, Oatmeal raisin	2 2" diam.	26	122	1.5	5	1.3	1	18	9	0.6	74	20	0.04	0.04	0.5	0
162.	Cookies, Peanut butter, homemade	2 cookies	24	123	2.0	7	2.0	11	14	10	0.5	71	12	0.03	0.03	0.9	0
163.	Cookies, sandwich, all	4 cookies	40	195	2.0	8	2.0	0	29	12	1.4	189	0	0.90	0.07	0.8	0
164.	Cookies, Shortbread	4 cookies	32	155	2.0	8	2.9	27	20	13	0.8	123	40	0.10	0.09	0.9	0
165.	Cookies, Vanilla	5 1¾" diam.	20	93	1.0	3	0.8	10	15	8	0.1	50	25	0.00	0.01	0.0	0
166.	Cookies, Vanilla wafers	10 wafers	40	185	2.0	7	1.8	25	29	16	0.8	150	70	0.07	0.10	1.0	0
167.	Corn, boiled on cob	1 ear 5" long	140	70	2.5	1	0.0	0	16	2	0.5	1	310	0.09	0.08	1.1	7
168.	Corn, canned, drained	1/2 c	83	70	2.2	1	0.0	0	16	4	0.4	195	290	0.03	0.04	0.8	4
169.	Corn chips	1 oz.	28	155	2.0	9	1.8	0	16	35	0.5	233	110	0.04	0.05	0.4	1
170.	Cornmeal, degermed, yellow, enriched, cooked	1/2 c	120	60	1.3	0	0.0	0	13	1	0.5	264	70	0.07	0.05	0.6	0
171.	Crab, canned	1 c	135	135	23.0	3	0.5	135	1	61	1.1	1,350	70	0.11	0.11	2.6	0
172.	Crackers, Cheese	10 crackers	10	50	1.0	3	0.9	6	5	11	0.4	112	25	0.05	0.04	0.4	0
173.	Crackers, Graham	2 squares	14	55	1.1	1	0.3	0	10	6	0.2	95	0	0.01	0.03	0.2	0
174.	Crackers, Ritz	1 cracker	3	15	0.2	1	0.2	0	2	3	0.1	30	0	0.01	0.01	0.1	0
175.	Crackers, Ryewafers, whole grain	2 crackers	14	55	1.0	0	0.3	0	10	7	0.5	115	0	0.06	0.03	0.5	0
176.	Crackers, Saltines	4 squares	11	48	1.0	1	0.3	1	8	2	0.1	123	0	0.00	0.00	0.1	0
177.	Crackers, Soda	1	3	13	0.3	0	0.1	0	2	1	0.1	39	0	0.02	0.01	0.1	0

Code	Food	Amount	Weight gm	Calories	Protein gm	Fat gm	Sat. Fat gm	Cholesterol mg	Carbohydrate gm	Calcium mg	Iron mg	Sodium mg	Vit A I.U.	Thiamin (Vit B$_1$) mg	Riboflavin (Vit B$_2$) mg	Niacin mg	Vit C mg
178.	Crackers, Triscuits	1	5	23	0.4	1	0.3	0	3	0	0.0	0	0	0.00	0.00	0.0	0
179.	Crackers, Wheat Thins	1	2	9	0.2	0	0.1	0	1	1	0.1	17	0	0.01	0.01	0.1	0
180.	Cranberry juice	1 c	253	145	0.1	0	0.0	0	36	8	0.4	5	5	0.02	0.02	0.1	90
181.	Cream, light coffee or table	1 tbsp	15	20	0.5	2	0.5	5	1	16	0.0	7	70	0.00	0.02	0.0	0
182.	Cream, heavy whipping	1 tbsp	15	53	0.3	6	1.3	12	1	11	0.0	5	230	0.00	0.02	0.0	0
183.	Croissant	1	57	235	4.7	12	4.0	13	27	20	2.1	452	50	0.17	0.13	1.3	0
184.	Croissants (Sara Lee)	1 roll	18	59	1.6	2	0.3	0	8	22	0.6	105	0	0.14	0.09	0.8	0
185.	Croissan'wich, egg, cheese Burger King	1 sandwich	110	315	13.0	20	7.0	222	19	112	1.8	607	500	0.22	0.37	1.4	0
186.	Cucumbers, raw pared	9 sm slices	28	4	0.3	0	0.0	0	1	7	0.3	2	70	0.01	0.01	0.1	3
187.	Danish, Apple, McDonald's	1	115	390	6	17	11.0	25	51	0	1.0	370	0	0.30	0.18	2.0	15
188.	Danish, Cinnamon Raisin	1	110	440	6	21	13.0	34	58	48	0.1	430	0	0.30	0.27	3.0	4
189.	Dates hydrated	5	46	110	0.9	0	0.0	0	29	24	1.2	1	20	0.04	0.04	0.9	0
190.	Doughnut, plain	1	42	164	1.9	8	2.0	19	22	17	0.6	210	30	0.07	0.07	0.5	0
191.	Doughnut, yeast raised	1	27	235	4.0	13	5.2	21	26	17	1.4	222	2	0.28	0.12	1.8	0
192.	Dressing, Bleu cheese	1 tbsp	15	77	0.7	8	1.9	4	1	12	0.0	8	32	0.00	0.02	0.0	0
193.	Dressing, French	1 tbsp	16	83	0.1	9	1.4	0	1	2	0.1	184	0	0.00	0.00	0.0	0
194.	Dressing, French, low cal	1 tbsp.	15	24	0.0	2	0.2	0	2	6	0.1	306	0	0.00	0.00	0.0	0
195.	Dressing, Italian	1 tbsp.)	15	69	0.1	9	1.3	0	2	1	0.0	73	29	0.00	0.00	0.0	0
196.	Dressing, Italian, low cal	1 tbsp.	15	10	0.0	1	0.0	0	0	1	0.0	136	1	0.00	0.00	0.0	0
197.	Dressing, Ranch style	1 tbsp.	15	54	0.4	6	0.9	6	1	15	0.0	65	36	0.01	0.02	0.0	1
198.	Dressing, Thousand Island	1 tbsp.	15	60	0.2	6	1.0	4	2	2	0.1	110	75	0.00	0.01	0.0	0
199.	Dressing, Thousand Island, low cal	1 tbsp.	15	25	0.1	2	0.2	2	3	2	0.1	153	70	0.00	0.00	0.0	0
200.	Egg, hard cooked	1 large	50	72	6.0	5	1.8	250	1	24	1.0	113	520	0.05	0.13	0.0	0
201.	Egg, fried with butter	1	46	95	5.4	6	2.4	278	1	28	0.9	162	320	0.04	0.13	0.0	0
202.	Egg McMuffin	1	138	327	18.5	15	5.9	259	31	226	2.9	885	591	0.47	0.44	3.8	1
203.	Egg salad sandwich	1	111	325	10.0	19	3.9	215	28	95	2.5	461	242	0.29	0.29	2.1	0
204.	Egg, scrambled, with milk, butter	1 egg	64	95	6.0	7	3.0	282	1	54	0.9	176	510	0.04	0.18	0.0	0
205.	Egg, white	1 large	33	17	3.6	0	0.0	0	0	3	0.0	48	0	0.00	0.09	0.0	0
206.	Egg, yolk, raw	1 yolk	17	63	2.8	6	1.7	248	0	26	1.0	8	390	0.04	0.07	0.0	0
207.	Enchilada, beef	1	200	487	21.8	23	8.8	63	26	425	2.9	262	595	0.02	0.27	3.5	5
208.	Enchilada, cheese	1	230	632	25.3	34	17.6	82	31	876	2.6	596	1,672	0.13	0.40	1.2	15
209.	Figs, dried	1 large	21	60	1.0	0	0.0	0	15	26	0.6	1	20	0.16	0.17	3.9	0
210.	Filet of Fish, McDonald's	1	131	402	15.0	23	7.9	43	34	105	1.8	709	152	0.28	0.28	3.9	4
211.	Fish sandwich, Wendy's	1	182	460	16	25	5.0	55	42	120	1.8	780	0	0.60	0.45	4.0	1
212.	Fish, sticks	2	56	140	12.0	6	1.6	52	8	22	0.6	106	40	0.06	0.10	1.2	0
213.	Flounder	3 oz.	85	171	25.5	7	1.0	60	0	21	1.2	201	0	0.06	0.06	2.1	3
214.	Flour, all purpose enriched	1 c	125	455	13.0	1	0.0	0	95	20	3.6	3	0	0.55	0.33	4.4	0
215.	Flour, whole wheat	1 c	120	400	16.0	2	0.0	0	85	49	4.0	4	0	0.66	0.14	5.2	0
216.	Frankfurter, cooked	1	57	176	7.0	16	5.6	45	1	4	1.1	627	0	0.09	0.11	1.5	0
217.	Frankfurter, turkey, cooked	1	45	102	6.4	8	2.7	39	1	58	0.8	454	60	0.04	0.08	1.7	0
218.	French Dip, Arby's	1	154	368	22	15	5.6	43	35	60	2.8	1,018	0	0.20	0.50	8.4	0
219.	French toast	1 piece	65	123	4.9	4	1.1	73	15	79	1.1	189	285	0.15	0.17	1.1	0
220.	Fries, Curly, Arby's	1 small	99	337	4	18	7.4	0	43	24	1.0	167	0	0.06	0.07	2.0	0
221.	Fruit cocktail	1 c	245	91	1.0	0	0.0	0	24	22	1.0	12	370	0.05	0.02	1.2	5
222.	Fruit cocktail, juice pack	1 c	248	115	1.1	0	0.0	0	29	20	0.5	10	380	0.03	0.04	1.0	7
223.	Grapefruit, raw white	1/2 med	301	56	1.0	0	0.0	0	15	22	0.5	1	10	0.05	0.03	0.3	52

APPENDIX A ▼ *Nutritive Value of Selected Foods*

#	Food	Serving	124	50	0.6	0	0.0	0	12	11	0.2	2	10	0.05	0.03	0.3	46
224.	Grapefruit, juice unsweetened canned	1/2 c	50	34	0.3	0	0.0	0	9	6	0.2	2	50	0.03	0.03	0.2	2
225.	Grapes, seedless, European	10 grapes	127	84	0.3	0	0.0	0	21	14	0.4	3	0	0.05	0.03	0.3	0
226.	Grape juice, unsweetened bottled	1/2 c															
227.	Gravy, beef, homemade	1 tbsp	17	19	0.3	2	1.0	1	1	1	0.1	49	0	0.01	0.01	0.2	0
228.	Haddock, fried (dipped in egg, milk, bread crumbs)	3 oz.	85	141	17.0	5	1.0	54	5	33	0.9	150	0	0.03	0.06	2.7	3
229.	Halibut, broiled with butter or margarine	3 oz.	85	144	21.0	6	2.1	55	0	15	0.6	114	570	0.03	0.06	7.2	1
230.	Ham (cured pork)	3 oz.	85	318	20.0	26	9.4	77	0	9	2.6	48	0	0.43	0.20	3.8	0
231.	Ham, lunch meat	1 slice	28	37	5.5	1	0.5	13	0	2	0.2	405	0	0.26	0.06	1.4	7
232.	Hamburger, Big Classic, Wendy's	1	251	480	27	23	7.0	75	44	180	4.2	850	300	0.45	0.27	7.0	12
233.	Hamburger, Big Mac	1	204	581	25.1	36	12.0	85	40	207	5.0	999	388	0.49	0.39	7.3	3
234.	Hamburger bun	1 bun	40	129	3.7	2	1.0	0	23	61	1.3	271	2	0.22	0.15	1.8	0
235.	Hamburger, Jr. Bacon Cheeseburger, Wendy's	1	170	440	22	25	8.0	65	33	240	3.0	870	300	0.45	0.27	6.0	9
236.	Hamburger, McDonald's	1	99	257	13.0	9	3.7	26	30	63	3.0	526	231	0.23	0.23	5.1	2
237.	Hamburger, McLean Deluxe	1	206	320	22	10	5.0	60	35	180	2.4	670	500	0.38	0.36	7.0	6
238.	Hamburger, McLean Deluxe, w/cheese	1	219	370	24	14	8.0	75	35	240	2.4	890	750	0.38	0.36	7.0	6
239.	Hamburger, Quarter pounder	1 burger	160	427	24.6	24	9.1	80	29	98	4.3	718	115	0.35	0.32	7.2	3
240.	Hamburger, Quarter pounder, with cheese	1 burger	186	525	29.6	32	12.8	107	31	255	4.8	1,195	640	0.37	0.41	7.1	3
241.	Hamburger, Wendy's	1	219	440	26	23	7.0	75	36	120	3.6	850	300	0.38	0.18	7.0	9
242.	Ham N' Cheese, Arby's	1	169	355	25	14	5.1	55	35	204	1.8	1400	0	0.83	0.40	7.8	0
243.	Honey	1 tbsp	21	64	0.0	0	0.0	0	17	1	0.1	1	0	0.00	0.01	0.1	0
244.	Honeydew melon	1 slice (1/10 melon)	129	45	0.6	0	0.0	0	12	8	0.1	13	25	0.10	0.02	0.8	32
245.	Horsey Sauce, Arby's	.5 oz.	14	55	0	5	2.0	0	3	24	0.0	105	0	0.00	0.00	0.0	0
246.	Hotcakes w/Margarine & Syrup, McDonald's	1 serving	174	440	8	12	5.0	8	74	120	1.2	685	200	0.30	0.36	3.0	0
247.	Hotdog bun	1 bun	40	115	3.3	2	1.0	2	20	54	1.2	241	2	0.20	0.13	1.6	0
248.	Ice cream, vanilla	1/2 c	67	135	3.0	7	4.4	27	14	97	0.1	42	295	0.03	0.14	0.1	1
249.	Ice cream cone	1 small	115	185	4.3	5	2.2	24	30	183	0.1	109	218	0.06	0.36	0.4	0
250.	Ice cream cone, Dairy Queen	medium	142	230	6.0	7	4.6	15	35	200	0.0	150	300	0.09	0.26	0.0	1
251.	Ice cream, hot fudge sundae	1	164	357	7.0	11	5.4	27	58	215	0.6	170	233	0.07	0.31	1.1	2
252.	Ice milk, vanilla	1/2 c	61	100	3.0	3	1.8	13	15	102	0.1	45	140	0.04	0.15	0.1	1
253.	Instant breakfast, whole milk	1 c	281	280	15.0	8	5.1	33	34	301	8.0	286	2,057	0.39	0.46	5.2	29
254.	Instant breakfast, skim milk	1 c	282	216	15.4	0	0.0	4	35	312	8.0	292	1,635	0.39	0.41	5.2	29
255.	Jams or preserves	1 tbsp	7	18	0.0	0	0.0	0	5	1	0.1	1	1	0.00	0.00	0.0	0
256.	Jelly	1 tbsp	18	49	0.0	0	0.0	0	13	4	0.3	3	0	0.00	0.01	0.0	1
257.	Kale, fresh cooked, drained	1/2 c	55	22	2.5	0	0.0	0	3	103	0.9	24	4,565	0.06	0.10	0.9	51
258.	Kiwi fruit, raw	1 med	76	46	1.0	0	0.0	0	11	20	0.3	4	65	0.02	0.04	0.4	75
259.	Kool Aid, with sugar	1 c	240	100	0.0	0	0.0	0	25	0	0.0	0	0	0.00	0.00	0.0	6
260.	Lamb leg, roast, trimmed	3 oz.	85	237	22.0	16	7.3	60	0	9	1.4	53	0	0.13	0.23	4.7	0
261.	Lamb loin chop, broiled, lean	3 oz.	84	183	25.0	8	3.4	78	0	16	1.7	70	7	0.10	0.23	5.7	0
262.	Lasagna, homemade	1 piece	220	357	23.6	18	8.3	50	27	413	2.8	703	1,008	0.19	0.30	3.3	6
263.	Lemon juice, fresh	1 tbsp	15	4	0.1	0	0.0	0	1	1	0.0	0	0	0.00	0.00	0.0	7
264.	Lemonade (concentrate)	12 oz.	340	137	0.2	0	0.1	0	36	11	0.6	11	73	0.02	0.07	0.1	13
265.	Lentils, cooked	1/2 c	100	106	8.0	0	0.1	0	19	25	2.1	0	20	0.07	0.06	0.6	0
266.	Lettuce, crisp head	1 c sm chunks	75	10	0.7	0	0.0	0	2	15	0.4	7	250	0.05	0.05	0.2	5
267.	Lettuce, cos or romaine	1 c chopped	55	10	0.7	0	0.0	0	2	37	0.8	5	1,050	0.08	0.04	0.2	10
268.	Liver, beef, fried	1 slice 3 oz.	85	195	22.0	9	2.5	345	5	9	7.5	156	45,390	0.22	3.56	14.0	23

Code	Food	Amount	Weight gm	Calories	Protein gm	Fat gm	Sat. Fat gm	Cholesterol mg	Carbohydrate gm	Calcium mg	Iron mg	Sodium mg	Vit A I.U.	Thiamin (Vit B₁) mg	Riboflavin (Vit B₂) mg	Niacin mg	Vit C mg
269.	Liverwurst, fresh	1 slice 1 oz.	28	87	5.0	7	3.5	50	0	3	1.5	0	1,800	0.06	0.37	1.6	0
270.	Lobster	1 c	145	138	27.0	2	1.0	293	0	94	1.2	305	0	0.15	0.10	0.0	0
271.	M&M's, Chocolate, plain	1 oz.	28	140	1.9	6	3.3	0	19	47	0.5	24	30	0.01	0.07	0.2	0
272.	M&M's, Chocolate, w/peanuts	1 oz.	28	145	3.2	7	3.2	0	17	36	0.4	17	15	0.02	0.05	0.9	0
273.	Macaroni, enriched, cooked	1/2 c	70	78	2.4	0	0.0	0	16	6	0.7	1	0	0.10	0.06	0.8	0
274.	Macaroni and cheese	1/2 c	100	215	8.2	11	4.0	21	20	181	0.9	543	430	0.10	0.20	0.9	0
275.	Margarine	1 tsp	5	34	0.0	4	0.7	0	0	1	0.0	46	160	0.00	0.00	0.0	0
276.	Mars bar	1 bar	50	240	4.0	11	4.8	2	30	85	0.6	85	1	0.02	0.16	0.5	0
277.	Matzo	1 piece	30	117	3.0	0	0.0	0	25	*	0.0	0	*	*	*	*	*
278.	Mayonnaise	1 tsp	5	36	0.0	4	0.7	3	0	1	0.0	28	13	0.00	0.00	0.0	0
279.	Milk, chocolate, 2%	1 c	250	180	8.0	5	3.1	17	26	284	0.6	151	143	0.09	0.41	0.3	2
280.	Milk, evaporated whole	1/2 c	126	172	9.0	10	5.8	40	13	329	0.2	149	405	0.05	0.43	0.2	2
281.	Milk, lowfat 2% fat	1 c	246	145	10	5	3.1	5	15	352	0.1	150	200	0.10	0.52	0.2	2
282.	Milk shake, chocolate	1 (10 fluid oz.)	340	433	11.5	13	7.8	45	70	383	1.1	328	312	0.20	0.83	0.5	0
283.	Milk shake, Frosty, Wendy's	16 oz.	324	460	13	13	7.0	55	76	480	1.0	260	500	0.15	1.08	0.8	0
284.	Milk shake, strawberry	1 (10 fluid oz.)	340	383	11.4	10	6.0	37	64	384	0.4	281	418	0.14	0.61	0.5	4
285.	Milk shake, vanilla, McDonald's	1	289	323	10	8	5.1	29	52	346	0.2	250	346	0.12	0.66	0.6	3
286.	Milk, skim	1 c	245	88	9.0	0	0.3	5	12	296	0.1	126	10	0.09	0.44	0.2	2
287.	Milk, whole 3.5% fat	1 c	244	159	9.0	9	5.1	34	12	288	0.1	120	350	0.07	0.40	0.2	2
288.	Milky Way bar	1 bar	60	260	3.2	9	5.4	14	43	86	0.5	140	125	0.03	0.15	0.2	1
289.	Molasses, medium	1 tbsp	20	50	0.0	0	0.0	0	13	33	0.9	3	0	0.01	0.01	0.0	0
290.	Muffin, apple bran, fat free, McDonald's	1	75	180	5	0	0.0	0	40	48	0.7	200	0	0.15	0.18	2.0	0
291.	Muffin, blueberry	1	45	135	3.0	5	1.5	19	20	54	0.9	198	40	0.10	0.11	0.9	1
292.	Muffin, bran	1	45	125	3.0	6	1.4	24	19	60	1.4	189	230	0.11	0.13	1.3	3
293.	Muffin, cornmeal	1	45	145	3.0	5	1.5	23	21	66	0.9	169	80	0.11	0.11	0.9	0
294.	Muffin, English, plain	1	57	140	4.5	1	0.3	0	26	96	1.7	378	0	0.26	0.18	2.1	0
295.	Muffin, English w/butter	1	63	186	5.0	5	2.3	15	30	117	1.5	310	164	0.28	0.49	2.6	1
296.	Mushrooms, fresh cultivated	1/2 c sliced	35	12	1.0	0	0.0	0	2	4	0.5	4	0	0.04	0.12	2.4	1
297.	Mustard greens, cooked drained	1/2 c	70	16	1.7	0	0.0	0	3	96	1.2	13	4,060	0.05	0.10	0.4	33
298.	Noodles, egg, enriched cooked	1/2 c	80	100	3.3	1	0.0	0	19	8	0.7	2	55	0.11	0.07	1.0	0
299.	Nuts, Brazil	1 oz. (6-8 nuts)	28	185	4.1	19	4.8	0	3	53	1.0	0	0	0.27	0.03	0.5	0
300.	Nuts, Pecans	1 oz.	28	195	2.6	20	1.4	0	4	21	0.7	0	40	0.24	0.04	0.3	1
301.	Nuts, Walnuts	1 oz. (14 halves)	28	185	4.2	18	1.0	0	5	28	0.9	1	10	0.09	0.04	0.3	1
302.	Oil, Corn	1 tbsp.	15	125	0.0	14	1.8	0	0	0	0.0	0	0	0.00	0.00	0.0	0
303.	Oil, Olive	1 tbsp.	15	125	0.0	14	1.9	0	0	0	0.0	0	0	0.00	0.00	0.0	0
304.	Oil, Safflower	1 tbsp.	15	125	0.0	14	1.3	0	0	0	0.0	0	0	0.00	0.00	0.0	0
305.	Oil, Soybean	1 tsp.	5	44	0.0	5	2.0	0	0	0	0.0	0	0	0.00	0.00	0.0	0
306.	Okra, cooked, drained	1/2 c	80	23	1.6	0	0.0	0	5	74	0.4	2	390	0.11	0.15	0.7	16
307.	Olives, black, ripe	10 extra large	55	61	0.5	7	1.0	0	1	40	0.8	385	30	0.00	0.00	0.0	0
308.	Onions, mature, cooked, drained	1/2 c sliced	105	31	1.3	0	0.0	0	7	25	0.4	8	40	0.03	0.03	0.2	8
309.	Onion rings, fried	3	30	122	1.6	8	2.3	0	11	9	0.5	113	68	0.08	0.04	1.1	0
310.	Onion rings (Brazier) Dairy Queen	1 serving	85	360	6.0	17	6.0	15	33	20	0.4	125	0	0.09	0.00	0.4	2
311.	Orange juice, froz. reconstituted	1/2 c	125	61	0.9	0	0.0	0	15	13	0.1	1	270	0.12	0.02	0.5	60

312. Orange, raw (medium skin)	1 med	180	64	1.3	0	0.0	0	16	54	0.5	1	260	0.13	0.05	0.5	66
313. Oysters, Eastern, breaded, fried	1 oyster	45	90	5.0	5	1.4	35	5	49	3.0	70	220	0.07	0.10	1.3	4
314. Oysters, raw, Eastern	1/2 c (6-9 med)	120	79	10.0	2	1.3	60	4	113	6.6	145	370	0.17	0.22	3.0	0
315. Pancakes	1 6" diam x 1/2" thick	73	169	5.2	5	1.0	36	25	74	0.9	310	90	0.12	0.16	0.9	0
316. Pancakes, buckwheat	1 4 in. diam.	27	55	2.0	2	0.9	20	6	59	0.4	125	17	0.04	0.05	0.2	0
317. Pancakes w/butter, syrup	1 large	100	250	4.0	5	1.9	24	47	1	1.1	535	160	0.13	0.18	1.1	2
318. Papaya, raw	1/2 med	227	60	0.9	0	0.0	0	15	31	0.5	5	2,660	0.06	0.06	0.5	85
319. Parsnips, cooked	1 large 9" long	160	106	2.4	1	0.0	0	24	72	1.0	13	50	0.11	0.13	0.2	16
320. Peaches, canned, heavy syrup	1 half 2⅛ tbsp liq.	96	75	0.4	0	0.0	0	19	4	0.3	2	410	0.01	0.02	0.6	3
321. Peaches, canned, juice pack	1 half	77	34	0.5	0	0.0	0	9	5	0.2	3	147	0.01	0.01	0.5	3
322. Peaches, raw, peeled	1 2¾" diam.	175	58	0.9	0	0.0	0	15	14	0.8	2	2,030	0.03	0.08	1.5	11
323. Peanut butter	2 tbsp	32	188	8.0	16	1.0	0	6	18	0.6	194	0	0.04	0.04	4.8	0
324. Peanut butter, jam sandwich	1	100	340	11.4	14	2.6	0	45	87	2.3	414	1	0.32	0.22	5.3	0
325. Peanuts, roasted	1 oz.	28	166	7.0	14	1.0	0	5	21	0.6	119	0	0.09	0.04	4.9	0
326. Pears, canned, heavy syrup	1 half 2¼ tbsp liq.	103	78	0.2	0	0.0	0	20	5	0.2	1	0	0.01	0.02	0.1	1
327. Pears, canned, juice pack	1 half	77	38	0.3	0	0.0	0	10	7	0.2	3	3	0.01	0.01	0.2	1
328. Pears, raw	1 pear	180	100	1.1	1	0.0	0	25	13	0.5	2	30	0.03	0.07	0.2	7
329. Peas, canned, drained	1/2 c	85	75	4.0	0	0.0	0	14	22	1.6	200	585	0.08	0.05	0.7	7
330. Peas, frozen, cooked drained	1/2 c	80	55	4.1	0	0.0	0	10	15	1.5	92	480	0.22	0.07	1.4	11
331. Peppers, sweet, raw	1 pepper 3¼" x 3" diam.	200	36	2.0	0	0.0	0	8	15	1.1	21	690	0.13	0.13	0.8	210
332. Pickles, dill	1 large 4" long	135	15	0.9	0	0.0	0	3	35	1.4	1,928	140	0.00	0.03	0.0	8
333. Pickles, sweet	1 large 3" long	35	51	0.2	0	0.0	0	13	4	0.4	0	30	0.00	0.01	0.0	2
334. Pie, Apple	1 piece (3½")	118	302	2.6	13	3.5	120	45	9	0.4	355	40	0.02	0.02	0.5	1
335. Pie, Apple, fried	1 pie	85	255	2.2	14	5.8	14	32	12	0.9	326	15	0.09	0.06	1.0	1
336. Pie, Blueberry	1 piece (3½")	158	380	4.0	17	4.0	0	55	26	2.1	423	140	0.17	0.14	1.7	6
337. Pie, Cherry	1 piece (3½")	118	308	3.1	13	5.0	137	45	17	0.4	355	40	0.02	0.02	0.5	1
338. Pie, Cherry, fried	1 pie	85	250	2.0	14	5.8	13	32	11	0.7	371	95	0.06	0.06	0.6	1
339. Pie, Chocolate cream	1 piece (1/6 pie)	175	311	7.4	13	4.5	15	42	160	1.1	427	170	0.15	0.30	1.1	1
340. Pie, Lemon meringue	1 piece (1/6 pie)	140	355	4.7	14	3.5	137	53	25	1.4	395	330	0.10	0.14	0.8	4
341. Pie, Pecan	1 piece (1/6 pie)	138	583	6.3	24	3.9	13	92	35	1.9	304	206	0.22	0.17	1.1	0
342. Pie, Pumpkin	1 (3½")	114	241	4.6	13	3.0	70	28	58	0.6	244	2,810	0.03	0.11	0.6	0
343. Pineapple, canned, heavy syrup	1/2 c	128	95	0.4	0	0.0	0	25	14	0.4	2	65	0.10	0.03	0.3	9
344. Pineapple, canned, juice pack	1/2 c	125	75	0.5	0	0.0	0	20	17	0.3	1	24	0.12	0.24	0.3	12
345. Pineapple, raw	1/2 c diced	78	41	0.3	0	0.0	0	11	13	0.4	1	55	0.07	0.03	0.2	13
346. Pizza, Cheese, Thin 'n Crispy, Pizza Hut	1/2 10" pie	*	450	25.0	15	7.0	125	54	450	4.5	1,200	750	0.30	0.51	5.0	1
347. Pizza, Cheese, Thick 'n Chewy, Pizza Hut	1/2 10" pie	*	560	34.0	14	6.0	110	71	500	5.4	1,100	1,000	0.68	0.68	7.0	1
348. Plums, Japanese and hybrid, raw	1 plum 2⅛" diam.	70	32	0.3	0	0.0	0	8	8	0.3	1	160	0.02	0.02	0.3	4
349. Popcorn, cooked, oil	1 c	11	55	0.9	3	0.5	0	6	3	0.3	86	20	0.01	0.02	0.1	0
350. Popcorn, popped, plain, large kernel	1 c	6	12	0.8	0	0.0	0	5	1	0.2	0	0	0.00	0.01	0.1	0
351. Pork, roast, trimmed	2 slices 3 oz.	85	179	24.0	8	2.2	65	0	11	3.1	863	0	0.55	0.22	4.3	0
352. Pork, sausage, cooked	1 sm link	17	72	2.8	6	2.1	13	1	0	0.3	221	0	0.00	0.00	0.0	0
353. Potato, au gratin	1 c	245	228	5.6	10	6.3	12	32	203	0.8	1,076	380	0.05	0.20	2.3	8
354. Potato, baked in skin	1 potato 2⅓ x 4¼"	202	145	4.0	0	0.0	0	33	14	1.1	6	0	0.15	0.07	2.7	31
355. Potato chips	10 chips	20	114	1.1	8	2.1	0	10	8	0.4	150	0	0.04	0.01	1.0	3
356. Potato, French fried long	10 strips 3½-4"	78	214	3.4	10	1.7	0	28	12	1.0	5	0	0.10	0.06	2.4	16

Code	Food	Amount	Weight gm	Calories	Protein gm	Fat gm	Sat. Fat gm	Cholesterol mg	Carbohydrate gm	Calcium mg	Iron mg	Sodium mg	Vit A I.U.	Thiamin (Vit B$_1$) mg	Riboflavin (Vit B$_2$) mg	Niacin mg	Vit C mg
357.	Potato, Hashbrowns, McDonald's	1 patty	55	144	1.4	9	3.0	4	15	5	0.4	325	6	0.06	0.01	0.8	4
358.	Potato, mashed, milk added	1/2 c	105	69	2.2	1	0.4	8	14	25	0.4	316	20	0.09	0.06	1.1	11
359.	Potato salad w/eggs, mayo	1/2 c	125	179	3.4	10	7.8	85	14	24	0.8	662	262	0.10	0.08	1.1	12
360.	Potato, hash brown	1/2 c	78	170	2.5	9	3.5	0	22	12	1.2	27	0	0.09	0.02	1.9	5
361.	Pretzel, thin, twists	1 oz.	28	113	2.8	1	0.3	0	23	8	0.6	456	0	0.09	0.07	1.2	0
362.	Prunes, dried "softenized" without pits	5 prunes	61	137	1.1	0	0.0	0	36	26	0.1	4	860	0.05	0.09	0.9	2
363.	Prune juice, canned or bottled	1/2 c	128	99	0.5	0	0.0	0	24	18	5.3	3	0	0.02	0.02	0.5	3
364.	Pudding, Chocolate, canned	5 oz.	142	205	3	11	9.5	1	30	74	1.2	285	155	0.04	0.17	0.6	0
365.	Pudding, Tapioca, canned	5 oz.	142	160	3	5	4.8	1	28	119	0.3	252	5	0.03	0.14	0.4	0
366.	Pudding, Vanilla, canned	5 oz.	142	220	2	10	9.5	1	33	79	0.2	305	1	0.03	0.12	0.6	0
367.	Quiche, Lorraine	1 piece	242	825	18	66	31.9	392	40	290	1.9	898	2,250	0.15	0.44	1.7	1
368.	Raisins, unbleached, seedless	1 oz.	28	82	0.7	0	0.0	0	22	18	1.0	8	10	0.03	0.02	0.1	0
369.	Raspberries, fresh	1 c	123	60	1.1	1	0.0	0	14	27	0.7	0	80	0.04	0.11	1.1	31
370.	Raspberries, frozen	1 c	250	255	1.7	1	0.0	0	62	38	1.6	3	75	0.05	0.11	1.5	41
371.	Rice, brown, cooked	1/2 c	96	116	2.5	1	0.0	0	25	12	0.5	275	0	0.09	0.02	1.3	0
372.	Rice, white enriched, cooked	1/2 c	103	113	2.1	0	0.0	0	25	11	0.9	384	0	0.12	0.01	1.1	0
373.	Rice, wild, cooked	1/2 c	100	92	3.6	0	0.0	0	19	5	1.1	2	0	0.11	0.16	1.6	0
374.	Roast Beef sand, Regular, Arby's	1	155	383	22	18	7.0	43	35	72	3.2	936	0	0.28	0.50	11.0	0
375.	Roast Beef Sub, Arby's	1	305	623	38	32	11.5	73	47	492	5.2	1,847	500	0.56	0.76	14.2	9
376.	Roll, hard, white	1 roll	50	155	5	2	0.0	0	30	24	1.4	313	0	0.20	0.12	1.7	0
377.	Rueben sandwich	1	237	488	28.7	28	10.4	85	30	364	5.3	1,685	461	0.25	0.44	3.9	12
378.	Salad, Caesar side, Wendy's	1	130	160	10	6	1.0	10	18	96	1.2	700	1,250	0.23	0.27	2.0	24
379.	Salad, Chef, Burger King	1 serving	273	178	17	9	4.0	103	7	128	1.6	568	4,750	0.35	0.26	3.6	15
380.	Salad, Chef, McDonald's	1	265	170	17	9	4.0	111	8	180	1.0	400	5,000	0.30	0.27	4.0	21
381.	Salad, Chicken, Burger King	1 serving	258	142	20	4	1.0	49	8	32	1.3	443	4,600	0.14	0.17	8.5	20
382.	Salad, Chicken w/celery	1/2 c	78	266	10.5	25	4.1	48	1	16	0.7	199	153	0.03	0.08	3.3	1
383.	Salad, Deluxe Garden, Wendy's	1	271	110	7	5	1.0	0	9	240	1.0	380	3,000	0.15	0.36	1.2	36
384.	Salad, Garden, Arby's	1	330	117	7	5	2.7	12	11	192	1.1	134	4,900	0.17	0.20	1.2	52
385.	Salad, Grilled Chicken, Wendy's	1	338	200	25	8	1.0	55	9	240	1.8	690	3,000	0.23	0.36	8.0	36
386.	Salad, Tuna	1 c	205	375	33	19	3.3	80	19	31	2.5	877	53	0.06	0.14	13.3	6
387.	Salami, dry	1 oz.	28	128	7.0	11	1.6	24	0	4	1.0	349	0	0.10	0.07	1.5	0
388.	Salmon, broiled with butter or margarine	3 oz.	85	156	23.0	6	2.2	53	0	0	0.9	99	150	0.15	0.06	8.4	0
389.	Salmon, canned Chinook	3 oz.	85	179	16.6	12	0.8	30	0	131	0.7	105	197	0.03	0.01	6.2	0
390.	Sardines, canned drained	1 oz.	28	58	7.0	3	1.0	20	0	124	0.8	233	60	0.01	0.06	1.5	0
391.	Sauerkraut, canned	1/2 c	118	21	1.2	0	0.0	0	5	43	0.6	878	60	0.04	0.05	0.3	17
392.	Sausage Biscuit w/Egg, McDonald's	1	175	505	19	33	20.0	260	33	120	2.4	1,210	300	0.45	0.36	4.0	0
393.	Sausage McMuffin, McDonald's	1	135	345	15	20	11.0	57	27	240	1.8	770	200	0.53	0.27	5.0	0
394.	Sausage McMuffin, w/Egg	1	159	430	21	25	14.0	270	27	300	2.4	920	500	0.53	0.45	5.0	0
395.	Sausage, smoked link, pork	1	68	265	15	22	7.7	46	1	20	0.8	1,020	0	1.04	0.29	5.0	14
396.	Scallops, breaded, cooked	6 pieces	90	195	15	10	2.5	70	10	39	2.0	298	105	0.11	0.11	1.6	0
397.	Sherbet	1/2 c	97	135	1.1	2	1.3	7	29	52	0.2	44	92	0.02	0.04	0.1	2
398.	Shrimp, boiled	3 oz.	85	99	18.0	1	0.1	128	1	99	2.7	0	60	0.00	0.03	1.5	0
399.	Shrimp, fried	7 medium	85	200	16.0	10	2.5	168	11	61	2.0	384	130	0.06	0.09	2.8	0
400.	Snickers bar	1 bar	61	290	6.6	4	5.4	0	37	70	0.5	170	25	0.03	0.11	1.8	0
401.	Soda pop, cola	12 oz.	369	144	0.0	0	0.0	0	37	27	0.0	30	0	0.00	0.00	0.0	0
402.	Soda pop, diet	12 oz.	340	2	0.1	0	0.0	0	0	13	0.1	31	0	0.00	0.00	0.0	0
403.	Soda pop, Ginger ale	12 oz.	366	113	0.0	0	0.0	0	29	0	0.0	45	0	0.00	0.00	0.0	0

APPENDIX A ▼ Nutritive Value of Selected Foods

#	Food	Serving												
404.	Soda pop, Lemon-lime	12 oz.	340	138	0.0	0	0.0	0	35	8	0.2	38	0	0.00	0.00	0.0	0
405.	Soda pop, Root beer	12 oz.	340	140	0.0	0	0.0	0	36	17	0.2	45	0	0.00	0.00	0.0	0
406.	Soup, Chicken, cream	1 c	248	191	7.5	12	4.6	27	15	180	0.7	1,046	710	0.07	0.26	0.9	1
407.	Soup, Chicken noodle	1 c	241	75	4.0	2	0.7	7	9	17	0.8	900	711	0.05	0.06	1.4	0
408.	Soup, Clam chowder, Manhattan	1 c	244	78	4.2	2	0.4	2	12	34	1.9	1,808	460	0.06	0.05	1.3	3
409.	Soup, Clam chowder, north east	1 c	248	163	9.5	7	3.0	22	16	187	1.5	992	160	0.07	0.24	1.0	4
410.	Soup, Cream of mushroom condensed, prepared with equal volume of milk	1 c	245	216	7.0	14	5.4	15	16	191	0.5	955	250	0.05	0.34	0.7	1
411.	Soup, Minestrone	1 c	241	80	4.3	3	0.5	2	11	34	0.9	911	1,170	0.05	0.04	0.9	1
412.	Soup, Split pea, condensed, prepared with equal volume of water	1 c	245	145	9.0	3	1.1	0	21	29	1.5	941	440	0.25	0.15	1.5	1
413.	Soup, Tomato, condensed, prepared with equal volume of water	1 c	245	88	2.0	3	0.5	0	16	15	0.7	970	1,000	0.05	0.05	1.2	12
414.	Soup, Tomato with milk	1 c	248	160	6.0	6	2.9	17	22	159	1.8	932	850	0.13	0.25	1.5	68
415.	Soup, vegetable beef, condensed, prepared with equal volume of water	1 c	245	78	5.0	2	0.0	0	10	12	0.7	1,046	2,700	0.05	0.05	1.0	0
416.	Soup, Vegetarian vegetable	1 c	250	70	2.1	2	0.3	0	12	21	1.1	823	1,505	0.05	0.05	0.9	1
417.	Sour cream	1 tbsp	14	30	0.4	3	1.8	6	1	16	0.0	8	135	0.01	0.02	0.0	0
418.	Soup cream, imitation	1 tbsp.	14	29	0.3	3	2.5	1	1	0	0.0	14	0	0.00	0.00	0.0	0
419.	Spaghetti, in tomato sauce with cheese	1 c	250	260	8.8	9	2.0	10	37	80	2.3	955	1,080	0.25	0.18	2.3	13
420.	Spaghetti, plain, cooked	1 c	140	155	5.0	1	0.1	0	32	11	1.7	1	0	0.20	0.11	1.5	0
421.	Spaghetti, whole wheat, cooked	1 c	125	151	6.6	1	0.1	0	32	19	1.1	16	0	0.21	0.09	1.5	0
422.	Spaghetti, with meatballs and tomato sauce	1 c	248	332	18.6	11.7	3.0	75	39	124	3.7	1,009	1,590	0.25	0.30	4.0	22
423.	Spareribs, cooked	3 oz.	85	377	17.8	33	12.0	73	0	8	2.2	31	0	0.37	0.18	2.9	0
424.	Spinach, canned, drained	1/2 c	103	25	2.3	1	0.0	0	4	121	2.6	242	8,200	0.02	0.12	0.3	15
425.	Spinach, frozen, cooked, drained	1/2 c	103	24	3.1	0	0.0	0	4	116	2.2	54	8,100	0.07	0.16	0.4	20
426.	Spinach, raw, chopped	1 c	55	14	1.8	0	0.0	0	2	51	1.7	39	4,460	0.06	0.11	0.3	28
427.	Squash, summer, cooked	1/2 c	90	13	0.8	0	0.0	0	3	23	0.4	1	350	0.05	0.07	0.7	9
428.	Squash, winter, baked mashed	1/2 c	103	70	1.9	0	0.0	0	18	41	1.0	1	6,560	0.05	0.14	0.7	8
429.	Strawberries, frozen, sweetened	1 c	250	245	1.4	0	0.0	0	66	28	1.5	8	31	0.04	0.13	1.0	106
430.	Strawberries, raw	1 c	149	55	1.0	1	0.0	0	13	31	1.5	1	90	0.04	0.10	0.9	88
431.	Stuffing, bread, prepared	1/2 c	70	250	4.6	15	3.1	0	25	46	1.1	627	4,460	0.09	0.10	1.3	0
432.	Sundae, choc. Dairy Queen	medium	184	300	6.0	7	4.9	79	53	200	1.1	175	455	0.06	0.26	0.0	0
433.	Sugar, brown granulated	1 tsp	5	17	0.0	0	0.0	0	5	4	0.1	0	300	0.00	0.00	0.1	0
434.	Sugar, white granulated	1 tsp	4	15	0.0	0	0.0	0	4	0	0.0	0	0	0.00	0.00	0.0	0
435.	Super Roast Beef, Arby's	1	254	552	24	28	7.6	43	54	108	4.3	1,174	150	0.39	0.61	12.4	9
436.	Sweet N' Sour Sauce, McDonald's	1.12 oz.	32	60	0	0.2	0.1	0	14	0	0.0	190	300	0.00	0.00	0.0	25
437.	Sweet potato, baked	1 potato 5" long	146	161	2.4	1	0.0	0	37	46	1.0	14	9,230	0.10	0.08	0.8	25
438.	Syrup (maple)	1 tbsp	20	50	0.0	0	0.0	0	13	33	0.2	3	0	0.00	0.00	0.0	0
439.	Taco Salad, Wendy's	1	510	640	34	30	12.0	80	70	540	5.4	960	1,750	0.23	0.45	3.0	27
440.	Taco shell	1 shell	10	60	1.1	3	0.3	0	9	26	0.3	62	36	0.00	0.01	0.3	0
441.	Taco, Taco Bell	1	83	186	15.0	8	0.0	0	14	120	2.4	79	120	0.09	0.16	2.9	0
442.	Tangerine	1 med 2⅜" diam.	116	39	0.7	0	0.0	0	10	34	0.3	2	360	0.05	0.02	0.1	27
443.	Tartar sauce	1 tbsp.	14	74	0.2	8	1.2	4	1	3	0.1	182	54	0.00	0.00	0.0	0
444.	Tea, brewed	1/4 c	180	0	0.0	0	0.0	0	0	0	0.0	0	0	0.00	0.00	0.0	0

Code	Food	Amount	Weight gm	Calories	Protein gm	Fat gm	Sat. Fat gm	Cholesterol mg	Carbohydrate gm	Calcium mg	Iron mg	Sodium mg	Vit A I.U.	Thiamin (Vit B$_1$) mg	Riboflavin (Vit B$_2$) mg	Niacin mg	Vit C mg
445.	Tomato juice, canned	1 c	244	42	1.9	0	0.1	0	10	22	1.4	881	1,357	0.12	0.08	1.6	45
446.	Tomato sauce (catsup)	1 tbsp	15	16	0.3	0	0.0	0	4	3	0.1	156	105	0.01	0.01	0.2	2
447.	Tomato, canned	1/2 c	121	26	1.2	0	0.0	0	5	7	0.6	157	1,085	0.06	0.04	0.9	21
448.	Tomato, raw	1 tomato 3½ oz.	100	20	1.0	0	0.0	0	4	12	0.5	3	820	0.05	0.04	0.6	21
449.	Tortilla chips	1 oz.	28	139	2.2	8	1.1	0	17	82	1.0	140	7	0.01	0.02	0.2	0
450.	Tortilla, corn, lime	1 6" diam.	30	63	1.5	1	0.0	0	14	60	0.9	0	6	0.04	0.02	0.3	0
451.	Tortilla, flour	1	35	105	2.6	3	0.4	0	19	21	0.5	134	0	0.13	0.08	1.2	0
452.	Tostada	1	148	206	9.2	18	3.0	14	25	167	1.8	200	445	0.06	0.13	0.8	6
453.	Trout, broiled w/butter, lemon	3 oz.	85	175	21.0	9	4.1	71	0	26	1.0	122	300	0.07	0.07	2.3	1
454.	Tuna, canned, oil pack, drained	3 oz.	85	167	25.0	7	1.7	60	0	7	1.6	0	70	0.04	0.10	10.1	0
455.	Tuna, canned, water pack, solids and liquid	3½ oz.	99	126	27.7	1	0.0	55	0	16	1.6	161	0	0.00	0.10	13.2	0
456.	Turkey, Lite Roast Deluxe, Arby'	1	195	260	20	6	1.6	33	33	156	2.3	1,262	200	0.29	0.43	15.4	12
457.	Turkey, roast (light and dark mixed)	3 oz.	85	162	27.0	5	1.5	73	0	7	1.5	111	0	0.04	0.15	6.5	0
458.	Turnip, cooked, drained	1/2 c cubed	78	18	0.6	0	0.0	0	4	27	0.3	27	0	0.03	0.04	0.3	17
459.	Turnip greens, cooked drained	1/2 c	73	19	2.1	0	0.0	0	3	98	1.3	14	5,695	0.04	0.08	0.4	16
460.	Veal, cooked loin	3 oz.	85	199	22.0	11	4.0	90	0	9	2.7	55	0	0.06	0.21	4.6	0
461.	Veal cutlet, braised, broiled	3 oz.	85	185	23.0	9	4.0	109	0	9	0.8	56	5	0.06	0.21	4.6	0
462.	Vegetables, mixed, cooked	1 c	182	116	5.8	0	0.0	0	24	46	2.4	348	4,505	0.02	0.13	2.0	15
463.	Waffles	1 waffle	75	205	6.9	8	2.7	59	27	179	1.2	515	49	0.14	0.23	0.9	0
464.	Watermelon	1 c diced	160	42	0.8	0	0.0	0	10	11	0.8	2	940	0.05	0.05	0.3	11
465.	Wheat germ, plain toasted	1 tbsp	6	23	1.8	1	0.0	0	3	3	0.5	0	10	0.11	0.05	0.3	1
466.	Whiskey, gin, rum, vodka 90 proof	1/2 11 oz (jigger)	42	110	0	0	0.0	0	0	0	0.0	0	0	0.00	0.00	0.0	0
467.	Whopper, Burger King	1 sandwich	270	614	27.0	36	12.0	90	45	64	4.9	865	550	0.34	0.41	6.1	12
468.	Whopper with cheese, Burger King	1 sandwich	294	706	32.0	44	16.0	115	47	176	4.9	1,177	950	0.34	0.48	6.1	12
469.	Whopper, double, Burger King	1 sandwich	351	844	46.0	53	19.0	169	45	72	7.2	933	550	0.35	0.56	9.4	12
470.	Wine, dry table 12% alc.	3½ fl. oz.	102	87	0.1	0	0.0	0	4	9	0.4	5	0	0.00	0.01	0.1	0
471.	Wine, red dry 18.8% alc.	2 oz.	59	81	0.1	0	0.0	0	5	5	0.0	4	0	0.01	0.02	0.2	0
472.	Yeast, brewers	1 tbsp	8	23	3.1	0	0.0	0	3	17	1.4	10	0	1.25	0.34	3.0	0
473.	Yogurt, fruit	1 c	227	231	9.9	2	1.6	10	43	345	0.2	125	104	0.08	0.40	0.2	2
474.	Yogurt, nonfat, TCBY	4 oz.	113	110	4	0	0.0	0	23	96	0	45	0	0.03	0.14	0	0
475.	Yogurt, plain low fat	8-oz. container	226	113	7.7	4	2.3	15	12	271	0.1	115	150	0.09	0.41	0.2	2
476.	Yogurt, regular, TCBY	4 oz.	113	120	4	3	2.0	13	23	180	0.5	60	0	0.06	0.18	0	0
477.	Yogurt, sugar free, TCBY	4 oz.	113	80	4	0	0	0	18	96	0	40	200	0.06	0.18	0	0
478.	Yogurt, vanilla lowfat, McDonald's	3 oz.	85	105	4	1	0.3	3	22	120	0	80	100	0.03	0.18	0.4	0

"0" represents both less than 1 and 0

Sources:

Nutritive Value of American Foods in Common Units. *Agriculture Handbook No. 456*. U.S. Dept. of Agriculture. Washington, D.C. 1988.

Young, E. A., E. H. Brennan, and C. L. Irving, Guest Eds. Perspectives on Fast Foods. *Public Health Currents*, 19(1), 1979, Published by Ross Laboratories, Columbus, OH.

Dennison, D. *The Dine System: the Nutrition Plan For Better Health*. C. V. Mosby Company St. Louis, Missouri, 1982.

Pennington, S. A. T. and H. N. Church. *Food Values of Portions Commonly Used*. Harper and Row Publishers, New York, 1985.

Kullman, D. A. *ABC Milligram Cholesterol Diet Guide*. Merit Publications, Inc. North Miami Beach, Florida 1978.

Food Processor nutrient analysis software by Esha Corporation, P.O. Box 13028, Salem, Oregon, 97309. With permission.

GLOSSARY

A

Abstinence To refrain completely from engaging in a particular behavior.

Accommodating resistance Strength-training program that requires the use of special equipment with mechanical devices that provide a variable resistance, with the intent of overloading the muscle group maximally through the entire range of motion.

Acquired immunodeficiency syndrome (AIDS) Virus (HIV) that destroys the immune system.

Addiction Compulsive and uncontrollable behavior(s) or use of substance(s), most frequently drugs.

Adenosine triphosphate (ATP) A high-energy chemical compound used for immediate energy by the body.

Adipose tissue Fat cells.

Aerobic exercise Exercise that requires oxygen to produce the necessary energy (ATP) to carry out the activity.

AIDS See acquired immunodeficiency syndrome.

Alcohol (drinking alcohol) Known as ethyl alcohol, a depressant drug that affects the brain and slows down central nervous system activity.

Alcoholism Disease in which an individual loses control over drinking alcoholic-containing beverages.

Altruism The act of giving of oneself out of a genuine concern for other people.

Alveoli Air sacs in the lungs where gas exchange (oxygen and carbon dioxide) takes place.

Amenorrhea Cessation of regular menstrual flow.

Amino acids Chemical compounds that contain nitrogen, carbon, hydrogen, and oxygen. Amino acids are the basic building blocks that the body uses to build different types of protein.

Anabolic steroids Synthetic versions of the male sex hormone testosterone which promotes muscle development and hypertrophy.

Anabolism Process whereby simple substances are formed into more complex substances.

Anaerobic exercise Exercise which does not require oxygen to produce the necessary energy (ATP) to carry out the activity.

Aneurysm Weakness in the arterial wall allowing the formation of a balloon-like pouch.

Angina pectoris Chest pain.

Anorexia nervosa An eating disorder characterized by self-imposed starvation to lose and maintain very low body weight.

Antioxidants Compounds such as the vitamins C, E, beta-carotene (a precursor to vitamin A) and the mineral selenium which prevent oxygen from combining with other substances to which it may cause damage. Antioxidants are thought to play a key role in the prevention of heart disease and cancer.

Arteries Major vessels that carry blood away from the heart to bodily tissues.

Arteriosclerosis Hardening of the arteries.

Atherosclerosis Type of arteriosclerosis characterized by plaque formation or the buildup of fatty tissue in the inner layers of the wall of the arteries.

ATP See adenosine triphosphate.

Atrophy A decrease in the size of a cell.

Autogenics A stress management technique. It is a form of self-suggestion where an individual is able to place him/herself in an autohypnotic state by repeating and concentrating on feelings of heaviness and warmth in the extremities.

Autoimmune disease Illness in which the body's immune system turns against the body.

B

Ballistic or dynamic stretching (flexibility) Stretching exercises that are performed using jerky, rapid, and bouncy movements.

Basal cell carcinoma Type of skin cancer that occurs primarily on the face. It grows slow and rarely spreads to other parts of the body.

Basal metabolic rate The lowest level of oxygen consumption (uptake) necessary to sustain life.

Behavior modification A process to permanently change destructive or negative behaviors for positive behaviors that will lead to better health and well-being.

Benign Noncancerous.

Bereavement The process of disbonding from a person that had played an important role in one's life and is now gone.

Beta-carotene A precursor to vitamin A.

Bioelectrical impedance Technique to assess body composition, including percent body fat, by running a weak electrical current (totally painless) through the body.

Biofeedback Stress management technique. A process in which a person learns to reliably influence physiological responses of two kinds: either responses which are not ordinarily under voluntary control or responses which ordinarily are easily regulated but for which regulation has broken down due to trauma or disease.

Blood pressure   The pressure of the blood exerted against the walls of the arteries.

BMI   See body mass index.

Body composition   Term used in reference to the fat and nonfat components of the human body. Body composition is important in the assessment of recommended or "ideal" body weight.

Body density   The weight of the body per unit volume.

Body mass index (BMI)   Ratio of weight to height, usually expressed in kg/(mts)2.

Breathing techniques for relaxation   Stress management technique where the individual concentrates on "breathing away" the tension and inhaling fresh air to the entire body.

Brown fat cells   Cells that produce body heat by burning fat.

Bulimia   An eating disorder characterized by a pattern of binge eating and purging to attempt to lose and maintain low body weight.

Burnout   A state of physical and mental exhaustion.

C

CAD   Coronary artery disease, see coronary heart disease.

Caffeine   A central nervous system stimulating drug most frequently found in coffee, tea, and colas.

Calorie   A unit to measure heat energy. A calorie (also referred to as small calorie) is the amount of heat necessary to raise the temperature of one gram of water one degree Centigrade. Short term for kilocalorie and it is used to measure the energy value of food and cost of physical activity.

Calorimeter   Equipment used to measure the caloric value of food or heat production of animals and humans.

Cancer   Group of diseases characterized by uncontrolled growth and spread of abnormal cells into malignant tumors.

Cancer-prone personality   Behavior pattern characterized by little demonstration of emotion, ambivalence toward self and others, and "distance" from others, including parents.

Cannabis sativa   Hemp plant from which marijuana and hashish are derived.

Capillary   Smallest blood vessels carrying oxygenated blood in the body.

Carbohydrates   Compounds containing carbon, hydrogen, and oxygen. Carbohydrates are the major source of energy for the human body.

Carbon monoxide   The carcinogenic gas emitted in automobile exhaust.

Carcinogens   Substances that contribute to the formation of cancers.

Cardiac output   Amount of blood ejected by the heart in one minute.

Cardiovascular diseases   Diseases that affects the heart and the circulatory system (blood vessels). Examples of cardiovascular diseases are coronary heart disease, peripheral vascular disease, congenital heart disease, rheumatic heart disease, atherosclerosis, strokes, high blood pressure, and congestive heart failure.

Cardiovascular endurance   The ability of the lungs, heart, and blood vessels to deliver adequate amounts of oxygen to the cells to meet the demands of prolonged (aerobic) physical activity.

Catabolism   Process whereby complex substances are broken down into more simple substances.

Catecholamines   Hormones, includes epinephrine and norepinephrine.

Cellulite   Term frequently used in reference to fat deposits that "bulge out." These deposits are nothing but enlarged fat cells due to excessive accumulation of body fat.

CHD   See coronary heart disease.

Chlamydia   A sexually transmitted disease caused by a bacterial infection that can cause significant damage to the reproductive system and may occur without symptoms.

Cholesterol   A waxy substance that is technically a steroid alcohol found only in animal fats and oil.

Chronic diseases   Diseases that develop over a prolonged period of time, usually associated to unhealthy lifestyle factors (hypertension, atherosclerosis, coronary disease, strokes, diabetes, and cancer).

Chronic obstructive pulmonary disease (COPD)   An air flow limiting disease that includes diseases such as chronic bronchitis and emphysema.

Chronological age   Actual age of the individual (also see functional age).

Cocaine   2-beta-carbomethoxy-3-betabenozoxytropane the primary psychoactive ingredient derived from coca plant leaves. Also referred to as coke, C, snow, blow, toot, flake, Peruvian lady, white girl, and happy dust.

Coenzyme   Nonprotein molecule required in enzyme reactions.

Complex carbohydrates   Carbohydrates formed by three or more simple sugar molecules linked together, also referred to as polysaccharides. Commonly used to designate foods high in starch.

Compound fats   A combination of simple fats with other chemicals. Examples of compound fats are phospholipids, glucolipids, and lipoproteins.

Concentric muscle contraction   Shortening of fibers during muscle contraction.

Congenital heart disease   Heart defects present at birth.

Coronary arteries   Arteries that supply the myocardium or heart muscle with oxygen and nutrients.

Coronary heart disease   Disease caused by the obstruction of the coronary arteries by plaque formation (also see atherosclerosis).

Crack   Cocaine mixed with ammonia, baking soda, and water then heated and smoked; freebasing.

Cruciferous vegetables   Plants that produce cross-shaped leaves (cauliflower, broccoli, cabbage, Brussels sprouts, and kohlrabi). These vegetables seem to have a protective effect against cancer.

D

Daily Values Standard nutrition values developed by the Food and Drug Administration (FDA) for use on food labels.

Dehydration A loss of body water below normal volume.

Delta-9-tetrahydrocannabinol The addictive psychoactive drug found in marijuana.

Deoxyribonucleic acid (DNA) Genetic material, substance of which genes are made.

Derived fats A combination of simple and compound fats.

Diabetes mellitus Condition where the blood glucose is unable to enter the cells because the pancreas either totally stops producing insulin or produces an insufficient amount for the body's needs.

Diastolic blood pressure Pressure exerted by the blood against the walls of the arteries during the relaxation phase (diastole) of the heart.

Dietary fiber Fiber in plant foods that cannot be digested by the human body.

Dietary induced thermogenesis (DIT) Extra amount of heat production caused by the metabolism of food.

Disaccharides Simple carbohydrates formed by two monosaccharide units linked together, one of which is glucose. The major disaccharides are sucrose, lactose, and maltose.

Distress Negative stress. Refers to unpleasant or harmful stress under which health and performance begin to deteriorate.

DIT See dietary induced thermogenesis.

DNA See deoxyribonucleic acid.

DRV (Daily Reference Values) Standards for nutrients and food components that do not have an established RDA (carbohydrate, fat, saturated fat, fiber, cholesterol, and sodium).

Drug chemical substance that has the potential to alter the structure and functioning of a living organism.

Dysmenorrhea Painful menstruation.

E

Eccentric muscle contraction Lengthening of fibers during muscle contraction.

ECG See electrocardiogram.

EKG See electrocardiogram.

Elastic elongation (flexibility) Refers to an elastic or temporary lengthening of soft tissue (muscles, tendons, and ligaments).

Electrocardiogram (ECG or EKG) A recording of the electrical activity of the heart.

Emphysema Pulmonary disease caused by distention (overinflation) of the alveoli.

Endorphines Morphine-like substances released from the pituitary gland in the brain during prolonged aerobic exercise. They are thought to induce feelings of euphoria and natural well-being.

Endurance See cardiovascular endurance and muscular endurance.

Energy The ability to do work.

Enzyme A catalyst that facilitates chemical reactions.

Epidemiology Science that studies the relationship between diverse factors (lifestyle and environmental) and the occurrence of disease.

Essential amino acids Amino acids that must be obtained in the diet because they cannot be produced in the body.

Essential fat Minimal amount of body fat needed for normal physiological functions. It constitutes about 3 percent of the total fat in men and 12 percent in women.

Estrogen Female sex hormone. Essential for bone formation and bone density conservation.

Eumenorrhea Normal menstrual cycle.

Eustress Positive stress: health and performance continue to improve, even as stress increases.

Exercise adherence Initiating and participating in an exercise program for life.

Exercise electrocardiogram An exercise test during which the workload is gradually increased (until the subject reaches maximal fatigue) with blood pressure and twelve-lead electrocardiographic monitoring throughout the test.

Exercise intolerance Exercise conducted at intensity levels well beyond a person functional capacity leading to symptoms such as very rapid or irregular heart rate, labored breathing, nausea, vomiting, light-headedness, headaches, dizziness, pale skin, flushness, excessive weakness, lack of energy, shakiness, sore muscles, cramps, and tightness in the chest.

Exercise tolerance test See exercise electrocardiogram.

Explanatory style A belief system; the way people perceive the events in their lives — i.e., optimistically or pessimistically.

F

Fatigue The inability to maintain a given workload.

Fats Compounds made by a combination of triglycerides.

Fiber A form of complex carbohydrate made up of plant material that cannot be digested by the human body.

Fight or flight mechanism Physiological response of the body to stress which prepares the individual to take action by stimulating the vital defense systems.

Flexibility The ability of a joint to move freely through its full range of motion.

Fraud See quackery.

Freebasing *See* Crack.

Free fatty acids (FFA) Fatty acids released by the breakdown of triglycerides.

Free radicals See oxygen free radicals.

Functional age Physiological age of the individual. Usually lower than the chronological (actual) age in fit people and vice versa in unfit people.

G

General adaptation syndrome The stress response, or "fight or flight," in which the body manifests a series of biological changes in response to a stressor.

Genetics Science that studies genetic or hereditary conditions.

Genital warts A sexually transmitted disease caused by a viral infection. Genital warts increase the risk of cervical cancer. Enlargement and spread of the warts leads to obstruction of the urethra, vagina, and anus.

Girth measurements technique Technique to assess body composition, including percent body fat, by measuring circumferences at various body sites.

Glucose Blood sugar, type of carbohydrate (monosaccharide), a primary source of energy for the human body.

Glucose intolerance Inability to properly metabolize glucose.

Glycogen Form of carbohydrate (polysaccharide) storage in muscle.

Glycolysis Breakdown of glucose to pyruvic or lactic acid.

Gonorrhea A sexually transmitted disease caused by a bacterial infection that can lead to pelvic inflammation in women, infertility, widespread bacterial infection, heart damage, arthritis in men and women, and blindness in children born to infected women.

H

Hardiness The ability to resist the negative effects of stress.

HDL See high density lipoprotein.

Health The balance of the physical, emotional, social, and spiritual aspects of personality that is conducive to optimal well-being.

Health promotion Programs aimed at helping people develop healthy lifestyle behaviors that will lead to a higher state of wellness.

Health-related fitness Refers to fitness components that when enhanced lead to better health (cardiovascular endurance, body composition, muscular strength and endurance, and muscular flexibility).

Heart attack See myocardial infarct

Heart rate reserve The difference between the maximal heart rate and the resting heart rate.

Heat cramps Muscle cramps caused by heat-induced changes in electrolyte balance in muscle cells.

Heat exhaustion Heat-related condition; symptoms include fainting, dizziness, profuse sweating, cold clammy skin, headaches and a rapid, weak pulse.

Heat stroke Heat-related emergency; symptoms include serious disorientation, warm dry skin, no sweating, rapid full pulse, vomiting, diarrhea, unconsciousness, and high body temperature.

Hemoglobin Protein-iron compound in red blood cells that transports oxygen in the blood.

Herpes A sexually transmitted disease caused by a viral infection (herpes simplex virus types I and II). No known cure is available for the disease. The disease is characterized by the appearance of sores on the mouth, genitals, rectum, or other parts of the body.

Hidden fat Fat in food that can not be readily observed (lean meats contain about 30 to 40 percent fat calories).

High density lipoprotein (HDL) Cholesterol-transporting molecules in the blood. High HDL-cholesterol (good cholesterol) seems to offer protection against some forms of cardiovascular disease.

HIV See human immunodeficiency virus.

Homeostasis State of balance within body systems that allows a person to react to stressors in a healthful manner.

Human immunodeficiency virus (HIV) Virus that causes acquired immunodeficiency syndrome (AIDS).

Human papilloma virus (HPV) Genital warts: a sexually transmitted disease.

Hydrostatic weighing Underwater weighing technique to assess body composition, including percent body fat.

Hyperglycemia Elevated blood sugar (glucose).

Hyperlipidemia Elevated blood fats or lipids.

Hyperplasia An increase in the number of cells.

Hypertension Chronically elevated blood pressure.

Hypertrophy An increase in the size of the cell (for example, muscle hypertrophy).

Hypoglycemia Low blood sugar (glucose).

Hypokinetic disease Diseases associated with a lack of physical activity (for example, hypertension, coronary heart disease, obesity, and diabetes).

I

Imagery Vivid mental visualization.

Insulin Hormone secreted by the pancreas that increases the absorption and utilization of glucose by the body.

Interval training Training method with repeated bouts of exercise with rest intervals between each exercise bout.

Ischemia Lack of blood flow.

Isokinetic contraction Muscular contraction at a constant velocity.

Isokinetic training Strength-training method where the speed of the muscle contraction is kept constant because the equipment (machine) provides an accommodating resistance to match the user's force (maximal) through the range of motion.

Isometric training Strength-training method that refers to a muscle contraction producing little or no movement, such as pushing or pulling against immovable objects.

Isotonic training Strength-training method that refers to a muscle contraction with movement, such as lifting an object over the head.

K

Kilocalorie A unit to measure heat energy. A kilocalorie (kcal) or large calorie is the amount of heat necessary to raise the temperature of one kilogram of water one degree Centigrade. One kcal equals 1,000 calories.

L

Lactic acid Strong acid, end product of anaerobic glycolysis (metabolism).

Lactovegetarians Vegetarians who also eat foods from the milk group.

LDL See low density lipoprotein.

Lean body mass Body weight without body fat.

Life experiences survey Questionnaire used to assess sources of stress in life.

Loneliness The result of a breakdown of a person's network of social relationships.

Locus of control A person's perception of how much influence he or she has over life events; at extreme ends of the continuum are *external* and *internal*.

Low density lipoprotein (LDL) Cholesterol-transporting molecules in the blood. High LDL-cholesterol (bad cholesterol) seems to increase the risk for some forms of cardiovascular disease.

M

Malignant melanoma Deadliest of all types of skin cancer. Tumors grow at a rapid rate and readily spread to other parts of the body if not treated at an early stage.

Marijuana A psychoactive drug prepared from a mixture of crushed leaves, flowers, small branches, stems, and seeds from the hemp plant cannabis sativa. Also referred to as pot and grass.

Max VO$_2$ See maximal oxygen uptake

Maximal oxygen uptake (Max VO$_2$) The maximal amount of oxygen that the body is able to utilize per minute of physical activity, commonly expressed in ml/kg/min. The best indicator of cardiovascular or aerobic fitness.

Meditation Stress management technique used to gain control over one's attention, clearing the mind and blocking out the stressor(s) responsible for the increased tension.

Megadose (of vitamins) Large amount of vitamin(s) intake. For most vitamins, a megadose is ten times the RDA or more.

Metabolism All energy and material transformations that occur within living cells necessary to sustain life.

Metastasis The spread of cancer that occurs when cancer cells from a growth breaks off and enter other parts of the body through the blood or lymph system.

METS (metabolic equivalents) A measurement unit of resting energy expenditure. One MET is the equivalent of 3.5 ml/kg/min.

Minerals Inorganic elements found in the body and in food which are essential for normal body functions.

Mitochondria Structures within the cells where energy transformations take place.

Monosaccharides The simplest carbohydrates (sugars) formed by five- or six-carbon skeletons. The three most common monosaccharides are glucose, fructose, and galactose.

Monounsaturated fat Fatty acids with only one double bond found along the carbon atom chain.

Motor skill-related fitness Refers to fitness components that when improved lead to enhanced athletic performance (agility, balance, coordination, power, reaction time, and speed).

Motor unit The combination of a motor neuron and the muscle fibers that it innervates.

Muscle fiber A muscle cell.

Muscular endurance (localized muscular endurance) The ability of a muscle to exert submaximal force repeatedly over a period of time (for example, 30 repetitions on a bench press exercise). It usually implies a specific muscle group (chest, thighs, abdominals).

Muscular strength The ability of a muscle to exert maximum force against resistance (for example, 1 repetition maximum or 1 RM on the bench press exercise).

Myocardial infarct Death of part of the myocardium.

Myocardium Heart muscle.

Myoglobin Iron-containing compound that holds oxygen in muscle tissue.

N

Neuron A nerve cell.

Nicotine Poisonous compound found in tobacco leaves.

Nonessential amino acids Amino acids that can be manufactured in the body, therefore, the do not have to be obtained in the diet.

Nulliparity Never having had a child.

Nutrient density Ratio of nutrients to calories in food.

Nutrient Substance found in food that provide energy, regulate metabolism, and help with growth and repair of body tissues.

Nutrition Science that studies the relationship of foods to optimal health and performance.

O

Obesity Refers to an excessive accumulation of body fat, usually about 30 percent above recommended body weight according to body size.

Oligomenorrhea Irregular menstrual cycles.

Omega-3 fatty acids Polyunsaturated fatty acids found primarily in cold water seafood and are thought to be effective in lowering blood cholesterol and triglycerides.

One repetition maximum (1 RM) The maximal amount of resistance (weight) that an individual is able to lift in a single effort.

Osteoporosis Softening, deterioration, or loss of total body bone.

Overload principle Key training concept stating that the demands placed on a system (cardiovascular, muscular) must be systematically and progressively increased over time to cause physiologic adaptation (development or improvement).

Ovolactovegetarians Vegetarians who include egg and milk products in their diet.

Ovovegetarians Vegetarians who allow eggs in their diet.

Oxygen free radicals Substances formed during metabolism which attack and damage proteins and lipids, in particular the cell membrane and DNA; leading to the development of diseases such as heart disease, cancer, and emphysema. Antioxidants are believed to exert a protective effect by absorbing free radicals before they can cause damage and also by interrupting the sequence of reactions once damage has begun.

P

Pelvic Inflammatory Disease Severe infection of the lining of the abdominal cavity most commonly caused by chlamydia and gonorrhea.

Percent body fat Term used in body composition assessment. It represents the total amount of fat in the body based on the person's weight. It includes both essential and storage fat.

Peripheral vascular disease Narrowing of the peripheral blood vessels (it excludes the cerebral and coronary arteries).

Personality The whole of one's personal characteristics; the pattern of behavior that distinguishes a person.

Physical fitness (health-related) The general capacity to adapt and respond favorably to physical effort, implying that individuals are physically fit when they can meet the ordinary as well as the unusual demands of daily life safely and effectively without being overly fatigued, and still have energy left for leisure and recreational activities.

Plastic elongation (flexibility) Refers to a permanent lengthening of soft tissue (capsules, tendons, and ligaments).

PNF See proprioceptive neuromuscular facilitation.

Polyunsaturated fat Fatty acids with two or more double bonds along the carbon atom chain.

Prevention index An annual measure of the effort Americans are making to prevent disease and accidents and to promote good health and longevity. The index is based on the 21 most significant health-promoting behaviors in the United States.

Progressive muscle relaxation Stress management technique. It involves progressive contraction and relaxation of muscle groups throughout the body.

Proprioceptive neuromuscular facilitation (PNF for flexibility development) Stretching technique in which muscles are progressively stretched out with intermittent isometric contractions.

Protein Complex organic compounds containing nitrogen and formed by combinations of amino acids. Proteins are the main substances used in the body to build and repair tissues such as muscles, blood, internal organs, skin, hair, nails, and bones. They are also part of hormones, antibodies, and enzymes.

Psychoneuroimmunology The scientific investigation of how the brain affects the body's system.

PSA test Protein-specific antigen blood test used to help diagnose prostate cancer.

Q

Quackery (fraud) The conscious promotion of unproven claims for profit.

R

Rate of perceived exertion (RPE) A perception scale to monitor or interpret the intensity of aerobic exercise.

RDA See recommended dietary allowances.

RDI (Reference Daily Intakes) Reference values and minerals for protein, vitamins.

Recommended dietary allowances (RDA) Daily recommended intakes of nutrients for normal, healthy people in the United States.

Red muscle fibers (slow-twitch or type I) Muscle fibers with greater aerobic potential and slow speed of contraction.

Reframing Changing the way one looks at the world.

Relaxation response An innate bodily reaction that counteracts the harmful effects of stress.

Repetition (in strength training) The number of times that a given resistance is performed (for example, 12 repetitions on the bench press exercise).

Repetition maximum (in strength training) The maximum number of repetitions (RM) that can be performed with a specific resistance or weight (for example, 10 RM with 150 pounds).

Residual volume Volume of air left in the lungs following complete exhalation.

Resistance (in strength training) The amount of weight that is lifted.

Ribonucleic acid (RNA) Genetic material involved in the formation of cell proteins.

Risk factors Lifestyle and genetic factors that may lead to disease.

RNA See ribonucleic acid.

RPE See rate of perceived exertion.

S

Saturated fat Fatty acids with carbon atoms fully saturated with hydrogens, therefore only single bonds link the carbon atoms on the chain. High intake of saturated fats increases the risk for coronary heart disease.

Self-esteem A sense of positive self-regard.

Self-efficacy One's perception of his or her ability to do specific things.

Serum cholesterol Blood cholesterol level.

Set (in strength training) A number of repetitions (1 set of 12 repetitions).

Setpoint theory The weight control theory that indicates that the body has an established weight and strongly attempts to maintain that weight.

Sexually transmitted diseases (STDs) Diseases spread through sexual contact.

Shin Splints Injury to the lower leg characterized by pain and irritation in the shin region or front of the leg.

Simple carbohydrates Carbohydrates formed by simple or double sugar units with little nutritive value (for example, candy, pop, cakes, etc.), frequently denoted as sugars. Simple carbohydrates are divided into monosaccharides and disaccharides.

Simple fats A glyceride molecule linked to one, two, or three units of fatty acids (monoglycerides, diglycerides, and triglycerides).

Skinfold thickness Technique to assess body composition, including percent body fat, by measuring the thickness of a double fold of skin at different body sites.

Slow-sustained or static stretching (flexibility) Stretching technique where the muscles are gradually lengthened through a joint's complete range of motion and the final position is held for a few seconds.

Specificity of training Training programs must be specifically aimed at the desired outcome. This is accomplished by training with the specific activity that the person is attempting to improve (aerobic, anaerobic, strength, flexibility).

Sphygmomanometer Equipment used to measure blood pressure. Consists of an inflatable bladder contained within a cuff and a mercury gravity manometer or an aneroid manometer from which the pressure is read.

Spiritual well-being An affirmation of life in a relationship with God, self, community, and environment that nurtures and celebrates wholeness.

Spot reducing Theory that claims that exercising a specific body part (for example, abdominal or midsection of the body) will result in significant fat reduction in that area. It does not work! (See Chapter 7 — Exercise: The Key to Successful Weight Loss and Weight Maintenance).

Squamous cell carcinoma Type of skin cancer that grows at a faster rate that basal cell carcinomas and seems to grow on sun-damaged areas. Squamous cell tumors spread to other parts of the body if not treated at an early stage.

STDs See sexually transmitted diseases

Storage fat Body fat in excess of the essential fat. It is stored in adipose tissue.

Strength See muscular strength.

Strength training A conditioning program that requires the use of weights to help increase muscular strength, endurance, power, and/or body size.

Stress The nonspecific response of the human organism to any demand that is placed upon it.

Stress buffers Factors that alleviate the deleterious effects of stress such as social support, a sense of control, physical fitness, a sense of humor, self-esteem, optimism, advantageous coping styles, and hardiness.

Stress test See exercise electrocardiogram.

Stressor Reaction of the organism to a stress-causing event.

Stroke volume Amount of blood ejected by the heart in one beat.

Structured Interview Assessment tool used in determining behavioral patterns (Type A and B personality).

Syphilis A sexually transmitted disease caused by a bacterial infection. During the last stage of the disease, some people will suffer from paralysis, crippling, blindness, heart disease, brain damage, insanity, and even death.

Systolic blood pressure Pressure exerted by the blood against the walls of the arteries during the forceful contraction (systole) of the heart.

T

Tar Chemical compound that forms during the burning of tobacco leaves.

Testosterone Male sex hormone.

Triglycerides Fats formed by glycerol and three fatty acids.

Type A (personality) Behavior pattern characteristic of a hard-driving, overambitious, aggressive, at times hostile, and overly competitive person.

Type B (personality) Behavior pattern characteristic of a calmed, casual, relaxed, and easy-going individual.

Type C (personality) Behavior pattern of individuals who are just as highly stressed as the Type A but do not seem to be at higher risk for disease than the Type B.

U

U.S. RDA The United States recommended daily allowances used between the late 1960s and the early 1990s. Derived from the RDA and developed as a standard for nutrition labeling.

V

Vasoconstriction Narrowing or clamping down of blood vessels.

Vasodilation Widening or opening up of blood vessels.

Vegans Vegetarians who eat no animal products at all.

Vegetarian Individuals whose diet is of vegetable or plant origin.

Veins Major vessels that carry blood back to the heart.

Very low density lipoprotein (VLDL) Triglyceride, cholesterol and phospholipid-transporting molecules in the blood. Only a small amount of cholesterol is carried by the VLDL molecules.

Viral hepatitis An infection that causes inflammation of the liver; has four identified types.

Vitamins Organic substances essential for normal metabolism, growth, and development of the body.

VLDL See very low density lipoprotein.

W

Waist-to-Hip Ratio Test designed by a panel of scientists appointed by the National Academy of Sciences and the Dietary Guidelines Advisory Council for the U.S. Departments of Agriculture and Health and Human Services to assess potential risk for diseases associated with obesity.

Weight training A conditioning program that requires the use of weights to help increase muscular strength, endurance, power, and/or body size.

Weight-regulating mechanism Mechanism located in the hypothalamus of the brain that regulates how much the body should weigh (also see setpoint theory).

Wellness The complete integration of physical, mental, emotional, social, and spiritual well-being — a complex interaction of the factors that lead to a quality life.

White muscle fibers (fast-twitch or type II) Muscle fibers with greater anaerobic potential and fast speed of contraction.

Work The ability to utilize energy.

Workload A given level of exercise intensity or physical performance.

Y

Yellow fat cells Cells used for fat storage (stores of energy in the form of fat).

Yoga An exercise technique known to induce calm and invigorate the mind as well as improve strength, flexibility, and endurance.

INDEX

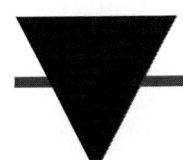

Absenteeism, work, 117, 278
Addiction, 75, 192, 223
    to caffeine, 282
    definition of, 278
    managing, 295–296
    overcoming, 300–302
    and personality, 279–281
    risk factors of, 281
Adipose tissue, 181, 225. *See also* Fat, body
Adler, Robert, 46
Adrenaline, 23, 29, 61
Aerobic exercise, 29, 30, 121, 134–135, 139, 146, 151, 191, 218, 246, 248
    and cardiovascular system, 240, 242, 243, 247–249
    and weight management, 225, 227, 228
Affirmations, 98, 100
Affleck, Glenn, 97
Age and aging, 145, 226–227, 247
    and cancer, 261, 262, 264
AIDS, 311-312
    and self–esteem, 98
    treatment, 315–316
    as a virus, 255
Alcohol consumption, 10, 82, 187, 190, 191, 192, 195, 295, 319
    addiction to, 284, 287–289, 298–300
    and cancer, 252, 254, 262, 264, 266, 267
    and heart disease, 244–248, 249
    and pregnancy, 289
Allergies, 25, 49
Altruism, 104–106
American Cancer Society, 248, 252, 258, 264, 266, 270
American College of Sports Medicine, 115, 121, 136, 137, 144
American Council on Science and Health, 10, 174
American Digestive Disease Society, 50
American Heart Association, 176, 179, 238, 239, 240–241, 245, 248
American Institute on Stress, 20, 21
American Lung Association, 248
American Medical Association, 46, 107, 118
American Psychological Association, 50
Amino acids, 175, 192. *See also* Proteins
Amphetamines, 225
Anaerobic exercise, 135, 191
Andrews, Howard, 105
Anemia, 187, 223, 289
Angell, Marcia, 50
Anger, 8, 51, 55, 94, 102
    definition of, 56
    and health, 56–58
Anorexia nervosa, 86, 223–224
Anson, Carol, 50
Anthropometric measurement, 207, 219
Antibodies, 48, 90
Antioxidants, 184, 191–192, 243, 248

Anxiety, 60–61, 94, 98, 106
Appetite, 181, 225
Ardell, Donald, 5
Arrowsmith - Lowe, Janet, 316
Arteries, coronary, 24, 239
Arthritis, rheumatoid, 55–56
Asthma, 22, 50, 86
Atherosclerosis, 76, 95, 114, 222, 238, 242, 244, 245, 247
Athletes, diet for, 198
ATP, 190–191
Atrophy, muscular, 140
Attitude, 56, 66, 75, 94, 95, 98, 100, 108, 252, 318
Autogenics, 35
Autoimmune disorders, 49, 55, 95

Back pain, 22, 106, 124, 135, 145, 147
    exercises to relieve, 148, 168–172
Ballistic stretching, 145–146
Barnard, James, 243
Benson, Herbert, 25, 33, 102, 106
Bereavement, 89–90
Bernikow, Louise, 75
Beta–carotene, 184, 191, 243, 248
Bioelectrical impedance technique, 212, 216
Biofeedback, 35–36
Blair, Steve, 114
Blood pressure, 136, 240, 241, 247
    control, 248–249
    high, 24, 61, 71, 80, 83, 84, 97, 106, 176, 189, 192, 239, 240, 244, 245, 248, 282, 289, 294
    measuring, 245, 249–250, 285
Blumberg, Eugene, 53–54
Body composition, 119, 120, 141, 227, 232, 246
    assessing, 207–208, 212, 216–217, 218
    definition of, 206
Body fat, 115, 136, 141, 147, 206, 246
    essential, 115, 136, 141, 147, 206
    storage, 206
Body mass, lean, 141, 206, 218, 226–227. *See also* Body composition
Body Mass Index (BMI), 216–217, 218, 220
Body weight, recommended, 10, 135, 192, 206, 217–218, 222, 246, 248
    and cancer, 266
Booth–Kewley, Stephanie, 50
Boredom, 67, 75, 281, 302
Borg, Gunner, 138
Borysenko, Joan, 55, 102
Brain, 23–24, 46, 47–48, 95, 108, 225
Breathing exercises, 34–35
Bro, Harmon, 105
Brody, Jane, 175
Brown, Jonathon,, 29–30
Bulimia, 224

Burnout, 105
    preventing, 32–33
Byrd, Randy, 102

Caffeine, 24, 29, 187, 189, 190, 249, 282
Calcium, 175, 184, 186–187, 192, 267
Califano, Joseph, 2, 3
Calipers, for measuring skinfold thickness, 207, 218
Calisthenics, 139, 145, 146
Calories, 28, 114, 139, 140–141, 175
    fat, 175–176, 192, 193, 243, 266
    and weight management, 222, 224–225, 226, 227–228, 229, 230–231, 246
Cancer, 72, 114, 192, 243
    bladder, 253, 263, 285
    breast, 58, 95, 97, 100, 106, 261–262, 267, 289
    cervical, 255, 262, 298, 307, 308, 309;
    colon, 182, 254, 256, 261
    definition of, 252
    and dietary fat, 175, 176
    and emotions, 86
    and explanatory style, 95
    and a fighting spirit, 100
    and hope, 108, 110
    incidence of, 252–253
    leukemia, 255
    and loneliness, 77
    and loss, 87-88
    lung, 110, 253, 260–261, 264, 284
    and marriage, 84
    and obesity, 222
    oral, 264, 285, 298
    ovarian, 262
    pancreatic, 263–264, 285
    preventing, 264–267
    prostate, 263
    risk factors for, 252, 258–259
    skin, 54, 94–95, 257, 260, 264–266, 312
    and smoking/ tobacco, 244, 253–254
    types of, 256–257
    uterine, 262
Cancer–prone personality, 50, 53–55, 256
Capillaries, 136
Carbohydrates, 174, 181, 182–184, 192, 195, 225, 230, 231, 243, 246
Carcinogens, 253, 254, 264, 291
Carcinomas, 256–257
Cardiac output, 136
Cardiovascular: endurance, 119, 120–121, 134–136, 137, 239–240
    fitness, 114–115, 139, 230, 240, 250
    system, 24, 136, 137, 138, 139–140, 247
Cardiovascular disease, 22, 25, 90, 103, 114, 222, 230. *See also* Heart disease
    and cholesterol, 242–243
    incidence of, 238
    preventing, 247–249

341

risk factors for, 238, 239, 240
and smoking, 244
Case, Robert, 76
Catecholamines, 61, 247, 249
Cellulite, 228
Centanni, Russell, 316
Center for Drug Evaluation and Research, 316
Challenge, 26, 31, 66–67
Chlamydia, 305-306
Cholesterol, 2, 10, 24, 115, 176, 179, 182, 192, 195, 239, 240, 241, 247, 248, 250, 267
    definition of, 242; HDL, 239, 240, 242–243, 244, 282
    LDL, 242–243, 244, 248
    VLDLs, 244
Church affiliation, 103–104
Chylomicrons, 244
Cigarette smoking, 10, 115, 186, 226
    and cancer, 252, 253–254, 260–261, 262, 263, 264, 267
    deaths from, 244
    and heart disease, 239, 240, 241, 242, 243
    quitting, 248, 249, 264, 285
    and second–hand smoke, 244, 261, 282, 284, 296–298
Circulatory system, 95, 120, 238
Clemons, Samuel, 98
Cobb, Sidney, 70
Cocaine, 291, 294
Cohen, Sheldon, 25
Cohn, Jeffrey, 85
Commitment, 9, 26, 55, 66, 232, 250
Common sense, 6
Communication, in families, 86
Community, sense of, 73, 83
Confidence, 8, 67
Confiding, 79
Control, 26, 66, 70, 71
    locus of, 96–98
Coronary heart disease (CHD), 239–242, 245, 246, 250. *See also* Cardiovascular; Heart disease
    and smoking, 248, 298
Cool down, 121, 139, 145
Cooper, Kenneth, 240
Coping, 97–98, 107
Coronary–prone personality, 50–52
Corticosteroids, 49, 90, 97
Cortisol, 76
Courtney, Joseph G., 256
Cousins, Norman, 8, 46–47, 96–97, 108, 110
Creativity, 6, 26, 280
Curiosity, 6, 20
Cyclamates, 254

Daradik, Irving, 30
Death. *See* Mortality
DeBusk, Robert, 139
Denial, 107, 108, 110
    in grief, 88
Depression, 61, 63, 83, 94, 105
    and divorce, 82
    and eating disorders, 223

and the heart, 62, 64
and hormones, 97
and the immune system, 62
and mother's effect on baby, 85
social support, 71
deSaint–Pierre, Michel, 94
Descartes, 47
Diabetes, 86, 114, 176, 181, 216, 222, 239, 240, 295
    and cancer, 262
    and heart disease, 246
Diet: anti–cancer, 266–267
    balanced, 27–29
    and cancer, 252, 253, 254, 261
    and cholesterol, 243–244
    and dieting, 225, 230, 246
    guidelines, 175, 176, 181, 182, 186, 192–193
    to prevent heart disease, 248–249
    industry, 222
    supplementation, 191–192
    typical, 174, 176
    for weight loss, 227
Direct gas analysis, 121
Disaccharides, 181
Disease: cardiovascular, 22, 25, 238
    chronic, 114, 238, 243
    gastrointestinal, 22, 25
    hypokinetic, 135
    musculoskeletal, 22
    and personality, 50, 67
    preventing, 46, 115, 238, 247
    recovering from, 100
    respiratory, 22, 25, 50
    and social support, 71
    and stress, 21–22
Distress, 20
Divorce, 82–83
    children of, 83
    and longevity, 84
DNA, 184, 243, 252
Duration of exercise, 136, 139
Duszynski, Karen, 75
Dysmenorrhea, 145
Dysphoria, 94

Eating disorders, 222, 223
    and explanatory style, 94
    and stress, 22
Economic impacts: of HIV and AIDS, 316
    of illness, 117
Edwards, Patrick, 85
Eisom, Wayne, 100
Electrocardiogram (ECG), 118, 137, 230, 239, 249–250
Electrolytes, 223
Emotions, 46, 48, 70
    and addiction, 278
    and cancer, 55, 86, 252
    and children of divorce, 82
    and divorce, 82
    positive, 94, 104
Endocrine system, 24
Endorphins, 48, 49, 97, 105
Endurance: cardiovascular, 119, 120–121, 134–136, 137
    muscular, 119, 124–126, 140, 143, 144

sports, 151
Energy, 190–191, 223, 243
Energy–balancing equation, 224–225
Engle, George, 90
Environmental influences/pollutants, 3, 4, 499, 255
    and cancer, 252, 255, 261, 262, 264
Enzymes, 136, 175, 230, 252
Epstein–Barr, 25, 76, 252, 255
Estrogen, and cancer, 252, 256, 261, 262
Eustress, 20
Exercise, 114, 120, 139, 186
    abdominal, 144
    aerobic, 29, 30, 121, 134–135, 139, 146, 151, 191, 218
    anaerobic, 135, 191
    benefits of, 115, 117
    and blood pressure, 240, 243
    duration of, 139
    equipment for, 151
    for flexibility, 162–168
    frequency of, 139, 144
    intensity, 137–139, 146–147
    intolerance, 149
    mode of, 139, 145–146
    regular, 10, 29–30, 115, 139, 151, 226, 232, 241
    for strength, 153–161
    and stress, 249
    stretching, 121
    tests, 121–123
    and weight loss, 226–229, 230
Explanatory style, 94–96
Eysenck, Hans, 49

Faith, 9, 100, 101, 106–107
Family, 7, 8, 10
    definition of, 84–85
    environment, 51, 55
    influence on health, 85–87
    as social support, 70, 72, 73
    stressed, 85–86
Fast foods, 174, 189
Fat: body, 115, 136, 141, 147, 206, 225, 239, 240, 243
    and cancer, 254, 263, 264
    essential, 206, 217
    storage, 206, 228
Fat: dietary, 2, 10, 28, 174, 175–176, 1192, 193, 195, 198, 225, 230, 231, 232, 243, 252
    monosaturated, 178, 243
    polyunsaturated, 178
    saturated, 176, 243
    unsaturated, 243
Fear, 60–61
Feelings, 8, 46, 70, 95. *See also* Emotions
Fetal alcohol syndrome (FAS), 289
Fiber, dietary, 2, 10, 28, 182–183, 192, 193, 195, 226
    and cancer, 254, 267
    and heart disease, 243, 246
Fight or flight, 22–23, 29, 46, 51, 247
Fighting spirit, 100–101, 314–315
Fish oil, 179
Fishman, Steve, 100
Fitness, 114, 141, 151, 238

cardiovascular, 115, 121, 138, 139–140, 149, 240, 247–249
  definition of, 118
  intensity of training, 138
  programs, individualized, 118
  standards, 119–120, 217
Flexibility, muscular, 119, 120, 127–128, 145–147
  exercises for, 162–168
Food and Drug Administration (FDA), 191, 193, 315
Food Guide Pyramid, 193
Forgiveness, 94, 102–103
Fosdick, Harry Emerson, 7
Framingham Heart Study, 97
Frequency of exercise, 136, 139, 144, 145, 147
Friedman, Howard, 49, 50
Friedman, Meyer, 51, 64
Friends, importance of, 10, 70, 71, 72, 77–79
Fructose, 181
Fruits, 183, 185, 190, 192, 193, 195, 198, 225, 232, 248, 267

Galactose, 181
Galen, 47
Gastrointestinal disease, 22, 24, 106
General adaptation syndrome, 22–23
Genetics/heredity, 49, 145, 223, 225, 280
  and addiction, 281
  and cancer, 252, 253, 255, 261
  and diabetes, 246
  and heart disease, 239, 242, 244–245
Genital warts, 307
Gershwin, Madeline, 98
Ghandi, Mahatma, 66, 101
Girth measurements, 212
Glucose, 181, 191, 230, 246, 247
Goals: health, 11, 12, 286, 289
  setting, 96, 151, 232, 280, 281
Gold, Philip, 62
Goleman, Daniel, 106
Gonorrhea, 306–307
Good, Robert, 95
Goodwin, Frederick, 62
Goodwin, James, 84
Goodyear Company, 117
Grief, 87–88
Gymnastics, 142

Happiness, 7, 104, 105
Hardiness, 25, 50, 64–67, 96
Hardison, James, 9
Harlow, Harry and Margaret, 74
Hassles, 20, 79
Hay fever, 22
Headache, 22, 57, 106, 282
Healing mechanism/process, 97, 98, 106, 110
Health, 114, 149, 151, 246
  and altruism, 105
  cardiovascular, 121
  and daily nutritional intake, 195
  definitions of, 2, 4, 5
  emotional, 6–8, 101
  and explanatory style, 94

  and a fighting spirit, 100–101
  fitness standards, 120, 133, 217
  and hope, 107, 108
  and locus of control, 97
  mental, 6, 75, 83,101
  and marriage, 81, 83–84
  and personality, 49–51
  physical, 5–6, 94, 101
  promotion, 11, 115
  protection, 11, 98
  screening, 118
  and self–esteem, 98–99
  social, 8–9
  and social support, 70–71
  and spirituality, 9, 101–104
Health care costs, 117
Healthy Eating Pyramid, 192, 196–197
Healthy People 2000. See Year 2000 National Health Objectives
Heart, 136, 137
Heart disease, 3, 114, 135
  and alcohol, 289, 295
  and anger, 57–58
  attacks, 239, 285
  and attitude, 95, 97
  and bereavement, 89
  and body fat, 216
  and caffeine, 282
  and cholesterol, 243
  and depression, 62, 64
  and dietary fat, 175, 176, 179, 189, 192, 238
  and family, 86
  and hostility, 60
  and loneliness, 75, 76–77
  and marijuana, 291
  and marriage vs. divorce, 83–84
  and personality, 49
  and pets, 80
  and smoking, 253
  and social ties, 72, 73
  and spirituality, 103
  and stress, 246–247
  and Type A, 51, 60
  and worry, 61
Heart rate, 24, 138, 139, 149
  maximal, 137
  resting, 136
Height/weight charts, 206
Helmrich, Susan, 246
Helplessness, 66, 67, 97, 100, 105, 108
Henker, Fred, 110
Hepatitis A, 309
Hepatitis B, 252, 309
Heredity. See Genetics
Herpes, 25, 308–309
Hippocrates, 47, 49
HIV, 255, 311–312, 313–314
  risk reduction, 319
  testing, 315
  treatment, 315–316
Homeostasis, 23
Honesty, 74
Hope, 8, 9, 107–108
  and hopelessness, 55, 100, 108
Hormones, 24, 46, 47, 55, 59, 76, 97, 102, 105, 106, 176, 184

  and cholesterol, 179
  estrogen, 252, 256, 261, 262
  and fear, 61
  and hostility, 60
  male, 141
  and protein, 175
  and stress, 247, 256
Hostility, 51, 52, 55, 83, 94
  characteristics of, 59, 60
  definition of, 58
  and hormones, 60
House, James, 70
Humor, 64, 280
Hydrostatic weighing, 207
Hypertension, 10, 22, 25, 75, 106, 114, 115, 135, 216, 238. See also Blood pressure
  essential, 248–249
  and heart disease, 245–246
Hypertrophy, 140, 141, 143, 144
Hypokinetic diseases, 135
Hypotension, 245
Hypothalamus, 49, 225

Iker, Howard, 110
Imagery, 35
Immune system, 8, 47, 48–49, 175
  and altruism, 104, 105
  and bereavement, 89–90
  and cancer, 252
  and depression, 62
  and explanatory style, 94, 95, 98
  and divorce, 83
  and a fighting spirit, 100
  and helplessness, 67
  and hope, 108
  and immunity, 46, 97, 98, 289, 291–318
  and loneliness, 76, 77, 79
  and marriage, 84
  and personality, 50
  and social support, 73
  and STDs, 305, 312
  and stress, 20, 23, 24–27, 256
Immunization, 11
Infectious diseases, 2, 25, 46, 94, 114, 238, 304
Injury and accidents, 11, 140, 143, 145, 146, 151, 192, 222, 230, 287
  treating, 149, 150
Insight, 8
Intensity of exercise, 136, 137–140, 145, 146–147, 228
Institute for the Advancement of Health, 46
Institute for Aerobics Research, 240
Insulin, 246. See also Diabetes
Internalizing, 94
Intimacy, 8, 74, 105
Iron, 184, 187, 189, 191
Isokinetic training, 143
Isometric training, 142, 146
Isotonic training, 142, 143

Jacobson, Edmund, 34
Jefferson, Thomas, 7
Joints: dislocation, 146
  range of motion, 127, 142, 143, 145, 147, 190

Kahn, Robert, 70
Kiecolt–Glaser, Janice, 27
Kiefer, Christie, 105
Killer cells, 89–90, 95, 97, 98. *See also* Lymphocytes
Klopfer, Bruno, 107
Knapp, Peter, 22
Koop, C. Everett, 10, 264, 284
Kosaba, Suzanne, 25–26, 31, 66, 96
Kubler–Ross, Elisabeth, 107
Label reading, 176, 181, 193, 195
Lactic acid, 191
Lactose, 181
Langer, Ellen, 97
Laughter, 7, 81, 96
Lazarus, Richard, 110
Lecithin, 192
Legumes, 193, 267
Leisure time, 149, 151
Lerner, Michael, 95
LeShan, Lawrence, 55
Leukemia, 255, 257
Levine, Alexandra, 108
Levy, Arnold, 50
Levy, Sandra, 95
Lice, pubic, 310–311
Lifestyle, 4, 10, 239
    active/positive, 5, 250–319
    and cancer, 252, 264
    changes, 27, 95–96
    and heart disease, 242, 245, 247, 250
    sedentary, 2, 114, 117, 141, 150, 206, 226, 229, 231, 238
    unhealthy, 3, 242
Lindbergh, Anne Morrow, 75
Lipids, blood, 136, 184, 222, 240, 244, 246, 248, 249
Listening, 86
Locke, Steven, 48
Locus of control, 96–98
Logic, 6
Longevity, 64, 240
    and divorce, 83
    and family, 85
    and loneliness, 72, 76
    and spirituality, 103, 104, 105
Loneliness, 72–73, 103
    and cancer, 55, 79
    definition of, 74–75
    and divorce, 82
    and heart function, 76–77
    and immune function, 76
    and longevity, 76
Loss. *See* Grief
Lourdes, 106–107
Love, 8, 72, 81, 94, 101, 105, 280, 317
Luks, Allan, 105
Lymphocytes, 25, 48, 49, 83, 89–90, 95, 97, 105
Lymphomas, 257
Lynch, James, 72, 75, 76, 82

Maddi, Salvatore, 36, 96
Maltose, 181
Marijuana, 289, 291
Marriage, 81
    and cancer, 84

    happy, 83–84
    and heart disease, 83–84
    and longevity, 84–85
    unhappy, 83
Maturity, 8, 280
Maximal oxygen uptake, 119, 121
Meaning, 9, 101
Meditation, 33–34
Memory, 6, 48
Melanoma, 54, 94–95, 257, 260
Mental: disorders, 75, 83, 278
    health, 6, 101
Metabolism, 28, 33, 124, 136, 140–141, 243, 246, 247, 249, 309
    and caffeine, 282
    and cancer, 252
    and nutrition, 174, 184, 191
    and weight management, 222, 225, 226, 227–228, 230, 232
Metastasis, 252, 257
Minerals, 28, 174, 182, 184, 186–189, 191–192, 195, 199, 201, 254
Minnesota Multiphasic Personality Inventory (MMPI), 50
Mitochondria, 136
Mode of exercise, 136, 139, 142, 145–145
Monosaccharides, 181
Mortality, 2, 46, 73, 102, 115, 151
    from AIDS, 314
    and bereavement, 90
    from cancer, 252, 253
    cardiovascular, 138, 179, 238, 240
    and church involvement, 103–104
    and depression, 62
    and fitness, 120
    and high blood pressure, 245
    infant, 10, 11
    leading causes of, 114
    and marriage, 84
    and obesity, 217, 222
    from smoking, 244
    and social support, 72
Mother Teresa, 104
Motor skills, 119, 145
Motivation, 108, 151
Movement, 114
Muscles/muscular: abdominal, 147, 154
    endurance, 119, 124, 140, 144
    fatigue, 140, 145
    flexibility, 119, 127–128, 140, 145–147
    hypertrophy, 140, 141, 143
    mass, 141
    soreness/stiffness, 144, 145, 146, 149
    strength, 119, 123–124, 136, 140–144

National Academy of Sciences, 184, 189, 191, 192, 193, 199, 200, 216, 253, 266
National AIDS hotline, 315
National Cancer Institute, 84, 183, 267
National Center for Health Statistics, 83
National Cholesterol Education Program (NCEP), 242, 243
National Council on Compensation Insurance, 21
National Institute on Aging, 90
National Institute on Alcohol Abuse and Alcoholism, 287–288

National Institute of Allergy and Infectious Diseases, 315
National Institute on Drug Abuse, 291, 315
National Institute of Mental Mealth, 61, 62
National Institutes of Health, 46, 48
National Library of Medicine, 315
National Research Council, 176, 192
Naval Health Research Center, 50
Nervous system, 47, 48, 55, 59, 60, 62, 104, 184, 257, 291
Neuroblastomas, 257
Nicotine, 29, 244, 264, 282, 297, 298. *See also* Cigarette smoking
1949 Conference on Life and Stress and Heart Disease, 20
Nutrition/nutrients, 174, 190, 192, 193, 194, 195. *See also* Diet
    deficiency, 223, 225
    and the heart, 248
    supplementation, 191–192

Obesity, 135, 141, 181, 195, 206, 216, 217, 222, 229
    and cancer, 261, 262, 266
    and diabetes, 246
    and heart disease, 246
    and stress, 22
Old, Lloyd, 100
Oliner, Samuel and Pearl, 104
1.0 mile walk, 121, 123
1.5 mile run, 121
Optimism, 7–8, 9, 30, 64, 100, 105, 280
    as explanatory style, 94–96
Ornstein, Robert, 58, 107
Osteoporosis, 175, 186, 188, 256
Overload principle, 136, 142, 145
Overtraining, 144
Oxygen, 120, 134–135, 136, 184, 190, 191, 227, 239, 240, 243, 244
Oxygen free radicals, 184, 243

Paffenbarger, Ralph, 114, 241–242
Pain, 98, 146–147
Panic attacks, 106
PAR–Q screening, 118
Paul, Steven, 61
Pavlou, Konstantin, 227
Peer pressure, 280, 281, 317
Pelletier, Kenneth, 101
Pelvic inflammatory disease, 309–310
Peptides, 48
Percent body fat, 206, 207, 208, 212, 216, 217, 218, 228
Personality, 4, 98
    addictive, 279–280
    altruistic, 104–105
    and anger, 55–56
    cancer–prone, 53–55
    coronary–prone, 50, 51–52
    definition of, 49
    disease–prone, 50
    disease–resistant, 64–67
    and hostility, 58–60
    immune–prone, 50
    and rheumatoid arthritis, 55–56
    Type A, 50, 51
    Type B, 73

Type C, 50, 51
and ulcers, 56
Pessimism, 94–95
Peterson, Christopher, 94
Pets, importance of, 79–81
Physical: health, 5–6, 94, 101, 114–115. *See also* Fitness; Health
inactivity, 239–242
therapy, 147
Play, 81
Post–Gordon, Joan, 67
Posture, 123, 145, 147
Prayer, 101, 102
President's Council on Physical Fitness and Sports, 115
Prevention: AIDs, 315
disease and injury, 2, 3, 10, 11, 46, 118, 145, 149
Productivity, 21, 238
and fitness, 117, 145
Progressive relaxation, 34
Proprioceptive neuromuscular facilitation (PNF), 145–146
Proteins, 28, 174, 175, 182, 184, 190, 192, 193, 195, 222–223, 243
Prudential Insurance Company, 117
Pruzinsky, Thomas, 60
Psychoneuroimmunology (PNI), 96, 108
definition of, 46–47
Public Health Department, 315
Pulse, 123, 137, 138

Rate of perceived exertion (RPE), 138–139
Recommended dietary allowance (RDA), 186, 191, 192–193, 195, 200
Recovery: heart rate, 149
time from exercise, 136, 144
Reframing thoughts, 31
Relaxation: response, 102
techniques, 33–36, 249, 298
Religion. *See* Spirituality
Remen, Naomi, 46
Remission, spontaneous, 100
Renshaw, Domeena, 46
Repetitions, 124, 143–144, 145, 147
Resistance: fixed, 144
in strength training, 124, 142, 143–145
variable
Respect, 8, 86
Respiratory disease/failure, 22, 25, 50, 70, 222, 294
Responsibility, 8, 86
Retinoblastoma, 255
Retroviruses, 255
Rheumatoid arthritis, 55–56
Rice, Phillip, 96
Risk factors, wellness, 9–10
Role playing, 31
Rolls, Barbara, 190
Rosch, Paul, 20
Rosenman, Ray, 51
Rotter, Julian, 96

Sagan, Leonard, 27, 85
Salber, Eva, 71
Salt, 29, 189, 190, 192, 195, 248, 249, 267
Sarcomas, 256

Sedentary living, 2, 114, 117, 141, 150, 206, 226, 229, 231
Seligman, Martin, 94
Sand, George, 106
Scabies, 310
Schmale, Arthur, 87, 110
Schweitzer, Albert, 104
Self-esteem, 81
definition of, 98
and eating disorders, 223, 224
and health, 98–100
low, 281
Self-exams: breast, 270–271
skin, 267
testicular, 270, 272
Self-image, 8
Selye, Hans, 20
Setpoint theory, 225, 227, 230
Sets, exercise, 143–145
Sexually transmitted diseases, 304–305
preventing, 316–318
Shoes, proper, 149, 151
Shultz, Johannes, 35
Siegel, Bernie, 8, 27, 67, 88–89, 94, 100, 101–102, 105, 108
Silverman, Samuel, 76
Skinfold thickness technique, 207–208, 218
Sleep (and insomnia), 10, 30–31, 106
Sobel, David, 58, 107
Social/support, 30, 64, 70, 83, 103
interaction, 151
wellness, 8–9, 20, 278
Society of Psychosomatic Medicine, 70
Sodium, 189–190, 192, 195, 249
Solomon, George, 101
Specificity of training, 142, 143, 145
Spiegel, David, 73–74
Spingarn, Natalie Davis, 107
Spirituality, 9, 20
and addiction, 279
and church affiliation, 103–104
and forgiveness, 102–103
and health, 101–102
and prayer, 102
Stanwych, Douglas, 50
Starches, *See* Carbohydrates
Staub, Ervin, 104
Strength, muscular, 119, 120, 123–124, 136, 140
tests to measure, 153–161
training, 143, 144, 227–228
Stress: and addiction, 281
and arthritis, 55
buffers, 64, 70, 79, 97, 101, 103, 105, 106
and cancer, 256
coping with, 7, 27
definition of, 20
and diet, 27–29
ECG, 118
and exercise, 145, 240
and explanatory style, 94
in family, 85–86
and gastrointestinal disease, 22, 24, 106
and heart disease, 22, 24, 239, 242, 246–247

and hypertension, 245
and immune system, 24–27, 97
and loneliness, 75, 76
management, 248–249
and musculoskeletal disorders, 22
and respiratory distress, 22
response, 22–23, 49, 247
and pets, 80
and social support, 72
and weight loss, 233
Stretching, 127, 139, 145–146, 147
Strokes, 22, 25, 72, 114, 176, 216, 222, 238, 245, 253, 285, 294, 298
Success, 7, 9
Sucrose, 181
Sudden death, 90
Sudden infant death (SID), 285
Sugar, 28–29, 181, 190, 192, 193, 195, 225, 244, 246, 248
Suicide, 62, 75, 82, 89
Sun exposure/sunscreens/sunburn, 264–266, 267
Swimming, 230
Syme, Loenard, 77
Syphilis, 311–312

T-cells, 252. *See also* Immune system
Target training zone, 138, 140, 149, 243
Tavris, Carol, 56–57
Teamwork, 9
Temoshok, Lydia, 54–55
Tenderloin Senior Outreach Project, 71
Tenneco, Inc., 117
Tension. *See* Stress
Thomas, Caroline Bedell, 50, 75
Thompson, S. C., 66
Time management, 31–32
Tobacco use, 253, 264, 282–286. *See also* Cigarette smoking
Toffler, Alvin, 20
Tolerance, 8
Training zone, cardiovascular, 137
Touch, 74
Transcendental meditation (TM), 33
Triglycerides, 136, 239, 244
Tronick, Edward, 85
Trust, 86
Twain, Mark, 98
Type A personality, 22, 50, 60, 73
Type B personality, 73
Type C personality, 50, 55, 256

Ulcers, 22, 25, 50, 56, 244, 285, 298
Uncertainty, 61
Underweight, 217, 222, 223
U.S. Centers for Disease Control and Prevention, 115, 135, 261, 304, 305, 308, 314, 315, 316
U.S. Department of Agriculture, 192, 216
U.S. Department of Health and Human Services, 3, 176, 192, 216, 260
U.S. Olympic Sports Medicine Council, 30
U.S. Public Health Service, 11, 118
U.S. Restaurant Association, 174
U.S. Surgeon General, 2, 10, 284, 296–297, 298

Vegetables, 177, 183, 187, 192, 193, 195, 198, 225, 232, 248, 267
Vegetarians, 191, 198
Vickers, Ross, 50
Viruses, 252, 255, 305, 309, 312, 314
Visual imagery/visualization, 233, 295
Vitamins, 28, 243
    and cancer, 262, 267
    in diet, 174, 176, 179, 182, 184, 201, 248, 254
Volunteerism, 96, 105–106, 302
VO_{2max}, 121, 123, 134, 135–136, 137, 139, 191

Waist-to-hip ratio, 216, 217, 218, 220
Walking, 248
Warm-up, 144, 145, 146

Water: exercise, 230
    loss in dieting, 222–223, 229
    and hypertension, 249
    as nutrient, 174, 232
Weight: healthy/recommended, 10, 135, 192, 206, 217–218, 222, 246, 248
    loss, 223, 224–226, 227–229, 230–232, 243, 249
    management/control, 139, 140, 230–232, 243, 249
    regulating mechanism (WRM), 225
Weight training, 228. *See also* Strength
Well-being, 2, 8, 70, 98, 217
Wellness, 98, 114, 115, 119, 151, 238, 246
    and addiction, 278–279
    definition of, 4–5
    dimensions, 5–9

    and nutrition, 195, 198
    risk factors, 9–10
Westcott, Wayne, 227
Williams, Jesse, 4
Williams, Redford, 51, 53, 58–59
Wolf, Stewart, 73
Workaholic, 66
World Health Organization, 10, 314
    definition of health, 2
Worry, 60–61

Year 2000 National Health Objectives, 11, 12, 286, 289
Yoga, 36
Yogi, Maharishi, Mahesh, 33

Zone, target, of training, 138–140, 149, 243